Eosinophils

A Comprehensive Review, and Guide to the Scientific and Medical Literature

Christopher J. F. Spry

British Heart Foundation Professor of Cardiovascular Immunology,
St. George's Hospital Medical School, University of London;
Hon. Consultant in Medicine,
St. George's Hospital, London

OXFORD NEW YORK TOKYO
OXFORD UNIVERSITY PRESS
1988

Oxford University Press, Walton Street, Oxford OX2 6DP
Oxford New York Toronto
Delhi Bombay Calcutta Madras Karachi
Petaling Jaya Singapore Hong Kong Tokyo
Nairobi Dar es Salaam Cape Town
Melbourne Auckland
and associated companies in
Berlin Ibadan

Oxford is a trade mark of Oxford University Press

Published in the United States
by Oxford University Press, New York

British Library Cataloguing in Publication Data
Spry, Christopher J. F.
Eosinophils: a comprehensive review, and guide to the scientific and medical literature.
1. Man. Blood. Eosinophils
I. Title
612'.112
ISBN 0-19-261408-8

Library of Congress Cataloging in Publication Data
Spry, Christopher J. F.
Eosinophils: a comprehensive review, and guide to the scientific and medical literature.
Christopher J. F. Spry.
(Oxford medical publications)
Bibliography, Includes index.
1. Eosinophilia. 2. Eosinophils. 3. Eosinophil disorders.
I. Title. II. Series.
[DNLM: 1. Eosinophils. WH 200 S771e]
RB145.S67 1988 616.1'54—dc19 88-15231
ISBN 0-19-261408-8

Set by CentraCet, Cambridge
Printed in Great Britain
at the University Printing House, Oxford
by David Stanford
Printer to the University

The EOS – REFS Database

Over 5500 scientific references on eosinophils, and eosinophilic diseases, which are kept fully up to date and which were used to write the book *Eosinophils,* are available as an indexed and searchable 5.5 Mb database called EOS–REFS for use on IBM-compatible microcomputers. About 30% of the articles are also provided with abstracts and other related information.

The database is provided complete with a read-only version of the well known Cardbox-Plus program* and a short guide to its use. Comprehensive direct search protocol is provided for authors, titles of article, keywords, etc., and data can be output to screen, printer, or disk.

Further details and copies of EOS–REFS are available from the author, Professor C. J. F. Spry, Department of Immunology, St George's Hospital Medical School, London SW17 0RE, U.K., telephone (01) 672 9944 Extension 55819.

Please use the lower portion of this card for orders and enquiries.

ENQUIRY/ORDER FORM

To Professor C. J. F. Spry, St. George's Hospital Medical School.

From:

Name & position: ____________________

Organization: ____________________

Address: ____________________

____________________ Telephone: ____________________

Pleae supply further details of the EOS–REFS database ______

Please supply ______ copies of the EOS–REFS database at £75.00 (plus £11.25 VAT in the UK) or US$150.00 on 3.5″/5.25″ disks*

*Payment of __________ is enclosed.

*Please invoice my organization quoting Order No. ______

*Debit my American Express/Visa/Mastercard No. ______

Signature: ____________________ Date: __________

**Please complete as appropriate.*

About Cardbox-Plus

Cardbox-Plus is an interactive, free-text, data storage and retrieval system which handles records as screen images in any user-defined format. With a limit of over 500 000 records per database, 36 rows by 132 columns are available for the main record 'card', where any word, number, or date can be indexed for fast retrieval, plus up to 8000 characters of extra text per record. Multiple retrieval criteria can be used, with wildcard facilities and range searches, on-line sorting and multi-record display. Selections can be combined and output to disk or printer in any user-defined format, including fully mailmerged letters and documents. Printer support for special attributes and international characters is included. Cardbox-Plus links to most other programs and word-processing systems for both input and output of data. Multi-user and networking versions are available.

The *Read-Only* version of Cardbox-Plus has all the facilities of the standard version with the exception of the commands which enable you to add or amend records from the keyboard. A facility is, however, provided for loading future updates of the EOS-REFS database.

Operating system: MS-DOS, PC-DOS. Memory requirements: 230K.

Please
affix
postage
stamp.

Professor C. J. F. Spry
Department of Immunology
St. George's Hospital Medical School
London SW17 0RE
England

OXFORD MEDICAL PUBLICATIONS

Eosinophils

Foreword

Professor Paul B. Beeson KBE

For more than a century the eosinophil has been easy to recognize, by microscopic examination of blood, marrow, and other tissues. Inasmuch as this cell is found in all vertebrates one seems justified in assuming that it must play some useful role (or roles). But despite countless observations and studies, the function of the eosinophil is only grudgingly being disclosed.

This cell resembles the neutrophil in morphology; it has the same site of origin; and it is capable of phagocytosis. But despite these similarities the two leucocytes manifest widely divergent behaviour in their responses to hormonal stimuli, or to the presence of foreign microbes, plant particles, or chemical substances. In many ways the eosinophil seems to belong to a different family of cells – those which make up the immune system – in contrast to those which digest and dispose of foreign materials.

A massive accumulation of clinical reports on the phenomenon of eosinophilia provides only a confusion of clues and inconsistencies, an example being the eosinophilia that is occasionally observed in neoplastic disorders.

Nonetheless, some progress in our knowledge of the eosinophil is being made. A substantial body of worthwhile information is emerging from reductionist scientific investigations, using improved systems for morphological study, together with better techniques of cell separation and cell fractionation. Consequently it has been possible to isolate and identify unique components such as the major basic protein and the cationic protein, and to catalogue enzymic constituents. Admittedly, much remains to be determined regarding the parts played by these products, in the turbulent settings of inflammatory reactions.

Some products of the eosinophil have been shown to be capable of injuring metazoan parasites, especially their larval forms; thus there are grounds for asserting that the cell benefits its host by combating diseases caused by such parasites. On the 'other side of the coin' we now have good evidence that eosinophil-derived agents can cause serious damage to host tissues.

The work presented here by Professor Spry results from his steady concentration on the eosinophil over a span of two decades. His own investigations have been carried out in the clinic and in the laboratory, particular attention being given to the ways in which eosinophils can damage the heart, or can combat certain parasites. His work and his wide reading have made it possible to accomplish a prodigious task in collating and critically reviewing much new work. By doing so he has produced an invaluable resource, for clinicians and cell biologists.

Preface

This books is designed to provide a comprehensive overview of eosinophils in man and animals. It includes a review of over 2000 selected scientific and medical references in this area, published up to the end of 1987. The book covers the cell biology of eosinophils, and the clinical disorders in which eosinophils are important. The sources database of 5298 references, which was derived from 4125 Medline entries listed between January 1977 and January 1988, and an additional 1173 references from other sources, is available as a supplement to the book for IBM compatible microcomputers, on direct application to the author.

Some of the significant advances in our knowledge of eosinophils during the past decade have come from the development of reproducible methods for purifying and culturing them, the cloning of the eosinopoietic factors, the discovery of eosinophil activation, and the isolation and characterization of many of the molecules synthesized and secreted by eosinophils. Their role as effector cells in disease is now accepted, and they are now seen as specialized cells, with several unique constituents, which give them a distinctive range of effector functions in disease. The applications of this knowledge to human diseases are already showing promise, in the study, and in treatment of several haematological, cardiac, respiratory, dermatological, parasitic, and other diseases. Current research is aimed at finding out what induces eosinophils to become activated and degranulated, and the effects that their secretion products have on cells and tissues.

This book has been written as a guide to the literature on eosinophils, and to the diseases where eosinophils may have a role. I hope that it will stimulate new approaches to this field, the questioning of dogmas about how eosinophils localize *in vivo* and interact with other cells, parasites, and allergens, so that more can be learnt about how eosinophils contribute to the beneficial or harmful effects of allergic reactions. I also hope that it will enable newcomers to the field to obtain an overview of eosinophils, and will provide specialists at the bench or in the clinic with a ready source of information to help them in their work.

I owe my apprenticeship, and what success I may have had in this field, to Professor Paul Beeson, and to my clinical and scientific colleagues in Oxford and London. The book could not have been written without the help of Dr Po-Chun Tai, Peter Ison, Kathy Maguire, and the librarians in the Wellcome Library at the Royal Postgraduate Medical School, St. George's Hospital Medical School Library, and the library of the Royal Society of Medicine, London. I am also grateful to the staff at Oxford University Press, and many others who have contributed to the preparation of this volume.

London
January 1988

C.J.F.S.

Contents

List of figures xv

List of plates xvii

PART I Cellular biology of eosinophils

1. Introduction and history 3
- 1.1. Discovery and description of eosinophils 4
- 1.2. The structure, cell biology, and effector functions of eosinophils 6
- 1.3. The roles of eosinophils in disease 8

2. Eosinopoiesis 10
- 2.1. Ontogeny of eosinophils 10
- 2.2. The eosinophil lineage 11
- 2.3. Morphology of eosinophil differentiation 12
- 2.4. Kinetics of eosinophil production 14
- 2.5. Assays for eosinopoietic factors 14
- 2.6. Eosinopoietic factors 17
- 2.7. Drugs and eosinophil production 24
- 2.8. Suppressor cells and eosinophil production 24
- 2.9. Eosinophil suppression of granulocytopoiesis 24
- 2.10. Genetic factors affecting human eosinophil production 25
- 2.11. Eosinophil cell lines 26
- 2.12. Blood eosinophil kinetics 27
- 2.13. Kinetics of eosinophils in tissues 28

3. Methods: eosinophil structure, constituents, and metabolism 29
- 3.1. Eosinophil counts 29
- 3.2. Leukapheresis 32
- 3.3. Cell separation 32
- 3.4. Culture of mature eosinophils 35
- 3.5. Staining techniques 36
- 3.6. Eosinophil structure 38
- 3.7. Eosinophil constituents and their properties 40
- 3.8. The metabolism of resting and stimulated eosinophils 66

4. The eosinophil cell membrane and receptors 74
- 4.1. Scanning electronmicroscopy 74
- 4.2. Freeze-fracture studies on eosinophil membranes 74
- 5.3. Membrane proteins 75

4.4. Membrane carbohydrates 83
4.5. Eosinophil membrane antigens 84
4.6. Alterations in the eosinophil plasma membrane 88
4.7. Antigen presentation by eosinophils 88

5. Endocytosis, secretion, and motility 89
5.1. Endocytosis 89
5.2. Secretion 90
5.3. Motility 95

6. Eosinophil activation, cytotoxicity, and interactions 103
6.1. Activation 103
6.2. Cytotoxicity 111
6.3. Interactions of secreted products with normal cells and tissues 121

7. Eosinophils in animals other than man 123
7.1. Phylogeny of eosinophils 123
7.2. Eosinophils in amphibia, birds, and fishes 124
7.3. Eosinophils in mammals other than man 125
7.4. Eosinophils in reptiles 127

PART II Eosinophils in disease

8. Bacterial, fungal, and richettsial infections 131
8.1. Bacterial infections 131
8.2. Mycoses 132
8.3. Rickettsial infections 133
8.4. Yeast infections, cryptococcosis 134

9. Viral diseases 135

10. Parasitic diseases 136
10.1. Helminthiasis 136
10.2. Protozoan infections 148
10.3. Ectoparasitic infestations and insect bites 149

11. Neoplasms 150
11.1. Leukaemias 150
11.2. Lymphomas 162
11.3. Reticuloendotheliosis 164
11.4. Neoplasms of vascular tissue 166
11.5. Neoplasms of solid tissues 169

12. Musculo-skeletal diseases 176
12.1. Bone and joint diseases 176
12.2. Muscle diseases 179

12.3. Fasciitis syndromes 180
12.4. Sjögren's syndrome 182

13. Digestive system diseases 183
13.1. Oesophageal diseases 183
13.2. Disease of the stomach and peptic ulcers 184
13.3. Eosinophilic gastroenteritis 184
13.4. Inflammatory fibroid polyps 186
13.5. Chronic eosinophilic pseudotumours in the abdominal cavity 187
13.6. Enteritis and enterocolitis 188
13.7. Crohn's disease 189
13.8. Colonic diseases 189
13.9. Rectal diseases 190
13.10. Liver and biliary tract diseases 190
13.11. Pancreatic diseases 191

14. Diseases of the mouth 192

15. Respiratory tract diseases 193
15.1. Sputum eosinophils 194
15.2. Bronchoalveolar lavage 194
15.3. Bronchial diseases 195
15.4. Lung diseases 205
15.5. Pleural diseases 212

16. Disease of the ear, nose, and throat 213
16.1. Diseases of the ear 213
16.2. Diseases of the nose 213
16.3. Pharyngeal and laryngeal diseases 214

17. Diseases of the nervous system 216
17.1. Central nervous system diseases 216
17.2. Peripheral nerve diseases 217
17.3. Schizophrenia 217

18. Eye diseases 218
18.1. Conjunctival diseases 218
18.2. Corneal diseases 219
18.3. Retinal diseases 219
18.4. Diseases of the orbit 219

19. Urological diseases 220
19.1. Kidney and ureteral diseases 220
19.2. Renal dialysis and eosinophils 220
19.3. Eosinophilic cystitis 223
19.4. Eosinophils in the urine 224
19.5. Prostatic diseases 224
19.6. Renal allograft rejection 224

20. Female genital tract diseases and pregnancy 226
20.1. The uterus and uterine diseases 226
21.2. Pregnancy 227

21. Cardiovascular diseases 228
21.1. Diseases of the heart, and pericardium 228
21.2. Vascular diseases 230
21.3. Vasculitis 230

22. Endomyocardial fibrosis 232
22.1. History 232
22.2. Eosinophilic endomyocardial fibrosis 235
22.3. Tropical endomyocardial fibrosis 249
22.4. Animal models of endomyocardial fibrosis 257
22.5. Comparisons of E-EMF and T-EMF 257

23. Diseases of the blood 259
23.1. Inherited diseases affecting eosinophils 259
23.2. Fanconi's anaemia 261
23.3. Cyclical haematopoiesis and eosinophils 261
23.4. Acquired platelet dysfunction with eosinophilia 262

24. The idiopathic hypereosinophilic syndrome (HES): Clinical features 263
24.1. Disease processes underlying HES 266
24.2. Variants of HES 266
24.3. Animal models of HES 267
24.4. Patients affected 268
24.5. Presentation 270
24.6. Nonspecific symptoms 270
24.7. Cardiovascular complications 271
24.8. Thromboembolic complications 271
24.9. Respiratory tract complications 272
24.10. Digestive system complications 272
24.11. Skin complications 273
24.12. Nervous system involvement 274
24.13. Musculoskeletal complications 276
24.14. Renal complications and hypertension 276
24.15. Breast involvement 277

25. The idiopathic hypereosinophilic syndrome (HES): Investigations 278
25.1. Blood eosinophils in HES 278
25.2. Serum and plasma constituents in HES 284
25.3. Bone marrow features of HES 284
25.4. Immunological investigations in HES 286
25.5. Coagulation studies in HES 286

26. The idiopathic hypereosinophilic syndrome (HES): Course of the disease, and treatment 288
26.1. Treatment of HES 289

27. Diseases in neonates and infants 294
27.1. Premature infants 294
27.2. Familial, and genetic diseases 295
27.3. Eosinophilic diseases in infants 295

28. Skin diseases 297
28.1. Dermatitis 297
28.2. Episodic angioedema with eosinophilia 299
28.3. Skin eruptions in pregnancy and in infancy 302
28.4. Scleroderma syndromes 302
28.5. Bullous skin diseases 302
28.6. Incontinentia pigmenti 303
28.7. Eosinophilic pustular folliculitis 304
28.8. Psoriasis 304
28.9. Erythema nodosum 304
28.10. Lymphomatoid papulosis 304
28.11. Erythema annulare 305

29. Immunological diseases 306
29.1. Autoimmune diseases 306
29.2. Drug hypersensitivity reactions 306
29.3. Graft-versus-host disease 314
29.4. Immunological deficiency syndromes 314
29.5. Absence of eosinophils 315
29.6. Hypergammaglobulinaemia E and infection syndrome 316

Appendix A: Research Groups working on eosinophils and eosinophilic diseases 318
Appendix B: The scientific literature on eosinophils 321

References 327

Index 451

Figures

2.1 Factors affecting eosinophil differentiation 21
3.1 Eosinophil purification 33
3.2 The structure of eosinophils 39
3.3 The synthesis of eosinophil granule proteins 41
3.4 The localizations of eosinophil granule proteins 43
4.1 Eosinophil plasma membrane receptors 76
4.2 Monoclonal antibodies to eosinophil membrane antigens 86
5.1 Eosinophil maturation, and secretion 90
5.2 The effects of different stimuli on eosinophil secretion 92
5.3 Eosinophil localization in tissues 98
6.1 The effector functions of eosinophils 104
6.2 Eosinophil activating factors 106
6.3 Eosinophil-dependent cytotoxic mechanisms 112
6.4 The interaction of eosinophils with other cells 122
10.1 Parasitic diseases and the tissues they affect 137
11.1 Malignant diseases, and eosinophils 151
13.1 Eosinophilic gastroenteritis 185
15.1 Eosinophils and asthma 196
19.1 Eosinophils in urological diseases 221
22.1 Eosinophilic endomyocardial fibrosis 233
22.2 Degranulating eosinophil in a cardiac biopsy 247
22.3 A comparison of eosinophilic, and tropical endomyocardial fibrosis 258
24.1 The principal complications of the idiopathic hypereosinophilic syndrome 264
28.1 Eosinophils in skin diseases 298
29.1 Drug-induced hypersensitivity reactions with an eosinophilia 308

Plates

(*Plates fall between pp. 254–255 of the text.*)

1. A normal human blood eosinophil forming a complement rosette.
2. Autoradiograph of a radiolabelled rat bone marrow eosinophil metaphase.
3. An activated human blood eosinophil stained immunocytochemically.
4. Vacuolated human blood eosinophils stained immunocytochemically.
5. Hypogranular blood eosinophils stained with Giemsa's stain.
6. A lymphoma containing activated eosinophils.
7. The heart from a patient with eosinophilic endomyocardial fibrosis.
8. The heart from a patient with tropical endomyocardial fibrosis.
9. Resected fibrotic endomyocardium.
10. A blood count bottle containing many eosinophils.
11. The retina of a patient with a retinal artery occlusion.
12. A Churg–Strauss granuloma in the heart containing activated eosinophils.
13. A skin lesion in lymphomatoid papulosis.
14. Episodic angioedema with eosinophilia with skin lesions, and ridged finger nails.

Part I

Cellular biology of eosinophils

1. Introduction and history

Eosinophils are cells which are produced in the bone marrow and migrate through the blood to the tissues, where they carry out a wide range of different functions. They are a well-defined and distinct cell type and are prominent in histological sections, as they stain strongly with eosin, which is used with haematoxylin to define cytoplasmic structures and nuclei in cells. They have been found in all vertebrate species which have so far been examined, and they are usually classified as polymorphonuclear leucocytes because the nucleus in the blood form of the cell has two or three lobes, similar to neutrophils. Like neutrophils, they possess characteristic granules, which suggests that the two cell types have much in common. However, this apparent relationship is misleading, as eosinophils are derived from a different progenitor cell than neutrophils, and they should be considered as distinct from neutrophils as they are from macrophages.

The complex life history of eosinophils is only beginning to be unravelled with the availability of special techniques for studying them *in vivo*. They develop from primitive stem cells which are present in the bone marrow and blood. These stem cells divide and differentiate, acquiring the distinct granules which are the special feature of eosinophils. After a few hours maturing further in the bone marrow, they enter the blood stream and are distributed throughout the body, where they first attach to vascular endothelium, and then migrate into perivascular sites. This is their normal place of residence in tissues, although in many diseases they migrate further into areas of inflammation. There are normally very few eosinophils in the blood (less than 0.6×10^9/l), and tissues, but in certain diseases they can be produced in enormous numbers. The highest reported blood eosinophil count in man is 326.4×10^9/l in a Nigerian patient with eosinophilic leukaemia described in 1970.[208]

Eosinophils are stimulated by one or more of a range of signals from adjacent cells, including reticular cells, endothelial cells, lymphocytes, macrophages, and other cells, which induce them to differentiate further and to become activated. Further stimulation with complexed IgG, IgE and/or C3b, and other products of inflammation, causes them to secrete their stored granule contents, and to synthesize and secrete membrane-associated components, especially lipid mediators. These events take place over several hours, and can continue for as long as they remain alive, which may be for only a few hours in some settings, or many days or weeks in others.

The principal function of eosinophils is to synthesize and deposit their stored and newly formed molecules in areas of acute and chronic inflammation. They are also able to ingest particles, such as bacteria, after they have become activated, although this function is more often carried out by neutrophils and other phagocytic cells.

A comparison of eosinophils and neutrophils in general terms is as follows: eosinophils are mainly perivascular (tissue) cells, whereas neutrophils defend intravascular sites; eosinophils respond to IgG, IgE, and complement components, whereas neutrophils do not respond to IgE stimulation; eosinophils 'secrete' whereas neutrophils 'ingest'; eosinophils mostly take part in acute and chronic hypersensitivity reactions, and are often found close to other intact cells, whereas neutrophils are most commonly present in areas of acute necrosis, where they are the main component of pus. Eosinophils are mainly associated with allergic, parasitic, and chronic inflammatory responses, whereas neutrophils are primarily found in acute bacterial infections, ischaemic lesions, and reactions to damaged cells and tissues.

1.1 Discovery and description of eosinophils

At the beginning of the nineteenth century, compound microscopes were used to examine many different tissues, including blood samples. In 1846 Wharton-Jones, an anatomist at Charing Cross Hospital, London, was able to distinguish granulated cells from red cells in the blood of several species, including the frog, the elephant, and man. He added water or acids to the preparations to make the cells swell, so that he could see the nuclei.[1921] With these simple microscopes, and without a staining method, it is unlikely that early microscopists could have distinguished eosinophils from other granulated cells. However, eosinophils may have been seen in the blood of two patients with eosinophilic leukaemia in 1861 and 1876, and in bone marrow samples in 1862 and 1869, according to T. R. Brown (1898).[219]

The best known characteristic of eosinophils was discovered by Paul Ehrlich in 1879, when he was a young doctor in Leipzig; he found that they could be stained with negatively charged chemicals, especially eosin. His paper on this subject, 'Ueber die specifischen Granulationen des Blutes', was presented to the Berlin Physiological Society on 17 January 1879.[498] The history of Paul Ehrlich's discovery of the staining properties of eosinophils was described by the Hirschs in 1979, on the centenary.[801] His technique was to make a blood smear, and to fix it by heating at 110° for 60 to 90 minutes. Then the smear was stained with a mixture of orange

G, acid fuchsin, and methyl green (Ehrlich's triple stain). Tissue sections were stained with haematoxylin, and eosin.

Eosin is a bromeinated fluorescein derivative, and not an aniline dye. Its general use, with haematoxylin, as the standard stain for tissue sections, was one of the main reasons why eosinophils were so easily noticed in disease, as there are few cells and structures which stain as prominently. We now know that eosin stains eosinophils because they possess granules which contain markedly cationic proteins which preferentially bind eosin and other negatively charged stains.

In 1879 Ehrlich suggested that the bone marrow was the site of origin for eosinophils.[497] He published a number of papers in German, and later wrote a monograph in English,[499] which shows the high quality of his work, and the remarkable insight he had into the nature and importance of eosinophils. For example, in 1900 he suggested that 'eosinophils exert their functions in tissues'.[499] Initially, there was opposition from many physicians to his proposal that it was useful to stain blood cells. However, his methods soon became widely recognized as of great benefit in general medicine, and this led to the discovery of many eosinophil-disease associations. These findings dominated much of the literature on eosinophils during the subsequent thirty years and included descriptions of eosinophils in asthma in 1889,[693] ankylostomiasis in 1891,[372] skin diseases including prurigo, urticaria, psoriasis, and pemphigus in 1892,[266, 1272] malignant diseases in 1893,[1485] and trichinosis in 1898.[219]

The standard methods for studying eosinophils at the turn of the century was to stain either tissue sections or blood smears. Differential blood counts were then carried out, and the results were given as a percentage of the total white cell count. Absolute counts were often provided as well, but many doctors thought that percentage data was more useful than absolute counts. We now know that percentage data on its own is of no clinical value.

In 1910, hypotonic solutions were introduced to lyse red cells in blood samples, so that eosin could be used to count the number of eosinophils directly.[475] From this grew the standard methods used today, in which an acetone/water/eosin solution, or a comparable mixture, is used to count eosinophils in suspension.

An important technical difficulty in this field is that eosinophils are predominantly tissue cells, and large numbers can be present in the tissues, when there are only a few in the blood. Blood counts reflect a complex relationship between cells leaving the marrow, marginating, and leaving the blood. There is no significant recirculation of eosinophils back from the tissues to blood. For this reason, blood eosinophil counts are of most value when there is a steady state. Single blood counts cannot be used either as a measure of the number which are being produced by the marrow, or the number being deposited in tissues.

1.2 The structure, cell biology, and effector functions of eosinophils

Present day knowledge of eosinophils began with the research programmes set up in the early 1960s by James Hirsch at the Rockefeller Institute, New York, in which he and G. T. Archer isolated horse blood eosinophils, and studied their granule enzymes, their capacity to phagocytose, and to degranulate in vitro.[55] Cine films were made, and high quality photomicrographs were taken of this process. It was noted that cells often degranulated, releasing lysosmal enzymes and large amounts of a peroxidase.[56] This work was followed by high resolution electronmicrographs of the crystalloid structures inside human and rat eosinophils, and changes within the cell undergoing phagocytosis. On his return to Australia, G. T. Archer began to look at the interactions between eosinophils and parasites, and demonstrated that this induced eosinophil degranulation. He postulated that eosinophils might be involved in parasite killing, and possibly in other disease processes, such as mucus production in the bronchial epithelium in asthma.

During the early 1960s it was thought that one of the main roles for eosinophils was to ingest and remove foreign proteins.[1536] This concept was supported by experiments in rodents, which showed that within five minutes of injecting immune complexes into the foot pad of rats, eosinophils appeared in the medulla of draining lymph nodes.[1085, 1086] Another hypothesis was that eosinophils processed antigens, and presented them to lymphocytes. Unfortunately these experiments did not throw light on the functions of human eosinophils, which seemed to have a much more limited phagocytic capacity than rodent eosinophils.

One of the major functions of eosinophils was thought to be the inactivation of histamine. In 1968, R. K. Archer published a review of what was then known about eosinophils, their biochemistry, numbers in tissues, methods for isolation, and their possible roles in antigen-antibody reactions.[60]

The discovery that basophils and mast cells, but not eosinophils, contain histamine, then led to the suggestion that eosinophils might inhibit the functions of mast cells, by degrading mast-cell-derived mediators in tissues.[684] Experiments in K. Frank Austen's laboratory in Boston using the latest techniques of protein chemistry, began to define the constituents and properties of eosinophils in acute hypersensitivity responses, especially their capacity to interact with and inhibit mast cell products. Their initial findings supported the concept that eosinophils could inhibit several mediators from mast cells, especially histamine, the slow reacting substance of anaphylaxis (SRS-A), which had not then been characterized, platelet activating factor (PAF-acether), and heparin.

In the mid 1960s two research projects, one in Oxford and the other in Cambridge, looked at eosinophils in animal models of disease. In Cambridge, A. Barry Kay and his colleagues started to work on the hypothesis that eosinophil localization in guinea pig tissues was due to the production of specific chemotactic factors. He continued this work in Austen's laboratory, and reported in 1971 the discovery of an 'eosinophil chemotactic factor of anaphylaxis' (ECF-A).[933] Since then, with ECF-A as a model system, many chemotactic factors have been extracted in various degrees of purity from cells, tissues, and parasites, and shown to affect eosinophil directional movement *in vitro*.

In Oxford, Professor Paul Beeson and a small group, myself among them, studied the mechanisms of eosinophilia in rats. By 1968 Anthony Basten and Paul Beeson had shown that T-lymphocytes regulated eosinophil production in rats injected intravenously with *Trichinella spiralis* larvae. They concluded that eosinophilia was an integral part of an immunological response, which was T-cell dependent.[136] Subsequent work has expanded, and built on this, and the T-lymphocyte dependency of the response to many molecules which stimulate and affect eosinophil function has become an area of increasing importance.

In the early seventies, Sheldon Wolff and colleagues at the National Institutes of Health, Bethesda, USA, who were interested in studying vasculitic diseases, began to be referred patients with marked eosinophilia. They were found to have distinct clinical features which set them apart from patients with other vasculitic disorders, such as polyarteritis nodosa. No causes for their eosinophilia were found, so they were classified under the general term of the 'idiopathic hypereosinophilic syndrome' (HES). Their findings in 14 patients with HES were published in 1975.[325] This group of patients increased in number over the subsequent decade, and it is now the largest group of patients with this disease.

In 1972 Inge Olsson and colleagues in Lund, Sweden, who were interested in the biochemistry of granulocytes in patients with leukaemia, first isolated eosinophil cationic protein (ECP) from the blood cells of a patient with chronic myeloid leukaemia.[1328] By the end of the 1970s it became apparent that ECP was one of the principal mediators of eosinophil-dependent effects on tissues and cells.

In 1973 Gerald Gleich, and colleagues at the Mayo Clinic, Rochester, USA, isolated the eosinophil major basic protein (MBP) from guinea pig eosinophils.[664] In 1976 his group showed that MBP was also present in human eosinophils.[665] The main thrust of this work, during the late 1970s and early 1980s, was to determine the importance of MBP in immunobiology, including its capacity to injure parasites and other cells.

In 1971 it first became possible to grow human eosinophils as colonies *in vitro*.[312, 844] The finding that they were distinct from neutrophil and mixed neutrophil/macrophage colonies showed that they belonged to a different lineage. It soon became clear that eosinophils were also different from neutrophils in many other respects. Subsequent work on eosinophil production *in vitro* was slow, due to the difficulties in preparing pure eosinopoietic factors. However by 1987, three of the principal eosinophil colony stimulating factors, IL-3, GM-CSF, and IL-5, had been cloned, and studied as recombinant molecules.

In the mid 1970s I became interested in looking after and studying patients with marked eosinophilia, and I began to collect together patients with HES, and eosinophilic leukaemia. As many of these patients had endomycardial fibrosis, I then began to work on the association between eosinophils and heart damage. With colleagues in the clinic and laboratory, we were able to show that eosinophils were responsible for causing this serious cardiomyopathy. At this time experiments also began to be done which have led to the concept that eosinophils are predominantly secretory cells. This was shown using a variety of immunological stimuli, and assays for each of the granule constituents, which had then become available.

Although several people in the late 1960s and early 1970s had raised the possibility that eosinophils might be involved in parasite immunity, it was not until a paper was published by Butterworth and colleagues in 1975 on eosinophil-dependent killing of the schistosomula of *Schistosoma mansoni*,[255] that major studies began in this area. This assay was then adapted to study how eosinophils might function. By 1977 it became clear that eosinophils were pro-inflammatory cells, and the concept of mast cell 'down regulation' by eosinophils had become less attractive. Although there was some evidence that enzymes in eosinophils could degrade basophil, and mast cell products in vitro, it was found that neutrophils contained larger amounts of histaminase than eosinophils, that eosinophil arysulphatase could not break down SRS-A, and that eosinophils themselves produce large amounts of PAF-acether and leukotriene C4.

1.3 The roles of eosinophils in disease

Most of the hypotheses about the roles of eosinophils in disease have been based on particular properties which they were thought to possess at the time, which made them distinct from other cell types. At the turn of the century, it was thought that they had a protective role in removing debris, and detoxifying components of tissue reactions in allergic and granulomatous diseases.[1580] This view persisted, with minor variations, and was adapted in the 1960s, to include roles in histamine effects, and antigen presentation for antibody synthesis.[1669] In the mid 1970s most work on the roles of eosinophils in disease was based on the hypothesis that eosinophils 'down regulated' mast cell mediated responses.[80] Other possible roles for eosinophils have also been proposed over the last one hundred years. These include the remodelling of tissues, for example by stimulating connective tissue catabolism in the uterus of animals undergoing oestrus,[133] acceleration of repair mechanisms following trauma,[101, 135] and the stimulation of mucus production in glandular epithelium.[52]

By the mid 1970s, the modern view of eosinophils and their functions had come to the fore: that they are 'pro-inflammatory' cells involved in defence against large potentially harmful organisms, such as nematodes. They are also known to have a marked capacity to secrete their stored granule components, newly formed lipid mediators, and products of oxygen metabolism, which affect adjacent cells and tissues in inflammation. These effects may be reversible. For example, they may induce a permeability change in rat uterine blood vessels,[1761] and produce angio-edema in man.[919] Occasionally eosinophils can damage, and even kill adjacent cells.

My own approach to the issue of the functions of eosinophils, which has support of others,[124] is to assess the roles of eosinophils in each setting in which they are found, in an unprejudiced way. There is no good reason for thinking that they have only one function. Just as it is no longer possible to provide a unifying concept of the 'role' of macrophages in disease, I feel that eosinophils also have no single function. They affect cells and tissues in many different ways, according to the settings in which they find themselves, and the range of stimuli which act on them. For these reasons I suggest that no unifying hypothesis is possible, or even necessary, when one considers the remarkable variety of diseases in which eosinophils are present.

2. Eosinopoiesis

The morphological features of human eosinophil differentiation in the marrow have been known for many years. This involves their development from the promyelocyte stage, through the myelocyte stage, to the metamyelocyte stage, when eosinophils can no longer divide, although they continue to mature. Light microscopy and ultrastructural studies have shown the changes which occur in the crystalloid granules as the cells mature. The granule proteins are synthesized on the rough endoplasmic reticulum, and are transported to the Golgi apparatus, where they undergo several changes which have yet to be defined, but presumably involve glycosylation, and changes in tertiary structure. Then they are transported to the crystalloid granules, which gradually take on the characteristics found in peripheral blood eosinophils.

The microenvironment in which eosinophils develop in the marrow is important in determining the rate and the number of cell divisions that they undergo. Reticulum cells, which may have a 'nurse' function, have been seen in electronmicrographs of rat bone marrow,[1541] but the way in which these cells might interact with eosinophil precursors is not known. Present day work on eosinopoiesis and eosinopoietic factors is limited to studies on the effects of cloned stable molecules. The possible effects of factors with a short half-life, and direct stimulation by cell-to-cell contact remains to be explored.

Eosinopoiesis only occurs outside the human bone marrow in disease. However, in rodents, eosinophil colonies containing dividing eosinophils are occasionally found in the spleen, and this is also the site in which rodent eosinophils mature after leaving the bone marrow, before they re-enter the blood.

2.1 Ontogeny of eosinophils

In man, eosinophils and basophils appear together in the early fetus, and increase in number in the blood during the first and second trimester. This was documented in 1985, in blood samples from 99 normal fetuses which had undergone direct vision fetoscopy.[1211] In man, unlike other species, myelopoiesis does not take place in the liver, and it is confined to the marrow at birth.

The ontogeny of blood cells in cats has been studied in detail. Myelopoiesis occurs in the yolk sac longer than in other mammals, and in this site recognizable eosinophils appear after neutrophils, concomitantly with the first production of lymphocytes. The proportions of leucocytes which are eosinophils remain unchanged during embryogenesis. In cats, eosinophils are produced in the liver during the second half of embryogenesis, but this changes to the bone marrow. Some eosinopoiesis can be found in cat lymphoid tissues at birth.[1782] This sequence of events is also seen in the horse, where eosinopoiesis also occurs in the thymus for some time after birth.

2.2 The eosinophil lineage

There are a number of reasons for believing that eosinophils, basophils, and occasionally erythrocytes, and lymphocytes, can develop from a common precursor cell. The relationship of these cells to neutrophils, monocytes, and megakaryocytes is more distant. Lineage pathways have been proposed for progenitor cell differentiation into mature blood cells. However, it is more likely that progenitor cells are susceptible to the differential effects of lineage-directing growth factors for much longer in their life history than lineage pathways suggest. This was shown in 1985 when the two progeny of single progenitor cells were able to develop into two different colonies, including eosinophil colonies.[1044] Single progenitor cells from umbilical cord blood were also found to be able to develop into mixed colonies.[1263]

2.2.1 *Common origins with basophils*

Clinical evidence to link the differentiation of eosinophils with basophils and not neutrophils has come from several sources:

1. Defects in both eosinophils and basophils have been seen.[899, 1793]

2. In patients with chronic myeloid leukaemia, a variable proportion of the immature and more mature leukaemic cells contain both eosinophilic and basophilic granules.[1947, 1896] In a study from Essen, West Germany published in 1986, leukaemic cells with both types of granule were detected in all 13 patients studied, when care was taken to look for them with special staining techniques.[1227] Doubly granulated cells have also been seen in patients with myelofibrosis, and in cultured cord blood cells.[433]

3. A patient was described in 1983, who had cyclical depression of neutrophil and monocyte production in the marrow, with normal eosinopoiesis.[16] Neutrophil promyelocytes disappeared from the marrow during these episodes.

4. A patient was described in 1980 with transformation of chronic myeloid leukaemia to a disease in which blood basophil counts rose to more than 100×10^9/l, with large numbers of eosinophils in the tissues.[1281]

Biochemical studies on eosinophils, and basophils are equally convincing. Both cell types contain MBP, and the Charcot–Leyden crystal (CLC) protein, although eosinophils do not contain histamine. However, MBP and histamine are present together in 'eosinophil-type', or 'type II' colonies grown from human blood, which contain basophils.[432] In 1984 it was shown that basophils and eosinophils can develop in agar cultures from a common progenitor cell.[1042] In 1985 the plating efficiency, and the glucose 6 phosphate dehydrogenase isoenzyme content of type II colonies also showed that they were clonally derived.[433]

2.2.2 *Common origins with some lymphocytes*

There is clinical evidence that lymphocytes and eosinophils can develop from a common precursor cell. In 1977, a 41-year-old man in Copenhagen, Denmark, was reported with a T-cell lymphoma, and hypereosinophilia with atypical eosinophil granules, which suggested that both cell types were involved in the malignant process.[1151] In 1979, a two-and-a-half-year-old boy was seen in London, who had a lymphocytic leukaemia with increased numbers of eosinophils and basophils,[1360] and we have seen several patients who had lymphomatoid papulosis (a paraneoplastic disease affecting T-cells) and the idiopathic hypereosinophilic syndrome (HES).[1926] I have also seen two patients with eosinophilic leukaemia, who had bony deposits of undifferentiated leukaemic cells which had several phenotypic features of lymphoid cells. Several patients with a biclonal leukaemia, involving lymphocytes and eosinophils were described between 1984 and 1987.[154, 1923, 943, 995]

2.3 Morphology of eosinophil differentiation

There is little information on the nature of the cellular interactions that occur in the bone marrow at the sites of eosinophil differentiation, although it is probable that short range interactions are important.[332] Weiss has shown that reticulum cells are often present in the bone marrow of rodents, adjacent to developing eosinophils.[1541] These may be sources of eosinopoietic factors.

A number of electronmicroscope (EM) studies have been carried out on the development of eosinophil granules in human bone marrow. EM studies in 1970 showed that condensation of the early granule contents transformed them into typical mature crystalloid granues.[1584] This was confirmed in 1976.[204] In 1977, EMs of bone marrow from a patient with a marked eosinophilia led to the suggestion that granule formation begins in the endoplasmic reticulum. The granules appeared to become progressively more dense, possibly due to interaction with the Golgi vesicles, producing dense immature granules. Some granules were found within large vacuoles, and as the vacuole membranes were seen to fuse with the plasma membrane, it was suggested that some of the granule material was being secreted during their development.[42] The work of Zucker-Franklin on developing eosinophils in agar cultures suggested that there was continued transport of new granule material from the Golgi vesicles to the crystalloid granules during the promyelocyte stage.[2007]

In 1987, morphometric EM studies in Israel on normal rat bone marrow and peritoneal eosinophils showed that the volumes of eosinophil granules in both sites were multiples of the smallest sized granules. This suggested that larger granules were formed by the fusion of smaller ones, and not by continuous growth in size of each granule.[508] This has not yet been studied in human eosinophil development.

There is ultrastructural evidence that eosinophil granules, and their protein contents, are secreted during eosinophil differentiation. Some newly synthesized lysosomal granule ensymes, which have been phosphorylated, but which fail to bind to mannose 6-phosphate receptors for transport and packaging in granules, are known to be secreted.[999] However, it is not known if the basic proteins in eosinophils are treated as lysozomal enzymes, or whether there is some other way in which they are packaged in the granules. Scott and Horn first reported in 1970 that immature normal human bone marrow eosinophils sometimes contained tubular sinusoids filled with dense material, which often communicated with the extracellular space. Electron dense material, which resembled sinusoidal contents, was found on adjacent cell surfaces.[1584] This process could account for the reduced number of granules which can be seen in blood eosinophils from some patients with a marked eosinophilia, such as HES. In one patient with 'eosinophilic leukaemia', eosinophil granules were shown to be secreted at the promyelocyte stage of differentiation.[42]

This topic was studied further at the Mayo Clinic in 1984.[242] Serial samples of blood were collected from bone marrow biopsy needles put in the posterior iliac crest of 15 normal individuals. Measurements of the concentrations of MBP and CLC protein showed that initially high MBP levels decreased until they were the same as in the peripheral blood. On the other hand, although CLC protein levels also fell, they remained at over twice the serum level. Supernatants from their marrow cultures contained both MPB and CLC in quantities which were related to the amount of eosinophil colony growth that had occurred. Electromicrographs of the colonies also suggested that there was some release of eosinophil granule constituents from immature eosinophils.

2.4 Kinetics of eosinophil production

Normal adult human bone marrow contains 3 to 3.5 per cent eosinophils, of which 37 per cent are myelocytes, 26 per cent metamyelocytes, and 37 per cent granulocytes. Sixteen per cent of the myelocytes are undergoing DNA synthesis at any one time, and can be 'flash' labelled with radioactive nucleotides. The emergence time of eosinophils (the time from the end of the last cell division until they appear in the blood) in normal people is 2.5 days. In 1979 two studies were reported from Germany on the kinetics of eosinophil production, which was assessed using ^{3}H-thymidine labelling. Flash labelling in three normal subjects showed a mean turnover of eosinophils of 0.22×10^{9} cell/kg per day, and a mean post-mitotic eosinophil reserve capacity of the bone marrow of 0.14×10^{9} cells/kg.[1871] The large reserve capacity could contribute to the rapid rise in blood eosinophil counts which occurs in some circumstances. Labelling by continuous infusions for 3 to 10 days in 2 patients with normal blood eosinophil counts, and 6 with chronic lymphocytic leukaemia showed that the mean eosinophil intramedullary maturation and storage time was 103 hours.[1707]

In 1971 I published details of the kinetics of eosinophil production in normal rats and rats which were induced to produce an eosinophilia.[1676, 1677] The percentage of labelled eosinophil mataphases was assayed at intervals after a single injection of ^{3}H-thymidine into each animal (Plate 2). I noted that large sized eosinophils were cells which were about to undergo cell division, but that size alone did not define their stage of maturation. The cell cycle time for stimulated eosinophils was much shorter than that for unstimulated eosinophils. In rats with an eosinophilia, the number of cell divisions which took place before definable eosinophils entered the blood increased from three to five. In inflammatory diseases with eosinophilia, there is usually an increase in neutrophil as well as eosinophil counts in the blood, but there seems to be no competition for a precursor cell, i.e., eosinopoietic factors do not appear to divert cells from neutrophil synthesis. On the other hand, there is some evidence, from studies on neutropenic patients with eosinophilia, that mature eosinophils may suppress the formation of neutrophils, by releasing prostaglandins.[1764]

2.5 Assays for eosinopoietic factors

A number of assay systems have been developed to study eosinophil development *in vivo*. These include assays with peritoneal chambers, and assays for the number of eosinophil colonies which develop in rodent spleens after intravenous injection of marrow cells. Alterations in eosinophil labelling index have also been used to study the effects of eosinopoietic factors *in vivo*. None of these techniques has been very satisfactory, reflecting our ignorance of *in vivo* events in eosinopoiesis. All of the reproducible and sensitive assays for human eosinopoiesis involve the culture of eosinophil progenitor cells in semi-solid or liquid culture systems. The semi-solid agar technique was developed in the late 1960s, to assay marrow myeloid progenitor cells. Most of the *in vitro* colonies were derived from granulocyte-macrophage (GM) progenitor cells. The colony stimulating factor (CSF), which increased the number and the size of these colonies is now known as GM-CSF.

Four types of colonies can be formed by progenitor cells (CFUc) in double layer agar cultures: eosinophil, granulocyte, macrophage, and mixed granulocyte-macrophage. In 1980, a comparison of the numbers of colonies which grew from 5×10^5 normal human bone marrow cells, and an equal number of lymphocyte-enriched blood cells, and of cord blood cells, showed that there were a total of 89, 39, and 65 colonies respectively, of which 72 per cent, 48 per cent, and 23 per cent were eosinophil colonies.[972]

2.5.1 *Agar colony cultures*

The first descriptions of the *in vitro* growth of eosinophil colonies from human peripheral blood[312] and bone marrow[844] were published in 1971. Eosinophil colonies were separate from GM colonies, and grew more slowly. This was the first decisive evidence that eosinophils have a different origin in marrow from neutrophils. It was soon noted that eosinophil progenitor cells were present in surprisingly large numbers in human blood, and that they could be induced to form distinct colonies in agar cultures stimulated with certain types of conditioned media. Under optimal conditions, one third of the agar colonies which grow from human blood in conditioned medium were eosinophil colonies. These colonies were small, and they were usually distinguished by their special staining properties with dyes such as Biebrich scarlet, or Luxol fast blue.[879, 569] A peroxidase-based method for distinguishing eosinophil colonies was described in 1985.[472]

Eosinophil colonies were usually pure, although they occasionally contained small numbers of neutrophils or macrophages.[1043] Details of this technique for growing eosinophil colonies in agar are now well described, e.g.[175]

The EM appearances of eosinophils in soft agar colonies were reviewed in 1980, and it was noted that they did not form the characteristic granule crystalloid.[2007] It would be interesting to know if they would stain with anti-MBP antibodies.

The progenitor cells for eosinophil agar colonies have been shown to possess membrane HLA-DR antigens, and they did not have other membrane markers found on blood T- or B-lymphocytes.[244] Bone marrow eosinophils are heavier than other cells. In a comparative study on the density of marrow cells in Percoll gradients, eosinophils had the highest density: 1.0904 g/ml.[1312]

In patients with an eosinophilia the number of circulating eosinophil progenitor cells may increase. This was seen in a study of eosinophil progenitor cells in 12 Egyptians with schistosomiasis and an eosinophilia, and 8 healthy controls. The total number of colonies was doubled in the patients' blood samples, although there was no increase in the proportion which were eosinophilic.[903] The number of marrow-derived eosinophil progenitor cells may also increase: this was reported in a study on eosinophil colony development in bone marrow cultures, done in patients with the graft-versus-host disease.[1280] However, as another study in 1984 on 17 patients with eosinophilia found no increase in eosinophil progenitor cells in the blood or marrow,[952] this topic remains unsettled.

Several studies have been carried out on the possible effects of drugs and different disease processes on eosinophil development in agar cultures. It was found that eosinophil colony growth could be inhibited by cytotoxic drugs, and that steroids inhibited eosinophil progenitor cells directly, rather than through an effect on T-lymphocyte-derived colony stimulating factors.[177]

2.5.2 *Bone marrow liquid cultures*

Liquid culture systems were introduced in 1976 for the study of bone marrow eosinophil development.[1530] Initially they were used to study mouse marrow eosinophil development, and because they only maintained dividing eosinophils for a few days, they were most useful for defining factors which had a rapid effect on eosinophil proliferation, such as eosinophil growth stimulating factor (eosinophil-GSF),[118] and eosinophilopoietin (EPP)[1138, 1140]

Longer term liquid culture systems were then developed. These contained 0.9 per cent methylcellulose, and 30 per cent serum, and maintained marrow eosinophil growth for up to three weeks, providing that they were also stimulated with conditioned medium from lymphocytes or certain cell lines, such as the EL-4 murine thymoma cell line.[1820] In 1985, it was shown that eosinophils in mouse (but not human) cultures could be assessed conveniently by assaying eosinophil peroxidase.[1715]

In 1986 a two step culture system was developed which enabled eosinophil progenitor cells to grow from human bone marrow into large colonies containing up to 3000 cells, after three weeks' culture. In the first step, Percoll-separated interface cells, which were nonadherent, were cultured for four days with EL-4 conditioned medium. Then the cells were separated on a Percoll gradient again, and cultured in 0.9 per cent methylcellulose with 30 per cent serum, and 10 per cent EL-4 conditioned medium.[247]

2.5.3 *Assays* in vivo

The search for eosinophil specific growth factors which act *in vivo* has been a long one, and several groups have claimed success. In 1953, Samter showed that extracts from the lungs of guinea pigs which had previously been injected intraperitoneally with antigen–antibody complexes, when injected into normal guinea pigs, would produce an eosinophilia, suggesting that the lungs could be a site of formation of eosinopoietic substances.[1549] The main difficulty with this type of experiment has been to produce a reliable assay system.

In a series of papers between 1977 and 1980, Mahmoud and colleagues defined a low molecular weight pronase-sensitive substance called eosinophilopoietin (EPP), from mice, which increased the number of dividing marrow eosinophils *in vivo*, and raised the blood eosinophil counts of normal, and nu/nu mice.[1139, 1138, 1133] Mouse bone marrow cells in liquid culture were also stimulated by EPP to develop into eosinophils, and similar effects were produced with products from antigenically stimulated spleen cells, with the maximal response occurring at two days.[119] Some activity was found in mice infected with *S. mansoni* or *T. spiralis*,[1140] but none was seen in sera from patients with HES.[1135]

2.6 Eosinopoietic factors

Three different ways have been tried to find and characterize the factors which might stimulate the production of bone marrow eosinophils. The first was based on the knowledge that T-lymphocytes were required for animals to develop eosinophilia. In these studies, eosinophil growth-promoting factors were purified from supernatants of stimulated or cloned lymphocytes. The second approach, which has only been used in one centre, was to deplete circulating eosinophils with specific antibodies, and to examine the sera from these animals to see if an eosinopoietin was produced, by analogy with the production of erythropoietin following acute anaemia. The third method, which has been outstandingly successful, was to screen purified and recombinant colony stimulating factors (CSFs) for possible eosinopoietic activity. The results of this work are now providing a comprehensive picture of how eosinophil production may be increased in disease. Two stages in eosinopoiesis can now be postulated:

(1) an early event in which several CSFs, from adjacent cells in the marrow, stimulate eosinophil precursor cells to divide, and

(2) a later process in which helper T-lymphocytes, which are taking part in immunological responses, produce interleukin 5 (IL-5), which amplifies this proliferative response specifically.

The relative roles of the different CSFs and interleukins should soon become clearer, now that they have been isolated as recombinant proteins, although they may not have the full biological activity of the native molecule.

All of the purified factors which regulate eosinophil production are CSFs. Others, which remain to be defined, have been described in cultures of tumour cells, in the complement system, and in parasites. No common basis for this wide range of stimuli has yet been defined, and it is not known whether they act directly on eosinophil precursors, or via another cell type in the culture vessel. Little is known about the factors which induce the production of CSFs *in vivo*. Unstimulated cultured human vascular endothelial cells, which produced several molecules which could induce erythrocyte or macrophage/granulocyte colony formation *in vitro*, did not stimulate eosinophil development.[71] It has been known since 1976 that stimulated lymphocytes produce soluble factors, which increase the proliferation of eosinophils in several assay systems. They were called

(a) eosinophil-growth stimulating activity (GSF),[1530]

(b) eosinophil stimulation promoter (ESP),[342, 866] and

(c) eosinophilopoietin (EPP).[118, 1138, 1140]

It was later found that eosinophil-GSF and EPP were probably identical: they were both of low molecular weight, and had rapid effects on eosinophil proliferation.[119] This suggested that they were acting on a more differentiated eosinophil precursor than the CSFs,[124] which take several days to produce a noticeable change in the number of eosinophils in culture.

2.6.1 *Factors from T-lymphocytes*

By 1970 it had been shown that T-lymphocytes were involved in the regulation of eosinophil production, at least in rats.[136, 147] In 1976, Ruscetti and colleagues found that primed mouse lymphocytes stimulated with *T. spiralis* extracts produced a supernatant, which increased the proportion of eosinophilic colonies in methycellulose cultures of femoral bone marrow cells, and produced a three- to fourfold increase in the number of eosinophils formed in liquid cultures. This response was antigen specific, as supernatants from BCG primed cells, which had been stimulated with the parasite antigens, were inactive.[1530] In 1976 Miller and McGarry also reported finding a soluble eosinopoietic factor released by mouse lymphocytes.[1212] Subsequent work confirmed that antigen-stimulated human T-cells produce an eosinopoietic activity, and aspergillus-sensitized human T-lymphocytes produced an eosinopoietic activity.[518] This stimulated the growth of eosinophils in both agar and liquid cultures.[519]

The types of lymphocytes involved in the induction of eosinopoiesis have been presumed to be helper T-cells, but experiments in mice suggest that suppressor T-cells may also be involved. It may not be limited to any one T-cell subset, as human cortical thymocytes may have this property; see reference 945.

Interleukin 5, IL-5, EDF In 1985 Sanderson and colleagues in London reported that a hybrid clone (NIMP-TH1) of a mouse thymoma cell line BW5147, and spleen cells from mice infected with *Mesocestoides corti*, produced an eosinophil-specific growth factor, after stimulation with phorbol myristate acetate (PMA).[1879] They also found that a high proportion of primary alloreactive T-cell clones from mice with an eosinophilia produce this eosinopoietic factor.[1555, 1553] This activity was called 'eosinophil differentiation factor' (EDF). In 1986 EDF was found to be able to stimulate human eosinophil differentiation.[1101] The hybrid clone was grown in bulk, and used for further characterization of the molecule, including its capacity to act as a B-cell growth factor.[1552] It was suggested that EDF should be called IL-4, but as the IL terminology is restricted to cloned molecules, this name for it was not generally accepted.

Mouse EDF had several properties which suggested that it could be a close analogue of the putative human eosinophil-specific CSF, as it was a selective stimulus for the clonal proliferation and differentiation of human bone marrow eosinophils.[1823]

In 1986, work by Honjo and colleagues in Japan led to the cloning of a murine T-cell factor which stimulated B-cell growth: B-cell growth factor II, which was given the internationally recognized name of IL-5.[966] It soon became clear that EDF and IL-5 were identical molecules. In 1987, the Japanese workers cloned the human gene for IL-5.[85] In 1987 a group in Australia and the UK[264] cloned, sequenced, and developed expression vectors for the gene for human IL-5. rHuIL-5 was found to be a unique molecule, specific for human eosinophil differentiation. Studies are now under way, to see how IL-5 affects human eosinophil differentiation, and whether IL-5 can be assayed in human samples, especially from patients with eosinophilia. It has been found to stimulate eosinophil development to the myelocyte stage in suspension cultures of human bone marrow and cord blood (Saito, H. 1988, personal communication), and to maturity (Clutterback, E. J. 1988, personal communication). It also activates and alters the morphology of mature eosinophils (Vadas, M. A. 1988, personal communication). Although recombinant IL-5 stimulated murine B-cells to express IL-2 receptors,[1108] and synthesize IgA, it did not appear to affect human B-cells (Sanderson 1987, personal communication).

Interleukin 2, IL-2 Injections of purified recombinant interleukin 2 (IL-2) into patients with malignant diseases can give rise to a marked eosinophilia.[586] However, it is not known yet whether this is a direct, or indirect effect of IL-2 itself on eosinophil production, or a secondary effect produced by GM-CSF released from IL-2 stimulated T-lymphocytes. It was not prevented by injections of dexamethasone.[1857] As IL-2 induced murine T-cell clones to secrete GM-CSF (CSF-α),[950] the effects of IL-2 on eosinopoiesis may be indirect. This possibility is supported by a study on 11 patients with an eosinophilia, due to many different causes, in whom 5 had a raised blood helper/suppressor T-cells ratio. In all 11 patients, culture of purified blood T-lymphocytes with IL-2 increased the amount of eosinophil and monocyte-macrophage CSF which was secreted into the medium during a 5-day culture. Surprisingly, this capacity persisted after eosinophilia had disappeared in 3 of the patients.[517] (See also page 301.)

2.6.2 *Colony stimulating factors*

The properties of CSFs from cultures of placental and other cells have been studied for nearly two decades by Metcalf, Nicola, and their colleagues in Australia and other centres.[1192] A summary of the principal CSFs affecting eosinophil colony growth is shown in Fig. 2.1. CSFs, with predominant effects on eosinophil colony growth in agar culture were described in several centres in the early 1970s. In 1974 Metcalf and colleagues showed that supernatants from pokeweed-mitogen-stimulated mouse spleen cells contained a separate factor which induced eosinophil development from mouse bone marrow. It was distinct from neutrophil and macrophage CSFs.[1196]

Two of the well-defined CSFs, GM-CSF (previously known as CSF-α), and multi-CSF (which is also called interleukin 3, IL-3), affect eosinophil proliferation especially.[1824] The gene for murine GM-CSF was cloned in 1984,[704] and a cDNA expression product was produced from transfected monkey COS cells in 1986,[1787] but it was not as potent as the native molecule. GM-CSF is a 127 amino acid protein with two internal disulphide groups.

In a review on eosinophil activating factors in 1984, Vadas emphasized the importance of differential regulation of eosinophils and neutrophils with GM-CSF (CSF-α) and G-CSF (CSF-β).[1818]. GM-CSF stimulated both eosinophil- and neutrophil-mediated cytotoxicity, whereas G-CSF had a stimulatory effect only on neutrophils. It was reported in 1987 that recombinant G-CSF did not induce eosinophil colonies *in vitro* from

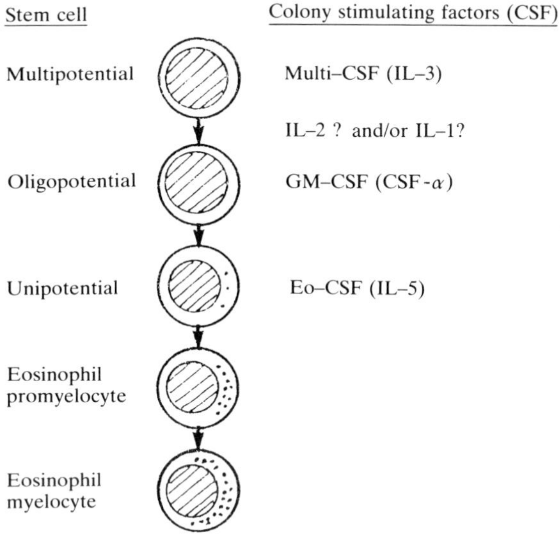

Fig. 2.1. Factors affecting eosinophil differentiation. The earlier cells are probably stimulated by multi-CSF, and possibly by IL-2. GM-CSF induces further differentiation, and in the final step, Eo-CSF induces the dividing cells to become eosinophils.

human marrow, or alter blood eosinophil counts in guinea pigs, although it gave them a neutrophil leukocytosis.[2005]

GM-CSF (CSF-α) In 1986, two groups showed that rGM-CSF induced the development of eosinophil colonies from normal marrow. Metcalf and colleagues in Australia used both rMuGM-CSF,[1195] and rHuGM-CSF.[1193] Tomonaga and colleagues in California used rHuGM-CSF.[1787] The work in California also showed that rHuGM-CSF induced eosinophil formation by HL-60 cells, although this has not been confirmed in other laboratories.

Earlier work from Australia had already shown that the activities of GM-CSF were identical to those of CSF-α, which had been previously purified from placental conditioned medium, and which increased the capacity of eosinophil to kill antibody-coated schistosomula.[232]

The effects of GM-CSF are not always concentration dependent. Low concentrations of human placental-conditioned medium containing GM-CSF were most effective in stimulating eosinophil colony growth in agar cultures of human bone marrow, whereas stimulation was concentration-independent in suspension liquid cultures.[954]

Injections of large amounts of recombinant GM-CSF give rise to a marked eosinophilia in man. This was first shown in a study on 16 patients with AIDS studied in Boston, and reported in 1987.[718] A bone marrow eosinophilia developed in 8 patients. In one patient given 1×10^4 u/kg/day as a bolus on day 1, and by continuous infusion from days 3 to 17, the blood eosinophil count reached 15.5×10^9/l, at day 17, after which the injections were stopped, and the eosinophil counts then fell rapidly towards normal. These results are consistent with the hypothesis that GM-CSF is a natural stimulus for eosinopoiesis in disease.

Interleukin 3 (IL-3), multi-CSF (M-CSF) In 1987 it was reported that cloned gibbon interleukin 3 stimulated the proliferation and differentiation of human bone marrow cells to produce eosinophil colonies in semisolid agar.[1103]

Purified recombinant murine multi-CSF (IL-3) induced normal murine bone marrow cells to develop into colonies. At high concentrations (above 50-100 u/l), eosinophil colonies developed. Similar findings were made with native multi-CSF. When 6 mg were injected into the peritoneum of Balb/c mice, more eosinophils were found at 6 days than in mice injected with serum-saline. This was dose-dependent. These results show that M-CSF affects a range of cell types. Although M-CSF has not been detected in serum, or organ extracts, it may be a stimulus for eosinophil production under some pathological conditions.[1194] Labelled murine M-CSF has been shown to bind to immature murine marrow eosinophils, but not to more mature eosinophils.[1277] Further studies with rM-CSF in man are awaited with interest.

2.6.3 *Factors in inflamed tissues*

In 1982, a GM-CSF-like activity was found in blister fluid of three out of five patients with bullous pemphigoid.[1840] Nasal polyp epithelial cells from patients with allergic rhinitis were reported in 1987 to be able to produce eosinophil colony-stimulating factors.[431]

2.6.4 *Factors from tumour cells, and cell lines*

A number of unsuccessful attempts have been made to find eosinopoietic factors in the serum of patients with an eosinophilia,[1866, 117] and in tumour cell extracts from patients with neoplasms and hypereosinophilia. However, in 1983 and 1984 eosinopoietic factor(s) were detected in the sera and tumour extracts from patients with carcinoma of the lung and marked eosinophilia.[1646, 986] Viruses with oncogenic potential can also stimulate the production of eosinopoietic factors. For example, supernatants from human lymphocytes infected with HTLV-1 retrovirus produce a number of lymphokines, including an eosinophil growth, and maturation activity.[1543] In 1983, a factor from a malignant fibrous histiocytoma was shown to have eosinopoietic activity.[1591]

Several cell lines produce eosinophil growth-promoting activities. In 1986 'pleuripoietin alpha' was described in the human bladder carcinoma cell line 5637.[614] In 1987 it was shown that a T-cell leukemia cell line (Mo) produced a conditioned medium containing an eosinophil growth-stimulating activity. This was heat stable, and could be partly separated by DEAE chromatography from a basophil growth-stimulating activity, when assayed by the methylcellulose technique with cord blood mononuclear cells.[1754] The properties of several growth-promoting factors from a number of other human cell lines were reviewed in 1987.[1754]

2.6.5 *Factors in serum from patients with eosinophilia*

The presence of eosinopoietic factors in the serum of patients has not been reported very often, possibly because most eosinopoietic substances act as paracrine substances, e.g., they act on adjacent cells only. In 1983 a weak CSF activity was detected in sera from a patient with a carcinoma-of-the-lung-induced eosinophilia.[1646] No comparable activity was found in sera from patients with acute lymphocytic leukaemia and hypereosinophilia.[806] In 1986, it was reported from Berlin that serum, and a crude extract of a malignant fibrous histiocytoma which had produced eosinophil counts up to 17.5×10^9/l in a 63-year-old woman, increased the number of eosinophil colonies grown from normal bone marrow cultured by a plasma clot technique. As much activity was found in 10 per cent patient's serum as in a 5 per cent solution of the tumour extract.[1591]

A study from Sydney, Australia in 1987 reported that sera from a group of patients with chronic myeloid leukaemia, two of whom were studied during blast cell transformation, contained an eosinopoietic activity, which increased the survival and growth of bone-marrow-derived 'persisting' eosinophil colonies in semi-solid agar. These colonies had grown for 35 days, or longer. It was suggested that this might be IL-3, and that it could be involved in inducing the transformed cells to proliferate.[217]

In 1986 it was reported that sera from IL-2 treated patients with AIDS who developed an eosinophilia, contained an 'eosinophil-producing activity' (EPA) in bone marrow liquid culture.[953] Similarly, sera from six other patients with HES, four with CML and eosinophilia, two with non-Hodgkin's lymphoma, and six with acute helminthic infections and eosinophilia were found to be able to increase the number of eosinophils in 12-day liquid cultures of human bone marrow from 0.1×10^5 eosinophils/250 μl, to 2.1×10^5/250 μl. Four normal sera and sera from eight people without eosinophilia had no effect. Serum was added at 5-40 vol per cent. Unfortunately, these experiments did not distinguish between differential survival of eosinophils in the cultures, and stimulation of eosinopoiesis. The activity was destroyed by heating at 65° for 20 minutes, and had an apparent molecular weight of 80–85 kDa on Sephadex G-100. Interestingly, active serum was ineffective in stimulating eosinophil colony growth in agar cultures.[954]

2.7 Drugs and eosinophil production

Injections of cyclophosphamide together with a parasitic or other eosinopoietic stimulus, have been shown to be able to induce marked eosinophilia in mice[1816, 1722] and rats.[1774] With this approach it was found in 1982 that genetic factors have a role in regulating eosinophil production in mice.[1817] There are no reports of a similar mechanism occurring in man.

A number of studies have found that steroids (hydrocortisone) inhibited the development of human eosinophil colonies *in vitro*. It was therefore surprising that experiments from Switzerland in 1987 showed that hydrocortisone can increase the capacity of human marrow or blood cells to form eosinophil colonies *in vitro*, either when the drug is added to the cultures, or when the blood cells are obtained from people given hydrocortisone. It was suggested that the acute effects of steroids in causing a fall in eosinophil counts *in vivo* are mainly a result of the redistribution of the cells in the blood.[115]

The addition of lithium, rubidium, and caesium salts to human bone marrow cultures increases the number of colonies, including eosinophils,[114] but there are no reports that patients taking lithium salts develop eosinophilia.

2.8 Suppressor cells and eosinophil production

Suppressor T-cells may be able to inhibit eosinopoiesis. This possibility was suggested when an excess of T-suppressor-cells were found in the blood of a patient with a thymoma, and a total absence of eosinophils.[1220] No experimental work has been done yet to test this possibility, which could be of clinical importance in patients with persistent eosinophilia, such as HES. However, in mice, suppressor T-cells, which reduced the numbers of eosinophils in the peritoneal cavity, have been found in the spleens of animals injected with high doses of tetanus toxoid, or tetanus toxoid in complete Freund's adjuvant. These cells inhibited the development of peritoneal eosinophilia in mice injected with tetanus toxoid with alum, following cyclophosphamide pretreatment.[1746]

2.9 Eosinophil suppression of granulocytopoiesis

As prostaglandins inhibit GM colony formation in agar cultures, it has been suggested that eosinophil-derived prostaglandins could act in this way. Experiments with mouse peritoneal eosinophils supported this idea:

they inhibited the formation of mouse bone marrow colonies in agar, and this effect was prevented with indomethacin.[626] However, although there are a few clinical conditions in which eosinophils persist longer than neutrophils when granulocytopoiesis is inhibited, in patients with marked eosinophilia, neutrophil numbers are almost invariably increased as well. There is also no evidence as yet that bone marrow eosinophils can secrete prostaglandins.

2.10 Genetic factors affecting human eosinophil production

There are three lines of evidence which suggest that genetic factors influence the number of eosinophils that are produced in response to stimulation. These are studies in man, which have shown that certain chromosomal abnormalities are associated with marked eosinophilia, and experiments in inbred rodents, some of which can produce marked eosinophilia to stimuli which only induce a small response in others. In addition there is a report that homozygous Sl/Sl and Wv/Wv mice had only 15 per cent of the number of blood eosinophils found in littermate controls. This was probably due to a defect in eosinophil production, as there were also less eosinophils in the bone marrow, spleen, and thymus.[1931]

2.10.1 *Cytogenetic studies*

Cytogenetic studies on patients with malignant haemopoietic diseases involving eosinophils have shown G banding abnormalities in several chromosomes which may be involved in eosinophil differentiation. These include abnormalities with:

(1) chromosome 5,[1980, 390] where the gene for GM-CSF, IL-3, IL-5, and M-CSF are located; IL-5 is at 5q31.

(2) chromosome 7, which was abnormal in two patients with myeloblastic leukaemia, and marked eosinophilia;[827, 1224]

(3) chromosome 8, which is abnormal in the eosinophil cell line EoL,[1537] and which was a trisomy in two patients with eosinophilic leukaemia.[1365, 1899] An 8;21 translocation affecting eosinophils was seen in a girl with eosinophilic leukaemia in Japan, in 1983.[904]

(4) chromosome 12, which was abnormal in a patient with a malignant proliferation of eosinophils;[943]

(5) chromosome 16, where rearrangements, and other alterations have been seen in patients with M4-Eo acute leukaemia with an eosinophilia (see page 158). An abnormality is present on the long arm of chromosome 16 in the HL-60 cell line, which has been induced to form eosinophil granules.[569]

There is no evidence that the c-fos proto-oncogene, which has been suggested to be important in the control of monocyte development, is involved in human eosinophil differentiation, as mRNA was not detected by *in situ* hybridization in blood eosinophils.[1004]

2.10.2 *Genetic studies in rodents*

In 1982, it was shown by Vasas and colleagues that the eosinophil response in inbred mice was genetically controlled. Evidence that the major histocompatibility complex was involved soon followed.[1593] High and low responsiveness were shown to be determined by the bone marrow, as the development of eosinophilia in radiation chimeric mice was related to the origin of the bone marrow used to make the chimeras.[1720]

2.11 Eosinophil cell lines

Several eosinophil cell lines have been developed, which are being used to study the synthesis of eosinophil constituents,[567, 13] and to prepare cDNA coding for eosinophil constituents. These have been derived from the HL-60 cell line, which was originally developed in the USA, and EoL cell line, which was derived from a patient with eosinophilic leukaemia in France.

The HL-60 cell line, which was developed from a patient with acute promyelocytic leukaemia in 1979,[617] has a chromosome 17 inversion. HL-60 cells have several characteristics in common with eosinophils found in patients with acute myelomonocytic leukaemia with eosinophilia (FAB class M4-eo). For example, in 1981 they were found to contain some luxol-fast-blue granules, a feature of eosinophils.[1116] In 1983 it was shown that a small percentage of HL-60 cells in culture matured into typical eosinophils, but this was not influenced by additional human eosinophil CSFs.[1191]

Fischkoff and colleagues continued to develop eosinophil cell lines from cloned HL-60 cells. They showed that in soft agar cultures, a few HL-60 cells differentiated into eosinophils, some of which became mature cells, containing small granules. Although crystalloids were rarely seen, they contained eosinophil peroxidase (EPO), MBP, CLC protein, arylsulphatase, and acid phosphatase.[569]

In 1985 they reported that more HL-60 cell lines were induced to synthesize eosinophil granules by culturing them at pH 7.4 with 0.5 mM butyric acid for seven days.[568] Neutrophil induction occurred with 176 mM dimethyl sulphoxide. Enzyme assays and electronmicroscopy showed that peroxidase was synthesized, and packaged in spherical granules, although the Golgi apparatus contained little peroxidase. Acid phosphatase, arylsulphatase, and lysophospholipase were synthesized in smaller amounts than in normal eosinophils.[567]

In 1986, it was reported that two stable eosinophil cell lines had been developed by serial subculture of HL-60 colonies which contained many eosinophils. They retained lineage fidelity even after stimulation with GM-CSF.[1786] It was suggested that these cell lines would be particularly useful for studying the production and functions of human eosinophils, and for analysing leukaemic cell differentiation, and stem cell commitment.

In 1984, an eosinophilic leukemia cell line was established in Paris from a 33-year-old man with a Phi-negative eosinophilic leukemia.[1537] This was obtained from separated white blood cells grown in suspension culture, and in 0.3 per cent agarose. The cells began to proliferate after two months' culture, and were subcultured at 10 weeks. Six clones were derived. Three clones, named 'EoL-1', 'EoL-2', and 'EoL-3' had eosinophilic features. Three other clones, 'Eo-B', had a B-cell phenotype. No feeder cells were used. EoL-1 grew in single cell suspension. EoL-2 and EoL-3 formed cell clusters. Occasional cells contained eosinophil granules, but after induction with alkaline medium or dimethylsulphoxide, 40 per cent contained granules. The EoL lines expressed Ia receptors, the myeloid antigens IF10, and MY9, and IL-2 receptors.

2.12 Blood eosinophil kinetics

Eosinophils leave the bone marrow and enter the blood sequentially, and leave it randomly. This is easily shown by injecting labelled cells which appear in tissues sites (such as nasal secretions) immediately, and continue to do so during the next few hours. In the bloodstream, many eosinophils are believed to be marginated at any one time, in exchange equilibrium with an equal number in the circulation.

The kinetics of human blood eosinophils were measured accurately by two groups in Germany in 1976 and 1979 using ^{3}H-thymidine autoradiography. In the first study it was found that the eosinophil emergence time was 3.5 days. The blood half-life was 13 hours, and the mean blood transit time 25 hours. The S phase was 13 hours, and myelocyte generation time about 34 hours. There was some evidence for two pools of proliferating eosinophils. Similar results were obtained for neutrophils' kinetics which were measured at the same time.[1371] The second study, in 1979, showed that the mean blood eosinophil relative turnover rate was 4.0 per cent per hour, the mean blood transit time (or blood sojourn time) was 26 $\pm$ 3 hours, and the blood half-life was 18.0 $\pm$ 2.1 hours.[1707]

The eosinophil blood half-life is prolonged when there is eosinophilia. This may be because the number of sites through which eosinophils can migrate into the tissues is limiting. The process of emigration from the bloodstream occurs in venules, and involves loose attachment to vascular endothelium, followed by migration between endothelial cells, and into the connective tissue around the blood vessels. (See page 97)

In many infectious diseases due to bacteria or viruses, the blood eosinophil count has been found to be low, or zero.[124] Although the eosinopenia of infection may be due partly to the production of steroids during the stress produced by inflammation, it has been shown that eosinopenia can occur in infected mice, without an increase in blood corticosterone levels.[121] Steroids, other than large amounts of dexamethasone, had little effect on human eosinophil colony growth from blood or marrow progenitor cells.[243]

The rapid decrease in blood eosinophil counts following infection or stress involves both an increased uptake of eosinophils into tissues, and a decreased output of eosinophils from the marrow.[122] A host component, which was present in inflammatory reactions in the mouse, appeared to be responsible for these effects.[123] Injections into rabbits of zymosan-activated serum, partially purified C5a, and f-Met-Leu-Phe caused an immediate eosinopenia, suggesting that these could also mediate the acute eosinopenia of infection.[125]

2.13 Kinetics of eosinophils in tissues

The survival time of eosinophils in tissues is not known, but it is likely that they can remain there for several days. As human eosinophils can live in culture for over 14 days with CSFs,[148] or endothelial cell conditioned medium,[1522] and there are often more eosinophils in chronic inflammatory sites than in the blood, their life span is likely to be at least two weeks.

3. Methods: eosinophil structure, constituents, and metabolism

3.1 Eosinophil counts

It is often necessary to be able to count the number of eosinophils in the blood and tissues. Unfortunately, there are no areas of the body where eosinophils are evenly distributed, although the blood comes closest to this. Even here, some eosinophils are marginated, and some in the circulating pool of cells. The best approach to this difficulty is to measure the number of eosinophils in several samples, and to use statistical methods to calculate their distribution. The amounts of eosinophil-specific constituents can be measured per unit mass of tissue, but most investigators count stained cells in suspension, or in sections. This is likely to underestimate the involvement of eosinophils in diseases, where degranulated eosinophils may not be stained as in normal tissues. Measurements of eosinophil numbers taken at a fixed time are also unable to provide any information about the flux or kinetics of eosinophil transit into and out of the tissues being studied.

Ottolenghi and colleagues have assessed the extent of eosinophil involvement in rats by assaying tissue levels of lysophospholipase. This approach was based on their finding in 1967 of large amounts of phospholipase (lysolecithinase) in rat tissues using histochemical methods.[1344] In 1970 this was related to their content of eosinophils,[1342] which led to the development of an enzyme-based assay for the involvement of eosinophils in inflammatory lesions produced by parasites in rats.[1343] This type of measurement has not yet been used to study the eosinophil content of human tissues, or their contribution to inflammatory reactions, and it would need careful validation before it could be used instead of cell counts.

Although the much criticized routine of using 'per cent eosinophils', as a crude measure of eosinophil counts, persists in many centres, fortunately most automated counting systems now provide printouts in which the total number of white blood cells is multiplied by the per cent eosinophils to provide clinically useful data. The term 'per cent eosinophils' should not be used unless there are specific reasons for knowing the proportions of eosinophils compared to other cells in a sample. It is no substitute for an accurate eosinophil count. There is no reason to continue a practice which began in the early part of the century when it was thought (incorrectly) that the presence of one cell type in the blood could affect the numbers of another cell type.

3.1.1 *Manual methods*

The most widely used, and one of the most accurate methods for measuring blood eosinophil counts in the internationally agreed SI notation (eosinophils $\times$ 10^9/l), is to use an improved Neubauer counting chamber, into which is pipetted the blood, diluted 1 in 10 (or 1 in 20, if the blood eosinophil count is greater than 1 $\times$ 10^9/l) with a stock solution of one of the bromeinated derivatives of fluorescein which stain eosinophils strongly, such as eosin (tetrabromo-fluorescein), or phloxin (tetrabromo-tetrachloro-fluorescein). In the eosin method, which is widely used outside the USA, the stock solution contains 1 per cent aqueous eosin-Y (five volumes), acetone (five volumes), and distilled water (90 volumes) to lyse the red cells. This is an adaptation of the counting method developed by Dunger in 1910.[475]

In the phloxin method, which was introduced in 1944 by Randolph in the USA, where it is still often used, propylene glycol is added to 'clear' the red cells, which are not lysed. Methylene blue is used to stain the nuclei of the white cells, and phloxin to stain the eosinophils.[1476] Randolph discussed the advantage of using propylene glycol to enable the eosinophil and white blood cell counts to be done in the same counting chamber.[1477] In both methods, an assessment is made of the volume of fluid in the counting chamber which contains 200 eosinophils, using both sides of the chamber if necessary, to ensure that the accuracy of the counts are consistent, and independent of the total eosinophil count. This is especially important when the count is less than 1 $\times$ 10^9/l.

Although total blood eosinophil counts can be calculated from differential blood counts done on blood smears, this is not recommended, as the accuracy is low.[564] This is because eosinophils are large cells, which tend to be pulled to the ends and sides of smears. Also, as eosinophils comprise only a proportion of the 200 white cells counted, the accuracy of the count is only acceptable if they make up more than half of the total white blood cells examined.

A statistical analysis of the chamber method has shown its superiority to differential counts.[454] Although smears can give accurate counts in expert hands,[1035] modern haematology laboratories now use automated counting methods, in which 2000 white cells are assessed.

3.1.2 *Automated methods*

The validity of automated differential counting systems for assessing the number of blood eosinophils has been shown by comparisons with manual counting methods in adults[65] and children.[366] Although most major laboratories find that automated counting systems are accurate[99, 618] they can produce errors in samples with high blood eosinophil counts.[98] Besides their speed and reproducibility, they have the added advantage that they may bring to light a patient with eosinophil peroxidase deficiency.[1748]

3.1.3 *Normal blood eosinophil counts*

In a study of my own on 100 adults of both sexes in Oxford, UK, blood eosinophil counts ranged from 0 to $0.55 \times 10^9/l$. I excluded people with allergic rhinitis, hayfever, and other mild allergic disorders whose counts were slightly higher than this. For practical reasons I consider blood eosinophil counts of between $0.55–1.5 \times 10^9/l$ as 'needing follow up', between $1.5–10 \times 10^9/l$, as 'needing investigation soon', and over $10 \times 10^9/l$ as 'needing urgent assessment'.

An analysis of a large number of blood eosinophil counts, which were done in the USA between 1971–75 for people aged 25–74 years, was published in 1982.[1174] However, these results were derived from differential counts, which is not very satisfactory for obtaining absolute values, as described above.

It was reported in 1987 that the blood eosinophil count in 740 medical students in Pittsburgh, USA, was $0.015–0.65 \times 10^9/l$ (95 per cent confidence limits).[1003]

In a group of normal children aged four to eight years, blood eosinophil counts were $0.206 \pm 0.270 \times 10^9/l$. Over 12 years of age they were lower: $0.096 \pm 0.140 \times 10^9/l$, and males were: 0.180 ± 0.160, and females $0.145 \pm 0.120 \times 10^9/l$.[374]

Blood eosinophil counts vary diurnally in normal people. The counts are inversely related to blood cortisol levels, e.g., the counts are lowest in the morning, and highest at night. In 1981 the mean variation in blood eosinophil counts were assessed in 21 normal adults, using the Hemalog-D automated counter. The intra-subject within-day variation was 27 per cent, and the diurnal variation was over 40 per cent.[1938] This showed the importance of doing serial blood counts at a fixed time of day.

In 1984, a comparative study of blood eosinophil counts in four ethnic groups living in Britain (Indian, black (African, and West Indian), white (Northern European), and oriental), showed no significant differences. This confirmed the generally accepted view that high eosinophil counts in tropical countries are related to parasitic infections, rather than genetic factors.[97] A similar conclusion was reached in a study in Kenya, in 1979.[1309]

It has been known for several years that exercise increases the blood eosinophil count,[317] which can be exploited when normal blood eosinophils are needed for experimental studies.

3.2 Leukapheresis

Obtaining large numbers of human eosinophils from the blood is straightforward when the eosinophil count is high, but leukapheresis has also been used successfully to obtain eosinophils from both normal and patient's blood. In this technique dextran, methylcellulose, or hydroxyethyl starch[671] are used to sediment the red cells before the white cells are aspirated from the collection bag. This technique has provided up to 2×10^{11} eosinophils from an individual with a blood eosinophil count of 50×10^{9}/l.[661]

In 1987, leukapheresis using hydroxyethyl starch was used to separate blood eosinophils for biochemical and ultrastructural studies from five patients with HES.[780] However in two patients, the presence of cytoplasmic Charcot–Leyden crystals in the purified eosinophils, which are never seen in freshly drawn blood, suggested that the procedure may have had a detrimental effect on the eosinophils.

3.3 Cell separation

Many different methods for separating eosinophils from other cells have been described in the past, but none of them proved satisfactory until non-toxic density gradient methods were devised, which were able to exploit the greater density of eosinophils (1.088 g/ml) compared to other leukocytes. These methods were reviewed in 1983,[655] and 1986.[1511] Most methods have used blood cells, but they can also be used to separate eosinophils in exudates, and even in normal tissues, such as the lungs.[1837]

Samples of blood are first anticoagulated. This can either be done with preservative-free heparin 5 u/ml, if functional studies are to be done, or EDTA pH 7.2 10 mM final concentration. The red blood cells should be removed before purifying eosinophils from other white cells. This can be done by sedimentation with 5 per cent dextran, although this usually leads to the loss of 30 per cent or more of the white blood cells within the sedimented red cells. A mixture of methylcellulose and Hypaque in place of the dextran gives a higher yield in this first step.[825] We use this routinely. The removal of residual contaminating erythrocytes is best done with isotonic ammonium chloride pH 7.2, at 4°.[1512] Other methods for red cell lysis, such as rapid lysis with distilled water, damage eosinophils.

3.3.1 *Differential binding to surfaces*

A method has been developed to separate human blood eosinophils from neutrophils on the basis of their different binding capacity to complexed IgG, using plastic dishes to which IgG was attached with carbodiimide.[1739]

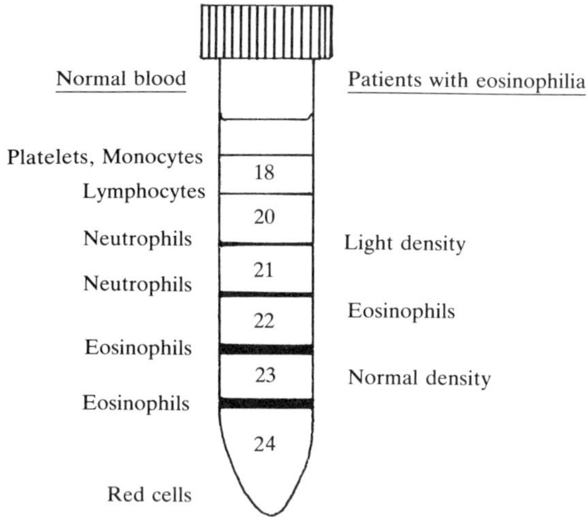

Fig. 3.1. The separation of human blood eosinophils by isopycnic density gradient centrifugation on discontinous metrizamide. Eosinophils are found between the denser bands. Blood eosinophils from patients with eosinophilia can be separated into light density and normal density eosinophils with this method.

3.3.2 *Density gradient separation*

The most commonly used density gradient solutions to separate eosinophil from blood are metrizamide and Percoll.

In 1979, Vadas and colleagues developed what has become the standard method for purifying eosinophils from human blood, using metrizamide.[1821] The key steps were the use of DNAase to prevent cell clumping, and the use of slightly hypertonic discontinuous gradients. Normal blood eosinophils equilibrate in the 23–24 per cent bands, but in many diseases with eosinophilia, lighter density eosinophils separate with neutrophils in the 22 per cent band (Fig. 3.1).

Percoll density gradients have been used to purify eosinophils since 1980.[628] A method for separating eosinophils from bone marrow or blood samples using discontinuous Percoll gradients was described in 1984.[504] Using this method, it was found that in gradients of 56 per cent, 64 per cent, 68 per cent, and 77 per cent Percoll, eosinophils were obtained in highest purity in the 77 per cent layer.[1539]

A variety of other methods for using Percoll to isolate eosinophils have also been described. These include a method described from Rome in 1982,[420] and a method described at the NIH Bethesda, USA, in which fMLP was used to activate neutrophils, which then became lighter, and easier to separate.[1497] However, as eosinophils are also stimulated by fMLP,[1604, 1970] this method is not recommended. A method was described in 1987, from Amsterdam, in which eosinophils were separated over two successive Percoll gradients.[1969]

In our hands, Percoll gradient separation of eosinophils has given less consistent results than metrizamide gradients, and there appears to be no method for removing the Percoll particles from the purified cells. However, as the Percoll separation technique is carried out in isosmolar conditions, it can be used to measure the differences in density between eosinophils in normal blood (normal density, or normodense eosinophils), and patients' eosinophils some of which may be of lighter density (light density, or hypodense cells).[1389]

The finding of light density eosinophils in patients' blood was first discussed in 1980 by Bass and colleagues. They used gradients of metrizamide and Hypaque, and found that in patients with eosinophilia, eosinophils were often present in the lighter bands with the neutrophils, instead of in the denser layers where eosinophils from normal individuals always separated.[127] This was also noted by other groups in 1982[1944, 420] and 1983.[1452]

Several years earlier, we had noted that many degranulated eosinophils in patients with HES had a similar density to neutrophils. The presence of contaminating neutrophils prevented us from comparing their functional properties with eosinophils of normal density. This problem persists, as there is no effective method for separating viable light density eosinophils from neutrophils. This type of study can only be done when patients are found who have low blood neutrophil counts. Percoll density gradients have been used to determine the density of light density eosinophils. The peak density of normal eosinophils is 1.088 g/ml, and light density eosinophils 1.076 g/ml.[611] Fractions containing light density eosinophils were seen to have a number of properties which suggested that they had been activated. Light density eosinophils were first called 'hypodense' cells in France. There are semantic and scientific objections to the use of this hybrid Greek-cum-Latin word, in place of the better term 'light density'. 'Hypodense' also suggests, incorrectly, that there may be two populations of eosinophils: eosinophil density is a continuum. There are many diseases in which light density eosinophils have been detected in the blood, including asthma,[611] allergic diseases, HES, and experimental hookworm infections.[1925] Light density eosinophils have been found in samples taken from outside the blood stream, including bronchoalveolar eosinophils. This was first demonstrated in 1984 in bronchoalveolar lavage (BAL) fluid from three patients with pulmonary infiltrates,[1453] and confirmed in a study in 1987 in Kyoto, Japan, where it was found that 93 per cent of the eosinophils in BAL fluid from patients with PIE syndromes were of lower density than normal. This was a higher proportion than in other diseases with eosinophils in BAL fluid.[316]

The presence of light density eosinophils in patients with eosinophilia is still not explained. It is not known whether they result from accelerated eosinophil production giving rise to smaller and lighter granules, or whether they are produced by an effect of some component of the blood stream, or vasculature on normal density eosinophils.

3.3.3 *Elutriation centrifugation*

There have been no reports of the successful use of elutriation centrifugation to separate blood eosinophils, although several laboratories are assessing its potential value.[1511]

3.4 Culture of mature eosinophils

Although there has been anecdotal information for many years that eosinophils can survive in tissue culture for over 10 days, it is only since 1985 that this has been studied formally, using conditioned medium from lymphocytes and endothelial cells.

3.4.1 *Lymphocyte products*

In 1985, during a study on the culture of HES blood eosinophils, we found that they would survive intact for three weeks in the presence of lymphocyte conditioned medium (Lai, P. and Spry, C. J. 1985, unpublished). The light density, degranulated eosinophils appeared to survive as well as, if not better than, the normal granulated cells, suggesting that degranulation was not inevitably associated with eosinophil death.

3.4.2 *Endothelial cell products*

In 1987 it was shown that normal human blood eosinophils could be maintained for several weeks by co-culturing them with bovine aortic endothelial cells, or conditioned medium from endothelial cells.[1522] Under these conditions it was found that most of the surviving eosinophils were of light density.

3.4.3 *Colony stimulating factors, CSFs*

It was first reported in 1986 that several CSFs can prolong the survival of human blood eosinophils in culture for up to nine hours. These factors were recombinant human GM-CSF[1105] and partially purified preparations of murine GM-CSF, and murine IL-5, which increased the survival of blood eosinophils in culture from a mean of 28 to 38 hours, but had no action on blood neutrophil survival.[1823] Interestingly, recombinant human GM-CSF also enhanced the survival of neutrophils for six hours, but murine GM-CSF, and its human analogue CSF-β, only prolonged the survival of neutrophils, suggesting that there was cell lineage specificity for the actions of these CSFs on mature granulocytes.[148]

Owen and colleagues in Boston, USA were the first to show in 1987 that normal blood eosinophils can survive in culture for one or two weeks in the presence of recombinant GM-CSF, providing it is replenished at each change of the culture medium. Sixty per cent of the innoculum survived. As GM-CSF can be produced by endothelial cells, which gave even better survival percentages *in vitro*, it was suggested that blood vessels might provide GM-CSF to enable perivascular eosinophils to survive for many weeks *in vivo*.[1346]

3.5 Staining techniques

There are many ways to stain eosinophils in sections, or when smeared or centrifuged onto glass slides. As their granules are the most characteristic component of the cell, most staining methods detect these in fixed material. They can be fixed in air, absolute alcohol, methanol, or formalin, but care needs to be taken that their granule basic proteins are not extracted in weak acids before they have been properly fixed.

3.5.1 *Eosin, phloxin, and other fluorescein derivatives*

Because eosinophil granules contain basic proteins which are acidophilic, they can be stained with acidic dyes, such as eosin-Y and phloxin. The component(s) in the granules which take up the acidic dyes have not been defined, but as Ehrlich noted that the periphery of the granule was stained more than the centre,[499] and as EPO-deficient eosinophils stain normally with eosin,[1437] it is possible that ECP and EDN/EPX are responsible.

The capacity of eosin-Y, and the Romanowsky stains to stain eosinophil granules from man, pig, and horse is increased up to six times by pretreatment with 0.2 M EDTA, or 2 per cent sodium citrate for up to eight hours. This is believed to be due to chelation of metals which mask the reactive sites on the granule basic proteins for these stains. The absorption maximum of eosin is at 530 nm, and there is an additional component at 600–650 nm when Romanowsky stains are used. Both are increased by chelation treatment.[694]

In addition to eosin staining of eosinophils, other fluorescein derivatives, such as fluorescein-isothiocyanate (FITC), can also stain eosinophil granules in immunocytochemical preparations, in man, and in many other animals. This has often led to the incorrect impression that FITC-linked antibodies can stain eosinophil granules specifically,[581] and can cause confusion when immunofluorescent studies are done on samples rich in eosinophils.[447]

The non-specific staining of eosinophils with fluorescein-labelled antibodies can be prevented by prior treatment with either

(1) Lendrum's stain (chromotrope 2-R),[882] or

(2) H_2O_2 and diaminobenzidine, which block the binding sites on the granules for the fluorescent conjugate;[1829, 969] azide may also be required or

(3) o-benzoquinone.[599]

Eosinophil autofluorescence It has been known, at least since the mid 1960s, that alcohol-fixed eosinophils in bone marrow smears show intense autofluorescence when excited with green light, although some variation has been noted from patient to patient.[607] In 1987, this property was used to study the deposition of eosinophil granules in the bone marrow of patients with a variety of malignant diseases.[1546]

In 1981, it was found that unfixed blood eosinophils could be separated from neutrophils in a fluorescent activated cell sorter, on the basis of their larger size and greater autofluorescence.[1895] An attempt was made to isolate the fluorescent component in eosinophils, but this was not successful. We have also examined this property of human eosinophils. We found that light density eosinophils in patients with an eosinophilia were of similar size and fluorescence as neutrophils, so that they could not be distinguished by this technique. In 1982, blister fluids from six patients with bullous pemphigoid were found to increase human blood eosinophil autofluorescence,[1840] but the significance of this is not known.

3.5.2 *Romanowsky stains*

The Romanowsky staining technique is the most commonly used method for detecting eosinophils in blood smears. Their morphology is best seen in cytocentrifuge preparations (See Plate 1). The basis of this staining method was reviewed in 1987.[816] In urine, Hansel's stain is said to be preferable to Wright's stain for detecting eosinophils.[1284]

3.5.3 *Chromotrope 2R*

As eosin (or phloxin) is not a specific stain for eosinophils, Lendrum (1944) developed a method for staining fixed eosinophils using chromotrope 2R dissolved in phenol (carbol-chromotrope). Sections are stained first with haematoxylin, then with carbol chromotrope for 30 minutes. Other cells and tissues either do not stain red, or they develop a brown colour, which is easily distinguished from the bright red eosinophils.[1056]

3.5.4 *Biebrich scarlet*

Some acidophilic dyes can be made to stain eosinophils with great specificity, as they are only retained in eosinophils (and a few other cells with highly cationic constituents, such as spermatozoa, and Paneth cells), after washing in strong alkali solutions. Biebrich scarlet is one of the most useful stains to exploit this approach, as it provides a familiar red colour for eosinophils.[1671, 1564] Adams' stain has been reported to be equally specific.[1225]

3.5.5 *Other stains*

A number of other acidophilic staining methods can be used to define eosinophils in tissue sections. These include basic orcein, ninhydrin, Luxol fast blue alkaline erithrosin B, aniline blue,[162] Congo red,[720] and triazo dye Chlorazol black E,[915] p-dimethylaminobenzaldehyde-nitrite,[1045] and the xanthene dye C.I. acid red 52 (C.I. 45100) which stains eosinophil granules dark red.[916] Mercurochrome has been suggested as a useful eosinophil stain on the grounds that it stains eosinophils, and is also fluorescent, and electron dense.[559] In electronmicroscopy, two per cent palladium chloride has been recommended to provide high quality contrasting images of eosinophil granules.[560] In 1987 it was reported that certain fluorescent-labelled lectins from *Griffonia simplicifolia* and soybeans bound to human eosinophil granules, and could be used as specific markers for eosinophils in acetone-fixed cell smears, formalin-fixed, pepsin-treated tissue sections, and even eosinophils in suspension, after they had been made permeable with glycerol.[1047]

3.6 Eosinophil structure

The principal structures in human blood and tissue eosinophils are shown schematically in Fig. 3.2.

Eosinophils are usually oval in sections of tissues, although long pseudopodia can develop in culture, and these may be seen in samples of blood and tissues.[749]

The classical study on the ultrastructure of human blood eosinophil granules was reported from the Rockefeller University, New York, by Palade, and colleagues in 1966.[1213] They produced fine pictures of the crystals in human eosinophils, and showed that they were more varied in shape than those in rat eosinophils. A regular structure was seen within about one third of human blood eosinophil granule crystals. These gave interference patterns characteristic of cubic lattice crystals with a periodicity of 4.1 μm, and occasionally 2.8 μm. In addition, the granule matrices frequently contained small membrane-bounded vesicles, which have not

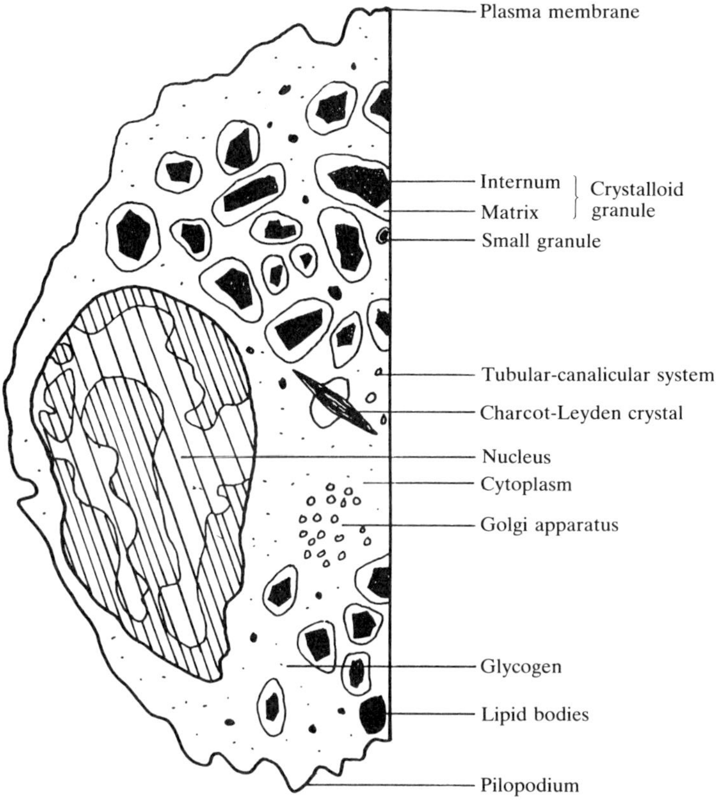

Fig. 3.2. The principal structures seen in electronmicrographs of mature human eosinophils. This schematic cell has not yet been stimulated to secrete its granule contents, which remain packaged in the granules. The Charcot–Leyden crystal and the lipid body are mainly seen in stimulated or tissue eosinophils.

been discussed in later work, although they are commonly seen in eosinophils which have degranulated.

In the late 1960s, questions were raised about the possible significance (in normal eosinophils) of dense crystalloids in a lighter staining matrix, as compared to the presence of light staining crystalloids and a darker matrix. This was resolved by careful work in 1966, which showed that the crystalline core of the normal eosinophil granule is darker when stained with uranyl acetate and lead citrate. However, this can be reversed by adding precipitating substances such as phosphotungstic acid, or molybdic acid during the alcohol dehydration stage.[537]

In 1986, morphometric studies on electronmicrographs made from normal blood eosinophils from six people showed that eosinophils have a volume of 275 fl, and a diameter of 8 μm. The nucleus occupies one-fifth of the cell volume, and the specific granules one-fifth of the cytoplasm.[1659] The same group reported similar findings in eosinophils from nine men and nine women in 1987.[1660] Electronmicrographs of human blood eosinophils show that they can often contain lipid droplets.[340]

3.7 Eosinophil constituents and their properties

Eosinophils are difficult cells to break down into their component granules, nuclei, and membrane components, by traditional mechanical methods. They are usually suspended in 0.34 M sucrose, and either repeatedly passed through an 18 gauge needle,[1918] or homogenized in a glass homogenizer. After 20 or 30 strokes, a small number of eosinophils are ruptured, and this is only slightly increased as more strokes are made. The use of a Waring blender increases the number of eosinophils that are ruptured, but this also breaks the nuclei. An efficient method for obtaining human blood eosinophil cytoplasts containing their granules was reported in 1985.[1991] This technique uses saponin to rupture the plasm membrane, followed by Percoll gradient separation of the cytoplasts.

3.7.1 *Cell nucleus*

In 1967, the number of nuclear lobes in blood eosinophils was measured in 14 normal individuals, 15 with asthma, 10 with ulcerative colitis, and 6 others. The 'lobe index' in normals was 2.05, and 2.3 in the others. Occasional blood eosinophils had three, or even four lobes, but there was no correlation between the lobe index and the blood eosinophil count.[1668] In 1987 it was shown that there were more nuclear segments in bronchoalveolar lavage fluid eosinophils in patients with pulmonary infiltrates than in other diseases with pulmonary eosinophilia, and eosinophils with four segments were only seen in these patients.[316] This suggests that segmentation increases as eosinophils reach maturity in tissues. The causes or the consequence for cell function of the increase in nuclear lobes is not known.

Although individual chromosomes can be seen in dividing eosinophils in the marrow of patients with eosinophilia, there has been no formal attempt to study the nature of the nuclear constituents in human eosinophils. The main classes of histones have been seen in extracts of human blood eosinophils. These are highly basic proteins, and as some have molecular weights comparable with those of the basic proteins in eosinophil granules, they could be a cause of confusion if their presence is not recognized in crude eosinophil extracts.

For over twenty years antinuclear antibodies have been noted in the serum of some patients which reacted with fixed human eosinophil nuclei,

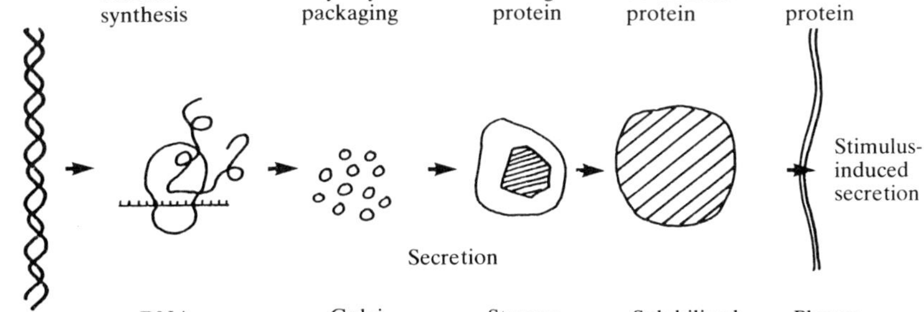

Fig. 3.3. The synthesis of eosinophil granule constituents. The proteins undergo a complex series of alterations, from the time that they are synthesized, to when they are secreted from the cell. At present most is known about the storage proteins, as these can be extracted easily.

but not with neutrophil nuclei. Their significance, and the way in which they are induced are unknown. In a study which was reported in 1985,[1517] this unusual antibody specificity was found in low titres only (less than 1/250) in 4 (4 per cent) of 112 children with juvenile chronic polyarthritis, and 14 (27 per cent) of 38 adults with rheumatoid arthritis. Their blood eosinophil counts were normal. A related antibody which only bound to the nuclei of neutrophils has been described in the serum of patients with rheumatoid arthritis and chronic active hepatitis in Australia.[1927]

3.7.2 *Cytoplasmic constituents*

The cytoplast of adherent human blood eosinophils has been studied by stereo high-voltage electronmicroscopy in 1987 at Chapel Hill, USA.[1455] This showed the presence of a highly organized cytoplast, containing an intricate network of strands: the microtrabecular lattice. This lattice can alter the shape of granules. In stimulated cells, there was reorganization of the cytoplast, so that the granules became more central, and a framework was formed for the granules. The cytoplasm of human eosinophils contains a wide variety of components. Only a few of these have been well characterized, and their biosynthesis, structure, and functions in eosinophil biology are largely unknown. A summary of the probable biosynthetic pathways for the crystalloid granule proteins, and their secretion from the cell, is shown in Fig. 3.3.

Lipid bodies Lipid bodies are often present in blood eosinophils from patients with eosinophilia, including patients with the Spanish toxic oil syndrome,[613] and in tissue eosinophils. In light microscopy they can be confused with endocytotic vesicles, and altered granules, but as they do not have a surrounding bilaminar membrane they are quite distinct in electronmicrographs. The lipid contents are removed by fixation, or washing in alcohol. They are also found in mast cells, and some macrophages. In 1985 lipid bodies were studied in blood eosinophils from two patients with eosinophilia, by autoradiography, after incubation of the separated cells with ^{3}H-arachidonic acid. It was found that the labelled unsaturated fatty acid was esterified to form phospholipids, which were retained almost entirely within lipid bodies. This suggested that lipid bodies may be an important site for the metabolism of arachidonic acid in eosinophils.[1911] Lipid bodies may be storage sites for plasma membrane lipids, which need to be internalized, and replaced in the plasma membrane as the cell alters its shape, and hence its surface area.

Ribonucleic acid The RNA content of human marrow eosinophils decreases as they mature, and none can be found in blood eosinophils using standard histochemical methods.[59] Nucleic acid synthesis in human marrow eosinophils was studied in samples from seven patients, by incubating marrow aspirates with ^{3}H-uridine. Autoradiographs showed that some of the radiolabel had become associated with the crystalloid granules, suggesting that RNA might be synthesized (or may accumulate) on the surface of these granules.[1929] ^{3}H-thymidine-5-triphosphate has been found to attach to the cytoplasm of human eosinophils. Neutrophils were not labelled.[1874] The significance of this is not known.

3.7.3 *Golgi apparatus*

The Golgi apparatus is prominent in blood eosinophils, distinguishing them from neutrophils. It has been known since 1968 that this is a major site for the processing of newly formed eosinophil granule components, when it was shown that ^{3}H-lysine was incorporated into bone marrow eosinophils *in vitro*, and transported through the Golgi apparatus to the crystalloid granules.[552] Microtubules probably link the Golgi apparatus to adjacent granules, although no direct connection has yet been shown in electronmicrographs.

3.7.4 *Mitochondria*

Blood eosinophils contain more mitochondria than blood neutrophils. There has been no work on their properties, but there is no reason to think that they might be different from mitochondria in other cells.

3.7.5 *Cytoplasmic granules*

Blood and tissue eosinophils contain crystalloid granules which develop from immature granules, and first appear at the promyelocyte stage. A

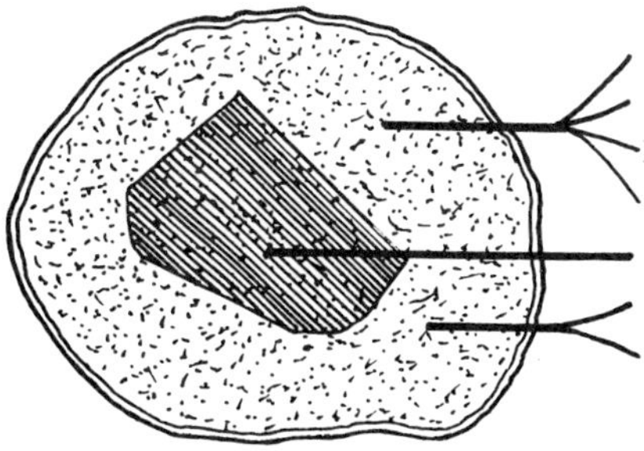

Fig. 3.4. The localization of different eosinophil granule constituents within the granule. The crystalloid is comprised of MBP, and the remaining components are present in the surrounding matrix.

diagram of the localization of the main granule constituents is shown in Fig. 3.4.

Crystalloid granules In 1975, eosinophils from the blood of five patients with HES at the N.I.H. Bethesda, USA were assayed for their enzyme content, and the results were compared with similar measurements on neutrophils. Eosinophil lysates had more total protein, and β-glycerophosphate than neutrophil lysates. Larger amounts of peroxidase, and β-glucuronidase activity were also found, which were present in extracts of isolated eosinophil granules, which had a density of 1.24 g/ml. No lysozyme or alkaline phosphatase was detected in eosinophils.[1918]

Eosinophils in the rat contain many of the enzymes described in human eosinophils, and these have been shown histochemically.[1409] Ultrastructural studies have also shown the presence of alkaline phosphatase in rat eosinophils.[1932]

Rat crystalloid granules also contain peroxisomal enzymes,[1975, 1977] which may be involved in the production of H_2O_2.[1976] For this reason, rat eosinophil granules can be classified as having features of both lysosomal and peroxisomal granules. It is not known if this is also true for human eosinophils.

'Small' granules In electronmicrographs of blood and tissue eosinophils, some small granules are visible. These were commented on by Parmley and Spicer in 1974.[1362] The eosinophil small granule has a round or elongated profile, 0.1–0.5 μm in diameter. They are moderately but homogeneously stained in standard electronmicrographs, and contain uniform acid phosphatase activity which is unmasked and resists fixation. They stain strongly for arylsulphatase, although peroxidase activity is equivocal. Eosinophil promyelocytes and myelocytes do not contain small

granules. Blood eosinophils have 2–8 small granules per section. They are increased in number in tissue eosinophils, especially in Hodgkin's disease.[1363] They have structural similarities with tertiary granules in rabbit heterophils, and some granules seen in mononuclear cells and platelets. They were mainly found around the Golgi zone and peripheral cytoplasm. It was suggested that they could fuse with pinocytotic vesicles, or supplement products in crystalloid granules. Small granules have also been seen in rat uterine eosinophils,[1761] and as rat peritoneal eosinophils were found to take up gold particles within small granules, it was suggested that these could be small heterophagic organelles.[996]

I suspect that small granules in human eosinophils are the remains of crystalloid granules which have secreted most of their contents. My reasons for suggesting this are that:

(1) they contain similar components to the crystalloid granules;

(2) the acid phosphatase in small granules is unmasked, as it is in granules without crystalloids, in contrast with crystalloid granules where acid phosphatase is mostly masked;[520]

(3) they are most prominent in eosinophils which are in sites where they might be expected to be secreting their contents;

(4) the localization of arylsulphatase, which has been considered to be confined to the small granule, has only been assessed by histochemistry, and it may well be present as an inactive complex in the crystalloid matrix.

Support for this would come from experiments showing that antibodies to arylsulphatase bound to both the crystalloid, and small granule components, but this has yet to be carried out.

'Microgranules' In 1973, electronmicrographs of eosinophils from 20 different species were said to show the presence of 'microgranules', which were dumb-bell in shape.[1566] However, Zucker-Franklin in 1980 considered that these were small profiles of endoplasmic reticulum, and not specific granules, and that they were part of the cell's secretory machinery. This would explain their presence in dividing eosinophils (which are known to secrete their granule contents) and their peripheral location in the cell.[2007]

Comparisons with neutrophil granules There are several types of granules in human blood neutrophils: azurophil (primary) granules, which are lysosomal granules; specific (secondary) granules, which contain lactoferrin and B12-binding protein; and the newly discovered tertiary granules, which are lighter than specific granules and contain a gelatinase.[1147] It is probable that many lysozomal enzymes are common to both neutrophils and eosinophils. This is supported by the finding that an antibody (Leu M1)[1878] recognized a common component in eosinophil and neutrophil granules.

Comparisons with basophil granules Eosinophil crystalloid granules have several features in common with basophil granules. When eosinophil granules are first formed in the marrow they are basophilic, but they lose this property as they mature. MBP is present in both eosinophil crystalloids, and in the heparin-containing granules of human basophils. In one study, normal basophils contained on average 140 ng MBP/10^6 cells, whereas purified eosinophils from normal donors and patients with the hypereosinophilic syndrome had 4979 and 824 ng MBP/10^6 cells, respectively.[7] MBP was not detected in mast cells,[1053] although it may be synthesized by a mast cell line (Gleich 1987, personal communication).

Although guinea pig basophils can ingest horse eosinophil peroxidase (EPO) *in vitro*, which becomes associated with their granules,[486] and human basophil colonies can incorporate EPO in a similar way,[485] this is unlikely to provide a functionally significant quantity of EPO in basophils *in vivo*.

Basophils have also been shown to possess large amounts of CLC protein (lysophospholipase). In a study of this property, basophils were purified from the blood of normal people by flow microfluoremetry with fluorescent anti-IgE antibodies. Charcot–Leyden crystals formed after incubation for 24 or 48 hours. As there was staining of the basophil cell membrane with a polyclonal anti-CLC protein antibody, it was suggested that basophils, like eosinophils, have large amounts of this protein at their surface.[11] The finding of CLC protein within basophils shows that the presence of this crystal type in tissues cannot be solely ascribed to eosinophils, but may represent basophil involvement in some instances. Mast cells do not contain CLC protein.[1053]

Comparisons with mast cell granules Mast cells appear to be quite distinct from eosinophils. They do not contain MBP, or the CLC protein,[1053] and eosinophils do not contain mast cell tryptase.[287]

3.7.6 *Eosinophil major basic protein*

MBP has been detected and characterized in eosinophils in a number of animals, including guinea pigs, rats, cattle, horses, and man. It is believed to be an important mediator of eosinophil-dependent damage to parasites and host tissues. The properties of MBP were reviewed by Gleich and Adolphson in 1986.[656] There is no published work on the biosynthesis of MBP.

Purification and structure MBP was first isolated from guinea pig peritoneal eosinophils in 1973[664] and subsequently from rats.[1066] It was first purified from human eosinophils in 1976.[665] The main method for purifying MBP involves its extraction in weak acids from isolated blood eosinophil granules, and partial purification on Sephadex G-50 columns followed by weak ion exchange chromatography.[665]

Early work on MBP centred on animal eosinophils. Guinea pig MBP was shown to have a molecular weight of about 11 kDa.[663] After electrophoresis in 8 per cent polyacrylamide gels it migrated as a single band. It contained 10 or 11 arginine residues, 6 half-cystine residues, and 0.8 per cent carbohydrate. When it was reduced and carboxymethylated it was more stable in solution, and so easier to handle and store. It had a pI of over 10.5. As MBP contains tryptophan it is not a histone-like protein.

The amino acid composition of MBP is different from ECP.[665] In 1987, the amino-terminal sequence of MBP from a patient with HES was reported to be unique: ?-?-Arg-Tyr-Leu-Leu-Va-Arg-Ser-Leu-Gln-Thr-Phe-Ser-Gln-Ala-?-Phe-Thr-?[1906], and sequence studies on purified and mRNA translated human MBP showed it had 117 amino acids, with 8 half cysteines, with hydrophilic and hydrophobic domains (Gleich 1987, personal communication). No work has yet been reported on possible differences between the storage, and secreted forms of MBP.

Assays for MBP Human MPB is homologous with guinea pig MBP, and antibodies to guinea pig MBP[1065] cross-react with human MBP. Antibodies to human and rat MBP do not cross-react. MBP can be assayed in serum, or other solutions with a radioimmunoassay.[1888] MBP can be visualized in paraffin-embedded tissues, using a rabbit antibody after trypsin digestion.[562] The amount of MBP in blood eosinophils from 10 normal people was found to be 8.62 ± 1.45 μg/10^6 eosinophils,[1389] and it was thought to account for over half of the granule protein.

In 1978 MBP was shown to make up the crystalline core of guinea pig eosinophil granules, using peroxidase immunoelectronmicroscopy, and extraction from purified crystalloids.[1064] In 1986, immunoelectronmicroscopy was used to localize MBP in human eosinophils. In studies with human blood eosinophils using gold-labelled rabbit antibody, MBP was shown to be present in the crystalloid granule cores of eosinophils from four normal individuals.[495] MBP in nasal polyps was found to be predominantly within eosinophil granule cores, and not within other eosinophil organelles, plasma cells, mast cells, lymphocytes, or neutrophils.[1390]

In 10 normal subjects who were studied at the Mayo Clinic, Rochester, Minnesota, USA, the plasma MBP level was 0.307 ± 0.038 μg/ml (mean ± SD). In this group of normal people, and in patients with eosinophilia, plasma MBP levels were related directly to the blood eosinophil counts, the per cent light density eosinophils, and the mean blood eosinophil MBP content.[1389] It was shown previously that the serum MBP levels were related to blood eosinophil counts in a variety of diseases,[1889] although in some skin diseases the serum MBP levels were higher than was expected from the counts. In some eosinophilic diseases there can be very high levels of MBP: up to 14 μg/ml (1.5×10^{-6}M) in serum; 30 μg/ml (3.2×10^{-6}M) in pleural fluid; and 93 μg/ml (1×10^{-5}M) in sputum.[656]

Functional properties of MBP The main effects of MBP are to damage and/or kill parasites and normal human cells and tissues. It does not have any enzymatic activity. It became of particular interest to parasitologists when it was discovered in 1979 that MBP was highly toxic to the schistosomula of *S. mansoni*.[257] MBP is secreted from human blood eosinophils onto the surface of IgG-antibody-coated schistosomula, which are killed within a few hours. This was inhibited by heparin. Purified MBP induced a detachment and ballooning of the tegumental membrane of schistosomula *in vitro*.[5]

In 1987 it was found that the reduced and alkylated form of MBP was more effective than native MBP in killing newborn larvae of *T. spiralis*, which were killed rapidly.[747] However, MBP can also have a protective effect by acting as a scavenger for $HClO^-$ ions. This reduced the toxicity of $HClO^-$ ions for newborn *T. spiralis* larvae.[259] MBP is also toxic for amastigotes and epimastigotes of *Trypanosoma cruzi in vitro*.[1864]

In 1980, a bovine equivalent of MBP was described. This was a 16 kDa protein, but poor in arginine. It was able to kill juvenile *Fasciola hepatica in vitro*.[473]

The initial studies with MBP in 1976 showed that it did not affect vascular permeability, or cause smooth muscle contraction.[665] However in 1984, it was reported that injections of MBP into the skin of normal subjects produced a wheal-and-flare reaction.[672]

MBP is also thought to be an important mediator of inflammation in the respiratory tract, especially in asthma. This was reviewed by Gleich and colleagues in 1983.[662] Evidence in favour of this suggestion came from the finding in 1979 that 10^{-7} to 10^{-5}M MBP killed tracheal epithelial cells in 3 to 23 hours.[658] MBP can kill some pneumocytes,[83] and guinea-pig tracheal epithelium.[605] Although 10^{-5}M MBP was unable to kill cultured type II pneumocytes, EPO can do so in the presence of H_2O_2 and a halide.[24]

Purified human MBP reduced ciliary movement in rabbit tracheal explants, directly inhibited isolated porcine tracheal ciliary axonemes,[768] and altered fluid dynamics in the dog trachea, suggesting that it could be responsible for mucus impaction, which is a prominent feature of severe asthma.

MBP is nearly as potent as poly-L-arginine in inducing a non-cytolytic release of histamine from human basophils. This is a slow response, taking place over 40 minutes, with half-maximal release at 17 minutes. Native MBP is more potent than reduced and alkylated MBP.[1294] There was day-to-day variation in the amounts of histamine released by MBP *in vitro* from blood leucocytes (basophils) of patients with allergic disease, but there was no evidence that patients with allergic diseases released more histamine than normal.[1997] Other work on MBP-induced effects on basophils was reported from Uppsala, Sweden in 1985,[161] and Chicago, USA, in 1986.[1785]

In contrast MBP caused the release of histamine from rat peritoneal mast cells within one minute.[1294]

Guinea pig MBP, which was reduced and alkylated to make it stable in solution, has been shown to be toxic for a number of cells *in vitro*. 10^{-7} to 10^{-5}M killed spleen cells, mononuclear cells, intestinal, skin, and tracheal cells in 3 to 23 hours. 5×10^{-5}M MBP destroyed endothelial cells in 24 hours, and inhibited their growth at concentrations as low as 10^{-9}M.[658]

In 1974 it was shown that guinea pig MBP increased clotting time,[663] but its site of action in the coagulation system has not been determined.

In 1986 an abstract of work on the properties of MBP on the human complement system stated that MBP can bind irreversibly to EAC4b3b, and inhibit the generation of the alternative pathway convertase. These activities may have been related to the strong charge on MBP, as reduced and alkylated MBP was less effective than native MBP.[1897]

3.7.7 *Eosinophil cationic protein*

Eosinophil cationic protein is another of the principal basic proteins found within human eosinophils. It was first described in 1974 by Olsson and Venge in Sweden.[1329] It is not known whether eosinophils in other species contain ECP or related ribonucleases.

ECP is synthesized as a larger molecular weight precursor which is processed to become the storage form of the protein.[1325] Its biosynthesis was assayed by culturing bone marrow eosinophils from patients with eosinophilia with ^{14}C-leucine, followed by immunoprecipitation, PAGE electrophoresis, and fluorography. A 22 kDa ECP precursor protein was produced initially, which was processed into an 18-19 kDa molecule. This was inhibited by monensin.[1327]

Purification ECP is usually prepared from isolated eosinophil granules which have been solubilized with weak acids. It is then chromatographed by molecular sieve, and ion exchange chromatography.[1331] Nowadays, this can be done easily using fast protein liquid chromatography.[1327] ECP has also been purified from eosinophil granules by sequential chromatography on Sephadex G-50, and heparin-sepharose, where it was eluted in a broad peak at a higher salt concentration than EDN/EPX. This separated two forms in an early eluting (ECP-1) and a later eluting (ECP-2) fraction. In Uppsala, Sweden, Peterson and colleagues have developed a method for purifying ECP on a zinc-chelate Sepharose 6B column.[1395]

Structure ECP exists as several molecules of molecular weights 18.5 to 22 kDa, but can dimerize. The smallest form is the most basic. These forms contain different amounts of carbohydrate. The isoelectric points of ECP are greater than pH 11, and it contains 11 per cent arginine, and 10 half-cysteines. It is a single polypeptide chain in SDS–PAGE gels, and contains 2.5 moles of zinc per mole of protein.[1331] When purified ECP was eluted isocratically from a high-resolution cation exchange resin, it showed considerable heterogeneity. There were five components probably differing in their hydrophobicity. It was suggested that these could have different biological activities. The components had molecular weights of 16.7–19.5 kDa, and virtually identical amino acid composition. The amino terminal sequence of the first 33 amino acids of ECP was determined in 1986.[1327]

SDS-acrylamide electrophoresis of ECP-1 showed a major band at 18.3 kDa, and a minor band at 21.4 kDa. ECP-2 gave a doublet at 16 kDa, and a band at 16.9 kDa. In two-dimensional gels, ECP-1 migrated as a single spot with a heterogeneous tail in the acidic direction. ECP-2 migrated as a major spot, more acidic than ECP-1, with a heterogeneous tail in the basic direction. A minor spot of higher molecular weight showed comparable charge heterogeneity to the major band. Digestion of ECP-1 with Endo-F (which removes high-mannose, and complex obligosaccharides), reduced its size close to the two smaller forms of ECP-2. Endo-F digestion of ECP-2 removed the largest form. As Endo-F did not convert ECP-1 or ECP-2 to a single band, there may have been an O-linked oligosaccharide, or an amino acid difference at the C-terminal end of these two forms of ECP.[661]

The N-terminal 59 amino acid residues of ECP-1 and ECP-2 were sequenced in 1986.[661] These showed marked sequence homologies with human pancreatic ribonucleases, which was sequenced in 1984,[149] and ribonuclease from several other species.

ECP has an affinity for zinc, which may account for the high levels of zinc in eosinophil granules. This enables the protein to be separated by zinc-affinity chromatography. If the association with zinc is linked with its ribonuclease activity, ECP can be classified as a metalloenzyme.

The secreted form of ECP Following solubilization, ECP undergoes further structural changes which have been demonstrated using monoclonal antibodies, one of which was shown to bind to the secreted form of the protein.[1742] This antibody (EG2) has shown the presence of the secreted form of ECP in areas of eosinophil degranulation in the skin, gut, heart, and spleen.[1697] (See Plates 6, and 12) The secreted form of ECP has greater molecular weight heterogeneity than the storage form.[1395]

Assays for ECP ECP in serum is usually assayed by a radioassay with either rabbit antibodies,[1851] or with monoclonal antibodies. The method which we use employs monoclonal antibodies EG1 and EG2. (These can be purchased from SANBIO bv. Heinsbergenstraat 50, 5402 EG Uden, Postbus 540, 5400 AM Uden, The Netherlands, Phone: 04132 51115, Telex: 74827.) In our technique, antibody EG1 first concentrates ECP on to the floor of the reaction microwell, and then labelled antibody EG2 is added, which binds to the fixed antigen through a separate epitope. A commercial ECP assay kit which uses rabbit antibody is being developed by Pharmacia, Uppsala, Sweden, for sale in 1988. A competitive binding radioimmunoassay with a monoclonal antibody has been used in some studies in the USA.[661]

In 1987, a method was described for assaying ECP in urine, by an enzyme immunoassay with an antibody which was prepared against ECP from the urine of patients with interstitial cystitis. It was proposed as a useful assay for eosinophil involvement in this disease.[595] The cell content of ECP in normal human eosinophils is about 25 μg/10^6 cells.

The localization of ECP in eosinophils In 1986 it was reported by three groups, using immunogold electronmicroscopy, that ECP was present in the granule matrix of human eosinophils:

(1) This was shown with blood eosinophils from four normal people.[495] Small granules, which may correspond to those identified by Parmley and Spicer,[1362] were also positive.

(2) Sections of nasal polyps showed that ECP was mainly in the granule matrix, with small amounts in the crystalloids.[1390]

(3) We localized the secreted form of ECP to the granule matrix of eosinophils using monoclonal antibody EG2.[1115]

ECP has only been found in eosinophils, unlike MBP. In contrast with the EM localization of ECP, subcellular fractionation of blood eosinophils has shown ECP in four bands of different density (Fattah, D. *et al.* 1985, unpublished observations). This was noted by Peterson and colleagues,[1395] who also found that peroxidase was not present in three of these bands.

ECP in plasma and serum Small amounts of ECP are found in normal serum. In 93 people, aged 18-64 years, serum ECP was 15 μg/l (2–116, 2 SD).[737] It binds tightly to the fast form of α-2 macroglobulin *in vivo*,[1398] and this has been thought to inactivate its toxic properties, although this has not yet been tested. In 1977, serum ECP levels in normal people were found to correlate with their blood eosinophil counts.[1851]

Functional properties of ECP Like other strongly positive charged molecules, ECP binds to negatively charged surfaces, and this may localize its effects *in vivo*. Initial studies on ECP gave no clues about its roles in disease. It did not have bactericidal activity or esterolytic activity. It had no effect on histamine-induced, or guinea pig anaphylatoxin-induced contraction of ileal muscles,[1331] although it could augment the ingestion of immune complexes by phagocytic cells.

In 1986, it was found that ECP was a ribonuclease. Highly purified ECP completely degraded transfer RNA and ribosomal RNA at concentrations down to 1.4×10^{-8}M. No differences were found between the four ECP fractions which were separated by high resolution Mono-S cation resin exchange chromotography. However, the ECP ribonuclease activity was nonspecific, and less potent than the second ribonuclease in eosinophils, EDN/EPX.[729]

Both ECP, and EDN/EPX may belong to a ribonuclease family of proteins which are derived from a common ancestral gene. The present day proteins of this type may include pancreatic ribonuclease, ECP, EDN/EPX, and angiogenin, which was cloned,[1019] and sequenced in 1985.[1717] Although these proteins have differing ribonuclease activity, they have considerable structural and amino acid homology which supports this possibility.[657] If ECP is found to have angiogenin-like properties this could account for the presence of many blood vessels in areas where eosinophil degranulation is prominent, and in diseases such as angiolymphoid hyperplasia with eosinophilia, where there is a close relationship between eosinophils and abnormal vessel formation. It is unlikely that secreted ECP (or EDN/EPX) could enter intact cells or parasites and destroy their RNA, causing their death, as suggested in 1986,[729] although this may contribute to the final destruction of these targets. The toxicity of EDN/EPX and ECP does not correlate with their ribonuclease activity, and pancreatic ribonuclease is not toxic for *T. spiralis* newborn larvae.[747]

ECP is a potent cytotoxic molecule for a range of parasites, especially the schistosomula of *S. mansoni*.[1178] In a study on the relative toxicity of purified ECP, and MBP for the schistosomula of *S. mansoni in vitro*, it was found that ECP was eight to ten times more toxic than MBP. However as eosinophils in some patients with eosinophilia contain more MBP than ECP, it is possible that MBP may be more important under some circumstances.[5] *In vitro*, purified ECP caused the formation of blebs on the surface of schistosomula, followed by disruption of the surface, and extrusion of the parasite's contents.[1178, 5] ECP was able to paralyze the lung stage schistosomula of *S. mansoni in vitro*, but did not cause structural damage or parasite death.[1179]

In 1987, it was shown that ECP was as toxic as MBP in killing *T. spiralis* newborn larvae, although ECP killed more slowly.[747] ECP is also a powerful neurotoxin.[598] This was first discovered in 1982. 0.1–0.3 μg induced the Gordon phenomenon in guinea pigs, at concentrations 10–100 times less than those needed by the eosinophil neurotoxin, EDN/EPX, to produce a similar effect.[597] When 2–11 μg of purified ECP was injected into the cisterna magna of 17 rabbits, it produced paralysis in 5 animals. Minor symptoms were produced at doses below 2 μg. EDN/EPX had similar effects, but produced paralysis at doses less than 2 μg.[661]

When ECP was instilled into the trachea of rabbits, it caused the epithelium to strip off, and inflammatory cells to accumulate in the lumen, with plugs of mucus, as seen in severe asthma (Dahl, R. *et al.* 1985, personal communication).

Although Zheutlin and colleagues in the USA did not find in 1984 that partially purified ECP caused the release of histamine from blood mononuclear cells containing basophils,[1996] Bergstrand and colleagues in Sweden reported in 1985 that ECP, at concentrations of 10 and 30 μg/ml caused direct histamine release from human basophils, and that ECP also inhibited anti-IgE-induced histamine release from basophils. These experiments, which have not yet been published in full, raise the possibility that eosinophils may either augment or inhibit the effects of inflammatory stimuli in tissues giving rise to basophil secretion, and it might not be possible to predict how eosinophils would affect tissue responses in allergic diseases, such as the late phase IgE-mediated asthmatic responses.[161] Partially purified ECP caused the release of histamine from rat peritoneal mast cells.[1996]

Two groups have shown that eosinophils can inhibit lymphocyte-mediated responses *in vitro*. Experiments reported from Sweden using purified ECP and EDN/EPX showed that at 10^{-10} to 10^{-7}M, both of these proteins inhibited ^{3}H-thymidine incorporation into DNA, in cultures of human blood lymphocytes stimulated with PHA or allogeneic lymphocytes. ECP and EDN/EPX also appeared to increase the 'suppressor cell activity' generated by Con A.[1396] In the USA extracts of human blood eosinophils, and secretion products from stimulated eosinophils were also found to inhibit PHA-induced lymphocyte proliferation *in vitro*, and a newly synthesized product from eosinophils appeared to mediate the effect.[1471] However, as immunological assessment of patients with HES have failed to show any consistent defects in blood T-lymphocyte-mediated responses,[1369] and as there is no evidence that other patients with eosinophilic disorders have impaired T-cell responsiveness, the relevance of these findings is not clear.

There has been no formal study on the possible interactions of ECP with tumour cells.

ECP affects the coagulation system in several ways. Initially, it shortens the coagulation time of normal plasma, but after 10 minutes, the clotting time becomes prolonged.[1849] The recalcification time of plasma deficient in Factors V, VII, VIII, IX, X, and XI, is shortened by ECP, but the recalcification time of Factor-XII-deficient plasma is prolonged, suggesting that ECP mainly interacts with Factor XII. For this reason, kallikrein activation, which is Factor-XII-dependent, was increased by ECP.[1849] ECP also affects fibrinolysis. The hydrolysis of a plasmin-specific substrate by plasmin was increased by ECP, whereas ECP inhibited plasminogen activation by streptokinase, possibly because ECP bound to streptokinase.[381] Although plasminogen levels are normal in patients with eosinophilia, marked defects in other coagulation factors have been found in patients with HES, showing that there is likely to be a clinically significant effect of eosinophils on coagulation *in vivo*.

ECP inhibits the anticoagulant effect of commercially prepared heparin *in vitro*,[1850, 380] and therefore has the potential to inhibit this component from mast cell.

There have been no reports of the possible interactions of ECP with the complement system, although this is likely to occur, in view of the strong basic charge on ECP.

3.7.8 *The eosinophil-derived neurotoxin, or eosinophil protein-X*

In 1933 M. H. Gordon reported that the injection into the brains of rabbits of extracts of eosinophil-rich lymph nodes from patients with Hodgkin's disease produced paralysis.[699] He thought that this was due to a virus in Hodgkin's tissue. A similar effect was found in 1939, following the injection of bone marrow extracts.[968] Then it became clear that eosinophils in these tissues were the cause of the brain damage.[1802] This reaction is now called the Gordon phenomenon. The cause of the Gordon phenomenon began to be studied in the late 1970s in the USA, where the name 'eosinophil-derived neurotoxin' (EDN) was given to an activity in eosinophil extracts,[479] and in Sweden, where it was found to be due to a protein which had been called 'eosinophil protein-X' (EXP),[1397] because it was found in a column fraction which contained an unclassified protein (protein-X).

In 1982, work in Aarhus, Denmark, showed that EPX[1397] was probably identical with EDN.[1848] This review will use the term EDN/EPX for this protein, but clearly a better name is needed.

No work has been done on the biosynthesis of EDN/EPX, but it is likely to be similar to ECP, in view of their close structural homology, as described below.

Purification EDN/EPX was partially purified in 1979 by Durack and colleagues in Seattle, USA, by sequential sonication of blood eosinophils from three patients with HES, followed by ultracentrifugation, and fractionation on Sephadex G-50 at neutral pH. It was heat labile at 90°, but could be lyophilized.[479] Work on EDN/EPX was summarized in a report from the Mayo Clinic, USA in 1987.[657] It was purified from eosinophil granules by chromatography on Sephadex G-50, and heparin-sepharose, where it eluted at a lower salt concentration than ECP. In Sweden, EDN/EPX was purified by Bio Rex-70, and heparin-Sepharose chromatography.[1395]

Structure The results were published in 1981 of a collaborative study by Durack with Ackerman and colleagues at the Mayo Clinic, in which EDN/EPX was purified from extracts of whole eosinophils and granules by Sephadex G-50 chromatography. This showed that EDN had an estimated molecular weight of 17.7–19.2 kDa.[478] In 1986, it was reported that EDN/EPX, which was purified from eosinophil granules by chromatography on Sephadex G-50 and heparin-sepharose, produced a major band at 17.4 kDa, and a minor band at 20.3 kDa. In two-dimensional gels, EDN/EPX migrated as two spots differing in charge, but not in apparent molecular weight. Two minor spots of slightly higher molecular weights were seen above each major spot. Endo-F, which removes high-mannose and complex oligosaccharides, affected the larger form of EDN/EPX only. Endo-H, which only cleaves high-mannose-linked oligosaccharides, had no effect, suggesting that EDN/EPX possessed a single complex oligosaccharide with some additions. The amino acid composition of EDN from two patients was similar, suggesting that the protein is not polymorphic.[661] Similar findings, and confirmation of these results, were reported by Peterson in 1987.[1395] Like ECP, EDN/EPX undergoes a structural change when it is secreted, which can be detected with monoclonal antibodies. The nature of this alteration is not known.

Assays for EDN/EPX EDN/EPX can be assayed using rabbit antibodies or mouse monoclonal antibodies to human EDN/EPX. It is not known whether eosinophils in other animals contain EDN/EPX. A monoclonal antibody which is specific for EDN/EPX has been described, which inhibited its ribonuclease activity, and could be used in a competitive binding radioimmunoassay.[661]

The content of EDN/EPX in eosinophils has been estimated to be about 10 μg per 10^6 eosinophils, which is about 40 per cent of the amount of ECP in eosinophils.[1395] The serum levels of EDN/EPX in normal people, and patients with asthma were reported in 1977.[1853]

Localization of EDN/EPX in eosinophils EDN/EPX has been presumed to be an eosinophil granule matrix protein since it was shown in 1982 that it could be extracted from isolated human eosinophil granules,[478] and that MBP accounted for all of the protein in crystalloids. Its localization in eosinophils within nasal polyps was shown in 1986, using colloidal gold particles with immunoelectronmicroscopy. EDN/EPX was localized to the granule matrix, with small amounts in the crystalloids.[1390]

Functional properties of EDN/EPX In 1986 it was first reported by Gleich and colleagues at the Mayo Clinic, that EDN/EPX had marked homology with ECP and pancreatic ribonuclease.[661] Later that year, in Lund, Sweden, it was found that purified EDN/EPX completely degraded tRNA at concentrations down to 5.7×10^{-10}M.[729] Further work in the USA showed that ECP was 50 to 100 times less active as a ribonuclease than EDN/EPX. In addition, the ribonuclease activity associated with ECP was not significantly inhibited after exposure of ECP to polyclonal or monoclonal antibodies to EDN/EPX.[1645, 657]

There is some confusion as to whether EDN/EPX is toxic to schistosomula. One study showed that it had little effect.[5] Another study reported that EDN/EPX injured the schistosomula of *S. mansoni in vitro*, like ECP, and sub-lethal concentrations paralysed the lung stage, causing structural damage to the sub-tegumental musculature.[1179] EDN/EPX was 10 times less effective than either MBP or ECP in killing *T. spiralis* newborn larvae *in vitro*, and pancreatic ribonuclease was ineffective.[747]

It has been known since 1979 that intrathecal injections of partially purified EDN/EPX into rabbits caused stiffness in the fore-legs, and then the hind-legs. Ataxia and weakness developed progressively, which prevented the animals, which appeared to have normal higher functions, from feeding and drinking.[479] Histology showed lesions in the cerebellum, pons, and spinal cord, with loss of Purkinje cells of the cerebellum. The grey matter was normal, but the white matter in the spinal cord, cerebellum, and pons showed spongiform changes.[479]

In 1982, work in Aarhus, Denmark showed that EDN/EPX was highly toxic to the guinea pig brain, after intrathecal injection, and damaged all cells in proximity to the ventricular system. In these animals ECP was 100 times more toxic than EDN/EPX.[1848] On the other hand in rabbits, ECP and EDN/EPX had equivalent effects, which suggests that there is some species differences in the effects of the human eosinophil neurotoxins. In 1986 further work at the Mayo Clinic showed that as little as 0.15–7 μg EDN/EPX produced ataxia in rabbits after injection into the cisterna magna (five of eight rabbits). The onset of symptoms was three days at the higher doses, and seven days at the lower doses.[661]

The mechanism for this toxic effect has not yet been defined, but presumably involves binding to, and interference with Schwann cell functions. No studies have yet been published on the effects of purified eosinophil granule proteins on isolated neuronal cell, or glial cell function, although the growth of brain cells *in vitro* may be inhibited (Gleich, G. J. 1987, personal communication). Measurements of cerebrospinal ECP levels have begun to show that ECP may also be toxic to the human brain in patients with a variety of brain disorders.[740] Two groups have shown that partially purified EDN/EPX does not induce the release *in vitro* of histamine from blood mononuclear cells containing basophils.[1996, 161] In addition, partially purified EDN/EPX did not induce the release of histamine from rat peritoneal mast cells *in vitro*.[1996]

It was reported in 1986 that EDN/EPX at 10^{-10} to 10^{-7}M inhibited the uptake of ^{3}H-thymidine by PHA-blasts or MLR-blasts in a dose-dependent mechanism. This was irreversible, and it was not due to cytotoxic damage. It was suggested that the suppressive effect of EDN/EPX might involve suppressor cells, and it was proposed that EDN/EPX could have a regulatory role in immunological reactions.[1396]

There are no reports on the possible effects of EDN/EPX on the respiratory system, or its localization in respiratory diseases, and it is not known whether EDN/EPX is toxic for the heart or vasculature, or affects their function. No studies have been reported on the possible effects of EDN/EPX on the coagulation or complement systems.

3.7.9 *The relationship between ECP, and EDN/EPX*

In 1985 I suggested that ECP and EDN/EPX could be products of a common gene family,[1687] as they had similar physical and antigenic properties. Direct evidence to support this was produced in 1986, when sequence homology between these two proteins was first established.[661] Proof for this awaits sequencing of the genes for ECP and EDN/EPX. However they:

(1) have a similar amino acid content;

(2) have a closely related N-terminal sequence;

(3) possess at least one common antigenic epitope;[1742]

(4) have ribonuclease activity; and

(5) produce similar effects on brain cells and lymphocytes.[1396]

For these reasons, it might be preferable to call ECP and EDN/EPX by a common name, such as 'eosinophil ribonuclease', and to give each variant an internationally agreed enzyme classification term.

3.7.10 *Eosinophil peroxidase*

In 1963, G. T. Archer and colleagues first showed that EPO was distinct from myeloperoxidase, which had been studied in neutrophils. This conclusion was based on the finding that human and horse EPO were not inhibited by 10^{-3}M cyanide or azide, unlike myeloperoxidase.[61] Two years later it was shown that partially purified EPO from rat peritoneal eosinophils was a haemoprotein, with different reaction kinetics with guaiacol, and different spectral properties to myeloperoxidase.[53] In guinea pigs the substrate requirements for EPO have also been shown to differ from neutrophil myeloperoxidase.[528]

Biosynthesis The sites of peroxidase transport from ribosomes to the storage granules of rat and rabbit eosinophil myelocytes were studied in 1970 by a combination of cytochemistry and electronmicroscopy, and shown to occur along the endoplasmic reticulum, and to involve the Golgi cisternae, from where the enzyme became localized in primary and crystalloid granules. At a later stage in differentiation, the enzyme could only be detected in the granules. Acid phosphatase and arylsulphatase followed the same pattern, but were not detected in the mature granules by this technique.[100] In 1979, electronmicrographs of human bone marrow eosinophils also showed peroxidase to be present in the rough endoplasmic reticulum, in the Golgi apparatus, and in large homogeneous granules (0.6 to 1.2 μm) in early eosinophils. There was some structural evidence for secretion of peroxidase from these dividing eosinophils.[834]

Patients with a congenital absence of myeloperoxidase have eosinophils containing normal amounts of EPO. This proves that the genes responsible for the production of eosinophil peroxidase and myeloperoxidase are distinct.

The biosynthesis of human EPO in marrow samples from patients with eosinophilia was studied by pulse-chase experiments with ^{14}C-leucine in 1985. Three large molecular weight proteins of 78, 72, and 25 kDa were labelled, and the 53 kDa heavy chain of EPO was produced, by a pathway which was not inhibited by Monensin. As the antibody which was used in this study did not bind to the light chain of EPO, its biosynthesis from the labelled 25 kDa protein was only surmised.[1326]

Purification In 1965 rat peritoneal EPO was purified by electrophoresis, and shown to be a haemoprotein with several differences from myeloperoxidase, including its reaction kinetics with guaiacol, and its spectral properties. These were a Soret maximum of 403 nm for oxidized EPO, and 437 for its reduced form.[53] Guinea pig EPO was purified from bone marrow in 1972, and found to be a monomeric enzyme of 75 kDa, which could dimerize. It had a Soret maximum at 425 nm.[445] Horse EPO has been isolated from blood eosinophils,[895] and eosinophil granules.[894] They were very basic. Work on horse EPO, including its basic properties, was reviewed in 1983.[976] Human EPO was isolated from whole eosinophils in several studies reported between 1981 and 1984,[188, 1321, 1920] and from eosinophil granules in 1985.[280, 1326] In 1986, a method was developed which used granule-rich eosinophil cytosomes,[1189] to give EPO of high purity.

Structure EPO is a highly basic two-chain haemoprotein which loses much of its enzymatic activity when it is purified. The initial work on the enzymatic properties of EPO was done in rodents, and then horse EPO. Subsequent studies on human EPO have given a clear indication of its size, the nature of the haem component within the molecule, and its biophysical characteristics.

Human EPO has a molecular weight of between 71 kDa,[188] and 77 kDa.[280] It consists of a heavy chain of 50–58 kDa, and a light chain of 14–15 kDa, and it has a Soret band at 412 nm.[188]

Studies on the amino acid composition of EPO showed that it had a high content of arginine, leucine, and aspartic acid,[188, 280] and an isoelectric point greater than 11.[280] Carbohydrate is associated only with the heavy chain, and although the light chain is homologous with the MPO light chain, they are distinct.[1322]

In 1987, the partial N-terminal amino acid sequence of the smaller 14.45 kDa unit of peroxidase was shown to have a unique sequence of: ?-?-Ser-Asp-Lys-Try-Arg-Thr-Ile-Thr-Gly-?-?-Asn-Asn-Glu-?-?-Pro-Leu- . . . The larger chain was 49.250 kDa.[1906] So far neither component has been fully sequenced.

The haem prosthetic group in human EPO has been studied in detail.[188, 1622] This work showed that EPO is closely related to horseradish peroxidase, lactoperoxidase, and intestinal peroxidase, and unrelated to catalase.

No studies have been done to see whether EPO alters its antigenicity or size when it is secreted from eosinophils.

Assays for EPO Semi-quantitative measurements of EPO concentrations have been made for many years by enzyme cytochemistry. Quantitative assays for EPO are either enzymatic, which have the disadvantage that

EPO loses its activity relatively easily, or based on immunoassays with antibodies, which have the disadvantage that EPO can bind nonspecifically to surfaces, because of its basicity. Eosinophils contain 15 μg EPO per 10^6 eosinophils.[280]

EPO is commonly assayed by its ability to oxidize guaiacol, or o-phenylenediamine with H_2O_2. EPO is markedly inhibited by 3-amino-1,2,4-triazole, unlike myeloperoxidase, so that the two enzymes can be assayed when mixed together.[365] Conversely, EPO can be assayed when MPO has been inhibited.[192]

The histochemistry of human EPO has been studied extensively, see reference 750. EPO can be distinguished from myeloperoxidase because EPO is less easily inhibited by KCN in cell smears and sections. However, as MPO in neutrophil promyelocytes is less easily inhibited than blood neutrophil MPO, this can cause some difficulties with marrow samples.[1226]

A radioimmunoassay for EPO has been developed, with a specific rabbit antibody.[280] A monoclonal antibody to rat EPO has also been made, and used in immunocytochemical studies.[944]

A mouse monoclonal antibody has been produced, which binds to human EPO, and which has demonstrated the presence of large amounts of EPO in lymph nodes of patients with nodular sclerosing Hodgkins's disease.[1545]

The localization EPO in eosinophils Human and animal EPO is localized to the matrix of eosinophil crystalloid granules.[100, 520, 949, 1963] Lesser amounts are found in the small granules. Quantitation of the peroxidase-reaction product in ultrathin sections of murine eosinophils has been carried out by electronmicroscopy using a platinum technique.[412] EPO deficient human eosinophils have a thin matrix layer revealed in electronmicrographs.[1060]

Functional properties of EPO EPO has the property of catalyzing the formation of $HClO^-$ ions, and H_2O_2. It has been mainly studied for its capacity to act in the presence of hydrogen peroxide and a halide as a cytotoxic effector system. This is a potent mechanism for killing some parasites, bacteria, tumours and cells *in vitro*. In addition to this effector role, it can diminish the effector roles of inflammatory cells, by breaking down LTC4. It does not cause the Gordon phenomenon.

The principal role of EPO is to oxidize substances, by a catalytic action with H_2O_2, which is also generated by eosinophils.[975, 977] In the presence of iodide,[1411, 1209] bromide,[1902] or chloride,[890] this acts as an effective mechanism for killing a variety of organisms. EPO has a different pH optimum from MPO.[1919]

The EPO-H_2O_2-halide system is directly toxic to a number of parasites including schistosomula,[892] *T. spiralis* newborn larvae,[130] *Toxoplasma gondii*,[1089] and *T. cruzi*.[1283] EPO can also augment the capacity of neutrophils to kill schistosomula *in vitro*.[889] EPO is also able to kill newborn larvae of *T. spiralis* by generating $HClO^-$ ions, although it is less efficient than MPO in generating hypochlorite ions.[259]

In 1965, G. T. Archer found that purified rat EPO caused mast cells to disrupt *in vitro*.[57] This was confirmed in 1984, and studied by scanning electronmicroscopy.[315] In 1980, a similar process was seen using human EPO,[778] with the additional finding that a complex of EPO with mast cell products was more effective than EPO alone.

Unfortunately there are no studies on whether EPO can cause mast cell degranulation or disruption *in vivo*. EPO has been found to attach to the surface of isolated rat mast cell granules, where it retained its enzymatic properties.[781]

EPO appears to be able to 'arm' macrophages, so that they become more effective in killing staphylococci,[1475] toxoplasma,[1089] and trypanosoma.[1283]

In a study reported in 1987 on the uptake of EPO by human neutrophils, it was found that the enzyme was internalized, and held in microvesicular bodies. This did not occur with MPO.[1990] It is not known whether the uptake of EPO is a method for removing this potentially toxic molecule, or whether it increases the effector functions of inflammatory cells. EPO can bind to neoplastic cell line cells *in vitro*. This makes these cells susceptible to macrophage-mediated cytolysis, in the presence of H_2O_2 which is released from macrophages after contact with the coated cells.[1266]

Under certain conditions, EPO, like other peroxidases, can inactivate the leukotrienes LTB4, LTC4, and LTD4.[782] Its action on LTC4 is to produce biologically inactive isomers of LTB4,[679] and other molecules.[1799]

3.7.11 *Other cytoplasmic granule constituents*

Many different lysosomal enzymes and other components have been characterized in human blood eosinophils.

Phosphatases Large amounts of acid phosphatase have been extracted from human eosinophils, but in unstimulated eosinophils this enzymatic activity is masked, although the enzyme can be demonstrated with antibodies.[77] In 1966, cytochemical electronmicroscopy of normal human eosinophils showed that acid phosphatase was not detectable in granules containing cores, but was found both in the specific granules which did not possess crystalloids, and in small granules.[520, 639]

In 1980, Bass and colleagues noted that only 8 per cent of granules in blood eosinophils from normal individuals stained for acid phosphatase, when assessed by cytochemical electronmicroscopy, whereas in patients with eosinophilia, 49 per cent stained. The percentage stained could be increased by stimulating normal eosinophils with opsonized staphylococci, or the calcium ionophore A23187.[127] They studied the activation of this enzyme in detail, and showed that it occurred rapidly.[128] However, it is not known whether activation is due to an alteration in the permeability of granule membranes, dissociation of the enzyme from a glycosaminoglycan backbone, or some other mechanism.

Proteases, collagenase, and elastase Although neutrophils contain a potent collagenase, and this enzyme had been described in rat,[134] and guinea pig eosinophils,[794] it was not until 1984 that human eosinophils were also shown to contain an enzymatic activity which degrades collagen.[409] In this study, extracts of human eosinophils were shown to degrade collagen types 1 and 3. Some experiments suggested that the collagenase was different from neutrophil collagenase which cleaves type I collagen preferentially. This paper also showed that guinea pig eosinophil granule extracts contained a 'masked' collagenase, which was only revealed after trypsin treatment. Unlike macrophages and neutrophils, eosinophils were shown not to contain elastase or other types of nonspecific neutral protease.

Arylsulphatase B Eosinophils possess more arylsulphatase activity than other leukocytes, and the enzyme is present in the granules in an inactive form,[100] but it is active in small granules, most commonly in tissue eosinophils. In 1980, arylsulphatase B was purified from human eosinophils, and shown to have a molecular weight of about 60 kDa, and a pH optimum of 5.7, which is characteristic of type II arylsulphatase. It was suggested that arylsulphatase B was involved in the catabolism of proteoglycans, and glycosaminoglycans.[1917] In 1983, further work showed that it probably had a four-subunit structure, with a minimum molecular weight of 70 kDa. Its variable activity could be accounted for by changes in the association of its subunits.[1907]

Arylsulphatase B is inactivated by LTC4 *in vitro*.[1910] Suggestions, which were made between 1974 and 1976, that eosinophil arysulphatases could break down SRS-A[1334, 1884, 932] are incorrect. This activity was due to the presence of contaminants in the arylsulphatase preparations.[1359] In 1981 the content of arylsulphatase B in eosinophils was assayed, and shown to alter during the eosinophilia which occurred when bancroftian filariasis was treated with diethyl carbamazine.[1916]

Histaminase Histaminase (diamine oxidase) and histamine methyltransferase are the only constituents in granulocytes which degrade histamine in man. They have been shown to be secreted from human blood neutrophils after incubation with opsonized zymosan, or the calcium ionophore A23187.[1994] Eosinophils possess a histaminase, but this is present in smaller amounts than in neutrophils,[1995] although greater activity has been found in eosinophils from patients with eosinophilia.[789]

Eosinophil histaminase secretion has been studied by Colten and colleagues in Boston, USA, who compared it with the secretion of histaminase from neutrophils.[790] A number of differences were found. Histaminase and arylsulphatase were only secreted from purified blood eosinophils when they had phagocytosed C3b-, or cobra-venom-factor-coated particles, whereas attachment to C3b-particles was sufficient to stimulate neutrophils. Cytochalasin-B inhibited the release of histaminase from eosinophils, but increased neutrophil secretion. Components of the alternative pathway of the complement system also appeared to be required to induce eosinophils to secrete, as secretion did not occur when serum was depleted of factor B.

Phospholipase B and D It is not known whether human eosinophils contain phospholipase-B, although this enzyme has been found in eosinophils in other species, including the rat and horse. Phospholipase D was isolated from human eosinophil granules in 1976.[917] In 1980 it was shown to be able to liberate 0.3 nmol choline/hour/5 $\times$ 10^6 eosinophils, which is ten times more than that liberated from neutrophils. It had a molecular weight of 60 kDa.[1917] This enzyme is also able to degrade PAF-acether.

Catalase Human eosinophils contain catalase, which has been localized by immunoelectronmicroscopy.[842]

Nonspecific esterases Eosinophils contain nonspecific esterase activity,[1232] which is associated with the membranes of eosinophil granules, mitochondria, rough endoplasmic reticulum, and perinuclear cisternae.[1074]

Vitamin B12 binding proteins A vitamin B12 binding protein has been found in eosinophils.[1150] In 1984, measurements were made of serum unsaturated B12 binding proteins in nine patients with eosinophilia, four of whom had HES. The serum B12 levels, and/or the unsaturated B12 binding capacity, were markedly raised in all of them.[2002] In a further three patients with HES studied in India, normal levels of B12 binding proteins were found.[640]

Fibroblast growth factors Fibroblast growth factors have been described in supernatants, and cultures of many different cell types.[1770] The eosinophil appears to be no exception. Take has unpublished work showing that sepharose-C3b-stimulated human blood eosinophils released fibroblast growth-stimulatory factors of molecular weight 30–50 kDa. In 1987, Pincus and colleagues in Boston, USA detected a similar activity in human and guinea pig eosinophils.[1417] It was suggested that this might explain the occurrence of fibrosis in some lesions where eosinophils are found.

Glycosaminoglycans Glycosaminoglycans (acid mucopolysaccharides) have been demonstrated within the granules of immature, but not mature rat, and guinea pig eosinophils.[1256]

Metals A number of heavy metals are present in eosinophils.[1405] These include zinc, copper, manganese, magnesium, cobalt, and iron. They are probably bound through nitrogen ligands, especially the amine and imidazole groups of basic amino acids. The precise localization of zinc in eosinophils remains to be established. It could be determined by electron-probe scanning electronmicroscopy. It is not an integral part of lysophospholipase.[1914] as was considered at one time. However, in 1980 it was found with isolated ECP at 2.5 moles of zinc per mole of protein,[1850] so it is presumably a granule matrix constituent.

3.7.12 *The Charcot–Leyden crystal protein*

An unexplained feature of human eosinophils is the presence of large amounts of lysophospholipase (lysolecithin acylhydrolase, EC 3.1.1.5, or Charcot–Leyden crystal (CLC) protein) in eosinophils, and in sites where eosinophils have degranulated, where it forms into characteristic bipyramidal crystals: Charcot–Leyden crystals.

Biosynthesis In 1986, murine eosinophils were found to contain more lysophospholipase after culture with T-cells and macrophages with antigen, than when cultured alone, suggesting that cytokines could induce eosinophils to synthesize this protein.[19] The biosynthesis of CLC protein was studied in 1987, in human blood eosinophils and HL-60 cells after culture for 20 and 4 hours respectively, using ^{35}S-methionine. The newly synthesized labelled protein was found to be post-translationally modified by covalent attachment to myristic acid.[13]

Purification and structure of CLC protein A method for preparing large amounts of CLC protein was reported in 1980.[8] In the mid-1970s the CLC protein began to be studied at the Mayo Clinic, USA, and several of its biochemical characteristics were defined: it was shown to be a single hydrophobic polypeptide chain of 117–119 amino acids, with 18–19 residues of glutamic acid, 12 of valine, 6 residues of arginine, and 1.2 per cent carbohydrate. Later it was shown to have one sulphydryl group.[665] It could be solubilized at neutral pH after freeze drying, and had a pI of 5.7–5.1

and an apparent molecular weight of 13 kDa.[8] This molecular weight was subsequently revised to 17.4 kDa in 1984.[1909] CLC protein gave rise to several bands on electrophoresis in polyacrylamide gels and isoelectric focusing, but immunoprecipitation with antibodies and electrophoresis in SDS-polyacrylamide gels showed only one band.

Charcot–Leyden crystals *In vivo*, lysophospholipase forms into characteristic bipyramidal crystals, with a hexagonal cross section in tissues, sputum, and faeces where many eosinophils have accumulated and degranulated, and within eosinophils themselves. They can also be induced to form *in vitro*, using whole eosinophils or purified lysophospholipase.

Robin first described these crystals in Paris in 1853, in the heart blood, and spleen of a patient with a leukaemia, being looked after by Dr Charcot.[306] In 1872 Leyden noted them in the sputum of a patient with asthma.[1072] Since then, Charcot–Leyden crystals have been seen in the tissues of patients with a wide range of other diseases,[142] including eosinophilic pneumonia,[906] pulmonary ascariasis, tropical eosinophilia, ulcerative colitis, HES,[452] eosinophilic granuloma, histiocytosis X,[905] pemphigus vegetans,[1018] and pleural effusions of diverse causes.[1268] Their presence is believed to show sites of extensive eosinophil inflammation.

Experimental work on crystals from eosinophils began in 1922, when eosinophils from a patient with hypereosinophilia were seen to form crystals after incubation at 37°. These were soluble in hot water, 2 per cent acetic acid, and sodium hydroxide.[1172] Charcot–Leyden crystals were shown to consist of a small protein in 1956,[228] and 1962.[813] In 1963 G. T. Archer and Blackwood isolated blood eosinophils from a patient with 32.4×10^9/l eosinophil. After the cells had been left for 1-2 days in a refrigerator, Charcot–Leyden crystals were found to be present. Basophils which were suspended in hypotonic solutions also formed Charcot–Leyden crystals within two minutes. The crystals appeared in the cytoplasm and granules after the cells and their nuclei had become swollen. They also found that Charcot–Leyden crystals could be formed from protein extracts of eosinophils, and that they were soluble in acid solutions.[54] In 1971, it was noted that these crystals could form within the crystalloid granules, and electronmicrographs suggested that they formed by a rearrangement of the crystalloid constituents.[502] This is probably untrue, as the crystalloid consists only of MBP.

CL crystals also form *in vitro*, when either eosinophils or basophils have been left in hypotonic solutions, or after they have been treated with detergents. In tissues, although most crystals are probably derived from degranulated or lysed eosinophils, it has also been shown that they can form in intact eosinophils. For example, an electronmicrograph which was made in 1980 of a bone marrow eosinophil promyelocyte showed a CL crystal within the cell.[2007]

The persistence of CL crystals in tissues is probably due to their resistance to proteolytic digestion, and they may continue to function as lysophospholipases in the crystalline form.[1917] They are soluble in alcohol, and so leave characteristic spaces in conventionally processed tissue sections.

Assays for CLC protein A radioimmunoassay for CLC protein, using a rabbit antibody, was described in 1980[8] and 1983.[12] Eosinophils contain more than two and a half times the amount of lysophospholipase as mononuclear cells, and eight times as much as neutrophils.[1917] Initial work on the CLC protein in eosinophils suggested that it was only present in the plasma membrane, and not in granules or cytoplasm.[1917] This seems to be unlikely, as CL crystals have been seen to form within granules *in vivo* and *in vitro*, as described above. Normal human serum contains 37 ng/ml of CLC protein. High levels have been found in patients with raised blood eosinophil counts due to many different diseases (over 8 μg/ml in some patients). In these patients, the CLC protein levels were over twice as high as serum MBP levels.[8] Levels correlated (a) with peripheral blood eosinophil counts both in normals and patients with eosinophilia, and (b) with serum MBP levels. There was also a suggestion that CLC protein might exist in several forms in serum.[10]

Functional properties of CLC protein There is still no clear explanation for why eosinophils should contain so much lysophospholipase, or why it should be released from eosinophils to accumulate to form the characteristic crystals. Initial work on the CLC protein in 1976 showed that it did not alter vascular permeability, contract guinea pig ileum, or antagonize the effects of bradykinin or histamine;[665] nor does it cause the Gordon phenomenon.

In 1980, Weller and his colleagues in Boston, USA, first showed that the CLC protein had lysophospholipase activity,[1914] and that purified lysophospholipase formed into CL crystals.[1914] Evidence to support the identity of the CLC protein and lysophospholipase includes:

(1) that they both have this enzyme activity;

(2) that they co-migrate on SDS polyacrylamide gels;

(3) that they have antigenic identity;[1908]

(4) that they have the same Michaelis constant;

(5) that they have an identical amino acid composition, with blocked terminal amino acids; and

(6) that they are identical with faecal CLC protein.

CLC protein contains a single cysteine residue, and it may make up 10 per cent of the total proteins in eosinophils.[1909]

Lysophospholipase may protect eosinophils from the toxic effects of lysophospholipids,[1917] which have been shown to produce structural alterations in human eosinophils;[1741] or from toxic products released by parasites; or from metabolites generated in the plasma membrane itself, such as PAF-acether which would otherwise damage the cell.

CLC protein may also be involved in parasite killing. This has been suggested by Adewusi and colleagues, who have been studying lysophospholipase activity in mice infected with *T. spiralis*. They showed that antithymocyte serum reduced the eosinophil response and the tissue lysophospholopase activity in the tissues of infected mice. As the cuticle of *T. spiralis* contains phospholipids, it was suggested that lysophospholipase might have a hydrolytic action on the parasite cuticle,[21, 20] but this has not yet been tested directly.

3.8 The metabolism of resting and stimulated eosinophils

Much of the work on human eosinophil metabolism has been carried out with blood eosinophils isolated from patients with marked eosinophilia, especially patients with HES. As the metabolism of eosinophils can vary considerably from the resting to the stimulated stage, it has proved difficult to make relative assessments of the amount of glucose, oxygen, and other compounds utilized by eosinophils in normal and diseased states. However, measurements made by several groups show that eosinophils have a remarkably high capacity to develop a respiratory burst, to generate oxygen radicals, to metabolize glucose anaerobically, and to generate large amounts of leukotrienes and other products of arachidonic acid metabolism. Much of the energy for this work is stored in ATP, which is the principal nucleotide in eosinophils.[414]

3.8.1 *Glucose metabolism*

Blood eosinophils metabolize glucose. When blood samples containing about 100×10^9/l eosinophils were left without sodium fluoride, plasma glucose concentration fell from 140 to 5 mg/dl within three hours.[1051] When eosinophils are stimulated to produce a respiratory burst, there is a marked increase in glucose metabolism. This has been shown with radiolabelled glucose molecules, most of which are metabolized through the hexose-monophosphate-shunt.

In comparison with neutrophils, blood eosinophils in the resting state oxidize five times more ^{14}C-glucose, incorporate five times more ^{125}iodide, and contain six times more NADPH oxidase. They have a comparable capacity to reduce nitroblue tetrazolium salts. Similar differences have been shown between blood eosinophils and neutrophils when they are subjected to phagocytic stimuli. Eosinophils oxidized seven times more 1-^{14}C glucose than did neutrophils under these conditions. Nitroblue tetrazolium reduction, ^{125}I incorporation, and chemoluminescence were two times greater in eosinophils than in neutrophils, whereas superoxide anion production was similar.[427]

In tissues, eosinophils may have an even greater capacity to oxidize glucose when they have been activated. This possibility was first suggested in 1977, when peritoneal eosinophils from a 14-year old boy with eosinophilic gastroenteritis were isolated, and shown to have a marked increase in hexose monophosphate shunt activity, H_2O_2 formation, superoxide anion generation, chemoluminescence, thyroid hormone degradation, iodination, and oestrogen binding, as a result of ingesting particles. This metabolic burst following endocytosis was greater than for neutrophils.[975]

In 1972 the capacity of human eosinophils to oxidize glucose was studied using blood eosinophils from six patients with eosinophilia. In unstimulated eosinophils the oxidation of 1-^{14}C glucose, 6-^{14}C glucose, and ^{14}C fumarate was greater in eosinophils than in a comparable number of neutrophils. When the cells were induced to phagocytose particles, the oxidation of both 1-^{14}C glucose and 6-^{14}C glucose was also stimulated more in eosinophils than in neutrophils.[1207]

The carrier-facilitated transport of hexoses into blood eosinophils has been measured with ^{3}H-2-deoxyglucose. It was three times higher in eosinophils from patients with eosinophilia, and it could also be increased by stimulating the cells with zymosan activated serum,[127] and other chemotactic factors.[131] The addition of arachidonic acid, or its lipoxygenase products 5-HETE and 11-HETE, induced an increase in labelled deoxyglucose uptake into human eosinophils. Inhibitors of this pathway reduced the deoxyglucose uptake of blood eosinophils from patients with eosinophilia. These results suggest that lipoxygenase pathway metabolism and hexose transport are closely interrelated in eosinophils.[126]

In 1980 measurements were made of the hexose monophosphate shunt activity using the metabolism of 1-^{14}C glucose to $^{14}CO_2$ in normal blood eosinophils. Unstimulated eosinophils had the same activity as neutrophils, but whereas it was not significantly increased by stimulation of normal eosinophils, it increased seven- to tenfold in eosinophils from patients with eosinophilia.[127]

3.8.2 *Oxidative metabolism*

The capacity of eosinophils to respire is well known, and appropriately stimulated eosinophils produce a marked respiratory burst. This was first shown with eosinophils from the blood of patients with eosinophilia.

The respiratory burst In 1983, a comparitive study was reported on the oxygen uptake of blood eosinophils from five patients with malignant eosinophils, and six with reactive eosinophils.[373] This showed that malignant eosinophils had a greater respiratory burst in response to latex beads, or antibody- and complement-coated bacteria. No difference was found in their response to antibody-coated bacteria or immune complexes. In 1987, it was found that purified human blood eosinophils stimulated with PMA consumed twice as much oxygen as neutrophils from the same individuals. Zymosan-C3b gave a 70 per cent oxidative response. The bacterial-derived stimulus, formyl methionyl-leucine-phenylalanine (fMLP), and the calcium ionophore A23187 induced only a small response.[1969] However, fMLP-stimulated eosinophils produced a marked respiratory burst after incubation with PMA or opsonized zymosan, which was twice as great as that in neutrophils, and more prolonged.[1400]

The capacity of eosinophil granule-free membrane-bound cytoplasm (eoplasts) to utilize oxygen was 20 per cent of the intact cell. However, after stimulation with A23187, they consumed more oxygen than the intact cell. This method for preparing granule-free cytoplasmic particles enables experiments to be carried out which compare the properties of granule constituents and other cytoplasmic components.[1969]

Chemoluminescence The remarkable capacity of stimulated blood eosinophils to produce chemoluminescence has been repeatedly confirmed. fMLP was twice as effective as LTB4 in producing this effect.[1355] In a study from Wisconsin, USA, in 1985, eosinophils were found to be as effective as neutrophils in producing luminol-dependent chemoluminescence, and superoxide generation, after stimulation with opsonized zymosan, and twice as effective as neutrophils after stimulation with PMA.[1621] Blood eosinophils from patients with allergic rhinitis produced more luminol-dependent chemoluminescence in response to opsonized zymosan, and PMA, than normal, and the response was greatest when the patients' symptoms were worst.[1620]

In 1984, work in Lille, France, showed that light density eosinophils from the blood and tissues of patients with eosinophilia had reduced PMA-induced chemoluminescence.[1453] Although this was confirmed by one other group, light density eosinophils may be 'activated', and respond with a greater production of luminol-dependent chemoluminescence. For example, the lighter density cells in patients with HES or symptomatic asthma had a greater capacity to develop chemoluminescence with PMA or PAF-acether stimulation, than intermediate or normal density eosinophils from patients with asymptomatic asthma or atopy (Chanez, P. *et al.* 1987, personal communication).

Reactive oxygen species The respiratory burst in eosinophils is accompanied by the release of potentially toxic oxygen metabolites,[94] including the superoxide anion O_2^-[1041] and H_2O_2.[1413] The amount of superoxide anion produced by eosinophil from two patients with eosinophilia, three hours after stimulation with opsonized zymosan, was twice the amount produced by neutrophils from normal individuals.[1757] Superoxide production was greater than normal in blood eosinophils from individuals with experimental hookworm infection,[1925] suggesting that superoxide formation increases in activated blood eosinophils. The respiratory burst is produced by an enzyme system which oxidizes NADPH, and reduces molecular oxygen to superoxide. The enzymes which do this are present in large amounts in eosinophils.[425] Cytochrome b-245, which is important in this process, has been shown to be present in the plasma membrane of human blood eosinophils.[1586]

3.8.3 *Unsaturated fatty acid metabolism*

Eosinophils can be distinguished from neutrophils by their marked capacity to produce large amounts of leukotriene C4 (LTC4) and D4 (LTD4), whereas neutrophils preferentially synthesize leukotriene B4 (LTB4). The importance of this is that LTC4 can cause bronchoconstriction, alterations in vascular permeability and tone, and increased mucus secretion in man.

15-lipoxygenase pathway products, HETEs The ability of human eosinophils to generate 15-HETE was first shown in 1982,[1800] and in murine eosinophils in 1983.[1801] This occurred when the eosinophils were stimulated in cultures containing arachidonic acid, which diverts synthesis away from LTC4 synthesis. In a study reported in 1987 on arachidonic acid metabolism in collagenase-separated polyp eosinophils, the main metabolite was 15-HETE.[1649] Although the functions of HETEs from eosinophils are unknown, it has been shown that 15-HETE can act as an internal regulator of 5-lipoxygenase activity, reducing the amount of LTC4 secreted after stimulation of human blood eosinophils.[220]

Leukotrienes Resting blood eosinophils do not synthesize significant quantities of leukotrienes. However, when they are stimulated by the calcium ionophore A23187, or opsonized zymosan, they make large amounts of LTC4. The capacity of stimulated horse eosinophils to produce leukotriene C4 was first reported in 1982[893] and 1983.[1998] Similar findings were made in 1983 using human eosinophils,[1915] where 38 ng LTC4/10^6 eosinophils was produced after stimulation with A23187. The amounts of LTC4 and LTB4, and 15-HETEs produced by human eosinophils has been found to depend on the amount of arachidonic acid available to the cells to convert into these metabolites.[779] It has been suggested that 15(S)-HETE is the monohydroxy acid which leads to the preferential synthesis of 15-HETE.[224]

LTC4 secretion by human eosinophils was also reported from Holland in 1984.[1855] In this study it was found that 87 per cent pure blood eosinophils secreted nearly 40 × 10^6 LTC4 molecules/cell, after stimulation with 10 μM A23187. Only small amounts of LTB4 were made by stimulated blood eosinophils. On the other hand, neutrophils made large amounts of LTB4, and only small amounts of LTC4.[1855]

In 1985 it was reported that light density eosinophils secreted more LTC4 than normal density eosinophils.[902] In another study in 1987, it was found that this was also true when the cells were stimulated with zymosan-C3b, but not A23187.[921]

LTC4 from eosinophils may be an important bronchoconstricting agent in late-phase asthmatic reactions where eosinophils are often found.[220] LTC4 has also been shown to induce mucus secretion from human lung cells *in vitro*.[1157] The stimulation of eosinophils to produce LTC4 has been shown to involve an initial transient intracellular accumulation of biologically active LTC4, extracellular release, and the apparent limitation of oxidative metabolism to the outside of the cell.[1347] The properties of LTC4 and other products of arachidonic metabolism were reviewed in 1987 by Austen.[81] The main effect of LTC4 is to cause the contraction of vascular and nonvascular smooth muscle. It also produces a wheal-and-flare when injected intradermally in normal people.

A number of different stimuli have been shown to be able to induce human blood eosinophils to secrete LTC4. However there is no good comparative study of their efficacy, and there is no consensus on whether only a few stimuli,[1855] or many stimuli have this effect. There is also no study showing that eosinophils make LTC4 *in vivo*. The range of stimuli which induce LTC4 secretion include:

(1) the calcium ionophore A23187, which has been one of the standard stimuli for producing this response since it was first reported in 1983.[1915] (In 1987 it was shown that another effect of A23187 was to induce eosinophils to make lipoxin A: 5(S), 6(R), 15(S)-trihydroxy-7,9,13-trans-11-cis-eicosatetraenoic acid;)[1590]

(2) opsonized zymosan;[220, 223]

(3) fMLP;[1604]

(4) PAF-acether;[223]

(5) IgG complexes on the surface of beads;[1604, 371]

(6) eosinophil activating factors.

The capacity of normal (but not light density) eosinophils to secrete LTC4 was increased when they were incubated with partially purified eosinophil activating factor (EAF),[571] and this effect was also shown when Ig-coated particles were used instead of complement-coated particles, or A23187.[570]

After addition of the eosinophil cytotoxicity enhancing factor (ECEF) (a 1:3 dilution of LPS-stimulated blood mononuclear cell culture supernatants) to human blood eosinophils, additional LTC4 was made when the calcium ionophore was added. However, this effect varied considerably between different individuals, and it never reached more than 140 ng/10^6 eosinophils. Preincubation in the factor for 1–2.5 minutes was essential for this enhancement, and it was abolished by washing the cells. Although the responses were variable and small, it was suggested that activation with this factor might be an important mechanism for affecting inflammatory responses.[441] Tumour necrosis factor (TNF) had no effect on A23187-induced secretion of LTC4.[1627] Leukotriene production by eosinophils was suppressed by E-prostaglandins (PGE), stimulators of adenylate cyclase, and phosphodiesterase inhibitors. The importance of this is relation to the treatment of asthma was discussed in 1987.[1011]

Prostaglandins and thromboxanes It was first shown in 1975 that human eosinophils could secrete prostaglandins E1 (PGE1) and E2 (PGE2).[823] It was not until 1986 that prostaglandin synthesis by eosinophils was examined again. This was a study on the capacity of human peritoneal fluid eosinophils to secrete thromboxane B2 (TXB2), PGE2, and 6-keto-prostaglandin F1 (6-keto-PGF1). The basal release and A23187-stimulated release of TXB2 was greater than PGE2 release. Very little 6-keto-PGF1 was released. When TXB2 release was inhibited, there was a corresponding increase in PGE2 and 6-keto-PGF1 secretion.[583] Stimulated guinea pig eosinophils and neutrophils also released PGE2, but in quantities which were too small to inhibit mast cell degranulation.[1242]

Platelet-activating factor Platelet-activating factor, which is also known as PAF, PAF-acether, AGEPC, and 1-O-akyl-2-acetyl sn-glycero-3-phospho-choline, is an inflammatory mediator with a wide range of biological activities. It was first identified in 1972 in supernatants from basophils stimulated with antigen. Its main effects are to cause bronchoconstriction, platelet and neutrophil activation, and inflammation. It is produced by many different cell types, including eosinophils, but on a cell basis, eosinophils are probably the most potent. Although normal density blood eosinophils release less than 5 pg PAF-acether, light density blood eosinophils produced 100 ng/10^6 cells after stimulation with the calcium ionophore A23187.[1049, 898] It is a puzzling feature that eosinophil are also strongly stimulated by added PAF-acether *in vitro*, but it is not known if eosinophil-derived PAF-acether can act as an autocrine molecule.

3.8.4 *Protein synthesis*

Although there has been some interesting work on the synthesis of the individual granule proteins in bone marrow eosinophils, there is little information of the possible biosynthetic capacity of more mature eosinophils. This may be due to the dogma that blood eosinophils are 'end' cells, which simply deliver their preformed constituents to tissues. In 1978, it was found that ^{3}H-uridine and ^{3}H-leucine were taken up by mature bone marrow eosinophils after one hour culture, and the label localized on the surface of crystalloid-containing granules.[1930]

In 1987, studies in Boston, USA showed that when blood eosinophils were incubated with ^{35}S-methionine, radioactivity was incorporated into a 43 kDa protein within 30 minutes, and this was maximal at four hours. Three other proteins of molecular weights 24, 46, and 60 kDa were synthesized when the cells were stimulated with opsonized zymosan. Surprisingly, fMLP, A23187, and PMA did not induce new protein synthesis. It was suggested that changes in the functions of eosinophils may be affected by alterations in protein synthesis.[1472] These findings suggest that measurement of the biosynthetic capacity of mature blood eosinophils could be an important area for future study, using the conditions which maximize the survival and responsiveness of eosinophils in culture.

3.8.5 *Proteoglycan synthesis*

The presence of carbohydrates in eosinophils was demonstrated with fluorescent lectin markers in 1980. Sialic acid, galactose, and mannose were localized to the plasmalemma, cytoplasm, nuclear membrane, and granules of eosinphils. Basophil granules also stained but neutrophil granules were negative.[1713] Complex carbohydrates have also been identified in immature granules in human bone marrow eosinophils by cytochemistry and autoradiography. Mature granules were not stained by these methods.[1364] Cultured blood eosinophils have been shown to incorporate labelled sulphate into complex glycosaminoglycans. They contained 70–81 per cent chondroitin 4-sulphate, 9–12 per cent chondroitin 6-sulphate, and 5–12 per cent dermatan sulphate.[1198] Chondroitin 4-sulphate is also found in human neutrophils and platelets.

4. The eosinophil cell membrane and receptors

The eosinophil cell membrane has a number of important features which distinguish it from other cell membranes, although it has many characteristics in common with neutrophils and other cells. The cell surface charge of normal human blood eosinophil is 2.45 ± 0.03 μmoles/sec/volt/cm, compared to 1.98 ± 0.01 for neutrophils. This charge is lower in blood eosinophils from patients with eosinophilia, and it can also be reduced by incubation in zymosan-activated serum.[127]

4.1 Scanning electronmicroscopy

Scanning electronmicrographs (SEMs) have been published of blood eosinophils from patients with hypereosinophilia, but these show no features to distinguish them from blood neutrophils and lymphocytes. Some cells appeared to be relatively smooth, some had small projections, and others had ridges characteristic of secretory cells.[1428] I have seen some blood eosinophils in SEMs, which appeared to bud off small amounts of their plasma membrane. Eosinophils also have the capacity to send out long cytoplasmic projections on glass surfaces. There may be crystalloid granules at the tips of these projections. The nature of the processes and the factors which cause them to be produced have yet to be determined. Their formation must be energy-dependent, and require new membrane synthesis.

SEM appearances have also been described of the surface of eosinophils on glass smears made from blood from normal cattle. The bulges made in the cell surface by underlying large granules enabled the cells to be recognized easily.[1403]

SEM studies of the surface of rat peritoneal eosinophils have shown two types of projection: finger-like microvilli, and flattened and ridge-like projections.[1407]

4.2 Freeze-fracture studies on eosinophil membranes

Freeze-fracture studies on human eosinophils have been done, both with eosinophils from patients with eosinophilia, and in *in vitro* studies on eosinophils secreting onto the surface of the schistosomula of *S. mansoni*. Studies on blood eosinophils from three patients with marked non-leukaemic eosinophilia showed that there were more intramembranous particles in the outer face of the plasma membrane than in the inner face, and that the particles in the membranes of the crystalloid granules were larger: 8–15 nm. Aggregates of particles were not seen.[463]

A freeze-fracture study on peritoneal eosinophils from Am-1(2)/Tor rats found that there were few intramembranous particles in the plasma membrane compared to other similar cell types (706 and 549/μm^2 in the P and E faces respectively), but there were many in the membrane of the specific granules (1720/μm^2 in the P face).[1407] The significance of this is not known.

In 1987, freeze-fracture photographs were published of human blood eosinophils stimulated with the calcium ionophore A23187, and opsonized zymosan. This showed aggregates of intramembranous particles, and the formation of membrane pits.[780] Similar intramembranous particles had been seen in the freeze-etch studies on human eosinophil granules in 1975.[235]

4.3 Membrane proteins

The plasma membrane of eosinophils contains many components, such as 5' nucleotidase, which are also found in the plasma membranes of other inflammatory cells. Studies on the membrane proteins which can be labelled with ^{125}I, or which bind antisera, show that they are most closely related to neutrophils in these respects, despite having a separate lineage. The proteins in the plasma membrane of murine peritoneal eosinophils were studied in 1980, using partially purified cells from BALB/c mice infected with *M. corti*. ^{125}I bound to an eosinophil membrane protein of molecular weight 79 kDa, and to four other proteins larger than 50 kDa. A 90 kDa component (a major constituent of mouse neutrophil plasma membranes) was not present.[233] Membrane components are important in the interactions among eosinophils, normal tissue components, and foreign molecules which induce them to spread out and degranulate. A summary of the main immunological receptors on eosinophils is shown in Fig. 4.1. The molecular basis for eosinophil attachment to particles and surfaces is not known. The complement and immunoglobulin receptors are clearly important, but other structures are also involved. This was suggested in experiments in which human eosinophils were found to attach to albumin-coated Sepharose beads and microtitre plates to a greater extent than neutrophils.[1943]

4.3.1 *Immunoglobulin and complement receptors*

As eosinophils mature in the bone marrow, they lose Ia antigens,[988] and gain complement receptors (CR) and immunoglobulin receptors (FcR), which are most strongly expressed in stimulated and activated eosinophils.

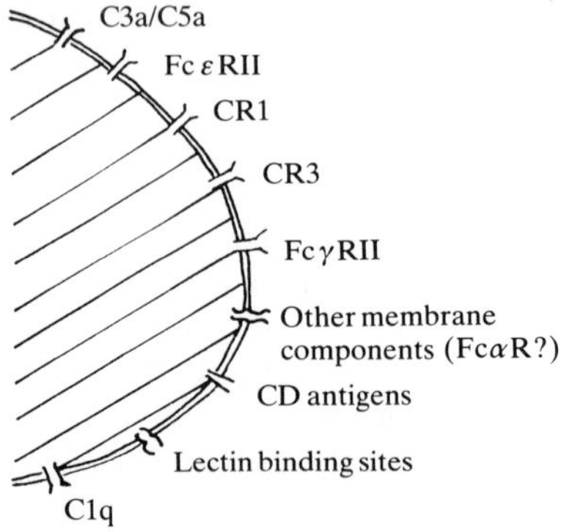

Fig. 4.1. The different types of immunological receptors found on human blood and tissue eosinophils. The spatial distribution of the receptors, and their relationship with each other remain to be determined.

Blood eosinophils from normal individuals bind immunoglobulins relatively poorly compared to neutrophils, and they generally express less CR than neutrophils and monocytes. This may be partly the result of masking of receptors by sialic acid containing membrane glycoproteins, as neuraminidase treatment leads to the increased expression of Fc-receptor binding capacity by normal blood eosinophils. There is also evidence that eosinophil CR are recycled (perhaps through coated pits) although this has not been formally demonstrated. We considered this possibility in 1976, after finding that CR were re-expressed within 30 minutes of digestion of these receptors from the surface of human blood eosinophils with proteolytic enzymes. Normal blood eosinophils do not have IgM receptors,[1340] although IgM binding to eosinophils can be induced by culturing them *in vitro*.[418] IgA can also bind and stimulate eosinophils under certain circumstances.

It was first claimed in 1976 that eosinophils can bind to sheep erythrocytes (E).[1609] In 1980, it was reported that a mean of 16 per cent of blood eosinophils from patients with parasitic diseases formed E rosettes, whereas they did not develop in normal individuals. It was suggested that this reflected an alteration in the membrane of patients' eosinophils.[419] However, it is possible that the separation techniques and culture conditions could have led to the release of cationic proteins which might bind erythrocytes to the eosinophil surface nonspecifically. Other groups, including ourselves, have not been able to detect the binding of sheep red cells to intact blood eosinophils.[1367]

Receptors for IgG (FcγR) Much of the early work on eosinophil IgG binding capacity was done using rosetting techniques. Guinea pig eosinophils were first shown to bind IgG-coated erythrocytes (EA) in 1969,[787] and we demonstrated that human eosinophils had receptors for IgG in 1976.[1738] They were found to bind complexed IgG almost as well as neutrophils; and eosinophils from the blood of patients with eosinophilia had an increased capacity to bind to complexed IgG, and form rosettes.[1696] We also showed that complexed IgG1 and IgG3 myeloma proteins inhibited IgG rosettes more effectively than IgG2 or IgG4 complexes.[1738] In 1978 Ottesen also found that eosinophils from the blood of seven patients with schistosomiasis, and four with filariasis had an increased binding capacity for mouse C3-, and rabbit-IgG-coated sheep erythrocytes.[1340]

Eosinophil FcγR first appears on dividing eosinophils in human bone marrow at the promyelocyte stage, earlier than in the mouse. In one study marrow aspirates were studied from five patients using rabbit-IgG-coated sheep erythrocytes. Twelve per cent of eosinophil myelocytes had detectable FcγR, the same as blood eosinophils studied with this technique.[788]

Subsequent work has involved the use of monoclonal antibodies to define and isolate the receptor proteins in the plasma membrane of phagocytic cells. At the Rockefeller University, monoclonal antibodies have been produced which distinguish between high affinity IgG receptors (FcγRhi or FcγRI), which are mainly found on immature granulocytes, and low affinity receptors (FcγRlo or FCγRII), which characterize more mature granulocytes. Using the monoclonal antibody (3G8) to FcγRlo, it was shown that there was a progressive loss of FcγRI during myeloid differentiation, with reciprocal expression of FcγRII. Mature eosinophils only expressed FcγRII.[577] Further studies with antibodies 3G8 and CLB-FcR-1 have shown that human blood eosinophils have less FcγRII than neutrophils.[1971] In 1984, a report was published in which two molecules of 16 and 18 kDa were isolated from human blood eosinophil surfaces labelled with ^{125}iodide by the lactoperoxidase method.[1775] These were thought to be components of FcγR because they were eluted from immobilized immune complexes. However, it is possible that these molecules were secreted ECP or EDN/EPX. In a careful study which was reported in 1984, and which set out to isolate FcγR from human blood eosinophils, it was found that they were more sensitive to proteolysis than neutrophil FcγR. The isolated eosinophil receptors had a molecular weight of 43 kDa, whereas neutrophils had receptors of 52 and 68 kDa. This work also gave some evidence that human IgG3 bound most effectively to eosinophil receptors,[1013] although studies by Walsh in 1986 using aggregates of myeloma IgG subclasses failed to show this.[1873]

In 1986 it was shown that human blood eosinophils have a 40 kDa IgG FcγR which is also found on neutrophils, monocytes, platelets, and K562 cells, and which was defined with monoclonal antibody IV3.[1099] This receptor may be the homologue of the murine macrophage FcRII, which is present on both neutrophils and eosinophils in that species.

Although these experiments suggested that there are two Fc receptors on human blood eosinophils, it is possible that the different epitopes recognized by antibodies 3G8 and IV3 are on the same Fc receptor which has varying degrees of glycosylation. This is supported by our experiments which showed that neuraminidase treatment of normal blood eosinophils increased their capacity to bind to complexed IgG.[1740] Many different stimuli, especially endotoxins, have been shown to increase the proportion of blood eosinophils which bind IgG-coated particles or complexes. It is probable that this event is an integral part of the 'activation' step which is the final stage in eosinophil differentiation and response to stimuli in tissues. Several factors increase the proportion of blood eosinophils which express FcγR, including ECF-A,[271, 78] and β-interferon (200 units/ml), which increased human blood eosinophil EA rosetting from 19 to 24 per cent after one hour incubation.[423]

The binding of eosinophils to IgG-coated surfaces can have several effects:

(a) If the particle is small, and if the eosinophils are activated, or come from the blood of patients with eosinophilia, they will be ingested. This difference between normal and patients' eosinophils was first shown in 1976.[1696]

(b) If the surface on which the IgG is deposited is large, then the eosinophils will attach firmly and generate LTC4, with a respiratory burst, and degranulate. This is the basis of the IgG-dependent cytotoxicity of eosinophils for antibody-coated parasites. Under these conditions eosinophils have been shown to synthesize new membrane proteins.[1776]

(c) If the IgG complex is in the blood, it will activate the complement system, and this will then bind to the eosinophil C3 receptors. This is probably the main way in which soluble IgG complexes induce eosinophil responses *in vivo*. As there is such a high concentration of IgG in tissue fluids and plasma, it is unlikely that soluble IgG complexes could bind to granulocyte FcγR directly.[1117] However, IgG immune complexes *in vitro* can interact with human eosinophils and produce morphological changes in the granules, including the development of tubulo-vesicular structures, which have been proposed as a route for granule secretion.[1311]

The enigma that basophil degranulation can be induced with anti-IgG4 antibodies may have been resolved with the finding in 1986 that this is a two-step process in which anti-IgG4 first cross-links IgG4 in eosinophil FcγR, resulting in the secretion of eosinophil cationic proteins, which then induce basophil degranulation. This may be a mechanism for amplifying eosinophil-dependent tissue injury in allergic diseases.[141]

Receptors for IgE (FcεR) The first experiments to show that human eosinophils can interact with complexed IgE were carried out by Arbesman and colleagues in 1974,[849] and 1975.[609] They showed that immune complexes of ragweed antigens, with IgE antibody in antigen excess, were taken up more by human eosinophils from nasal secretions than by neutrophils. IgE-antigen complexes in antigen or antibody excess were ingested to a greater degree by eosinophils than neutrophils, and the reverse was true for IgG antigen complexes. Although IgE was not found on the surface of these patients' eosinophils, Hubscher detected them in other patients' eosinophils in 1975, using immunoelectronmicroscopy with ferritin-conjugated anti-IgE.[822]

In 1981, Dr Monique Capron and colleagues in Lille, France first demonstrated that eosinophils had a low affinity receptor for IgE. In a series of studies they showed

(1) that human blood eosinophil formed rosettes with IgE-coated sheep erythrocytes;

(2) that they bound radiolabelled human IgE;[275]

(3) rabbit antibodies to IgE; and

(4) that they bound the monoclonal antibody BB10,[273] which recognizes the membrane signal site triggered by activation of cells by IgE[269] (Capron, M. 1987, personal communication).

In patients with eosinophilia, the proportion of eosinophils with IgE receptors was higher than in normal people, and the same was also found in rats infected with *S. mansoni*.[270] They showed that IgE was present in both circulating and tissue eosinophils in a number of diseases.[276]

The FcεR was found to be of the low affinity type, and was named the FcεR2 in 1986.[267] In 1987 it was found that the CR3 receptor is closely associated with the IgE receptor on eosinophils: Monoclonal antibodies to the α-chain (but not the β-chain) of the C3 receptor inhibited the binding and cytotoxicity of human light density eosinophils for IgE coated schistosomula.[274]

Light density eosinophils from patients with eosinophilia were more effective than normal density eosinophils in killing IgE-coated schistosomula. This killing was inhibited by preincubation of eosinophils with chemically-aggregated IgE, but not IgG, or anti-C3b receptor antibodies.[277] The IgE receptor may not be fully exposed on blood eosinophils, and other receptors may be also partly hidden in the plasma membrane. For example, IgG receptors are only partially exposed on normal blood eosinophils.[1740] The presence of an IgE receptor on mouse eosinophils was demonstrated in 1987.[990]

In 1984, Capron and colleagues demonstrated the presence of IgE on the surface of blood eosinophils of 17 out of 21 patients with a variety of eosinophilic disorders, including parasitic infections, HES, tumours, the Churg-Strauss syndrome, and asthma. In patients with IgE levels above 100 IU/ml, more eosinophils had surface IgE than when it was less than 100 IU/ml. Bronchoalveolar lavage eosinophils from five patients with respiratory disease (three with eosinophilic pneumonia, one with polyarteritis nodosa, and one with a drug hypersensitivity) had a greater proportion of IgE occupied receptors than blood eosinophils.[276] In 1986 they found that functional FcεR2 were restricted to light density (hypodense) eosinophils in patients' blood, although they could be detected by rosetting techniques on normal density eosinophils,[272] and this was confirmed elsewhere.[1873] The functional receptor may only appear as a result of eosinophil activation.

A possible role for IgE in eosinophil–parasite interactions has been considered at least since 1969, when G. T. Archer and colleagues in Australia reported that rat peritoneal eosinophils degranulated within 10 minutes of culture with immune complex formed from extracts of *Amplictacum robertsi* or ascaris body fluids and rat antibody. As the antibody was heat labile, they suggested that it might be IgE.[58] In 1984, Capron and her colleagues first showed that eosinophils could kill IgE coated parasites,[277] although an effect of the eosinophil CR3 receptor was also noted.[269] The killing of IgE-coated schistosomula took place in much the same way as IgG-dependent killing.[277] Rat eosinophils were also shown to have IgE receptors, and to be able to kill IgE-coated schistosomula.[268]

This was confirmed in studies from Japan in 1985, in which it was found that rat eosinophils bound to and killed dinitrophenol(DNP)-haptenated *S. japonicum* schistosomula when the parasites had been previously treated with a mouse IgE monoclonal anti-DNP antibody (B.53), but not when they had been pretreated with normal mouse serum. Eosinophils from the peritoneum of rats infected with *N. brasiliensis* were more adherent and toxic than normal, suggesting that they had an increased capacity to bind to IgE.[991, 992]

In 1977 it was first shown that human IgE-anti-IgE complexes could induce the release of EPO from human eosinophils *in vitro*.[1747] The effects of crosslinking the FcεR on human eosinophil secretion began to be studied by Capron and colleagues in 1985. They showed that the attachment of specific antigens to IgE antibodies in the FcεR2 receptor on human eosinophils induced the secretion of both EPO and MBP.[269] In the first of these experiments blood eosinophils were isolated from eight patients with filariasis and high serum IgE levels, and 10 patients with hypereosinophilia and normal IgE levels, and the quantity of EPO secreted in response to stimulation with anti-IgE, or specific filarial antigens was measured. Light density patients' eosinophils (but not normal density eosinophils) released large amounts of EPO, which was maximal one hour after incubation. As anti-IgG caused the release of equal amounts of EPO from normal and light density eosinophils, it was suggested that IgG-mediated secretion was independent of the cell density, whereas IgE effects were limited to the light density cells.[957] This was supported by their experiments in 1984 showing that light density eosinophils had a greater capacity to kill schistosomula of *S. mansoni* through an IgE-dependent mechanism.[277] IgE stimulation did not induce the release of ECP, and IgG stimulation had the reverse effect. This surprising observation has been confirmed, and it provides the first clear evidence that there may be differential control of eosinophil granule protein secretion.[957]

Complement receptors (CR1 and CR3) It was first shown in 1969 that guinea pig eosinophils could form rosettes with red cells coated with C3.[787] In 1976 we demonstrated the presence of complement receptors on human eosinophils using a similar technique.[1738] (See Plate 1) We also showed that human blood eosinophils did not have C3d (CR2) receptors, and that complement-receptor-dependent binding by blood eosinophils from patients with eosinophilia was greater than blood eosinophils from normals.[1696]

Human eosinophils possess C3b (CR1) and iC3b (CR3) receptors, which have been defined on other myelomonocytic cells. Binding to these receptors does not involve the cytoskeleton, unlike IgG Fc receptors, as attachment is not inhibited by cytochalasin B.[1740] Monoclonal antibodies to these two receptors bind to eosinophils, although eosinophils have half the number found on neutrophils.[1971, 566] The CR1 receptor is a polymorphic single chain glycoprotein of about 250 kDa, coded for by a gene with four alleles. Several stimuli increase the number of CR1 receptors on the plasma membrane, possibly by transferring them from intracellular site,[550] as our experiments suggested in 1980.[1740]

The adherence of neutrophils to surfaces depends on at least three plasma membrane glycoproteins, which share a common beta-subunit of 95 kDa, but distinct alpha-subunits of 150–180 kDa. These are the iC3b (CR3) receptor, the LFA-1 glycoprotein, and the p150,95 glycoprotein.

They are involved in cytoskeleton assembly following interaction with surfaces. Genetic defects in these proteins have been described, but it is not known if eosinophils were affected in these patients.[1147]

In 1977, Kay's group showed that the percentage of human eosinophils which formed rosettes with human-C3b-coated sheep erythrocytes was increased from 30 to 60 per cent by treatment with histamine or the two ECF-A tatrapeptides. No effect on IgG binding or on neutrophil-C3-binding was seen. Optimal conditions were at 10^{-4}M histamine, and following 80 minutes incubation.[45] It was suggested that this alteration could affect the functions of eosinophils. This effect of histamine was found to be H1-dependent.[46] In 1979, fMLP was also shown to increase eosinophil-C3b rosetting,[930] and both effects could be prevented with disodium cromoglycate.[934]

Eosinophil activating factors have the same effect: Mouse EDF increased the expression of the iC3b receptor in human eosinophils[1823] while supernatants from cultured human monocytes (mono-sup) increased the number of iC3b, but not C3b receptors on eosinophils.[1972] Several products of arachidonic metabolism increased the percentage of C3b receptors on blood eosinophils from four patients with eosinophilia. These were LTB4, 5-HETE, and 5 HPETE. LTC4 had no effect.[1257]

The binding of particles to the surface of eosinophils by the complement receptors CR1 and CR3 is a potent method for inducing them to secrete their granule contents *in vitro*. This has been confirmed by many groups, who used zymosan- or sepharose-C3b. See for example reference 1993. In 1977, a study using Sepharose particles showed a requirement for the alternative complement pathway components to be present, in order to produce the most effective stimulus for the secretion of arylsulphatase and β-glucuronidase.[1197]

Receptors for the anaphylatoxins C3a and C5a In 1977 it was found that peritoneal eosinophils from a 14-year-old boy with eosinophilic gastroenteritis responded to the chemotactic factor C5a,[975] suggesting that they also possessed receptors for C5a. In 1979, ^{125}I-labelled C3a and C5a were shown to bind to the surface of human eosinophils using autoradiography.[674] The C3a binding site was found to be of low affinity.[678]

Stimulation of eosinophil by C5a may also lead to the secretion of their granule contents. This was first suggested in 1986, when isolated human blood eosinophils were incubated with C5a, prepared by adding zymosan to serum. There was 60 per cent lysis of ^{51}Cr-labelled chicken red cells. As this was inhibited by catalase, sodium azide, and KCN, but not by superoxide dismutase, it was suggested that peroxidase and H_2O_2 rather than superoxide anions, were involved.[422]

Receptors for Clq Receptors for Clq were detected on normal human blood eosinophils in 1987, using radiolabelled Clq. Twice as many were found on eosinophils as on neutrophils. The binding of Clq took place through the collagen portion of the molecule. As Clq increased the cytotoxic capacity of eosinophils for schistosomula in the presence of small amounts of IgG antibody, it was suggested that the C1 receptor could have a role in the effector functions of eosinophil.[745]

4.3.2 *Steroid receptors*

In 1981, radiolabelled glucocorticoids were used to demonstrate that eosinophils have glucocorticoid receptors, and that the number of receptors per cell was similar on eosinophils and neutrophils.[1394] There have been many publications from Chile by the Tchernitchins and their colleagues on the interactions between oestrogens and eosinophils in the uterus of a number of species, including rats, guinea pigs, and man. Their work showed that rodent eosinophils can be stimulated by oestrogens to take part in the process of oestrus and implantation.[1763] In 1985, this group suggested that oestrogens could also induce rat eosinophils to degranulate in the blood and uterus.[1762] However, as experiments which were done in Seattle, USA in 1977 showed that radiolabelled oestradiol did not bind to human peritoneal eosinophils from a patient with eosinophilic gastroenteritis,[975] this work may not be applicable to man.

4.3.3 *Receptors for chemotactic factors*

In 1976 it was suggested that the ECF-A tetrapeptides bound to a specific receptor on human eosinophils,[194, 80] but this remains to be confirmed.

4.3.4 *Phospholipid-exchange protein*

A phospholipid exchange protein has been detected in human eosinophils. There were 199 units/5 × 10^6 eosinophils, compared to 7.5 units in the same number of neutrophils. It may transfer phospholipids or interact with phospholipids on other cells or organisms.[1917]

4.4 Membrane carbohydrates

Human blood eosinophils have a sialic-acid-rich-glycocalyx, which is reduced by incubation with neuraminidase.[1740] The plasma membrane of peritoneal eosinophils from rats also has a glycocalyx rich in carbohydrates, including concanavalin A binding sites, and acidic carbohydrates, as shown by ultrastructural cytochemistry.[1407] and by alterations in the electrophoretic migration of the cells after treatment with neuraminidase.[1406] There are no reports yet on whether human blood eosinophils possess the glycoproteins found on other blood cells, which have been defined by galactose-oxidase-tritiated borohydride labelling[37] and other methods. It is also not known whether human eosinophils can be agglutinated by wheat germ agglutinin, soybean lectin, or concanavalin A, as has been shown with guinea pig peritoneal eosinophils.[1413]

4.5 Eosinophil membrane antigens

Eosinophils, like neutrophils, do not have blood group antigens on their surface, although they express HLA antigens. In the mid 1970s a number of groups claimed to have raised rabbit antibodies which only bound to the surface of eosinophils. However, later work with monoclonal antibodies has shown that there are few qualitative differences in the membrane antigens expressed on eosinophils, compared to neutrophils.

4.5.1 *Polyclonal antibodies*

In the 1970s, Dr Adel Mahmoud and colleagues in Cleveland, USA, raised rabbit antibodies to murine and human eosinophils. Gleich and colleagues at the Mayo Clinic, raised rabbit antibodies to guinea pig eosinophils. These were used to 'ablate' eosinophils *in vivo*, with the hope that this would determine the function of eosinophils in parasitic and allergic diseases. Although a number of papers were published in this area showing some changes in resistance to parasitic infections (reviewed in reference 656), they were generally disappointing in their effects. The best results were seen with a combination of anti-basophil and anti-eosinophil sera in tick immunity in guinea pigs.[218] There has also been a suspicion that these rabbit antibodies to rodent eosinophils were not specific for eosinophils, although they caused a reduction in circulating and tissue eosinophils in experimental animals. Doubts have also been raised about whether the antibody to human eosinophils was eosinophil-specific.[124] No unique antigens have been detected on human eosinophils with mouse monoclonal antibodies.

Antibodies to mouse and guinea pig eosinophils A rabbit anti-mouse-eosinophil serum which did not bind to mouse neutrophils was described in 1973.[1141] It was used to study the role of eosinophils in resistance to *S. mansoni*,[1142] and *T. spiralis*.[722] In 1975, a rabbit antibody to guinea pig eosinophils was developed at the Mayo Clinic.[666] This was used to study the effects of depleting eosinophils in the blood and intestines on *Trichostrongylus colubriformis* infections,[668] and to study the immediate hypersensitivity reactions.[670] Neither anti-eosinophil serum, nor prednisolone reduced passive cutaneous or systemic anaphylaxis, but histamine release was reduced. This antiserum also reduced histamine replenishment in guinea pig skin after passive cutaneous anaphylaxis.[887]

Antibodies to human eosinophils Several rabbit antibodies which only bound to human eosinophils were reported in 1974 by Mahmoud and colleagues in Cleveland, USA. Sera from two rabbits immunized with blood eosinophils from a patient with schistosomiasis contained high titres of agglutinating and cytotoxic antibodies against human blood eosinophils. Absorption with red cells and white cells of different types was done to remove cross-reacting antibodies. Other antisera were produced against basophils, lymphocytes, and myeloblasts.[1136] Purified eosinophils from a patient with eosinophilia secondary to Hodgkin's disease, and a patient with eosinophilia in chronic granulocytic leukaemia, were purified and injected into rabbits. After absorption, these antibodies also appeared to be specific for eosinophils, causing agglutination and cytotoxicity.[1137]

4.5.2 *Monoclonal antibodies*

Monoclonal antibodies against eosinophil membrane constituents have been described by a number of groups. These fall into two broad categories: (a) antibodies which also bind to neutrophils, but not to other blood cells, lymphocytes, or platelets, and (b) antibodies which do not bind to neutrophils, but which also bind to platelets and some other cells. It should also be noted that there are antibodies to neutrophil plasma membrane antigens, which do not bind to eosinophils.[331] None of these antibodies are cell specific, e.g., only bind to one cell type. These antibodies are summarized in Fig. 4.2.

Antibodies which do not bind to neutrophils A monoclonal antibody (Eo-1) which binds eosinophils but not neutrophils was described in 1986 by Saito and colleagues, who raised it by immunizing a mouse with the eosinophil EoL cell line that they had developed. (See page 27). Eo-1 was shown to be a mouse IgG1 monoclonal antibody, which bound to the surface of 47 per cent of human blood eosinophils, dividing marrow eosinophils, 92 per cent of basophils, all platelets, and some lymphocytes, but not neutrophils. It recognized all cells of the pre-B cell lines NALM-1 and NALM-6 and (to a lesser extent) cells from other human haemopoietic cell lines. It bound to null ALL cells, and most pre-B-cell leukaemic cells, and cells of a basophilic leukaemia. In two patients with chronic myeloid leukaemia, a higher proportion than normal of blood and marrow eosinophils bound to the antibody. The antigen on platelets was a single chain polypeptide of 23 kDa, which was distinct from the Fcε receptor. A possible relationship was suggested between the antigen recognized by antibody Eo-1, and other 24 kDa antigens which are shared by platelets and pre-B-cells.[1539] In unpublished results by Tai, she has found that all light and normal density eosinophils from patients with HES bind this

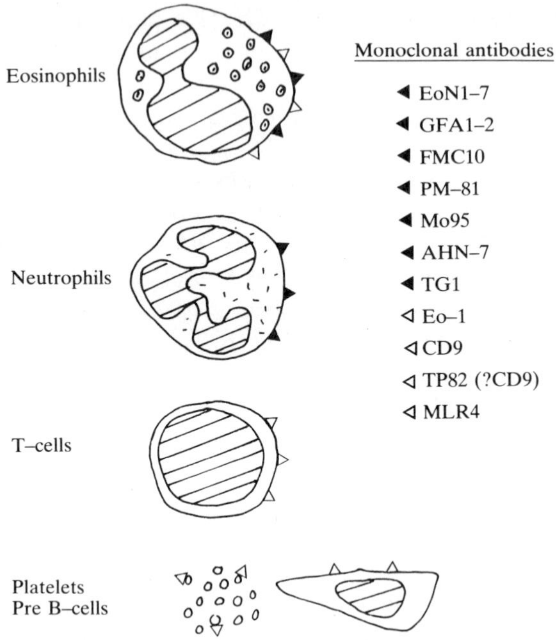

Fig. 4.2. Monoclonal antibodies to human eosinophil membrane antigens. Antibodies which bind to eosinophils and neutrophils, ▲, can be distinguished from antibodies which bind to eosinophils, T-cells, platelets, and pre-B-cells, △.

antibody, but there was greater uptake of labelled antibody by the HES light density cells.

A number of monoclonal antibodies have been described which recognize antigens on the surface of human leucocytes, and which are classified by international agreement as belonging to the cluster of differentiation 9 (CD9). Dr Jacqueline Breard has suggested that antibody Eo-1 may be of this type. We have tested 20 CD9 antibodies, and have confirmed this suggestion. Another closely related murine monoclonal antibody (TP82) which may also belong to the CD9 group was described in Tokyo in 1985. It binds to eosinophils and the platelet-C-ALL associated antigen p24.[1305]

The presence of shared membrane antigens on pre-B-cells, eosinophils, basophils, and platelets, is a feature which has been recognized

(a) in relation to Fcε binding;

(b) as a feature of the CD9 group of antibodies; and

(c) in relation to the capacity of IL-5 to stimulate eosinophil, pre-B-cell, and platelet production.

These associations, which may be accounted for by a common stem cell origin, may also point to a common set of membrane structures which are involved in the regulation of their maturation or their capacity to respond to haemopoietic stimulation.

Antibodies which also bind to neutrophils Dr Po-Chun Tai has been raising antibodies to membrane antigens on human blood eosinophils since 1981. It was hoped that some could be produced which would not bind to other haemopoietic cells. This assumption was based on the possibility that the earlier production of eosinophil-specific antibodies in rabbits would be applicable to the mouse. She screened her hybridomas with normal blood cells, and cloned those which (a) had strong reactivity with eosinophils, and (b) which failed to bind to one or more of the other blood leukocytes. However, over 100 of the anti-eosinophil antibodies which she developed also bound to blood neutrophils, although they stained less intensely than eosinophils. There was considerable variation in the percentages of blood eosinophils stained by her panel of antibodies. Alterations in the expression of these antigens were seen in patients with eosinophilia.

Tai immunized mice with isolated blood eosinophils from patients with HES. Six antibodies (EoN1-7) were finally selected. These also bound to blood neutrophils, eosinophil myelocytes, K562, and HL-60 cells. They differed in the proportions of normal and stimulated eosinophils which they stained. They bound to a higher proportion of intermediate and light density cells than to normal density eosinophils.[1734] These antibodies demonstrated that there is a marked capacity for eosinophils to alter their membrane constituents in disease, and several of them recognized antigens preferentially expressed on eosinophils during activation and degranulation.

Other reports have been published between 1981 and 1987 of monoclonal antibodies which are not CD9 antibodies or antibodies to the complement or immunoglobulin receptors, which bind to antigens in eosinophil and neutrophil plasma membranes. These include antibody FMC10;[2003] antibody PM-81,[107] which binds to a membrane glycolipid;[1132] antibody Mo95;[584, 1710] antibodies to granulocyte functional antigens GFA-1 and GFA-2 which binds to both human eosinophils and neutrophils, and stimulate the killing of schistosomula of *S. mansoni*;[1104, 1102] a mouse monoclonal antibody which binds to both bovine eosinophils and neutrophils;[1520] antibody AHN-7;[1640] and antibody TG1, which also binds to monocytes.[807]

Antibodies which also bind to T-lymphocytes In 1987, an abstract stated that 20 per cent of blood eosinophils from patients with eosinophilia formed rosettes with a monoclonal antibody (MLR4) which also bound to mixed lymphocyte-stimulated, but not mitogen-stimulated T-lymphocytes. This antigen was preferentially expressed on light density eosinophils, but was virtually absent from neutrophils.[417] We have unpublished work showing that a number of monoclonal antibodies against CD1–CD9 antigens expressed on human T-cells also bind to eosinophils.

4.6 Alterations in the eosinophil plasma membrane

The human eosinophil plasma membrane undergoes striking changes during development and following stimulation. This has been clearly shown in agar culture of mouse eosinophils, but it also occurs in cultured human eosinophils when the expression of Ia antigens is reduced, and they acquire additional C3b and Fc binding capacity.

Following activation, eosinophils also alter their membrane structures, as defined by monoclonal antibodies. For example, mouse EDF increased the expression of antigens GFA-1 and GFA-2 in human eosinophils.[1823] Stimulation of eosinophils with endotoxin and other stimuli which cause secretion of the lysosomal granule constituents, also alters the membrane, as they digest sialic-acid-rich components from membrane glycoproteins.[1740]

4.7 Antigen presentation by eosinophils

It has been suggested that eosinophils might be antigen-presenting cells. When antigens are injected into the footpad of rodents, they move rapidly to draining lymph nodes, and eosinophils are often found close these areas, initially in the cortex, and later in the medulla. However, there have been no formal attempts to show whether pure populations of eosinophils can present antigens to lymphocytes *in vitro*. This seems rather unlikely, in view of the occurrence of specialized antigen-presenting cells in the immune system.

5. Endocytosis, secretion, and motility

Eosinophils can ingest both small and large particles, and respond to a variety of stimuli by secreting their stored and newly formed constituents. This is under the control of a number of factors derived from adjacent cells in tissues (Fig. 5.1). Secretion in eosinophils appears to be finely regulated. These products of secretion can have a protective function, but they can also damage tissues, as I proposed in 1978.[1680]

5.1 Endocytosis

In vitro, normal blood eosinophils have only a quarter of the capacity of neutrophils to endocytose bacteria and other small particles, although they may be as effective as neutrophils when they have been purified from patients with hypereosinophilia. This was confirmed in 1987, when it was found that tissue eosinophils which were separated from colonic neoplasms by enzymatic dissociation and countercurrent centrifugation had a greater phagocytic capacity for *E. coli* than neutrophils or macrophages isolated at the same time. Sixty-seven per cent of mucosal eosinophils ingested a mean of 4.7 bacteria per cell.[146]

However, eosinophils, even when they have an impressive endocytic capacity, have a lower capability to kill staphylococci[229] and *E. coli*[426] than blood neutrophils. This was reviewed by Bass in 1982.[124] The ultrastructural events during eosinophil phagocytosis of mycoplasma[2009] and antibody-coated *Candida albicans*[848] have been described. Complement-coated particles, such as opsonized-zymosan and C3b-coated Sepharose particles can also induce a phagocytic response.

Surprisingly, the trypamastigotes of *T. cruzi* can be ingested by human eosinophils in serum-free medium, and killed.[962]

Most of the factors which induce endocytosis by eosinophils, such as complexes containing C3b, are similar to those involved in neutrophil phagocytosis. There is some confusion about the capacity of eosinophils to ingest IgE-coated particles. In 1974, it was found that immune complexes containing IgE were taken up to a greater extent by eosinophils than complexes containing IgM, IgG, or IgA,[849] athough in 1978 it was reported that IgG-coated latex beads were phagocytosed by eosinophils more

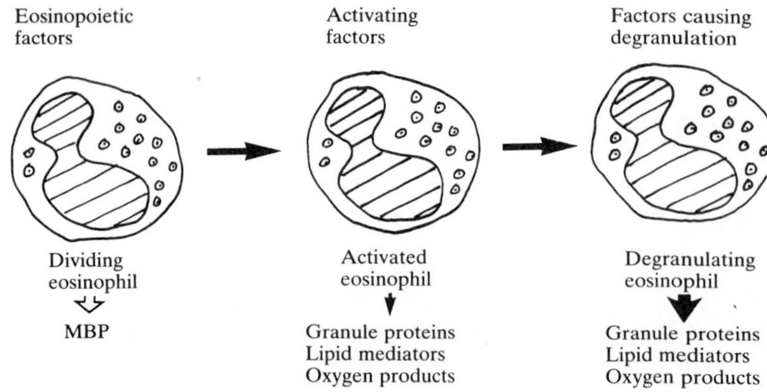

Fig. 5.1. Development of eosinophils, leading to their activation and degranulation. At each stage, eosinophils secrete some of their constituents. In the bone marrow, this occurs after they are synthesized, and possibly in response to CSFs. When non-dividing eosinophils are stimulated with activating factors, they secrete some granules and constituents, and become metabolically active, so that immunological signals can induce them to degranulate, and to synthesize and release newly-formed mediators.

effectively than IgE-coated beads, and blood eosinophils from ragweed sensitive patients had a lower phagocytic capacity than normal eosinophils.[723]

In 1975, rat peritoneal eosinophils were shown to have a marked capacity to carry out microendocytosis, as colloidal gold particles were taken up in large amounts.[996]

5.2 Secretion

In 1879, Paul Ehrlich suggested that eosinophil granules were storage depots of materials that were secreted into the environment as needed.[801] Kanthack and Hardy were the first to demonstrate this directly in 1895 in their studies on frog leukocytes.[907] They found that when anthrax bacilli were introduced into the dorsal lymph sac of the frog, eosinophils came in contact with the bacilli but did not ingest them. While they were attached together, eosinophils began to discharge their granules, so that after a time, their cytoplasm became relatively homogeneous, lacking granules.

In the 1960s, work on horse,[56] rat,[58] and guinea pig eosinophils[362] suggested that an important property of eosinophils was to mobilize and secrete their granule proteins into endocytic vacuoles like macrophages and neutrophils. However, this rarely happens with human eosinophils, which more commonly secrete their constituents to the outside of the cell.

Eosinophils in tissues rarely contain endocytozed particles, even in areas where other phagocytic cells have ingested large amounts of material. Until the mid-1970s, the only evidence for human eosinophil secretion came from electronmicrographs of the bone marrow or tissues from patients with a variety of eosinophilic disorders. These showed that their crystalline granules become disrupted with an altered electron density, as described by Kelenyi in 1968.[947] The factors which induce eosinophil secretion, the nature of the products which are secreted, and their effects on cells and tissues have become subjects of great interest, as they seem to provide the key to understanding the roles of eosinophils in disease.

A wide range of stimuli can induce human blood eosinophil secretion *in vitro*, but few of them induce eosinophils to release more than about 30 per cent of their stored granule components. This may be because multiple stimuli are required for eosinophils to respond effectively. This possibility is supported by the finding that pairs of monoclonal antibodies to eosinophil membrane antigens were more effective than individual antibodies in inducing secretion of ECP.[1735] Neutrophils also have a low capacity to secrete their azurophil granule contents in response to stimulation *in vitro*.[1147]

Activated eosinophils secrete more of their granule components than normal eosinophils, but no *in vitro* experiment has yet induced eosinophil to lose virtually all their granule proteins, as can be seen in blood eosinophils from some patients with HES. See also page 35.

Evidence is now being produced which supports the idea that there is control of eosinophil secretion of a far greater complexity than was originally thought. This control may extend to the selective release of individual components from the granules, with or without the generation of newly-formed products. In one study, complexed IgG induced the secretion of ECP, but not EPO, whereas complexed IgE induced the secretion of EPO, but not ECP.[957] Peterson and colleagues have also found that a synthetic glyceride (IpOCOC9) induced eosinophils to release 60 per cent of the stored ECP, but only 10 per cent of EDN/EPX, and 3–5.5 per cent of EPO after one hour incubation.[1395] If differential secretion does occur *in vivo*, this might explain why eosinophil granule proteins can be found in several different types of inflammatory response: either in chronic necrotic lesions, such as endomyocardial necrosis, or in acute inflammatory responses where necrosis does not occur, such as urticaria, where they may have reversible effects. See Fig. 5.2

5.2.1 *Secretory capacity in vitro*

The capacity of eosinophils to secrete their granule proteins in response to a variety of stimuli has been studied in many different laboratories. In 1981, the interaction of eosinophils with staphylococci was studied by

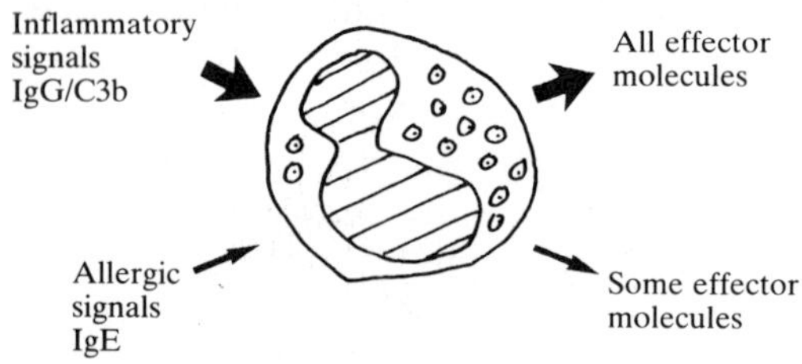

Fig. 5.2. Differential secretion by eosinophils. The 'strength' or the type of immunological stimuli applied to eosinophils, affects the type of molecules secreted. Inflammatory signals appear to cause the secretion of each of the main effector molecules, whereas IgE stimulation may only cause the secretion of some of these.

interference contrast microscopy. The granules marginated and were discharged.[1610] In the majority of studies on eosinophil secretion, the cells have been stimulated with either

(a) soluble stimuli, such as PMA, complement activation products, immune complexes, and sepharose-C3b;

(b) phagocytic stimuli, such as zymosan-C3b; or

(c) large, non-phagocytosable surfaces such as sepharose-C3b, or agar layers on glass, coated with complexes.[650]

Generally, about 15 per cent of each stored constituent is released within 40 minutes,[1942] although occasional reports have shown higher release. One reason for the low recovery of secreted proteins is that some of the secreted basic proteins may remain membrane-bound, or attached to adjacent surfaces. This may be an important mechanism for localizing and limiting the effects of these eosinophil secretion products *in vivo*. In 1987, a study was published on the capacity of purified normal blood eosinophils to secrete β-glucuronidase and arylsulfatase. Less than 9 per cent of the β-glucuronidase, and less than 20 per cent of the arylsulfatase were released under optimal, non-lytic conditions.[1969]

5.2.2 *Mechanisms of secretion*

It is important to know how stored eosinophil granule components are solubilized and exported to the outside of the cell. There are several possibilities. Granule-containing vacuoles may form and burst open on the outside of the cell, but this is less common with human than rodent eosinophils. The absence in most degranulating eosinophils, of tubules linking the granules to the outside of the cell, suggests that storage constituents are most commonly solubilized within the granule, transported through the cytoplasm as individual molecules, or via the endoplasmic reticulum, to be secreted at the cell surface. The energy required for this may be generated during the rapid respiratory burst that occurs when eosinophil are stimulated.

The routes taken by peroxidase from the storage granules to the outside of human eosinophils was studied by electronmicroscopy in nasal eosinophils and blood eosinophils stimulated in culture, in 1984. The calcium ionophore A23187 was used to stimulate these eosinophils to degranulate. This produced granule lysis, and the secretion of eosinophil peroxidase, which was dose-dependent. It required the presence of calcium in the incubation medium, and it was inhibited by pretreatment with the calcium antagonist TMB-8. Electronmicrographs of the stimulated eosinophils suggested that peroxidase secretion occurred (a) through the dilated endoplasmic reticulum and perinuclear space, and (b) by endoplasmic diffusion, and transudation through the cell membrane.[1540] It was suggested that these routes would enable the cell to protect itself from the toxic effects of peroxidase and other cationic granule constituents which may be secreted in the same way.[1310]

The ways in which the crystal of MBP is solubilized, and the processes which enable molar concentrations of highly insoluble cationic proteins to be brought to the cell surface, are important topics for future research. A configurational change in these molecules is likely to be involved, perhaps brought about by limited proteolysis, or digestion, altering the 3-dimensional structure of these proteins, so that hydrophobic residues are internalized, and other sites are exposed which enable these proteins to be transported through the cytoplasm. If this is the case, then a search for 'transport' molecules might be worthwhile. (Could MBP itself act as a transport protein for the other basic proteins?) Secretory processes are also potential sites of action for drugs which could affect eosinophil functions. Steroids, which are the most effective inhibitors of eosinophil secretion, may act in this way, although this has yet to be determined.

At least three steps are involved in secretion. In the first, cell stimulation leads to an alteration in the granules which begin to take up water, and form the characteristic vacuoles, which are refractile circular bodies seen in blood smears, but not in tissue sections. In the second step, the granule components are solubilized. Certain stimuli such as concanavalin A (con A), induce the granules to become solubilized, but they are not secreted.[1942] However, complement-coated particles, complexed immunoglobulins, and other stimuli such as the calcium ionophore A23187 cause the third stage to occur: the export of the proteins from the cell.

In 1983, Henderson and colleagues in Seattle, USA used A23187 to study the ultrastructural changes in secreting horse blood eosinophils. They showed that the granules moved to the cell periphery and fused with each other. Electron-dense granule material was released into large intracellular vacuoles, which opened to the outside of the cell through surface pores, and peroxidase was released. These events appeared to depend on calcium-dependent activation of phospholipase A2 and the generation of lipoxygenase products.[777]

In 1985, the same group reported that after incubation of human blood eosinophils with 10 μg/ml calcium ionophore A23187, there was an alteration in the structure of their granules within one minute. In the matrix of some of the granules, many vesicles were seen with loss of the electron dense crystalline core. Fusion of adjacent granules, and occasionally fusion of intact granules with the plasma membrane was noted, with probable secretion of whole granule contents to the outside. Large intracellular channels were found. These effects were most marked at 20 minutes, when many small granules were noted in the region of Golgi apparatus. Although the number of granules decreased and the size distribution of the granules was lowered, it was suggested that exocytosis of mature granules could be accompanied by the formation of new cytoplasmic granules.[776] This work contrasts with a separate study reported in 1985 from the Mayo Clinic, which showed that A23187 only induced the release of MBP from blood eosinophils by a cytolytic process.[610]

The time course of ECP solubilization from stimulated human blood eosinophils may take several hours. Kierszenbaum and colleagues incubated purified normal human blood eosinophils with *T. cruzi* amastigotes; the ultrastructural appearances of the phagocytozed parasites, and the changes in the granule correlated with the progressive increase in granule staining with monoclonal antibody EG2, which binds to the secreted form of ECP and EDN/EPX. Although no antibody or complement was present in the cultures, eosinophils ingested the amastigotes within 20 minutes, but the secreted form of ECP and EDN/EPX only began to appear in the granules at four hours, and in the phagosomes at five hours.[962] Experiments were not done with antibody or complement, which might have speeded up this process. Winqvist and colleagues have shown that Sephadex-C3b induced normal human blood eosinophils to begin to release ECP at 10 minutes,[1942] whereas unpublished experiments of Dr Po-Chun Tai have shown that IgG complexes only begin to stimulate release after two hours' incubation. The reasons for this are unknown, but may reflect the need for eosinophils to increase their membrane receptor density, or metabolism before they can respond to stimulation by several types of stimuli. Divalent cations are known to be involved in secretory events in most cells, and secretion does not occur in the presence of EDTA. Both calcium and magnesium are involved in the secretion of ECP from human eosinophils.[1945] Some secretagogues can alter the calcium content of eosinophils: fMLP (but not PMA) increased the eosinophil calcium content, as assessed with Fura2.[1419]

Experiments are now being done to see whether protein kinase C, and/or phospholipase C are involved. This possibility has some support from experiments in which certain triacylglycerides caused blood eosinophils to secrete 30–50 per cent of their ECP: more than was induced with opsonized particles.[1847] Preliminary experiments using supernatants from cultured monocytes which contain eosinophil activating factors have also suggested that these factors may induce the translocation of protein kinase C from the cytoplasm to the plasma membrane of eosinophils, priming the cell for subsequent stimulation.[1972]

5.2.3 *Drugs affecting secretion*

Steroids are amongst the most potent inhibitors of eosinophil secretion *in vitro*. In the first report of this effect in 1984, blood eosinophils from normal people and patients with eosinophilia, were stimulated with complement-coated Sephadex beads. This led to the secretion of 15 per cent of the ECP by 40 minutes, which was reduced by preincubating the eosinophils with 10^{-5}M hydrocortisone for 30 minutes.[1942]

Work has been carried out by Dr Harry Smith and colleagues at Beecham's Group Research, Epsom, UK into the potential use of a wide variety of drugs to inhibit eosinophil secretion, eosinophil accumulation in tissues, and eosinophil antibody-dependent cytotoxicity against a number of target cells.[356] Most of this work has been done with rodent eosinophils. The principal findings were that many steroids, a few membrane-active drugs, (which included some drugs with local anaesthetic activity, adenosine receptor antagonists, and histamine beta blockers), and a number of anti-allergic compounds were effective in these different assays. They included betamethasone, hydrocortisone, dexamethasone, propranolol, chlorpromazine, ketotifen, isoprenaline,[1670] chloradenosine, and dapsone. Sodium cromoglycate, nedocromil, and related drugs can also inhibit human eosinophil secretion *in vitro*.

Suramin may stabilize the granules of human eosinophils in patients with filariasis, reducing the proportion which are vaculolated, and degranulated.[1275]

5.3 Motility

Eosinophils, like other bone marrow-derived cells, are produced in one part of the body and function in another. For this reason they possess mechanisms which enable them to respond to signals, which induce them to leave the bone marrow, travel through the blood, attach to vascular endothelium, and emigrate into inflammatory lesions. At the end of the last century, the classical studies of Metchnikoff on inflammation in lower marine organisms imprinted the idea of chemotaxis into the minds of those interested in the mechanisms leading to the accumulation of cells in tissues. Ehrlich himself used the term 'chemotaxis' to describe this process. However, chemotaxis has not been shown to occur *in vivo* in vertebrates, and granulocytes move randomly in inflamed tissues. There is no work to show that concentration gradients are formed *in vivo*, of the kinds that are set up in chemotactic assays *in vitro*. Inflammatory cells move out of blood vessels in the same direction as the flow of freshly filtered interstitial fluids, which would flush away any chemotactic molecules as they were formed in inflamed tissues.

Those who work on chemotaxis have rarely assessed the biological effects of their reagents *in vivo*, and when they have done so, they have been largely unsuccessful in inducing cell accumulation without first damaging tissues to stimulate the normal processes which lead to cell localization. Despite these criticisms, a large, self-fulfilling literature has been built up around the concept of chemotaxis, some of which has come from respected laboratories. This has given the field a respectability which it does not deserve. Few workers have attempted to distinguish between directional migration (chemotaxis), and alterations in the rate of movement (chemokinesis).

There is an extensive literature on the capacity of isolated human blood eosinophils to show directional motility *in vitro* in response to a variety of stimuli. The main impetus for this work has been to account for the tissue localization of eosinophils *in vivo*, although few experiments have been done to assess this directly. Skin window studies in the rabbit, which were carried out to study the localization of monocytes and neutrophils, showed that directional movement after migration into injured tissues did not occur, and that accumulation of inflammatory cells was the result of the retention of cells in the lesion, and not directional migration towards it. It would be interesting to repeat these experiments with eosinophil, but there is no reason to suspect that they would be any different. The key events in the localization of blood-borne cells in tissues are margination and attachment to endothelial cells. Marginated cells migrate between endothelial cells and are retained in lesions, which they encounter during their random migration into the tissues. In any case, eosinophils probably do not travel very far in tissues once they have crossed the vessel wall. Surprisingly, no work has been carried out to see whether chemotactic factors induce eosinophil margination, and attachment to endothelium, as this would seem to be the most effective way for them to induce eosinophil to localize in tissues.

The main reason why so many studies have been done on eosinophil chemotaxis is that they are easy to perform, provide statistically significant results, and provide some insight into the kinds of stimuli which can affect eosinophil properties, in this case directional migration. It is unfortunate that these studies have not been extended to see how far other properties of eosinophils, such as activation, secretion, and cytotoxic capacity, are affected.

5.3.1 *Localization of eosinophilis in* vivo

As the uptake of eosinophils into diseased tissues can be very marked, a number of groups have attempted to reproduce this effect by isolating components of the response, and injecting them into the skin. For example, guinea pig IgGl (which is the anaphylactic antibody in this species) induced eosinophil accumulation in skin injection sites 12 to 24 hours after local passive anaphylaxis had been induced.[924] This type of experiment was done because it was hoped that there might be unique factors in these lesions which would cause eosinophils to accumulate. Differences in the number of eosinophils present in stimulated and control tissue sites have been reported with a wide range of substances, ranging from parasite extracts, to concanavalin A,[376] and individual components of the immune response.

Unfortunately much larger amounts of these substances have to be given than would be produced in disease, and the findings have often shown differences from the results of *in vitro* chemotactic experiments. For example:

1. PAF-acether is a potent chemotactic factor for eosinophils *in vitro*, but it does not induce eosinophil accumulation in normal human skin,[51] although it may do so in patients with atopy.[784]

2. 1 μg of LTB4, which has a weaker capacity to induce eosinophil chemotaxis than PAF-acether,[1626] does not cause significant eosinophil infiltration into the guinea pig eye after topical application, whereas 0.1 μg LTE4 and LTD4 induced an eosinophil infiltrate in the conjunctival epithelium.[1667]

However, as there are many technical difficulties in interpreting the results of injecting substances, other methods have been used, including topical application to the eye, the skin window technique,[500] and migration into peritoneal chambers and other implanted fluid-filled, cell-permeable vessels. Unfortunately, these experiments have provided little insight into the ways in which eosinophils localize in tissues, and the relative 'potency' of putative localizing substances is still disputed.

As outlined above, I think that future work on the localization of

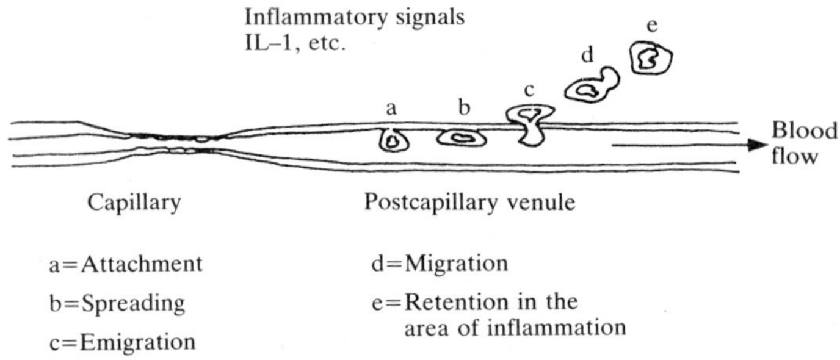

Fig. 5.3. Stages in the emigration of eosinophils from post-capillary venules into inflammatory lesions. Each of the stages 'a' to 'e' may be regulated separately. The first steps are probably the most important in determining the extent of eosinophil localization in tissues.

eosinophil in tissues is likely to be more fruitful if it is concerned with one or more families of molecules on the surface of endothelial cells and blood eosinophils. These molecules are now known to be involved in the initial attachment of leukocytes to endothelium in lymph nodes and areas of inflammation, and to be increased in response to inflammatory signals. A summary of this interesting potential area for future work is shown in Fig. 5.3.

In 1987, a glycoprotein antigen was described on the surface of murine leukocytes (including eosinophils) which was recognized by monoclonal antibody MEL–14. This antibody blocked the attachment of neutrophils to vascular endothelium in mice, *in vitro* and *in vivo*,[1063] but it was not tested on eosinophil attachment. Clearly it is important to know whether these antigens are induced to appear on post-capillary venules in areas of inflammation, as has been described in a large number of *in vitro* studies.[361, 1426, 165]

Four patients with ragweed sensitivity were induced to form blisters on their arms, by applying ragweed extracts. The blister fluid was removed, and after it was shown not to contain ragweed antigens, it was injected into other skin sites. Eosinophils were found in skin biopsies from challenged sites as early as 30 minutes after injection. Ragweed antigen itself took two to four hours to induce a significant blistering.[1784]

5.3.2 *Eosinophil motility* in vitro

The most widely used method for assaying eosinophil motility *in vitro* has been to use the Boyden chamber or its variants. Most work has measured chemotaxis, although chemokinesis is more likely to be relevant *in vivo* (where inflammatory cell movement is random), as cells which migrate the furthest are most likely to reach areas of inflammation.

Eosinophil chemotactic factors Over 180 papers (of very variable quality, and often with conflicting results) have been published on 'eosinophil chemotactic factors' since 1977. For this reason it is difficult to provide an overview of this work, although it seems that many of the substances secreted by eosinophils appear to be chemotactic for eosinophils themselves (LTC4, PAF-acether etc), and that a range of products from mast cells, parasites at different stages in their life cycles, T-lymphocytes, and tumour cells, besides complement components and many other stimuli, can induce eosinophil chemotaxis *in vitro*.

The difficulty in relating this work to *in vivo* events is borne out by the finding that eosinophils of different density have different chemotactic capacity, and that eosinophils can be 'deactivated' by prior incubation with many of these factors. This makes it difficult to know how to obtain 'normal' eosinophils for studies on eosinophil chemotaxis. It is also puzzling that stimuli which may have 'deactivated' eosinophils in the blood could then cause them to localize in tissues.

A large amount of research on eosinophils has been based on the hypothesis that stimulated mast cells release factors which attract eosinophils into tissues. In 1971 a search for this activity led to the description of an eosinophil-chemotactic factor of anaphylaxis (ECF-A).[933] Several molecules of varying size are now known to be included under this general term. In 1975, two of these were shown to be the tetrapeptides Val-Gly-Ser-Glu and Ala-Gly-Ser-Glu.[680] It was thought that these tetrapeptides and an intermediate weight ECF might attract eosinophils to sites of mast cell degranulation, where eosinophils would be retained by a process of 'deactivation'.[80] The properties of ECF-A were reviewed in 1977.[681]

It then became clear that these tetrapeptides had no significant biological effects on eosinophils *in vivo*.[225] Surprisingly, no critique has been published by the groups involved, or others. Later work to find other biologically active molecules which might have accounted for the earlier finding with 'ECF-A' has also been unsuccessful. It would be interesting to trace the origins and development of this concept, which dominated the work of several laboratories working on eosinophils in the 1970s. Its perceived importance at the time can be judged from the fact that so many papers were produced on the topic, that a separate heading of 'chemotactic factors, eosinophil' was created in 1980 in the Medline databases, and that ECF-A found its way into the eosinophil section of most textbooks.

There is an equally difficult series of papers to review on the effects of histamine on human blood eosinophils. Initially, histamine was found to be chemotactic and chemokinetic, and to interfere with the effects of ECF-A on eosinophil chemotaxis. Then it was suggested, on the basis of histamine-blocking experiments, that eosinophils had H1, H2, and a third type of receptor, each of which induced a different effect on eosinophil chemotaxis.[329] In 1982, further work using histamine and specific inhibitors was thought to show that eosinophils had H1 receptors for eosinophil-mediated cytotoxicity, and superoxide production,[1416] but not for chemotaxis or chemokinesis. However, in 1987, *in vivo* experiments showed that histamine was not involved in eosinophil localization, as injections of histamine into the normal skin of man and other primates did not give rise to an increased number of eosinophils in the test sites.[529] Some aspects of this confusing area were reviewed in 1982.[88]

There is often a close relationship between the development of a delayed hypersensitivity reaction and the presence of eosinophil-rich lesions in tissues. For example, studies done in 1963 on guinea pigs which had developed delayed hypersensitivity reactions to injected proteins, showed a striking accumulation of eosinophils in the sites where they were reinjected with heat-killed tubercle bacilli. Eosinophil infiltration began two hours after reinjection, and was maximal at six to eight hours. At four to eight hours the eosinophil was the most prominent cell, even though blood eosinophil counts were still normal.[66] Although *in vivo* studies could have been carried out, most subsequent work in this area centred on chemotaxis.

A T-lymphocyte chemotactic factor for eosinophils was first demonstrated in 1973 by Colley. In this study, lymphocytes from mice with schistosomiasis were found to produce a factor (eosinophil stimulation promotor, ESP) after stimulation with soluble schistosome egg antigens, which increased the migration of eosinophils from an agarose droplet.[342] In 1976–7, Colley's group defined the conditions for producing it,[343] and assayed its size as 25–31 kDa.[1067] A related factor from human lymphocytes was described by Parish in 1982.[1358] An unusual eosinophil chemotactic factor (ECF) was described in 1973 which was produced when a guinea pig lymphocyte-derived factor (ECFp) was incubated with immune complexes. It was thought to play some role in cellular immune processes.[1789] In 1987 another 15–20 kDa lymphokine was detected in supernatants from primed mouse spleen cells stimulated with *S. japonicum* soluble egg antigen. This factor increased the eosinophil chemotactic response to *S. japonicum* egg-derived eosinophil chemotactic factor.[1348]

A large number of eosinophil chemoattractants have been found in parasites which can infect man and animals. Some of these have been purified and partially characterized. Much of this work has been done in Japan and has used guinea pig eosinophils. Unfortunately there are no comparative studies on these factors or their properties. See for example, studies on a factor in extracts of *S. japonicum* eggs.[812] PAF-acether 10^{-6} to 10^{-9}M is both chemokinetic and chemotactic for human blood eosinophils of normal density, but affects neutrophils to the same extent. At these concentrations, LTB4, histamine, and the alanyl and valyl tetrapeptides had negligible effects on the movement of eosinophils.[1751, 1876]

There are conflicting reports about the chemotactic activity of PAF-acether on eosinophils of different density. In one study, PAF-acether at 10^{-5} to 10^{-8}M caused directional movement, and chemokinesis of light density eosinophils more than normal density eosinophils, while lyso-PAF was ineffective.[1877] In another study, the dense eosinophils were affected by concentrations of PAF-acether 100 times less than those which stimulated light density eosinophils.[1626]

LTB4, 5-HETE, and 5-HPETE were equally chemotactic to blood eosinophils from four patients with eosinophilia.[1257] Normal and light density eosinophils were both affected to the same extent by 30–100 nM LTB4.[1626] These findings suggest that eosinophils had receptors for LTB4 and analogues, although these have not yet been identified. However there is no evidence to suggest that LTB4 induces eosinophil localization *in vivo*. Injections or application of LTB4 in the skin of volunteers did not induce a significant eosinophil accumulation in two studies reported in 1986.[173, 1939]

Many different eosinophil chemotactic activities have been reported to come from neoplasms, by workers in the USA, UK, and Japan. The first of these was a 500 Da chemotactic peptide for eosinophils which was obtained in 1974 in Boston, USA, from a large cell carcinoma of the lung containing many eosinophils, in a patient who also had a blood eosinophilia.[1885] In 1978, the same group reported that serum from three patients with anaplastic carcinomas of the lung contained eosinophil chemotactic activity.[683] A factor was found in Hodgkin's diseases tissues in 1975.[931] In Japan, a factor was obtained from a squamous cell carcinoma in 1979,[1561] and a malignant cervical carcinoma in 1981.[841] In the USA in 1980, an acidic protein was isolated from a histiocytic lymphoma in the brain of a patient with eosinophilia of up to 8.0×10^9/l.[682] Large squamous cell cervical carcinomas were found to contain an eosinophil chemotactic factor, in Fukuoka, Japan in 1981.[841] In 1984, extracts of a large cell carcinoma of the lung in a Japanese patient were chemotactic for eosinophils,[986] and in 1986 a factor was derived from a malignant fibrous histiocytoma.[853]

C5a shows strong chemotactic activity for human eosinophils. This factor can be generated by many different surfaces and antigen-antibody reactions, via the classical and alternative pathways. Neutral proteases from human eosinophil granules can cleave C5 directly to produce an eosinophil chemotactic activity.[1299] Chemotactic factors for eosinophils have been produced from alveolar macrophages stimulated with anti-IgE or the corresponding allergen in patients with allergic asthma. This was described in 1984.[701] In 1987, histamine-stimulated blood mononuclear cells were shown to produce a number of factors of 2.5 and 13–25 kDa, which were also chemotactic for eosinophils.[1454]

In 1982, three eosinophil chemotactic activities were found in the serum of patients with idiopathic cold urticaria, in whom angioedema had been induced by immersion in ice water for three minutes.[1883] An eosinophil chemotactic activity was also detected in the sera of patients with eosinophilic fasciitis.[1886] In 1987 a heat-labile eosinophil chemotactic factor was described in the sera of patients with asthma, and the levels rose after antigen exposure.[1468]

A wide variety of skin lesions have been found to contain chemotactic factors for eosinophils. A low molecular weight factor was found in the skin of patients with bullous pemphigoid, atopic eczema, drug reactions, and contact sensitivity.[450]

6. Eosinophil activation, cytotoxicity, and interactions

Some of the most important discoveries about eosinophils in the period 1980–88 have been:

(1) that they are effector cells in inflammatory reactions, able to kill certain parasites and cells, and to secrete a range of biologically important molecules;

(2) and that their capacity to carry out these functions is only fully developed after they have been activated.

Many of the earlier misconceptions about the roles of eosinophils in disease have stemmed from a failure to appreciate the importance of these activation mechanisms. The range of diseases in which eosinophils may be involved in tissue injury is also under investigation. See Fig. 6.1.

6.1 Activation

A number of methods have been used to show whether eosinophils have been activated or not. They include antibody-dependent killing of schistosomula, LTC4 production, secretion of granule proteins, oxygen metabolism, etc. These assays have reflected the interests of the laboratories concerned, and there has been no attempt to see whether one type of assay is more sensitive than another, and whether all of these activities run in parallel. Activation may be a quantitative difference in effector function, rather than a qualitative difference in some aspect of the cell's ability to recognize and interact with environmental signals. This means that no single assay would be able to tell whether a cell was activated or not: it would simply demonstrate the extent to which a population of cells had become activated.

The development of a monoclonal antibody (EG2) which only binds to the secreted form of ECP and EDN/EPX has the particular advantage that it can be used to demonstrate individual activated cells. (See Plates 3, 4, 6 and 12)

There is no information about whether activation is reversible, or

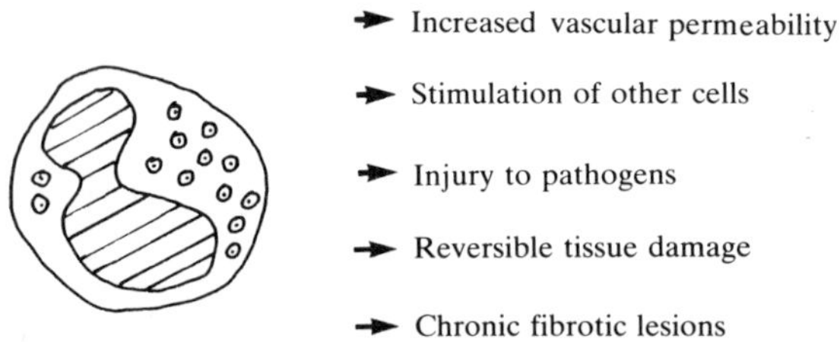

Fig. 6.1. The range of effector functions of eosinophils: an overview of the major areas in which eosinophils are believed to be involved in inflammation.

whether the various activating factors influence some or all of the effector functions of eosinophils.

So far, no unique functions of activated eosinophils have been detected which cannot be carried out by a larger number of non-activated eosinophils. If this proves to be generally true, then large numbers of nonactivated eosinophils should be able to carry out the functions of a smaller number of activated cells. It would be interesting to separate and study populations of eosinophils from the blood and tissues of patients, and to measure the amounts of each activating factor to which the cells had been exposed. This would show which of the many activating factors are important *in vivo*. This is of practical importance, as it could lead to the development of therapeutic methods for increasing or decreasing the effector functions of eosinophils in inflammatory reactions. These drugs would be of great benefit in the treatment of diseases in which eosinophils have protective, or harmful effects.

6.1.1 In vivo *studies*

In 1976, we showed that blood eosinophils from patients with an eosinophilia had several structural differences in their plasma membranes and granules, and in their functions, compared to eosinophils in normal people. We concluded that: 'blood eosinophils in patients with an eosinophilia may be functionally mature, or altered in response to unknown stimuli while they are in the blood'.[1696] This was one of the first pieces of evidence that eosinophils could be activated in disease.

In the same year, James and Colley in Nashville, USA, were the first to show that eosinophils from infected animals had an increased cytotoxic capacity for parasites. They reported that peritoneal eosinophils from mice infected with *T. spiralis* were more effective than eosinophils from uninfected mice in killing *S. mansoni* eggs *in vitro*.[867] In 1978 this group showed that eosinophil-rich peritoneal exudate cells from *S. mansoni*-infected mice were able to kill 20 per cent of *S. mansoni* eggs *in vitro*, which did not occur with eosinophils from uninfected mice. The culture of soluble products from isolated liver granulomas induced normal mouse eosinophils to become toxic to these eggs.[868]

Work in the rat, published in 1987, had confirmed that peritoneal eosinophils vary in their metabolic and effector functions, depending on the types of stimuli which are used to induce them *in vivo*.[355]

In 1980, an increased cytotoxic capacity for blood eosinophils in patients with eosinophilia was first demonstrated by David and colleagues. This study was done on blood samples from 30 patients in Brazil with a variety of disorders including infections with *S. mansoni*. Their eosinophil counts ranged between 2.2 and 3.2×10^9/l. Blood eosinophils from patients with the highest blood eosinophil counts had the greatest capacity to kill schostosomula of *S. mansoni in vitro* after 40 hours of culture. The extent of eosinophil antibody-dependent adherence to the parasites was also increased at 2 hours.[396] They showed that blood eosinophils from patients with the highest egg counts had more Fcγ receptors, and were more effective in killing schistosomula *in vitro*, than eosinophils from patients with low egg counts, or normal individuals.[1822]

In 1980, experiments by Bass and colleagues on the *in vitro* properties of eosinophils showed that there were alterations in the density, surface charge, metabolism, and other properties of blood eosinophils from patients with eosinophilia, compared to normal blood eosinophils. They interpreted this as evidence that the cells had been 'stimulated or activated' *in vivo*.[127]

Tissue eosinophils may have a much greater capacity to take part in inflammatory reactions than was previously thought possible, because they are activated in tissues. This was suggested in a study published in 1987, using human eosinophils isolated from colonic neoplasms by enzymatic dissociation and countercurrent centrifugation, which gave 1.8×10^6 eosinophils/g mucosa. C3b receptors were found on 75 per cent of these cells, and Fcγ receptors on 90 per cent. These eosinophils had a greater phagocytic capacity for *E. coli* than neutrophils or macrophages isolated at the same time.[146]

6.1.2 *Eosinophil activating factors*

Studies on eosinophil activation have followed similar lines to those taken during the investigation of macrophage activation, in which a small number of assay systems have been used to define the relative potencies of a wide range of potential activating factors.[1627] However, little is known about what activation is, how it comes about, and why all eosinophils are not normally activated in tissues. Most of the factors which cause eosinophil secretion are also activating factors, although there are some exceptions. For example lipopolysaccharides and PMA do not activate eosinophils for

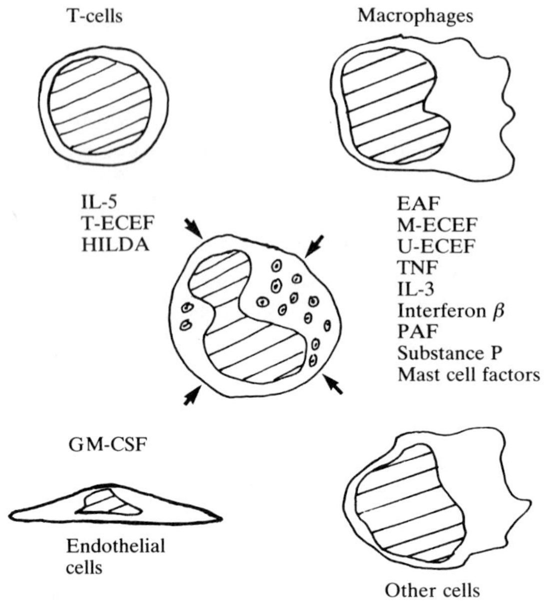

Fig. 6.2. Eosinophil activating factors. These are derived from adjacent cells in tissues. Several cell types produce each of these activating factors. The way in which they interact, and the importance of each one in different diseases has still to be determined.

antibody-dependent killing of schistosomula,[1779] although they are potent inducers of eosinophil secretion *in vitro*.

Endogenous factors Most of the molecules which are released from stimulated monocytes and lymphocytes, and which are loosely classified as cytokines, are able to augment several of the effector properties of human blood eosinophils. These factors were initially described in complex mixtures produced by stimulating T-cells or monocytes with different stimuli, or by culturing mononuclear cells without further stimulation. The availability of recombinant molecules, which have some of the properties of these impure preparations, is an important step forward. These have been used to show that eosinophils are receptive to most of the molecules which affect the properties of macrophages, and which stimulate lymphocytes to proliferate. Much of this area will become clearer as these different activating factors are cloned, and as techniques are developed for studying their occurrence, and relative importance *in vivo*, as well as *in vitro*. A summary of the principal eosinophil activating factors is shown in Fig. 6.2.

A highly purified 41 kDa glycoprotein interleukin (HILDA) released from a human alloreactive T-cell clone was chemotactic for mouse eosinophils in a tissue air sac, and induced blood eosinophils from four patients with HES to produce chemoluminescence, similar to that developed by PMA. It did not stimulate the growth and differentiation of eosinophil colonies from human bone marrow.[1239] Several features show that HILDA is distinct from EAF and EDF, although it has a similar molecular weight to EAF.

In Boston, USA, David, with Dessein, Silberstein, and other colleagues has worked for several years on the capacity of cultured human blood monocytes to generate factors which enhance the capacity of eosinophils to take part in cytotoxic and inflammatory reactions. These were initially called eosinophil cytotoxicity-enhancing activity (ECEA). This was distinguished from T-lymphocyte-derived factors, and called monocyte eosinophil cytotoxicity-enhancing factor (M-ECEF). Mononuclear cells from patients with chronic schistosomiasis in Brazil produced only 25 per cent of the amount of ECEA as matched controls, 84 per cent of whom produced ECEA.[443] It was thought possible that this defect occurred because these patients had altered immune responses to the parasite, which resulted in a failure of the mononuclear cells to produce ECEA.[442]

A principal effect of ECEA was shown to be an increase in the amount of eosinophil electron-dense material deposited onto the surface of schistosomula.[292] Dessein has summarized the work of the group which he subsequently set up in France, in a paper published in 1987.[510] In 1987, Silberstein and colleagues described the production of an ECEF by a human cell line (U937) with monocyte features, which was derived from a patient with a histiocytic lymphoma. This was produced after stimulation in serum-free medium with PMA for two days, and with LPS for a further two days. It had a subunit structure of about 9–10 kDa,[1627] and migrated in gels with apparent molecular weights of about 17 and 32 kDa, and isoelectric points 3.8–5.1. M-ECEF consisted of several components, including tumour necrosis factor (TNF) which accounts for part of its activity, and to which it may be related structurally.[1627] It was concluded that M-ECEF is one of several cytokines which enhance the toxicity of human blood eosinophils to schistosomula *in vitro*.[1628]

Butterworth, Thorne, and colleagues in Cambridge, UK have described an eosinophil activating factor (EAF) which is a 37 kDa protein, pI 4.4. It was partially purified from supernatants prepared by culturing unstimulated blood mononuclear cells from moderately eosinophilic people for 1–25 hours and from a cell line ESH 98. A smaller molecular weight activity was also produced, but this has yet to be characterized.[1779] Mononuclear cell supernatants from individuals with eosinophilia produced the most activity.[1845]

In 1986, EAF was shown to be distinct from TNF, ECEF, and GM-

CSF.[1779] EAF enchanced the capacity of human blood eosinophils to kill antibody-coated schistosomula, and cell line cells. It increased several properties of eosinophils: the expression of some membrane antigens; the adherence of eosinophils to schistosomula; degranulation; and the production of hydrogen peroxide, superoxide, and LTC4.[1780]

A similar eosinophil activating activity to EAF has been described in Amsterdam. This was detected in supernatants from cultured human monocytes (mono-sup), and increased the oxidative metabolism of human eosinophils in response to a variety of stimuli, except A23187.[1972]

Mast cells and basophils may produce factors which enhance the activities of eosinophils. This was suggested in a study in which stimulation of eosinophils with a F(ab')2 rabbit anti-human IgE increased their cytotoxic capacity against schistosomula, if there were human basophils also present in the cultures.[1234]

The discovery in 1982[444] that CSFs can also be activating factors raises the question of whether newly formed eosinophils are activated within the bone marrow, but lose this capacity when they enter the blood, or whether an additional tissue factor(s) is required for this final step in differentiation. These possibilities await measurements of eosinophil activation in different locations, and investigation of the possible role of the blood components in inhibiting (and reversing?) the activation process.

In 1986 it was reported that biosynthetic (recombinant) human T-lymphocyte GM-CSF enhanced eosinophil cytotoxicity toward schistosomula, and toward calcium ionophore A23187-induced generation of leukotriene C4 (LTC4). Augmentation of each eosinophil function by GM-CSF was time-and dose-dependent, which reached a plateau one hour after incubation, before stimulation with ionophore. There was an initial increase in intracellular levels of LTC4.[1629]

Colony stimulating factor α (CSF-α), derived from human placental conditioned medium, and which has identical activity to recombinant GM-CSF, was shown in 1982 to alter human blood eosinophils so that they adhered to antibody-coated schistosomula more rapidly *in vitro* by an irreversible binding machanism. This led to an increase in their capacity to kill the parasites at 24 hours.[444]

In 1987 it was reported that, after culture for up to two weeks in small quantities of recombinant human GM-CSF, normal human blood eosinophils became lighter in density, and had increased capacity to secrete LTC4, and to kill antibody-coated schistosomula.[1346] Both recombinant TNF and GM-CSF increased eosinophil antibody-dependent killing of schistosomula. Recombinant TNF was more potent than GM-CSF. The time course of activation by the two factors was different: eosinophils were maximally stimulated by GM-CSF at ten hours, whereas this was 30 hours using TNF.[1630] GM-CSF is produced by a number of cells, including endothelial cells, in response to stimulation with TNF,[1253] which is mainly produced by macrophages.

In 1987, mouse EDF (IL-5) was found to be an activating factor for human eosinophil antibody-dependent killing of some tumour cells, and phagocytosis of opsonized zymosan.[1823]

In the presence of bovine endothelial cells or their conditioned medium, cultured blood eosinophils developed an increased capacity to secrete LTC4 after stimulation with the calcium ionophore, and to kill antibody-coated schistosomula. In endothelial cell cultures, eosinophils of normal density also became lighter. It was suggested that endothelial cells could activate blood eosinophils during their passage into tissues.[1522] The molecules from endothelial cells which activate eosinophils may be both GM-CSF and G-CSF, as it has been found that human umbilical cord endothelial cells make both of these activating factors in response to stimulation with interleukin 1.[213] Substance P, which is released by sensory neurones in the lungs and gut and causes respiratory tract hyperreactivity, smooth muscle contraction, and urticaria, has been found to increase the expression of IgC and IgE receptors on isolated human blood eosinophils, and to increase their capacity to lyse rabbit-antibody-coated chicken red cells labelled with ^{51}Cr. This suggests that this undecapeptide may activate eosinophils and contribute to their effector roles in disease.[421] Eosinophils also contain substance P (Goetzl, E. J. 1988, personal communication).

PAF-acether, at concentrations of 10^{-7} to 10^{-9} M stimulated human blood eosinophils to kill complement- and antibody-coated schistosomula more than normal. It was 100 times more potent that histamine.[1236] Tumour necrosis factor can activate eosinophils for antibody-dependent killing of schistosomula. It has a lesser effect than GM-CSF, and unlike the 'all or nothing' effect of GM-CSF, it induces an increased cytotoxic response over a 10^4 concentration difference. These differences were thought to show that there are several different ways in which eosinophils respond to cytokines.[1627]

Interferon α did not activate human eosinophils in an antibody-dependent killing assay,[1779, 1627] although it increased the secretion of granule enzymes from eosinophils in response to zymosan-C3b stimulation.[1538] Injections of recombinant α-interferon into patients with solid tumours decreased the percentage of bone marrow cells that were eosinophils from 4.5 to 2.2 per cent.[524] β-Interferon enhanced the capacity of eosiniphils to lyse antibody-coated chicken red blood cells.[423]

IL-1 does not activate human eosinophils directly,[1779, 1627] but it has some effects on superoxide production and granule secretion in response to a number of stimuli.[1420] IL-2 does not activate human blood eosinophils.[1779] Cloned gibbon interleukin 3 (gIL-3) stimulated mature eosinophils to kill antibody-coated target cells, to produce superoxide anions, and to phagocytose opsonized yeast particles. It had more specificity as an activating factor than GM-CSF, as gIL-3 did not activate neutrophils.[1103]

Exogenous factors The possibility that schistosomula of *S. mansoni* produce activation factors for eosinophils was assessed in a study from Lille, France, in which secretion/excretion products from schistosomula were assessed for their capacity to induce rat and human eosinophil activation. These effects were compared with the capacity of ECF-A to induce activation of eosinophils from rats and man. The schistosome-released products (SRP) were of a larger molecular weight and different heat lability from ECF-A, and caused eosinophils to develop a greater cytotoxic capacity, more Fcγ receptor expression, and greater morphological changes after 4 hours incubation, than ECF-A. As SRP had less effect on human neutrophilis, it was proposed this could partly explain why eosinophils were more toxic for schistosomula than neutrophils, and how parasites themselves could influence the way in which inflammation developes in tissues.[78] It was later shown that rat eosinophil-dependent killing of schistosomula was enhanced by proteases released from schistosomes, and by collagenase. This suggested that the effect of SRP on rat and human eosinophil Fc receptors and antibody-dependent cytotoxicity involved eosinophil membrane structures which were changed by neutral proteases.[79]

Effects of activating factors on eosinophils Incubation of human blood eosinophils with EAF induced them to produce more lamellopodia, and their granules moved rapidly in phase-contrast preparations.[1778] A 25 kDa product from histamine-stimulated blood mononuclear cells also induced morphological changes in cultured blood eosinophils.[1454]

Activation signals can induce eosinophils to phosphorylate several proteins. This was seen when human blood eosinophils were cultured alone, or after stimulation with PMA, A23187, or opsonized zymosan. There was also dephosphorylation of a 21 kDa protein. Alterations in phosphorylation were not seen with fMLP. As each stimulus affected a different range of proteins of varying size, it was suggested that phosphorylation is not only an early event following cell activation, but that the proteins which are affected depend on the nature of the signal.[1473]

Cultures of partially purified mouse peritoneal eosinophils contained more lysophospholipase after incubation with mononuclear cells stimulated with parasite antigens to which they were sensitized, than control cultures. This suggested that mononuclear cell products can increase the amount of this enzyme synthesized by eosinophils. These findings also explain why higher levels of lysophospholipase are found in the tissues of parasitized mice than can be accounted for by the number of normal eosinophils.[20]

6.2 Cytotoxicity

It has been known for many years that eosinophils are less effective than neutrophils in killing bacteria. This is partly because less eosinophils ingest bacteria, and the number of bacteria ingested per cell is lower than for neutrophils. In addition it has been suggested that eosinophils have a less effective peroxidase-H_2O_2-halide killing system than neutrophils. The topic was reviewed by Bass in 1982.[124] The possibility that eosinophils might kill parasites was not seriously considered until the early 1970s, although there were earlier observations which might have suggested this. For example in 1968 it was shown that the ultrastructure of tissue eosinophils was altered by a parasitic infection, and it was shown that the central area of the granule had been affected. It was proposed then that the release of the central electron-opaque material could play some part in the reaction to the infestation. This work, by Casley-Smith in Australia, was done in rats infected with *Moniliformis dubius*.[285] He also compared this change in the crystalloid with changes in the matrix of eosinophil granules in patients with eosinophilia, which had been described in 1966 by Zucker-Franklin and her colleagues.[2009]

The capacity of eosinophils to kill the schistosomula of *S. mansoni in vitro*, which was discovered in 1975,[255] provided a major stimulus (and assay system) for the study of eosinophil-dependent cytotoxicity. Work in this area has led to the conclusion that eosinophils are major defensive cells in protection against certain helminthic and other parasitic infections. Some work on eosinophil-dependent killing of tumour cells *in vitro* has also shown their potential for protection in neoplastic diseases. This work has also raised the possibility that eosinophils could damage normal cells and tissues, and be responsible for several important clinical abnormalities, such as some forms of asthma, skin diseases, and endomyocardial fibrosis.

Most experiments in this field have been carried out using intact eosinophils, and targets coated with a molecule which can bind to one of the main receptors on eosinophils. In these experiments, several hundred eosinophils were required to kill each parasite, and the mechanism of killing was a three-step process in which the parasite was first recognized, then attached to, and finally killed by secretion products from the attached cells. Similar types of experiments have been carried out with mammalian cells coated with a variety of molecules which eosinophils can recognize. For example, in 1978 Sanderson and colleagues showed that August rat peritoneal eosinophils were able to cause the release of up to 30 per cent

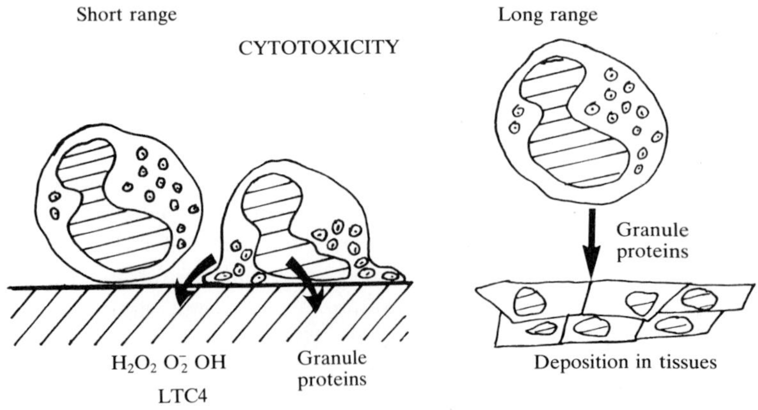

Fig. 6.3. Eosinophil-dependent cytotoxic mechanisms. These occur either at short range, with parasites, and at surfaces to which they have become attached, or at a distance, through the secretion of their granule proteins, which localize in sites of injury.

of the label from ^{51}Cr-labelled chicken red blood cells coated with rat antibody, after incubation in a 2.5:1 cell:target ratio for four hours. (This was less than the amount of ^{51}Cr released by neutrophils under the same conditions.) The ways in which eosinophils attached and partially ingested the labelled cells were different from neutrophil, as shown in a time-lapse film which they made.[1554]

Mammalian cells and tissues are probably killed in a different way. Normal cells and tissues are not coated with immunoglobulin or complement in the same way as invasive parasites, and in this case, the effects take place without a receptor-mediated attachment phase. In this model of eosinophil-dependent tissue injury, eosinophil products would be generated by soluble stimuli. Released products would attach to nearby structures and damage them. Long range interactions of secreted eosinophil products with cells and tissues could also occur. However, these are less likely in view of the basic properties of the eosinophil cationic proteins. See Fig. 6.3.

6.2.1 *Parasite killing*

During the past decade, the view that eosinophils provide a first line of defence against infection by a number of nematodes which induce the production of IgG and IgE antibodies, has gained wide acceptance. This was reviewed in 1984.[249] Antibodies coat certain stages in the tissue life cycle of the parasite, so that eosinophils can attach and degranulate onto their surface and kill them. Details of how this interaction takes place with schistosomula *in vitro* were published in 1979,[256] and 1980,[1819] and have provided the model system for this type of interaction.

One of the main effects of the attachment process was to cause the release of highly toxic cationic proteins onto the surface of the parasite. This has been studied by several groups using electronmicroscopy. Secreted EPO was found on the surface of the schistosomula,[1177] and *Angiostrongylus cantonensis* adults,[1983] and MBP on schistosomula,[257] and *Onchocerca volvulus* microfilariae.[951] However, the capacity of many parasites to alter their antigenic characteristics within a short time of invasion of the host, means that cell-mediated immunity can only act on certain stages in the parasite life cycle. A temporal and spatial association between eosinophilia and many parasites is often difficult to demonstrate in the early stages of an infection. Eosinophilia is usually more prominent in the later stages of the disease.[124] Even so, eosinophils do appear to have a role in limiting the number of invasive parasites which migrate to their final tissue locations. At the least, eosinophils provide a 'hostile' tissue environment for helminths, which are so common in man's environment.

Many nematodes may be able to resist or avoid eosinophil-dependent cytotoxicity, although there has been no formal study of the range of parasites which are susceptible to or resistant to this cytotoxic response. For example, the infective larvae of *Toxocara canis* were not killed *in vitro* by human blood eosinophils, even after they were activated *in vitro*. This was found to be due to the capacity of the larvae to shed their cuticles.[542]

Eosinophil-dependent killing may also act in tandem with other forms of cytotoxicity *in vivo*, but experiments to assess this *in vitro* are obviously more difficult to carry out. For example, an effect of EPO on the killing of *T. cruzi* epimastigotes by macrophages has been shown. Parasites are also susceptible to cytotoxic mechanisms when they lodge in sites where they are unable to develop further. For example, migrating larvae of *T. spiralis* are always killed in the heart, where they commonly localize in heavy infections. Eosinophils are a prominent component of this response.

In the case of parasites which produce eggs in their definitive tissue locations, eosinophils again may play an important role in host defence. In some instances this is beneficial, but the marked granulomatous response that can occur around ova in the gut, liver, and bladder wall can also be detrimental in the long term. The fibrotic reaction that occurs as a result of these granulomas may be partly due to products released during the tissue damage, or as a result of the release of fibrogenic molecules from inflammatory cells in these sites, including eosinophils. This possibility has still to be explored fully in the case of eosinophils, but the marked association of eosinophils with fibrotic reactions in many different tissues argues for their central role in this type of lesion.

Eosinophil killing of schistosomes Eosinophils may have a protective effect during penetration of the skin by schistosomula of *S. mansoni*. They may also kill migrating parasites in the lungs and other sites where the major depredation of migrating larvae is now known to take place. However, cultured schistosomula have the ability to alter their tegument, so that they no longer become susceptible to eosinophil-dependent killing mechanisms.[1287, 439] This protective change may also occur *in vivo*.

IgG antibody enables eosinophils to attach to the surface of the parasite. This is present in the serum of some patients with schistosomiasis. It has also been produced by immunizing animals with the haemocyanin glycoprotein from the keyhole limpet, giving some protection against infection.[726] Complement-mediated killing has also been reported using rat[1470] or human eosinophils.[48]

Most of the assays for eosinophil-dependent killing of schistosomula have been done using skin-penetrated parasites, although mechanically disrupted schistosomula have been used by some groups. Details of the techniques have been given in a number of the papers discussed below. The signs of parasite death are a reduction in motility, loss of their normal structure, and penetration of dyes such as methylene blue into the worm surface. Although ^{51}Cr release was used initially as an assay technique for eosinophil-dependent killing,[254] this was replaced by these other methods. In a review of this assay system in 1985, it was found that each of the components of the assay could affect the result, including the source of the eosinophils, the antibody, and even the reaction vessel.[253]

The biochemical events during the killing of *S. mansoni* eggs by mouse eosinophils were reported by James and Colley in 1978. They showed that inhibitors of eosinophil glycolysis (iodoacetate and 2 deoxy-D glucose) prevented eggs from being killed, and they also found that calcium and magnesium ions were needed. Aerobic metabolism was essential for satisfactory eosiniphil function *in vitro*, and there was also a requirement for microfilaments and serine esterases.[869] Histological evidence from liver biopsies of patients with *S. mansoni* supports the possibility that eosinophils can kill the miracidium in egg granulomas.[820]

Work with rodent cells continued in other laboratories in 1978, using rat eosinophils and schistosomula. Electronmicroscopy of the interaction of rat peritoneal eosinophils with schistosomula showed that eosinophils migrated under the tegument, and prised it away from the body of the worm. Eosinophils released many of their granules, and had begun to degenerate in these areas. In contrast, eosinophils adherent to complement-coated Sepharose beads did not show any evidence of specific granule secretion or vacuole formation, even after eight hours of culture.[1180] This is surprising, in view of previous studies in which complement-coated Sepharose has been shown to induce lysozomal enzyme release from eosinophils in man.[1197]

The interaction of eosinophils with the pentalaminar surface membrane of antibody-coated schistosomula is a close one, which was first studied in 1978 by phase-contrast and electronmicroscopy. The cells adhered and flattened; and then after fusion of the eosinophil granule membrane with the cell plasma membrane, electron-dense granule material was spread closely over the surface of the parasites. This was followed by evidence of damage to the tegument within the first five hours of incubation. Eosinophils continued to attach to the exposed deeper muscle layers, and ingested fragments of the parasites.[649]

In 1980, the interaction was studied using freeze fracture techniques. This showed that eosinophils did not fuse their plasma membrane with the outer membrane of the schistosomula, unlike neutrophils, but discharged their granule contents directly onto the surface of the parasite.[290] When eosinophils were detached from the surface of antibody-coated schistosomula, transmission EM and freeze fracture studies suggested that eosinophils adhered to the parasite surface by their discharged granule material.[291] This makes it probable that the toxicity of eosinophils for this parasite is linked to their capacity to secrete their granules and other components.

Although initial work in 1979 on eosinophil-dependent killing of schistosomula *in vitro* suggested that MBP was the most potent toxic component in eosinophils,[257] it is now known that on a molar basis, ECP is more toxic *in vitro*.[5] The capacity of ECP to kill schistosomula is greatly increased in the presence of oxygen metabolites. This was shown by incubating schistosomula with neutroplasts or eoplasts, which contain membrane oxidative enzymes but no granules. The importance of the respiratory burst was shown in experiments in which cytoplasts of granulocytes from patients with chronic granulomatous disease failed to synergize with ECP to kill schistosomula.[1973] For further discussion on the effects of individual eosinophil proteins on parasites *in vitro*, see Chapter 3.

Eosinophil killing of trichinella It was first shown in 1978 that *T. spiralis* newborn larvae could be killed by murine eosinophils *in vitro*.[942, 939] Human eosinophils and neutrophils were also shown to be able to kill these larvae.[129, 938] Studies done in Paris and reported in 1987 have shown that murine eosinophils are the main effector cells of *in vitro* antibody-dependent killing of larvae which are only 2 hours old, but that the parasite alters to become resistant by 20 hours.[620]

The mechanism of killing was initially ascribed to the generation by eosinophils of reactive oxygen species and hydrogen peroxide.[129] Then it was shown that MBP could kill newborn larvae[1887] but not muscle stage larvae.[246] A monoclonal antibody to newborn larvae, which could mediate eosinophil-dependent killing of the larvae *in vitro*, was able to reduce infectivity *in vivo*.[1336]

It was not until 1987 that the toxicity of three of the basic proteins in eosinophils, native MBP, and reduced and alkylated MBP, ECP, and EDN/EPX, was assayed in cultures of *T. spiralis* newborn larvae. MBP in its reduced and alkylated form was more toxic than the native molecule, and ECP was as toxic as MBP, but killed more slowly. EDN/EPX was about 10 times less active. Ribonuclease was ineffective.[747] As this parasite has lysolecithin within its tegument, it has been suggested that eosinophil lysophospholipase could also damage this parasite,[20] but this has not been tested.

Eosinophil killing of filariae Possible links between eosinophils and the pathology of onchocerciasis have been studied for several years, and there is a growing body of evidence that although eosinophils may have a protective role in this disease, they may also be responsible for some of the tissue lesions which produce permanent injury in the skin and eyes. IgE antibody may be involved, as sera from Sudanese patients with onchocerciasis was found to contain a heat-labile component which enabled blood eosinophils to adhere to third stage larvae of this parasite, during a three hour assay. Neutrophils did not adhere, and eosinophil binding to other filarial larvae was not seen. The most active sera came from patients with punctate keratitis.[1934]

Eosinophils can kill the microfilariae of *Onchocera volvulus*[714] and *Brugia malayi*[1632] *in vitro*. Eosinophils in the lymph nodes of patients with onchocerciasis who had been treated with diethylcarbamazine had features to suggest that they were destroying the microfilariae.[1465]

Eosinophil killing of trypanosomes In 1979 Thorne and colleagues found that human eosinophils could phagocytoze *Trypanosoma dionisii*, and kill the organism in endocytic vacuoles.[1777] In 1981 Kierszenbaum and colleagues also reported that trypomastigotes of *T. cruzi* were killed *in vitro* by reduced and alkylated MBP.[960] Killing was prevented with greater than 312 u/ml of heparin in cultures containing four eosinophils for each organism.[961] It has been shown that amastigotes of *T. cruzi* can be taken up and damaged by human blood eosinophils. Intact granules and MBP were also deposited onto extracellular organisms, and these may have been the cause of their death, as MBP was found to be directly toxic to epimastigotes[1863] and amastigotes.[1864]

Eosinophil killing of other parasites There is experimental work suggesting that eosinophils may be able to kill malaria parasites. This has come from studies in infected rodents, and from *in vitro* experiments with eosinophil secretion products.[1890] *Leishmania mexicana amazonensis* promastigotes and amastigotes were rapidly phagocytozed by rat peritoneal eosinophils, and destroyed both within endocytic vacuoles, and by secretion onto the surface of the parasites.[1408] This reaction was complement mediated.

In 1983, it was shown that human blood eosinophils were able to kill *Giardia lamblia* in an antibody-dependent cytotoxicity assay, although this effect was less than with neutrophils.[1653]

6.2.2 *Mammalian cell killing*

There are a wide range of non-parasitic diseases in which eosinophils are prominent and may have a toxic effect on cells and tissues. Examples include:

(1) atopic eczema, in which large amounts of eosinophil granule proteins are found in the dermis in areas where there are few eosinophils,

(2) eosinophilic cystitis,

(3) certain slow-growing tumours where eosinophils are found in, and around the tumour masses,

(4) in the gut in various inflammatory disorders such as Crohn's disease and allergic gastroenteritis and;

(5) granulomatous diseases where eosinophils deposit large amounts of their granule proteins.

Guinea pig MBP can damage a number of human cells *in vitro*, including spleen cells, mononuclear cells, intestinal, skin, and tracheal cells.[658] As the concentrations of MBP which had this effect could be reached *in vivo*, it has been suggested that this may be a cause of tissue injury in hypersensitivity diseases.[656]

Eosinophils and respiratory tract injury The finding of large numbers of eosinophils in the bronchial epithelium of patients dying with severe asthma prompted experiments to see whether eosinophils could be responsible for some of the pathology of this disease. Experiments using guinea-pig tracheal rings *in vitro* showed that MBP caused desquamation and damage to ciliated epithelial cells on the surface of the trachea, and reduced ciliary motility.

Eosinophil peroxidase which was purified from the blood of patients with HES killed cultured human A549 cells (which have some of the characteristics of type II pneumocytes) and rat type II alveolar pneumocytes, in the presence of an H_2O_2-generating system and a halide. It was suggested that at 10^{-5} mol/l did not cause lysis in this system, the EPO–H_2O_2–halide system may be an important cause of lung injury in patients with asthma and pulmonary eosinophilic syndromes.[24] Purified rat peritoneal eosinophils, either intact or after disruption, were able to prevent the confluent growth in culture of a human fetal lung fibroblast cell line, MRC-5. The inhibition was greater when the cells had been stimulated with PMA, and only then became as effective as neutrophil-dependent toxicity.[354]

Eosinophil killing of cell lines and tumour cells There is a body of experimental work which shows that eosinophils can kill tumour cells *in vitro*, raising the possibility that eosinophils may have a protective role against the growth of certain tumours. As mentioned above, during a two-hour incubation, EPO was toxic for cultured human lung A549 cells in the presence of an H_2O_2-generating and halide system.[24] Eosinophils in bronchoalveolar lavage samples from patients with respiratory diseases killed a cat lung diploid alveolar epithelial cell line (AK-D) spontaneously. Guinea pig eosinophils had the same effect and also killed a labelled human lung fibroblast cell line (HFL-1) spontaneously. Cultured fibroblasts, and mesothelial cells were killed, but less effectively. The mechanism of killing appeared to be through the production of oxygen radicals.[409]

Eosinophil killing of heart cells and vascular constituents The association of marked eosinophilia due to many different causes with the appearance of endymyocardial fibrosis has led several investigators to raise the possibility that eosinophils might be able to damage the heart. Since 1976, we have been investigating the role of eosinophils in cardiovascular injury in patients with hypereosinophilia. We have shown that eosinophil secretion products are highly toxic for isolated rat heart cells *in vitro*. Toxicity was due to damage to the sarcolemma, with secondary effects on mitochondrial enzymes which were inhibited stochiometrically. The most sensitivie enzymes were 2-oxoglutarate dehydrogenase and pyruvate dehydrogenase.[1736] Earlier studies using heart cell line cells and intact human blood eosinophils failed to show significant toxicity,[1367] but these experiments were done without prior activation of the eosinophils to enhance their potential cytotoxic capacities, and to cause them to secrete their contents. The intravenous injection of human eosinophil secretion products can also injure the right ventricular muscle of mice.[973] Isolated vascular endothelial cells can be killed by purified guinea pig MBP.[658]

6.2.3 *Mechanisms of eosinophil-dependent killing*

Eosinophils can damage target cells and multicellular organisms by both oxygen-dependent and oxygen-independent mechanisms. Oxygen-independent killing mechanisms affect cultured bronchial cells,[83] and schistosomula.[1414] Oxygen-dependent mechanisms are involved in schistosomula killing by eosinophils stimulated with activating factors.[1415] It is also interesting to note that eosinophils from patients with chronic granulomatous disease (CGD) are less effective than normal eosinophils in killing schistosomula.[941]

Cationic proteins Both eosinophils and neutrophils can damage targets by secreting their stored cationic proteins.

The toxic cationic proteins in neutrophils which kill some bacteria and fungi are of two types:

(1) small molecular weight cysteine-rich proteins containing only 29–30 amino acids, named defensins.[1589] (These can also kill tumour cells.);[1077]

(2) larger molecules of 37 and 57 kDa.[1594]

Eosinophil cytotoxic cationic proteins are probably unrelated to the neutrophil antimicrobial proteins, but their capacity to damage bacteria has not been as well defined. All these proteins appear to damage their targets through membrane interactions. In the case of the neutrophil defensins, this occurs within phagosomes, and less than 8 per cent is secreted after stimulation with PMA or opsonized zymosan.[621] The possibility that eosinophil basic proteins cause membrane damage by forming transmembrane lesions in target cells has been suggested on several occasions. Studies with purified human ECP have shown that it can form ion channels in liposomes,[1985] but these transmembrane pores were relatively voltage-insensitive and non-ion-selective.[1986] MBP may disrupt cell membranes in a way similar to mellitin,[1006] in which the basic N-terminal part of the molecule binds first, and the hydrophobic part then interacts with the cell membrane to damage it.[998]

Oxygen radicals Eosinophils may kill organisms by two oxygen-dependent mechanisms. One involves the generation of oxygen radicals (superoxide and O_2^-), and the other the production of $HI0_3$ or $HBrO_3$. These two events are linked, as newly formed superoxide is rapidly coverted to H_2O_2, which is highly toxic in the presence of a peroxidase and a halide. Superoxide and H_2O_2 can diffuse easily, but they are detoxified rapidly by superoxide dismutase, catalase, and glutathione peroxidase. Other reactive oxygen metabolites probably travel only a short distance.[94] The most toxic product of granulocyte oxygen metabolism is the hydroxyl radical.[1147]

Hydrogen peroxide and EPO There is an extensive literature on the capacity of products of oxidative metabolism from neutrophils to damage cells and tissues. This began with the classical study of Klebanoff, who showed in 1967 that myeloperoxidase with H_2O_2 and free iodine can iodinate and kill bacteria.[974] It has also been known since 1971 that eosinophils generate large amounts of H_2O_2.[92, 975]

The toxicity of the EPO + H_2O_2 + halide system in eosinophils is different from that in neutrophils, as iodide[1209] and bromide,[1902] but not chloride, are important in bacteria killing by eosinophils. The product generated may be HIO_3 or $HBrO_3$. However, when gelatin is absent from the reaction mixture, purified EPO can kill *E. coli* in the presence of H_2O_2 and chloride.[890]

The range of organisms which are killed in this way *in vitro* is impressive. It includes schistosomula,[940, 892] toxoplasma,[1089] trypanosoma,[1283] leprosy bacilli,[978] and other bacteria,[890] viruses,[150] mycobacteria, and fungi. However, it is not certain that eosinophils can mobilize this effector system very well. For example, phagocytozed *E. coli* are not destroyed by eosinophils as effectively as by neutrophils, although they appear to have the capacity to do so when purified peroxidase with H_2O_2 and a halide are used *in vitro*.[890] EPO can also kill mammalian cells *in vitro*. This has been shown with mast cells[778] and some tumour cells.[891]

6.2.4 *Factors which increase eosinophil-dependent cytotoxicity*

A large number of factors have been described which increase the cytotoxic capacity of eosinophils for target parasites, and cells. These include the following endogenous factors:

(1) GM-CSF (CSF-α);[1779]

(2) mast cell-derived factors, including ECF-A and histamine;[1235]

(3) ECF-A;[47, 271]

(4) leukotriene B4[1237] (a minimal effect);

(5) fMLP,[934] which is normally considered as a bacterial product, but which can also be generated by mitochondria;

(6) factors from stimulated T-lymphocytes including ESP[868] and EDF;

(7) IL-3;[1103]

(8) monocyte products including EAF[1779] and M-ECEF;

(9) recombinant TNF;[1779]

(10) β-interferon which increased ^{51}Cr release from antibody-coated chicken red blood cells from 24 to 30 per cent after 30 minutes, at an effector/target cell ratio of 25:1.[423]

6.3 Interactions of secreted products with normal cells and tissues

If the primary role of eosinophils is to release their granule components into areas of inflammation, it is clearly important to know what effects these secreted products have on other cells and tissues. With this in mind, several of the principal eosinophil constituents have been tested individually for their capacity to interact with other cells and tissues *in vitro* (see Chapter 3). However, most of these studies have used (partially) purified eosinophil extracts, which may possess different properties from naturally secreted proteins. In the case of ECP, antigenic differences between storage and secreted forms of the protein can be recognized with monoclonal antibodies. There may even be interactions between two or more of the secreted eosinophil proteins, giving rise to molecules with either increased or reduced capacity to interact with adjacent cells and proteins. Although experiments with complex mixtures of secretion products from eosinophils are 'messy', they are more likely to provide relevant information in this area, especially when they are carried out in the presence of blood and tissue components, which may modify their actions. Possible 'targets' for these effects of eosinophil secretion products are mast cells, basophils, lymphocytes, platelets, and other inflammatory cells, including other adjacent eosinophils.

In most of the *in vitro* studies in which individual eosinophil components have been tested on other cell types, their main effect has been to cause the target cell to release its own granule components, or to become 'deactivated', perhaps because important parts of the target cell membrane became covered with granule components. These effects would probably act at short range, as the eosinophil basic proteins would bind to surfaces and cells immediately adjacent to them. Heparin is the only endogenous inhibitor of eosinophil granule protein functions so far described,[1850] although others may exist, such as alpha 2-macroglobulin. They would also limit the range of action of these proteins. Eosinophil-derived reactive oxygen molecules could also have a very limited range of action. A summary of the possible actions of eosinophils on tissues is given in Fig. 6.4.

6.3.1 *Interactions with blood vessels*

It is likely that eosinophils affect vascular permeability, causing oedema, since the formation of a transudate is a common feature of many

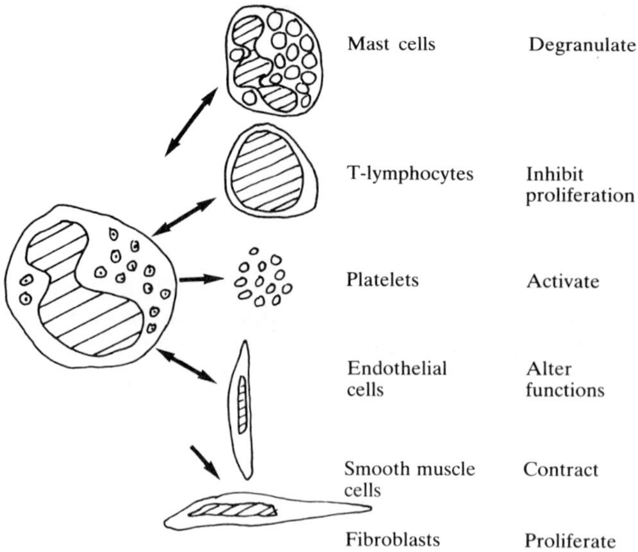

Fig. 6.4. The effects of eosinophils and their products on other cells. In some cases, the interaction occurs in both directions.

eosinophilic disorders. There are no details of how this could occur, although it has been stated that MBP causes a wheal-and-flare reaction when injected into human skin.[672] More is known about how neutrophils affect vessel permeability to small molecules: most of their effector mechanisms appear to be involved, ranging from granule enzymes and cationic proteins to products of arachidonic acid metabolism and products of oxygen metabolism.[1070]

7. Eosinophils in animals other than man

Eosinophils in animals have been studied by many people since Ehrlich noted in 1879 that eosinophils were present in all the species he examined, including frogs and birds.[801] Research on eosinophils in different species is important for several reasons. It offers the opportunity to determine the properties and roles of eosinophils *in vivo*, and to define the relationship between eosinophils and other cell types under controlled conditions. However, there are species differences which can cause difficulties if the findings in animals are to be related to man. For example, rodent peritoneal eosinophils have a phagocytic capacity which is usually greater than that of human eosinophils. In some animals, including members of the cat family, hyracoids, rhinoceros, hyenas, okapi, and some birds, there is no eosinophil peroxidase, and eosinophils in hyenas do not stain with eosin.[1810] Because eosinophil responses in animals are also often used in drug testing as a measure of an allergic reaction, the pharmaceutical industry has built up an extensive literature on eosinophils in different drug regimes. At the same time, the normal values of blood eosinophil counts have been established. A database of eosinophil counts (and other baseline measurements) in the most commonly used laboratory animals has been set up by the American Cyanamid Company, New York. This was summarized in 1986.[1949]

The morphology of eosinophils in different vertebrates shows considerable variation, both in the light and electronmicroscope, and they can be difficult to distinguish from other blood cells by their capacity to bind eosin. When molecular probes become available for the unique constituents in eosinophils (ECP, EDN/EPX, and EPO), it will be of great interest to determine the phylogeny of eosinophils in animals.

7.1 Phylogeny of eosinophils

All vertebrates appear to possess eosinophils. They have also been found in a number of cartilaginous fishes and more primitive organisms. It is not known whether an equivalent cell occurs in insects. No formal study has been done on the phylogeny of eosinophils, although this is an interesting area, which could be helpful in defining the biological role of eosinophils in normal and diseased organisms.

7.2 Eosinophils in amphibia, birds, and fishes

Eosinophils are present in the frog and triton, but their granules do not contain crystalloids.[948, 1190]

Eosinophil granules in chickens and pigeons do not have a crystalloid,[948] but Maxwell, in Roslyn, Scotland, has found crystalline cores in eosinophils from several other species of bird, including ducks.[1166, 1167] In 1986, he described a method of inducing large numbers of eosinophils to accumulate in the peritoneal cavity of chickens, using bovine serum albumin,[1168] and he had studied the morphology and enzyme content of avian eosinophils, including alterations in lipid bodies.

Eosinophils have been described in the blood and tissues of a number of different fishes, including lower vertebrates such as the elasmobranchs. They have been found in the nurse shark[833] and torpedoes (*Torpedo marmorata Risso* and *Torpedo ocellata Rafinisque*).[716] However, eosinophils are absent in hagfishes, which are Agnathan cyclostomes, and are direct descendants of the first fishes to emerge over four hundred million years ago. These are amongst the lowest living vertebrates, and have blood cells similar to neutrophils in higher organisms, but eosinophils and basophils were not detected in one electronmicroscopy study, which suggests that eosinophils may have appeared at a later stage in evolution.[1082]

The majority of fishes have eosinophils without crystalloids in the specific granules. This was shown in a study reported in 1986 on eosinophils from the peritoneum of the striped bass, *Morone saxatilis*.[184] However eosinophil granules with crystalloids are present in the tench[948] and a freshwater fish, the loach, *Misgurnus anguillicaudatus*,[850] in which eosinophils sometimes contain only one large granule, with separate small granules. One type of eosinophil granule in three teleosts (*Cyprinus carpio* L., *Tinca tinca* L., *Salmogairdneri* R.) has been shown to contain peroxidase, which varied in amount during development.[169] As the ultrastructure of eosinophil crystalloids in the loach was similar to man, it has been suggested that they might contain an analogous basic protein to human MBP.[850] The nurse shark, *Gingilymostoma cirratum*, also possesses eosinophils.[833]

The functional properties of fish eosinophils have been studied after separation by differential adhesion, or density gradient separation.[1143] Eosinophils from the peritoneum of the striped bass, *Morone saxatilis* were found to have lamellipodia, and were phagocytic.[184] Isolated eosinophils from the pronephros of the carp, *Cyprinus carpio* L., were also able to ingest bacteria, but unlike neutrophils in this species, the bacteria were not contained in endocytic vacuoles.[1766]

7.3 Eosinophils in mammals other than man

The majority of *in vivo* experimental studies on eosinophils have been carried out in inbred rodents, including mice, rats, and guinea pigs. Large animals, such as horses, cattle, and some primates, have also been used when greater quantities of eosinophils were needed.

7.3.1 *Buffalos, camels, cattle, goats, sheep, and swine (Artiodactyla)*

In this group of animals, there are reports of blood eosinophil counts in calves,[523] and wild fallow deer in Australia.[516] Blood eosinophil counts in the African buffalo (*Syncerus caffer caffer*) and in the red buffalo (*Syncerus caffer nanus*) were measured in 1985, and found to rise with age.[1433] Nematode infections in the yak, *Bos grunniens*, have been shown to produce eosinophilia.[771]

Cattle have provided large numbers of eosinophils by a technique in which antigen primed cows had antigens injected into their nipples, which they gave an inflammatory exudate rich in eosinophils.[473] Bovine eosinophils can be purified by density gradient centrifugation.[298]

7.3.2 *Cats, dogs, ferrets, mink, racoons (Carnivora)*

The general features of eosinophils in dogs and cats were reviewed in 1981.[2001] Eosinophils in cats have some of the most elegant crystalloids in the animal kingdom,[1442, 2007] although eosinophils in members of the cat family do not contain peroxidase.[1442, 1810] Eosinophils in dogs have been seen both in the blood, and in efferent lymph.[622] They can be purified by density gradient centrifugation in Percoll,[258] and they can form rosettes with human erythrocytes, in the same way as T-cells in this species.[1967]

7.3.3 *Rabbits (Lagomorpha)*

Although the rabbit has proved an important experimental animal for the raising of antisera, it has proved less successful for the preparation and study of the eosinophil, largely because heterophil granules in rabbits show some staining with eosin. Modern density gradient separation techniques have not been used to separate rabbit blood eosinophils, and this could be an interesting area for further work.

7.3.4 *Kangaroos and opossums (Marsupials)*

In a study on 112 opossums, although neutrophils were the commonest blood cell during the first few weeks of life, eosinophils increased rapidly so that they soon equalled or exceeded the number of neutrophils. After this period, eosinophils remained a prominent but smaller component of the blood.[375]

7.3.5 *Horses (Perissodactyla)*

In the 1960s horses were used as a major source of eosinophils, and their attractive large granules were thought to contain histamine. On the basis of this incorrect assumption, the role of eosinophils was thought to involve histamine-dependent processes. Horses have also been used in the preparation of large amounts of EPO. The ready availability of large numbers of eosinophils in individual horses still provides an important source for bulk separation of eosinophils and their components.

In 1984, the blood eosinophil counts in 474 healthy horses at Newmarket, UK, were assayed.[32] The counts were not normally distributed, but there was no difference in the blood eosinophil count in horses of different ages. The mean count was 0.2×10^9/l.

7.3.6 *Primates*

The majority of studies with eosinophils in primates have been carried out on anthropoidea. Many reports on eosinophils in primates have been given for the macaque monkey (*Macaca mulatta*) and baboons (*Papio*). In 1982, eosinophil counts were reported for a colony of 104 captive golden lion tamarins (*Leontopithecus rosalia*) in the Smithsonian Institute, Washington DC, USA.[236] In 1984, blood eosinophil counts in a captive group of 86 lesser mouse lemurs (*Microcebus murinus*) were reported as 0.54×10^9/l.[435]

7.3.7 *Rodentia*

Rodents have proved to be the most valuable experimental animals for studies on eosinophils *in vivo*, and the availability of inbred strains of many of these species has been particularly important for providing reproducible animal models of eosinophilic disorders. The genetic basis of eosinophilia in some species of *Rodentia* has also begun to be explored.

Chinese hamsters, gerbils, hamsters (Cricetidae) Eosinophil research has used these species only rarely, although there is a report in 1984 of the use of Chinese hamsters in the study of schistosomiasis.[364] The appearances of eosinophil in the bone marrow of the Mongolian gerbil were described in 1978,[1894] and acid phosphatase in hamster eosinophils in 1980.[496]

Guinea pigs Large numbers of eosinophils can be induced to localize in the peritoneal exudate of guinea pigs after repeated lavage with saline, or saline containing a wide range of protein antigens.[1410, 1081] This technique provides 'tissue' eosinophils, which can also be obtained by bronchoalveolar lavage of sensitized animals. No report has been published on the preparation of blood eosinophils from guinea pigs.

Rats and mice (Muridae) Mice and rats have been the most widely used experimental animals for studies on eosinophils, as they are available as inbred strains with reproducible and defined characteristics. Many strains of mice have been used for studies on eosinophils, especially BALB/C, C57B1, and CBA mice. Mice which have been infected with *Mesocestoides corti* produce large numbers of eosinophils in the peritoneal cavity, and this provides an excellent source of eosinophils for experimental studies.[880] Eosinophils have also be obtained from mice with toxocariasis.[1721]

Many inbred strains of rats have been used for studies on eosinophils. Normal blood eosinophils counts in rats have been well defined.[1948] A strain of August rat has been used extensively at the National Institute for Medical Research, London, as it has a spontaneously high level of eosinophils in its peritoneal cavity, which can be separated by density gradient centrifugation.[1124] Am-1(2)/Tor rats, which have been studied in Brazil, also have a spontaneously high number of these cells in peritoneal washings, and can be purified to over 90 per cent purity on metrizamide gradients.[1407] The largest numbers of eosinophils are obtained from rats which have been induced to develop eosinophilia. Two hundred fifty million eosinophils can be obtained from the peritoneum of a rat infected with *M. corti*, although the cells are in an activated state, with altered properties.[355] Rat and mouse peritoneal eosinophils can be purified using discontinuous metrizamide gradients.[870]

7.4 Eosinophils in reptiles

Eosinophils have been found in turtles and lizards, but they do not contain a crystalloid internum.[948] A primitive reptile, the tuatara *Sphenedon punctatus* (Gray), has eosinophils, but these do not have crystalloids.[446] The American alligator (*Alligator mississippiensis*) has blood eosinophil counts of about 0.6×10^9/l, which stain for alkaline phosphatase, and have some phagocytic capacity for bacteria *in vitro*.[1163]

Part II

Eosinophils in disease

8. Bacterial, fungal, and rickettsial infections

8.1 Bacterial infections

The majority of bacterial infections cause a rapid fall in blood eosinophil counts, and this has been used to help distinguish between allergic and infectious causes of, for example, inflammatory lung disease. This decrease in blood eosinophil counts is not always associated with an absence of eosinophils in the inflammatory lesions of bacterial infections, suggesting that some of the fall in blood counts is due to the uptake of eosinophils into the lesions. However, bone marrow production of eosinophils is reduced during most bacterial infections. Eosinophils may take part in bacterial infections, even though they may not be present in the blood. This possibility arises from the results of serial measurements which were made in 1978 of the serum concentrations of eosinophil granule-derived proteins in 12 patients with pneumonia, and 12 control subjects. Although patients with pneumonia had no circulating blood eosinophils, their serum ECP levels were raised on admission to hospital, and they only returned to normal after thirty days. This supported the possibility that, although eosinophils are not found in the blood during an infection, they may continue to secrete their granule proteins in tissues.[1852] The occurrence of eosinophilia with a bacterial infection is seen in certain immunodeficiencies in childhood, during drug hypersensitivity reactions, and occasionally as a response to the bacterial infection itself.

8.1.1 *Actinomycetales infections*

Eosinophilia may occasionally occur in patients with pulmonary mycobacterial infections, including *M. tuberculosis*,[580] atypical mycobacteria,[1954] *C. pseudotuberculosis*,[956] and avian tuberculosis.[752] More commonly, eosinophilia in patients with tuberculosis is due to a drug reaction to antibiotics.

8.1.2 *Enterobacteriaceae infections*

There are only a small number of reports of eosinophilia occurring in patients with bacterial infections of the gut, including bacillary dysentery and salmonella infections, emphasizing the importance of looking for parasites in patients who have a predominantly diarrhoeal illness.

8.1.3 *Staphylococcal and streptococcal infections*

Staphylococcal infections are not normally associated with eosinophilia, although there are a few reports of this unusual association; and although there were a number of earlier reports of eosinophilia in patients with chronic streptococcal infections, and during the recovery phase from scarlet fever, there are few reports of this today. This may be related to the reduced incidence in developed countries of some types of streptococcal infection, such as rheumatic fever and subacute bacterial endocarditis. However, a patient with a streptococcal sore throat and a blood eosinophil count of 56.3×10^9/l was reported from Athens in 1980.[494]

8.1.4 *Chlamydial infections*

A mild increase in blood eosinophil counts of 0.3×10^9/l or more is a feature of chlamydial pneumonia in infants. In 1982, 115 babies with this disease were reviewed in Berne, Switzerland.[1563] The infection is acquired during birth, and becomes manifested during the first three months as a respiratory infection with conjunctivitis and serous otitis.

8.2 Mycoses

Fungal infections are not normally associated with eosinophilia, except when they induce a hypersensitivity reaction. The components of fungi which produce this type of response have not yet been defined, although this could be studied, as fungal antigens produce eosinophilia after injection into the peritoneum of mice.[305] Occasionally, fungal infections in the skin can produce an eosinophilic pustular folliculitis.[1016]

8.2.1 *Aspergillosis and fungal lung diseases*

Aspergillosis is a well known cause of eosinophilia, both as a primary response to the fungus, and as a hypersensitivity reaction to fungal antigens in the respiratory tract of patients with asthma. The eosinophil response is most marked when a hypersensitivity reaction develops to antigens released from persisting fungal mycelia. This can occur in the absence of tissue invasion by the fungus. In bronchopulmonary aspergillosis a hypersensitivity response develops to this organism, which produces eosinophilia. A good review of this disease was published by R. G. Slavin in 1985.[1644] It was first described in 1952 in the UK, and in the USA in 1968. The American experience was reviewed in 1985.[160] Other reports have come from Australia, where 42 patients were described in Perth in 1981. Eleven of these patients did not have asthma, although they had blood eosinophil counts between 0.7 and 4.5×10^9/l. As three patients had other fungi in their lungs, it was suggested that the term 'allergic bronchopulmonary fungal disease' was a better name for the disease.[648] Ten other patients were described in Concord, Australia in 1984.[203] Other patients with chronic asthma and eosinophilia have fungi in their sputa. In these cases, it is difficult to know whether the fungus or the asthmatic process itself is responsible for the eosinophilia. The syndrome of allergic bronchopulmonary aspergillosis is characterized by episodes of fever, cough, purulent sputum, brown sputum plugs, and antibodies to aspergillus antigens. The basis of the disease is believed to be an immunological response to fungal antigens which gives rise to immediate hypersensitivity reactions, immune complex damage, and delayed hypersensitivity lesions. It is important to diagnose and treat this disease before irreversible changes have occurred which can be progressive without steroid treatment,[1208] or even fatal.[713] Occasionally other fungi, including *Curvularia lunata*,[744] can cause a similar syndrome.

Hypereosinophilic mucoid impaction is a disorder which is most commonly seen in allergic bronchopulmonary aspergillosis, but can occur in bronchocentric granulomatosis. It is characterized by bronchial mucous plugs filled with degenerating eosinophils, and is distinct from the mucous plugs seen in asthma.[873] It usually occurs in adults, but there are several case reports in young children, including one studied at post mortem.[318]

8.2.2 *Coccidioidomycosis*

Peripheral blood eosinophilia occurs in as many as 88 per cent of patients with primary coccidioidal infections.[467] Although eosinophils are not seen in the granulomas at sites of tissue invasion by this fungus, eosinophils are prominent in the tissue lesions when hypersensitivity reactions have developed to fungal antigens.[490] Two patients with pulmonary eosinophilia due to coccidioidal infections were reported from Stanford, USA in 1987,[1096] which emphasized the difficulties in distinguishing this disease from cryptogenic pulmonary eosinophilia, and suggested that skin testing and serological studies were important investigations to carry out in areas where *Coccidioides immitis* is endemic.

8.2.3 *Histoplasmosis*

Histoplasmosis produces eosinophilia in man. A clear account was given in a patient reported in 1979.[230] This was a man aged 21, who had a maximal eosinophil count of 1×10^9/l 18 days after his illness started, with many vacuolated and degranulated eosinophils.

8.3 Rickettsial infections

Although rickettsial infections are uncommon, they may be spreading in certain parts of western Europe and the east coast of the United

States, and eosinophilia has been described in a number of these patients.

8.4 Yeast infections: cryptococcosis

Crytococcal infections of the brain can give rise to eosinophilia in the cerebrospinal fluid.[1250]

9. Viral diseases

Viral diseases are not normally associated with eosinophilia, although they can occur occasionally when the respiratory tract is involved. It is not known why virus infections do not give rise to eosinophilia, especially as T-lymphocyte-dependent responses are a normal component of the immune response to viruses.

Herpes viruses can occasionally give rise to eosinophilia. Few reports have described viral hepatitis with eosinophilia. Only a handful of reports mention eosinophilia in patients with RNA virus infections. A 13-month-old boy with a silicon elastomere ventricular peritoneal shunt for porencephaly, developed a coxsackie B4 meningitis, and was found to have 45 eosinophils/μl in his cerebrospinal fluid. This disappeared when the infection resolved.[313] The only previous reports of a viral infection associated with eosinophils in the cerebrospinal fluid were in patients with chronic lymphocytic choriomeningitis meningitis.

Two patients with marked eosinophilia have been noted among the patients with AIDS looked after at St. George's Hospital Medical School, London (Lambert 1987, personal communication). This may be related to the capacity of HTLV-I to induce T-cells to produce an eosinophil growth and maturation factor *in vitro*.[1543] In Houston, USA, bone marrow samples from eight men with AIDS showed 4.5 per cent eosinophils compared to 2.7 per cent in controls.[819] A patient with AIDS and an eosinophilic temporal arteritis was described in 1986.[1579]

10. Parasitic diseases

Eosinophils are a striking feature of many parasitic diseases. As helminthic infections are so common, it is an essential part of the clinical assessment of patients with eosinophilia to look for parasites in the gut. In countries where parasitic infections are endemic, many asymptomatic patients have eosinophil counts of over $1 \times 10^9/l$. The study of Indochinese refugees from the Vietnam wars has provided a modern assessment of the parasite burden present in this part of South East Asia. Seventeen species of parasites were reported among 353 refugees examined in Japan in 1984.[1964] Similar findings were reported in 128 refugees with an eosinophilia who were studied in Bethesda, USA, in 1987.[1291]

Helminthic infections are the commonest parasitic diseases which produce eosinophilia, although ecto-parasitic diseases and protozoan infections can also induce eosinophilia. These diseases are largely confined to tropical and sub-tropical developing countries, but parasitic diseases are also common in visitors to these areas. In a retrospective study of 119 patients with eosinophilia after travel abroad from London, UK, a parasitic infection was diagnosed in 39 per cent, and eosinophilia disappeared after appropriate chemotherapy. In 66 patients, in whom no parasitic infection was demonstrated, and who had mean blood eosinophil counts of $1.8 \times 10^9/l$ (which was not significantly different from the patients who had a demonstrable parasitic infection), eosinophilia either resolved without therapy, or responded to empirical treatment with thiabendazole or mebendazole.[759]

10.1 Helminthiasis

These are the commonest cause of eosinophilia throughout the world. It is unusual for patients with helminthiasis not to have eosinophilia, but eosinophil counts can vary considerably during the course of the infection, with the highest counts occurring during the early invasive stage of the parasite life cycle, and waxing and waning of the counts during the subsequent weeks and months. Successful treatment of helminthic infection can produce a rapid rise in blood eosinophil counts, probably stimulated by the release of antigens from dead and dying parasites. A summary of the main parasitic diseases to consider in people with eosinophilia is shown in Fig. 10.1.

The question of why helminths induce eosinophilia has intrigued stu-

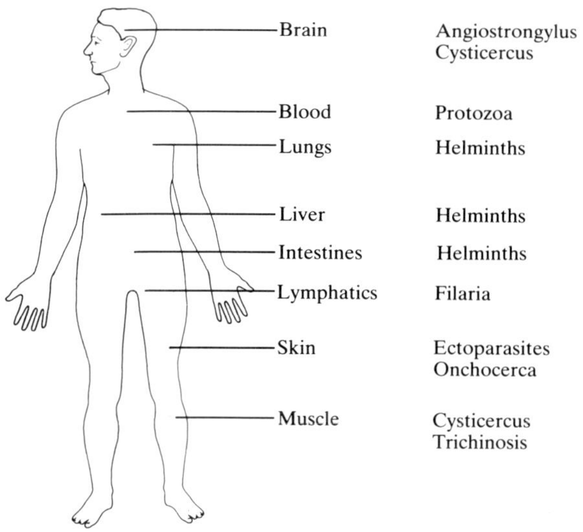

Fig. 10.1. The main types of parasitic diseases in man, and the tissues they affect.

dents for many years. In Paul Beeson's group in Oxford, UK, we showed that intact *T. spiralis* infective larvae had to be present within the vascular system for several hours or days, in order to produce eosinophilia. Larval extracts were ineffective, and larvae which were not injected into an artery or vein were less effective. This suggests that an endothelial cell product (possibly GM-CSF) may be at least partly responsible for the development of marked eosinophilia to this parasite. This could also explain why parasites which survive and migrate within blood and lymphatic vessels are such potent inducers of eosinophilia. Recirculating T-lymphocytes were a key component in the development of eosinophilia.[136] This may be because T-lymphocytes can produce IL-5.[1101] Now that so much has been learnt about the nature of eosinopoietic molecules in rodents and man, it would be interesting to re-examine these classical experiments with these possibilities in mind.

10.1.1 *Cestode infections*

Cestode infections give rise to eosinophilia less commonly than menatode or trematode infections. The reason for this could be due to the points discussed above. The principal organisms are *Taenia*, *Hymenolepsis*, *Dipylidium*, *Diphyllobothrium*, *Spirometra*,[263] and *Echinococcus*.

Echinococcosis Eosinophilia is found in about half of patients with hydatid disease, and it is most common in patients with hepatic and/or pulmonary involvement.

Taeniasis and cysticercosis *Taenia* infections are rarely associated with marked eosinophilia, possibly because of the mild nature of the infection. In a study from Poznan, East Germany in 1985, only 36 per cent of 296 patients with *T. saginata* infections had eosinophilia. Eleven per cent had an eosinophil count greater than 1×10^9.[985] However, the eggs of *T. solium*, but not *T. saginata*, can develop to the larval stage in man, and produce cysticercosis, in which there is often lodgement of larvae in the brain. This usually presents with epilepsy, but it does not often give rise to eosinophilia in the cerebrospinal fluid, possibly because it is diagnosed late in the course of the disease.[1846] In 1981, histological studies on a multi-lobulated mass of *Taenia* larvae in the brain of a 30-year-old woman showed a large number of eosinophils adjacent to the parasite. Previous reports of this rare disease were reviewed, and it was noted that eosinophilia is very variable, and may only follow surgical intervention and the release of antigenic material from the parasites.[28]

10.1.2 *Nematode infections*

Nematode infections account for the majority of patients with eosinophilia in tropical countries, especially in areas where filariasis is endemic. In many of these patients the infection is subclinical, and it is routine practice for patients in areas of endemic filarial, ascaris, and hookworm infections to take anti-parasite treatment once or twice a year. In western countries, nematode infections are often asymptomatic, coming to light only when a blood count is carried out.

Angiostrongyliasis Two main diseases are caused by *Angiostrongylus spp*. These are *A. costaricensis* and *A. cantonensis*. *A. costaricensis* infections are seen in the West Indies and parts of South America, where they produce abdominal complications, such as pain, appendicitis, and bowel wall lesions requiring surgical resection.[1106] *A. cantonensis* infections are common in many parts of the Pacific basin and South-East Asia, and are most noted for central nervous system involvement, meningitis with a marked eosinophil infiltrate into the cerebral spinal fluid, cranial nerve lesions, and a variety of focal signs.

Angiostrongylus cantonensis is the rat lung-worm. In man, a non-permissive host, it migrates to the brain, where the young adult worm dies. During this time there is marked eosinophilia in the brain, the meninges, the cerebrospinal fluid, and the blood, where eosinophil counts reach a peak two to three weeks after infection.

Experiments have shown that mice, which are also a non-permissive host for *A. cantonensis*, have many features which make them a useful animal for studying the immunology of this infection.[1723]

The number of reports of eosinophil meningitis are increasing in South East Asia, as it becomes more readily diagnosed, even when the parasite is not isolated. Details of 125 patients in southern Taiwan with eosinophil meningitis, or meningoencephalitis were published in 1976. Most of these patients had a mild or moderately severe illness, but 3 had permanent brain damage, and 4 died.[1974]

The disease is established in Samoa. Three New Zealand children who had visited Western Samoa and developed severe infections were reported in 1984,[1483] and a particularly severe outbreak occurred in 16 Korean fishermen in American Samoa in 1982, when 3 became comatose, and 1 died.[980]

In Thailand, cases of this disease have occurred after eating uncooked Pila snails, which are a local delicacy. It produces eosinophilic meningitis, which is usually a relatively benign disease, with a mortality of less than 1 per cent. Most patients present with headache, with or without signs of meningeal irritation. Blurred vision may develop, with swelling of the optic disc. The cerebrospinal fluid looks like coconut juice because it contain 0.5 to 5 $\times$ 10^9/l leukocytes, 70 per cent or more of which are eosinophils.[1846] Over a three year period up to 1968, 646 patients were seen with eosinophilic meningitis in one centre in Thailand.[1459] The post mortem findings in 3 patients were reported in 1978.[1663] These showed the tracks and cavities left by migrating worms in the brain and spinal cord.

Ascariasis Ascaris infections produce a higher blood eosinophil count in children than in adults, in whom infections are often asymptomatic and associated with mild or moderate eosinophilia, although a heavy infection can cause a serious illness.

Visceral larva migrans, which is due to the invasion of tissues with ascaris larvae gives rise to a moderately severe illness in childhood, associated with lung involvement and systemic features linked to the migration of larvae into different tissues. It has a low mortality, and patients recover over a few weeks, and can develop very high blood eosinophil counts. An ascarid of racoons, *Baylisascaris procyonis*, can produce visceral larva migrans and a severe or even fatal eosinophilic meningoencephalitis in children.[590]

Toxocara canis infections in man were identified as due to the infective, or second stage larvae of this nematode in 1952 by Beaver and colleagues.[143] About 5 per cent of children in New York have antibodies to *T. canis*, and there is some evidence that seropositive children have lower scores than controls, in neuropsychological tests.[1156]

The eggs from female adult worms in the intestines of puppies and pregnant bitches are deposited in soil, where they are ingested by young children who play in the same areas as the dogs defecate. The eggs then hatch into larvae in the stomach, and invade the tissues, where they become surrounded by a marked inflammatory reaction. Specific IgG and IgE antibodies develop at this stage.

Toxocariasis demonstrates a striking difference between children and adult infections, in that eosinophilia is most commonly seen in patients below the age of nine.[2000] In these children, who may have marked eosinophilia,[1686] the larvae are rapidly destroyed, although a few can persist in tissues where they usually cause little damage. In a controlled study on the use of thiabendazole in a group of Hispanic children with toxocariasis, reported in the USA in 1987, it had no effect on blood eosinophil counts or antibody levels.[132]

In older children, and adults, migratory larvae can lodge in the eye, where they may cause a localized inflammatory reaction, with gross appearances similar to those of a retinoblastoma. The eye damage is possibly partly the result of a toxic effect of eosinophils on the retina, while they take part in the protective inflammatory reaction against the parasite.[1508] *Toxocara* infections of the eye are best diagnosed by measuring serum antibody levels to secretory antigens from cultured *toxocara* larvae. If necessary, the aqueous humour can be aspirated to look for eosinophils.[1614]

Ocular toxocariasis can occasionally give rise to marked eosinophilia. One example was in a 19-year-old man, who presented with a blood eosinophil count of 3.72×10^9/l. Interestingly, a friend who appeared to have contracted this disease at the same time did not have eosinophilia.[970] Occasional reports have been made of marked eosinophilia in older patients with toxocariasis. An example of this in a 23-year-old woman was published in 1987.[1224]

Eosinophil-dependent killing mechanisms are probably less important than other components of the immune response in immunity to this parasite in man. This is surprising, as infected children can produce very high eosinophil counts. We found that although blood eosinophils were able to attach to antibody-and/or complement-coated infective larvae *in vitro*, and degranulate onto their surface, there was no evidence for parasite damage.[542] However, the parasites are destroyed after several weeks' residence in human tissues.

T. canis larvae can activate the alternative complement pathway directly, and fix C3 to their surface. Surface bound antibody can also cause the binding of guinea pig peritoneal eosinophils, which attach maximally in the presence of autologous IgG1, IgG2, and possibly IgE isotypes.[91]

Filariasis Filarial infections in man and animals invariably induce marked eosinophilia, which can produce some of the highest blood eosinophil counts found in any infectious disease. The high counts in *Loa loa* infections, especially in visitors to endemic areas, have been commented on many times. The reason for this marked host response is not known, but it may be related to the close spatial relationship that the adult parasite has with lymphocytes and endothelial cells in lymphatics and lymph nodes. The continued production of microfilariae, some of which are destroyed in capillaries in the lung and other tissues, probably accounts for the persistence of marked eosinophilia in untreated patients.

Biopsy specimens from 64 patients with filariasis, acquired while American troops were stationed in the Far East, have provided detailed histological information about the principal features of filarial infection in man. In patients with lymphadenitis, lymph nodes often contained many eosinophils in distended sinuses, lymphoid cords, and the connective tissue around the hilum. However, eosinophils were most prominent near adult worms, where they were the most conspicuous cell type. Eosinophils were also found in hydrocele fluid.[349]

Tropical (filarial) eosinophilia, which is often called tropical pulmonary eosinophilia (TPE), is a disease in which an immune response to microfilariae cause them to be sequestered in the lungs, where they are destroyed in multiple small inflammatory foci. These induce marked blood eosinophilia, with absent microfilariae in the blood. The disease was reviewed by Neva and Ottesen in 1978,[1273] and by us in 1982.[1695] Bronchoalveolar lavage has been done in TPE. This has shown large numbers of eosinophils in the lower airways, which return to normal after treatment.[1422]

As filariae of animal origin are often introduced by biting insects into people living in areas of endemic filarial infection, it has been suggested that tropical eosinophilia may be the result of a marked host response due to these nonpatent infections. This was supported by experiments in Malaysia, which showed that sera from patients with tropical eosinophilia (but not elephantiasis) were able to induce blood cells to attach to the surface of the third stage larvae of *Brugia pahangi*, and *Breinlia booliati*, which do not give rise to patent infections in man.[1633]

TPE was only recognized as being due to a filarial infection in the late 1950s, because of the difficulty to detecting microfilariae in the blood.[459] It is usually recognized by the asthmatic and coughing attacks that it produces, and the rapid response to treatment with diethylcarbamazine (DEC). Chest radiographs can show a variety of abnormalities, including diffuse mottling, pleural effusions, caviation, and even large areas of consolidation.[862] No relationship has been seen between the time of day when symptoms are worst and blood eosinophil counts, which are usually highest at 2 a.m. in these patients.[1637]

Sometimes the respiratory symptoms are not prominent, and marked eosinophilia is the main sign that the patient has this form of filarial infection. It is then often called tropical eosinophilia. This is commonest in male patients. It can occur in patients who have left filarial endemic regions several years previously. I have studied seven patients in London, and reported in 1981 the presence of prominent vacuoles in their blood eosinophils, an increase in their capacity to bind complexed IgG, and their response to treatment with DEC, including a fall in serum ECP levels.[1682]

Subsequent work has centered on the importance of IgE and IgG subclasses, especially IgG4[1339] in the disease.[831] In 1987, clinical details were published of a series of 50 patients with tropical pulmonary eosinophilia in the army in Kerala, South India, where the disease is hyperendemic. The commonest symptom was a nocturnal cough, in 72 per cent.[698]

In a study from India on patients with TPE, as many as 63 per cent of the blood eosinophils were found to contain vacuoles. The greatest number of vacuolated cells was found in midday blood samples, and the lowest number at midnight.[1557] The importance of this is that it suggests that eosinophils are releasing their constituents into the circulation of these patients.

In 1981, serum MBP and CLC protein concentrations were reported in 450 patients in a Pacific island where Bancroftian filariasis was endemic, to see whether the extent of eosinophil degranulation could be assessed before and during treatment with DEC. Following treatment, it was found that MBP levels increased as the eosinophil counts rose, so that they were still high at three weeks. Serum CLC levels rose at 14 days, and returned to normal at 21 days. Pretreatment serum MBP and CLC protein levels did not correlate with microfilaraemia, but serum MBP and CLC levels correlated with eosinophil counts. These findings suggested that eosinophil constituents were released following treatment, but that their levels were not useful in assessing the worm burden.[6]

Localized and dangerous systemic reactions produced by the treatment of filariasis with diethylcarbamazine (the Mazzotti reaction) may be mediated by the release of toxic granule proteins from eosinophils attached to dying microfilariae. This has been reviewed in 1987 by Ottesen.[1338]

Dirofilarial infections are common in many parts of Africa, but rarely give rise to disease or marked eosinophilia. However, a number of patients have been found to respond to treatment with a fall in blood eosinophil counts, so it seems certain that Dirofilarial infections can cause moderate eosinophilia, especially in Europeans returning from tropical countries.

Loa loa infections, like many filarial infections, are mainly found in rural areas in tropical countries, where there are few public health facilities. The migrating worms give rise to a tissue eosinophilia which seems unable to destroy the parasites, even though many eosinophils are found close to them. The main features in endemic regions are episodic angioedema, especially in the backs of the hands; the presence of migrating adults worms around the eyes; lymphadenopathy; microfilaraemia; and a moderate or marked increase in blood eosinophil counts. The lesions in lymph nodes in tissues affected by *Loa loa* have been shown to be distinct from those produced by other filarial infections.[1353]

Loaiasis is another cause of marked eosinophilia in Caucasians returning from visits to Africa. Two reports of this were published in 1986. In patients seen at the Hospital for Tropical Diseases, London, between 1978 and 1984, the mean blood eosinophil count was 6.4 × 10^9/l, and it responded to treatment with DEC.[759] In 20 with loaiasis who were reported from NIH, Bethesda, USA, in 1986,[1290] blood eosinophil counts were as high as 3 × 10^9/l, and most of them had developed a vigorous immunological response to the infection, so that only 3 had a microfilaraemia.

Onchocerciasis, which gives rise to a dermatitis, subcutaneous nodules, sclerosing lymphadenitis, and eye lesions, including punctate keratitis, is an important cause of a moderate or high blood eosinophil count in many tropical countries. Much of the pathology of the disease is the result of the host's response to dead microfilariae.[348] Patients with large numbers of living microfilariae have the least tissue injury, although this can become severe when the microfilariae are killed by chemotherapy.[1125]

Eosinophils play an important role in these tissue lesions, as they are induced to degranulate, releasing several eosinophil granule components. Following treatment with DEC, damage occurs in lymph nodes[1466] and the skin,[951] where dense deposits of MBP have been seen around dead or dying microfilariae. Some MBP was also seen in areas where there were few eosinophils, suggesting that eosinophils could have effects in sites were few eosinophils are seen by conventional histological techniques. Patients may develop a systemic reaction, the Mazzotti reaction, soon after treatment starts, and it has also been suggested that this may be due to the release of eosinophil granule components in the blood as a result of stimulation by parasite products released from dead or dying organisms.[727, 831]

Hookworm infections Hookworm infections which are common in both tropical and subtropical regions are usually found associated with other parasitic infections of the gut. Eosinophilia may be related to the worm burden, and to the extent of damage to the duodenum. The blood eosinophil count is usually lower in patients with profound anaemia than in patients who have been treated, but counts can rise as high as 50 × 10^9/l.[372] Ancylostomiasis is readily diagnosed by examining the stools, and successful treatment results in the return of blood eosinophil counts to normal. Hookworm is one of the main causes of eosinophilia in patients returning to Britain from tropical countries. In nine patients reported in 1986, the mean blood eosinophil count was 2.3 × 10^9/l,[759] but counts as high as 20 × 10^9/l have been reported.[984] In an experimental study on two volunteers in 1986, in Western Australia, who were infected percutaneously with 1200 larvae of *Ancylostoma ceylanicum*, eosinophilia was first detected at four weeks, and eggs appeared in the faeces at five weeks.[283] Prior immunity is unlikely to affect the eosinophil counts, as there was no difference in the blood eosinophil counts in a dog model of ankylostomiasis, in animals which had been partially protected from a second infection, by the presence of an earlier infection.[282]

The invasive stage of hookworm infections is associated with a systemic disorder in which there may be marked eosinophilia, itching, and respiratory symptoms, similar to that found with visceral larva migrans due to *Ascaris* invasion. Cutaneous larga migrans is usually caused by *A. braziliense*, the dog and cat hookworm. This was reviewed in 1985.[240]

Necator americanus produces clinical features very similar to *Ancylostomiasis*. It responds equally well to treatment, once it has been diagnosed from stool microscopy. A course of mebendazole, 200 mg daily for two days, is often sufficient to treat this infection. Details of an experimental study on necatoriasis in volunteers was published in 1986.[1925] The main effect of the infection was to produce a rise in blood eosinophils, with little effect on neutrophils. Preliminary work has been published on the interaction of human blood eosinophils with the infective larvae of *N. americanus*.[436]

The course of an experimental infection of five American volunteers with a small number of *N. americanus* third stage larvae was studied at NIH, Bethesda, and reported in 1987. After being infected in the skin with 50 larvae, they developed marked eosinophilia, which was maximal at the seventh week, with mean counts of 3.5×10^9/l. At this time egg laying was occurring in the intestinal tract, and this was associated with abdominal symptoms. Only small changes of other immunological measurements, including T-cell responses to larval antigens, were seen. Total and specific serum immunoglobulins, including IgE, bronchoalveolar washings at 8–21 days, when larval migration was taking place, and biopsies of the skin sites of larval penetration at day five, showed no alterations from normal. A surprising feature of this primary infection was the massive eosinophil response and the absence of significant changes in other measurements of the host response to this infection.[1165]

Capillaria *infections* *Capillaria* infections, which occur in carnivores such as cats and dogs, can give rise to marked eosinophilia in man, and this is one of the causes of a massive infiltration of eosinophils into the liver,[1341] and of pulmonary eosinophilia.[23]

Trichinosis Trichinosis is an underdiagnosed parasitic disease, largely because the persisting tissue form of the parasite can be asymptomatic following the initial disease process. Less than 200 cases are reported each year in the USA. Although the chronic stage of the disease in mildly infected people is of little clinical importance, a systematic illness, with widespread painful lesions can occur when a large number of larvae have been ingested. An outbreak of the latter type occurred outside Paris in 1979, affecting 125 people who had eaten contaminated horse meat;[197] and 29 people in Alaska were infected in 1975 from eating contaminated walrus meat.[1152] Occasionally, trichinosis can produce a hypersensitivity response, giving a necrotizing vasculitis which can affect the brain.[1535]

As the encapsulated worms can only encyst successfully in skeletal muscle, migratory larvae are destroyed when they settle in other tissues. Histology of the lesions in a fatal infection in a 46-year-old woman showed extensive ventricular endocardial damage with superimposed thrombi. It was suggested that eosinophils may have been partly responsible for the endocardial damage,[40] although dying parasites could also have injured adjacent heart cells. Interestingly, only 20 per cent of patients with fatal trichinosis have a blood eosinophilia, although it is one of the most useful investigations, with serum creatine phosphokinase and *Trichinella* antibody measurements, in making the diagnosis in less severe infections.[1634]

The introduction of compulsory methods for controlling trichinosis in animals for human consumption, has been successful in many parts of the world in reducing the spread of the disease to man. Individual outbreaks in temperate climates are usually linked to a failure to boil pig swill, or to cook infected meat adequately.

Trichuris infections Infections with *Trichuris trichiura*, which are limited to the colon, produce a moderate, or rarely a high blood eosinophil count. Results of blood eosinophil counts, and serum IgE levels were reported in 21 boys in an institution in Sao Paulo, Brazil, in 1982.[1515] The mean eosinophil count was 0.58 (range 0.14–1.58) $\times 10^9$/l. In 7 Caucasian patients seen in London, the mean blood eosinophil count was 1.4 $\times 10^9$/l.[759]

Strongyloidiasis Strongyloidiasis is another important parasitic infection to consider in patients in temperate or subtropical climates who have marked eosinophilia, especially when stool examinations are normal. Failure to make the diagnosis can lead to an incorrect diagnosis of HES, and if the patient is then treated with steroids, the parasite may become disseminated.[2019] It may be difficult to diagnose this parasitic infection on clinical criteria alone in areas where other intestinal parasites are common. This was clearly shown in a study on 88 patients with strongyloidaisis in Brazil.[415] As the infection can persist for over 20 years in patients who have left endemic areas, it is important to look for it in former servicemen, and others who have lived in endemic areas.[634]

Diagnosis is best carried out from duodenal aspirates, and biopsies. This should always be done in patients who are to be treated with immunosuppressive drugs who might have contracted this infection. Strongyloidiasis in otherwise healthy people produces only moderate eosinophilia: mean $1.0 \times 10^9/l$ in one group of 6 patients.[759] In another group of 152 patients, the mean percentage of eosinophils in the blood was 10 per cent, and serum IgE 2944 IU/ml.[1185] Occasionally, strongyloidiasis gives rise to appendicitis, as described in 1986 in a 47-year-old man in the USA. Histology showed a marked eosinophilic inflammatory reaction, containing Charcot–Leyden crystals within epitheloid cell granulomas, and parasite remnants in the appendix.[1595] Eosinophils may be involved in protection against disseminated strongyloides infections, as blood eosinophil counts were lower in 4 hyperinfected, immunosuppressed patients, than in 5 others who had severe infections without hyperinfection.[633]

Trichostrongyloidiasis Infections with this group of parasites is not very common, although it can give rise to marked eosinophilia.

Gnathostomiasis *Gnathostoma spinigerum* is a nematode which infects dogs and cats, and rarely man, to produce a severe and even fatal disease. It was first described in the stomach of a tiger in the London zoo. Most human reports have come from Thailand and other parts of South East Asia.[923] It was recognized in South America in 1984. The usual clinical presentation is with severe pain in the limbs or trunk, due to irritation of nerve roots by the migratory larvae. This may progress to urinary retention and paraplegia. The brainstem can be involved, and when this happens, the disease is usually fatal. Occasionally the presentation is with subarachnoid haemorrhage.[1846] The parasite is acquired by eating poorly cooked intermediate hosts for the parasite, including eels, frogs, fishes, and snakes. The parasite migrates to many parts of the body and produces two main clinical problems: recurrent skin swellings, and cerebral lesions, especially intracranial haemorrhage and eosinophilic meningoencephalitis. It usually gives rise to marked eosinophilia during the migratory phase, but the eosinophil count can be normal in some patients.[189]

Enterobiasis Infections with *Enterobius vermicularis* (the pin worm, or thread worm) cause few clinical problems other then pruritus ani in children, unless they invade the tissues, where they can give rise to salpingitis or acute appendicitis[1229] with eosinophilia.

10.1.3 *Trematode infections*

Two of the several trematode infections which give rise to eosinophilia in man are of particular interest: fascioliasis and schistosomiasis. These infections occur in temperate and tropical countries respectively. Work on the role of eosinophils in the killing of the schistosomula of *S. mansoni* has provided a great deal of insight into how eosinophils may function in parasitic infections. Although initial work suggested that they were important mediators of protection in both infections, this appears to be limited to certain stages in their life cycle, and they are only one of a number of effector mechanisms which partly control these infections and prevent reinfection.

Fascioliasis *Fasciola hepatica* is an important veterinary problem, and can occasionally occur in man where it is often misdiagnosed, leading to unnecessary investigations and surgery on the biliary tree. Eosinophilia and alterations in liver function are the commonest findings. In 1984, a report was published from Puerto Rico on the value of a variety of diagnostic approaches, including radionuclide imaging, in making the diagnosis.[1495]

Schistosomiasis The widespread occurrence of *Schistosoma mansoni*, *S. haematobium*, and *S. japonicum* accounts for the common finding of schistosomal infections, both in endemic areas, and in people who have returned from these areas to temperate climates. It is nearly always associated with eosinophilia[758] which may be remarkably high, especially after the parasite has first entered the skin (the Katayama syndrome),[1230] during diarrhoea produced by *S. mansoni*, when it can reach 18×10^9/l,[984] and when egg formation continues at a high rate.

The epidermal skin reaction induced by the cercariae of *S. mansoni* has been studied in Kenya in captured baboons with schistosomiasis. In animals which had been infected for eight months (but not less), many eosinophils surrounded schistosomula which were trapped and killed in the epidermis. Eosinophil-rich abscesses were also seen in the deeper dermis, but here many schistosomula appeared to have escaped injury, and were not surrounded by eosinophils. This study suggests that in primates with several months infection, the epidermal reaction involving eosinophils may be an important part of the protective response to further infection with *S. mansoni*.[1587]

As eosinophils can kill schistosomula *in vitro*, a search has been carried out to see whether this mechanism might be protective in patients with schistosomiasis mansoni. A group of 119 children were studied in Kenya, and some were found to have partial protection against reinfection following a course of treatment. The resistant children were two years older than susceptible children, but there was no difference in their blood eosinophil counts. Although differences were found in the capacity of blood mononuclear cells from different children to produce EAF (see page 107), this did not correlate with their susceptibility to reinfection.[251] No evidence was found that the possession of high-titre antibody to *S. mansoni* conferred resistance.[250] However, the possession of antibodies to egg antigens appeared to increase their susceptibility to reinfection, possibly by acting as 'blocking antibodies', which have been found to inhibit eosinophil-dependent killing of schistosomula *in vitro*. Three IgM monclonal antibodies which bound to an egg antigen, and to the surface of schistosomula, reduced the eosinophil killing in the presence of human infection serum.[476] A research programme is also underway in the Gambia to study the immune response to *S. haematobium*. One interesting finding, which was not seen in East Africans with *S. mansoni* infections, was that blood eosinophil counts correlated with resistance to reinfection, although eosinophil induced antibody- or complement-dependent killing of *S. haematobium* was barely detectable.[731]

10.2 Protozoan infections

Protozoan infections seldom give rise to eosinophilia during an uncomplicated infection, although there are occasional case reports which show that this group of parasites can induce eosinophilia. Amoebiasis due to *Entamoeba* is only rarely associated with eosinophilia.

Amoebic meningitis due to *Naegleria spp*. can be associated with an eosinophil infiltrate in the heart, even though the organism is not found in this site. This was shown in a histopathological study in 15 patients with primary amoebic meningoencephalitis. Seven had a focal or diffuse myocarditis consisting mainly of neutrophils, although there were scattered eosinophils and plasma cells, and myocardial necrosis was seen in two.[1154]

Although *Giardia lamblia* can give rise to marked tissue invasion and damage to the intestine, it is rarely associated with eosinophilia. Most leishmanial infections are not associated with eosinophilia, although eosinophilia may occasionally be seen in visceral leishmaniasis.

Patients with malaria who have eosinophilia are usually found to have other parasitic infections as well, and the blood eosinophil count usually falls during the acute stage of the illness. The possibility that eosinophils might protect against these infections has some experimental support.[1890]

Pneumocystis carinii pneumonia in infants can give rise to marked eosinophilia. An example of this was reported from Memphis, USA in 1987.[1380] The patient was a boy with hypogammaglobulinaemia, who developed *P. carinii* pneumonia at age five months. His blood eosinophil count was 14.2×10^9/l, and fell after treatment with gammaglobulin. Other previous patients with a T-cell deficiency have been described with a similar syndrome.

Toxoplasmosis is rarely associated with eosinophilia, although this has been described in a few patients, including a patient in South Africa who had a diffuse encephalopathy with marked eosinophilia. Treatment with pyrimethamine and sulphadiazine was effective in this patient, and there were negligible sequelae.[711]

Trypanosomiasis does not produce eosinophilia in African patients, although there are some patients in South America who appear to have developed eosinophilia.

10.3 Ectoparasitic infestations and insect bites

The human skin, and hair follicles are inhabited by mites in at least 10 per cent of normal people, but these seldom produce an inflammatory response. However, there are several ectoparasites which can produce irritating skin lesions, including head lice, and scabies. Other insects attack the skin to obtain blood and tissue fluids. Where breaches of the skin are produced, eosinophils and other inflammatory cells are often found in the lesions.

Many people have follicle mites in the skin of their face or other parts of their body, and their prevalence increases with age. Men are more commonly affected than women. Two species are involved: *Demodex folliculorum* and *D. brevis*.[84] Their importance in human disease has not been easy to define, and the nature of the eosinophilic material, which is often found adjacent to them in hair follicles, is not known.

Scabies usually produces an eosinophil-rich inflammatory response in the skin. In one study on 60 patients in Oslo, Norway, 10 had eosinophilia which related to the severity of the infestation,[536] and raised counts returned to normal after effective treatment had been given. The histological appearances of the skin lesions show a mixture of lymphocytes and histiocytes, with numerous eosinophils.[558]

11. Neoplasms

Eosinophilia may precede, or be found at presentation in a wide variety of malignancies. This has been known since before the turn of this century. For example, a report was published in 1893 of a 31-year-old woman who had a tumour in the neck, associated with a blood eosinophil count of 57.6×10^9/l.[1485]

Some tumours give rise to an increase in blood eosinophil counts, without a great increase in eosinophils within the tumour itself. Some patients have a normal blood eosinophil count with a heavy infiltrate of eosinophils into the tumour, and in some cases, both occur together. It is important to distinguish between blood and tissue eosinophilia in discussions about tumour-associated increases in eosinophils, as evidence is accumulating that tissue eosinophilia can be beneficial, whereas blood eosinophilia may be a sign of tumour dissemination.[1109] The commonest tumours which give rise to, or are associated with increased numbers of eosinophils in the blood or tissues are carcinomas of the lung, lymphoreticular malignancies (especially Hodgkin's disease), and lymphocytic leukaemia. (Fig. 11.1).

Several groups have attempted to isolate eosinopoietic substances from tumours, and some success has been reported with large cell carcinomas of the lung. No work has been done to see whether these tumours induce T-cells, endothelial cells, or other cells to generate eosinopoietic substances, such as IL-5 and GM-CSF.

11.1 Leukaemias

Eosinophilia can occur in patients with leukaemia, (a) as a 'reactive' phenomenon, or (b) as an integral part of the leukaemic process.[964] Few studies have distinguished between these two mechanisms, although it can be attempted to comparing clones of leukaemic and eosinophil colonies using cytogenetic and recombinant DNA techniques. However, this may be difficult in evolving leukaemias, and where there may be no detectable abnormality in the leukaemic clones.

11.1.1 *Eosinophilic leukaemia*

Over 100 cases reports of this unusual neoplasm have now been published, in which there is no doubt about the diagnosis. In 1960 Chen and Smith

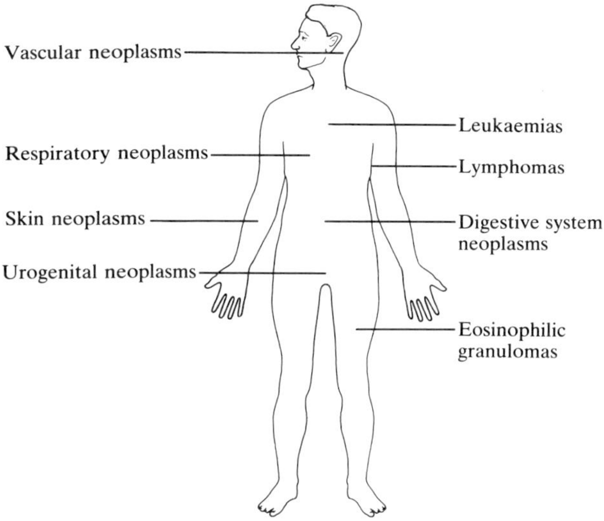

Fig. 11.1. The principal tumours which are associated with an increased number of eosinophils in the blood, or in the tumour, or in both.

reviewed twenty-nine patients with eosinophilic leukaemia and they reported a 36-year-old patient with a marked cough, and a blood eosinophil count of 43×10^9/l. He died one year later in heart failure, with endomyocardial lesions, and thrombi.[308] Five patients with eosinophilic leukaemia, among a group of 20 patients with hypereosinophilia, were reviewed by Bentley in 1961.[156] Since then there has been no comprehensive review of this disease.

The difficulties in distinguishing eosinophilic leukaemias from HES were best defined by Bousser in 1957,[198] who carried out a multi-centre investigation, in which the clinical features and prognosis of patients with eosinophilic leukaemia, and what is now known as HES, were clearly distinguished. A failure to recognize that most patients with a marked eosinophilia of unknown cause do not have a leukaemic process used to result in deaths from the incorrect prescriptions of cytotoxic drugs. Recognition of the non-malignant course of HES is most patients has been an important advance in this field.

Chronic eosinophilic leukaemia occurs either with the classical Philadelphia chromosome, or with a number of other chromosomal abnormalities which are also seen in other forms of chronic myeloid leukaemia. Here again, it has proved difficult to provide a single diagnostic group into which all these patients fall, and it may be impossible to distinguish patients with chronic eosinophilic leukaemia from patients with HES on clinical grounds alone.

Eosinophilic leukaemia has been reported to occur following radiotherapy of Hodgkin's disease, and the treatment of multiple myeloma with melphalan. In the latter patient, there was 5q-, and monosomy 7,[1130] which is a characteristic of other treatment-induced leukaemias.

Acute eosinophilic leukaemia Acute eosinophilic leukaemia can be distinguished most easily from the more aggressive forms of HES when there is a marked increase in the number of immature eosinophils in the blood and/or marrow, with more than 5 per cent blast forms in the marrow, infiltration of tissues with immature cells of predominantly eosinophilic type, and a clinical course similar to other defined types of acute leukaemia. The main complications are anaemia, thrombocytopenia with bleeding, and an increased susceptibility to infections, which usually results in the death of the patient within a few weeks or months.[1490] Occasionally, a marked eosinophilia may develop in patients who present with erythrocytosis. In one patient in whom this occurred, endocardial thrombi developed later in the illness.[1769]

An important feature of eosinophilic leukaemia is the propensity for the disease to produce myeloblastomas in bones, such as the sternum,[821] ribs,[638, 505], spine,[483, 572], head,[505], pelvic region,[1941] and tibia.[1960] We are looking after a patient with widespread lytic lesions, who also has hypercalcaemia. An abdominal mass may have been produced by an eosinophilic chloroma in a patient in Hong Kong.[687] Several other patients have been described with eosinophilic chloromas which had features to suggest that T-lymphocytes were also involved in the leukaemia process (see page 12).

Localization of eosinophil leukaemia cells in the central nervous system, and in cranial nerves, is another important feature in some patients. Infiltrates of tumour cells into the Gasserian ganglion were described in one patient in 1951,[1285] and into the cerebrospinal fluid in another in 1987.[995]

Chromosome studies and agar colony cultures of bone marrow should be part of the assessment of these patients. As eosinophilic leukaemia occurs in childhood, and there are very few cases of HES below the age of 14, all children with marked eosinophilia of unknown cause should have a particularly careful assessment for a leukaemic process, so that chemotherapy and bone marrow transplantation can be considered as early as possible. It can occur in infants as young as five months and seven months of age.

Examples of eosinophilic leukaemia in childhood include:

1. two infants, aged 5 and 7 months with eosinophilic leukaemia described in the UK in 1987.[390]

2. a one-year-old girl who died 3 months after presentation with widespread tissue infiltration by eosinophils, and thrombi.[424]

3. a three-year-old boy with an eosinophil count of 57×10^9/l, who was found to have acute eosinophilic leukaemia, and died 11 months later. Emphasis was placed on the isolation of *Mycoplasma orale* from his bone marrow, although the significance of this is unknown.[1749]

4. a five-year-old boy who had a blood eosinophil count of 157×10^9/l at presentation, and who died after 7 months, with blast cell infiltrates in his liver and spleen.[156]

5. a nine-year-old girl with an enlarged liver and spleen, and whose eosinophil counts reached 77×10^9/l.[904]

6. a 10-year-old boy with lymphadenopathy, enlarged liver and spleen, and endocardial fibrosis, whose eosinophil counts reached 95×10^9/l. He died after 5 months.[539]

7. an 11-year-old boy from Bangladesh who developed eosinophil counts of up to 120×10^9/l. The lymph nodes, liver, and spleen increased in size, and despite treatment with steroids and cytotoxic drugs he died in a blast cell crisis.[851]

8. an 11-year-old boy, who lived for a year after he presented with 31×10^9 eosinophils/l blood, and developed endomyocardial fibrosis, with multiple thrombi. Many blast cells were seen in tissues at post mortem.[1773]

9. a 12-year-old boy who had an eosinophil count of 51×10^9/l at presentation, with structurally abnormal blood eosinophils. He developed endomyocardial fibrosis, pulmonary infarction, skin and peripheral nerve lesions. When he died 4 months later, immature eosinophils and blast forms were found in his liver and lymphoid tissues.[1962]

10. a 14-year-old Austrian boy with T-ALL, in whom a shift in tumour cell phenotype occurred, both in the blood and cerebrosphinal fluid. Eosinophil myeloblasts were first found in the bone marrow, and although the cerebrospinal fluid initially contained only lymphoblasts, 4 weeks later cytotoxic drug treatment was started, 35 per cent were found to be eosinophil myelocytes, increasing to 75 per cent within 8 days.[995] This case report supports the suggestion that T-lymphocytes and eosinophils might have a common stem cell origin.

Examples of eosinophilic leukaemia in adults include:

1. a 34-year-old man with an eosinophil count of $7.9 \times 10^9/l$, up to 25 per cent blast cell in the blood, and 6 per cent in the bone marrow. His liver and spleen were enlarged and he had a petechial rash and cardiac involvement. He had a partial deletion of the long arm of chromosome 16 del(16)(q22) in 56 per cent of 68 metaphases. Treatment with hydroxyurea gave no improvement, and he died 2 months later from infections. Cyanide-resistant peroxidase was demonstrated in the blast cells, but they also contained naphtol–AS-D-chloroacetate esterase, which is a feature of neutrophils. The proportion of blast cells in tissues was greater than expected from the number in the blood.[168]

2. a 46-year-old Japanese man, in whom the blood eosinophil count was $234 \times 10^9/l$.[800] Initially, only mature eosinophils were seen, and there was a partial response to steroids. However, 2 months after presentation, he died with blast cells in many tissues, and eosinophilic endymyocardial fibrosis in the acute necrotic stage, with large endocardial thrombi. Cytogenetics had shown 45 XO/46 XY.

3. a 47-year-old woman, with a carcinoma of the breast, lymphocytic lymphoma, and a eosinophilic myeloproliferative disorder.[1658]

4. a 54-year-old man, with a three year history of alcohol intolerance, who then developed what appeared to be HES, with respiratory, lymphatic, liver, and endocardial disease, which became an acute eosinophilic leukaemia, with C group trisomy 3 months after presentation.[1351]

5. a 60-year-old Nigerian man who was described in 1970. He was anaemic, and had a total white cell count of $510 \times 10^9/l$, with $326.4 \times 10^9/l$ eosinophils, 9 per cent of which were blast cells. This appears to be the highest blood eosinophil count ever recorded. At post mortem there were renal and splenic infarcts. His heart was enlarged, with endomycardial disease, and the myocardium was infiltrated by leukaemia cells. This report also reviewed 19 previous patients who had marked eosinophilia and heart disease.[208]

6. a 65-year-old man, in whom the blood eosinophil counts rose over a 4 year period to $13 \times 10^9/l$. The serum B12 level increased, and the marrow contained some fribrosis. Finally, he developed a myeloblastoma involving the pleura.[638]

7. a 67-year-old man with a large cell carcinoma of the lung, cerebral meningioma, occult ademocarcinoma of the prostrate, and follicular adenoma of the thyroid, who developed hypereosinophilia, which progressed to eosinophilic leukaemia, with karyotype 45, X, 15q22-.[685]

The cytochemical appearances of eosinophils from patients with eosinophilic leukaemia have been reported in only a few patients since 1879, when Paul Ehrlich described the staining characteristics of eosinophils in a patient with large numbers of marrow eosinophils, many of which were immature.[801] In 1973, it was reported that leukaemic eosinophils stained for chloroacetate esterase, which is not present in normal eosinophils.[1565] The use of cyanide-resistant peroxidase as an eosinophil marker, when maturation is arrested at an early stage, was recommended in 1986. Four patients were studied in this way.[612] More details of histochemical reactions in eosinophils from two further patients with eosinophilic leukaemia were published in 1975.[1956] Four patients with eosinophilic leukaemia have been found to have increased serum levels of vitamin B12.[483, 572, 1222, 827]

As early as 1965, the finding of an abnormal acrocentric chromosome in some metaphase from two patients with eosinophilic leukaemia, suggested that it was not just a variant of chronic myeloid leukaemia.[686]. In 1975 an isochromosome 17 was found in a 50-year-old man with eosinophilic leukaemia. This patient had other features to suggest that he had a myeloid leukaemia, including raised serum B12 levels, a low alkaline phosphate score, and increased numbers of platelets. Fifteen months after presentation, the eosinophil count had risen from 0.9 to 30 × 10^9/l.[1222] A second patient with isochromosome 17 was described in 1979.[1097] In 1979 a review was made of published cytogenetic studies on 45 patients with marked eosinophilia.[821] Chromosomal abnormalities were found in 20, and an additional patient was reported: a man, aged 47, who had hypereosinophilia for five years, with malignant cells which had a hyperdiploid karyotype.

Cytogenetic studies in patients with eosinophilic leukaemia have shown a variety of abnormalities, involving particularly chromosomes 5, 7, 8, 12, 16, and 22. In 1986, we reviewed 13 reports of chromosome banding findings in patients with eosinophilic leukaemia,[1365] and in 1987 many of these findings were reviewed again, but emphasis was put on abnormalities seen in chromosome 12.[943] Sixteen earlier reports of G banding chromosome abnormalities in patients with eosinophilic leukaemia were listed, and the clinical and cytogenetic findings were provided of four other patients with marked eosinophilia, who had translocations affecting chromosome 12p13.

Two infants, aged 5 and 7 months with eosinophilic leukaemia were described in the UK in 1987, who had translocations of chromosomes 1 and 5: t(1:5)(q23:q33) and (q23:q33).[390] This translocation has not been reported previously in patients with haematological malignancies, although a t(5:14)(q31:32) has been reported in a patient with ALL, who had lymphoblasts in the marrow, and a blood eosinophil count of 120 × 10^9/l,[1788] and a t(5:11) (p15:q13) in 1984.[1980] The suggestion has been made that, as the GM-CSF gene is present on chromosome 5q31, and the c-fms oncogene is on 5q34, this region of chromosome 5 may be involved in the development of eosinophil malignancies.[390]

Patients with abnormal marrow eosinophils and nonlymphoblastic leukaemia, particularly of the myelomonocytic sybtype, have been found with abnormalities in chromosome 16, especially 16q22.[67, 1040, 1768] Because of this finding, it was suggested that chromosome 16q22 may contain gene sequences that are important in eosinophil differentiation.[1768]

In 1986, a 27-year-old woman with eosinophilic leukaemia was found to have the clonal chromosomal anomaly: t(10:11)(p14:q21).[214]

A 57-year-old man with a short Y chromosome was reported in 1972,[572] and a boy with monosomy 7 and marked eosinophilia complicating a myeloproliferative disorder, in 1981.[827]

In 1986, we described a patient with eosinophilic leukaemia and trisomy 8,[1365] and reviewed a similar previous case.[1899] Another patient with eosinophilic leukaemia, who had trisomy 8 and trisomy 7, was reported from Munich, West Germany in 1985.[1164] Two patients with t(8;21) have also been described.[904, 859]

In 1986, three patients with acute myeloid leukaemia and marked marrow eosinophilia were reported from New York.[1260] They were unique in having trisomy 22. One patient also had inversion of chromosome 16.

In 1984, a patient with acute myelomonocytic leukaemia and marked marrow eosinophilia was found with a 15;17 translocation.[1231]

Chemotherapy has not proved to be of any benefit in these patients, but the small number of patients involved has not enabled any clear studies to be carried out on the potential benefits of different forms of therapy. Bone marrow transplantation is of potential benefit to these patients, and a number of centres have considered this, but none has been carried out yet.

Chronic eosinophilic leukaemia There have been descriptions of patients with chronic myeloid leukaemia, in whom the majority of cells are eosinophils. This group of patients can be distinguished from others with acute myeloid leukaemia, or a secondary eosinophilia, by carrying out agar colony cultures, which show large numbers of eosinophil colonies in patients with chronic eosinophilic leukaemia, but normal numbers of eosinophil colonies in other diseases. This was first shown to be useful in 1975, during a detailed study on a elderly woman with the clinical features of chronic myeloid leukaemia. She had a high blood eosinophil count, and was shown to have chromosome 10 tetraploidy. Large numbers of colonies developed when her bone marrow cells were cultured in agar.[690]

Over 90 per cent of patients with well-defined chronic myeloid leukaemia have the classical cytogenetic features of a Philadelphia (Phi) chromosome (an abnormal chromosome 22),[1526] where there is a reciprocal translocation between chromosomes 9 and 22 t(9:22)(q34:q11), with the c-abl oncogene moving from chromosome 9, and fusing with the break cluster region (bcr) on chromosome 22, where an abl-bcr mRNA is transcribed.

Examples of patients with Phi-positive chronic myeloid leukaemia, in whom there was marked eosinophilia include two reported in 1965,[686, 725] one seen in 1975,[324] and a man of 59, described in 1980, who had a double Philadelphia chromosome, with eosinophilia of 21.2 × 10^9/l, and heart disease with widespread leukaemia deposits in his tissues.[1712]

Rarely, chronic myeloid leukaemias are Phi-negative. In a few of these cases of Phi-negative CML, a similar genomic event occurs as in Phi-positive disease, without the visible chromosomal alteration, and this gives rise to a clinically identical disease. Work is now being done to see if the remaining cases of Phi-negative CML, without c-abl translocation, have a different form of CML, or a variant of the myelodysplastic syndrome, such as chronic myelomonocytic leukaemia, which has a worse prognosis than Phi-positive CML. Against this background of information about neutrophil-predominant CML, it is possible that some of the problems in differentiating HES and eosinophil-predominant CML, would benefit from a similar search for abl-bcr juxtaposing, and the abnormal fusion product mRNA, and protein. No studies of this kind have been reported in patients with marked eosinophilia.

Eosinophilic leukaemia in animals Eosinophilic leukaemia has been described as a spontaneous disease in a pig[913] and in cats.[565, 1791] In 1985, it was reported that eosinophilic leukaemia was induced in one cat by the injection of a recombinant feline retrovirus PR8. This virus also induced marked eosinophilia in another cat, but did not induce a leukaemia. No T-cell tumours were produced in either of these animals, although they can occur in cats infected with this virus.[1069] Spontaneous eosinophilic leukaemia has been also described in a Syrian hamster[1430] and two horses.[1243] Acute eosinophilic leukaemia has not been reported in dogs, although there may be a marked increase in blood eosinophils in dogs with chronic myeloid leukaemia.[764]

11.1.2 *Myelocytic leukaemia*

Acute myeloid leukaemia (AML) and chronic myeloid leukaemia (CML) are occasionally associated with marked eosinophilia. A good example of 'reactive' eosinophilia is given in a report from Fukushima, Japan in 1987, in which eosinophil colonies which grew from the peripheral blood of a patient with AML were cytogenetically normal, even though he had a blood eosinophil count of 13.4 × 10^9/l, and GM colonies contained chromosomal abnormalities.[964] In other patients, who probably have reactive eosinophilia, the number of eosinophils in the bone marrow and blood varies during the course of their illness, and in response to treatment.

Myeloblastic leukaemia, acute nonlymphocytic leukaemia In 1982, a distinctive type of leukaemia was described. These patients had acute nonlymphocytic leukaemia (ANLL) with an increased number of marrow eosinophils, which were morphologically and cytochemically abnormal. The FAB classification for this group is M4Eo. It was soon found that they had a characteristic cytogenetic feature: rearrangements of chromosome 16, with breakpoints at 16p13 and 16q22. Many of these patients seemed to have a slightly better prognosis than others with classical ANLL, even though they had a high incidence of leptomeningeal disease, and occasional intracerebral myeloblastomas.[810] It occurs in 5 per cent of patients with acute nonlymphocytic leukaemia, and was reviewed in 1987.[987]

In 1983, 5 patients were found with this disease, among a group of 61 patients with ANLL at the University of Minnesota Hospitals, USA. They had partial deletion of the long arm of chromosome 16 del(16)(q22), and a marked increase in the percentage marrow eosinophils, which appeared to be part of the malignant clone, as they were structurally abnormal. Two patients who had blood eosinophil counts of 1.6 × 10^9/l, went into remission for two and three years after treatment was started.[67] A further 18 patients were reported by Le Beau and colleagues in 1983.[1040] In 1984, 6 patients were reported from Baltimore, USA,[808] and 3 from Boston, USA.[1756]

In 1985, there were reports of this disease in patients in Paris,[159] and 26 patients in Houston, USA.[810] Other reports were published that year from Tokyo,[1307] Kiel, West Germany,[1572] Leuven, Belgium,[1186] and Barcelona, Spain.[1947]

In 1986 6 further cases were described in Bordeaux, France,[378] who had an abnormal chromosome 16 which had a pericentric inversion inv(16)(p13:q22) in 4 patients. Two patients were in remission at 14 months, and four years, but relapsed 7, 9, and 20 months after diagnosis, and one died, suggesting that some patients did not have as good a prognosis as in the initial reports. Thirty-seven patients at the University of Chicago, USA, were also described in 1986, and the previous reports were reviewed.[1033] A nine-month-old baby girl in Japan with this disease was reported in 1987.[1304]

Difficulties in deciding whether the cytogenetic defect is an inversion or partial deletion of chromosome 16 were discussed in another paper in 1986.[762] FAB M2 acute myelocytic leukaemia with t(8;21) can be associated with a similar syndrome,[845] and M4-Eo leukaemia may develop in the absence of chromosome 16 abnormalities.[1703]

In 1984, 30 patients with the 8;21 translocation and 3 with closely related variants were described. Auer rods were present in eosinophil precursors in two cases, and in one patient, the marrow contained an excess of eosinophils with abnormally staining 'basophilic' granules.[1730] This suggested that the eosinophil cell line was involved in this malignant process. In 1987, there was a report of a 63-year-old man with myeloblastic leukaemia, and an eosinophil count of 5.7 × 10^9/l, with a variety of cytogenetic abnormalities, including chromosome 7 defects.[1224]

Chronic myelocytic leukaemia The blood and marrow eosinophil count is commonly raised in patients with chronic myeloid leukaemia (CML). In one series of 50 patients with Phi-positive CML reported in 1977, 46 had a mean blood eosinophil count of 5 × 10^9/l, ranging from 0.3 to 30 × 10^9/l. An equally high incidence of eosinophil myelocytes was found in the blood of these patients and some of the eosinophils were partly degranulated.[1672] Young patients with CML may have the highest marrow eosinophil counts, but this is unrelated to survival times.[1023] The eosinophils in CML are probably a component of the malignant process, as patients who are heterozygous for the glucose 6 phosphate dehydrogenase genes have eosinophils and eosinophil CFU of only one allotype. This has been shown with Phi-positive[989] and Phi-negative patients.[561] In patients with CML, eosinophils can show abnormal positive histochemical staining for chloroesterase activity, and have PAS and Astra blue staining with toluidine blue metachromasia.[1084]

An unique case report of Phi-negative CML with eosinophilia and multiple eosinophil chloromas in the spleen was described in 1984.[309]

11.1.3 *Lymphocytic leukaemia*

A small number of patients with acute lymphocytic leukaemia have been found to have a marked increase in eosinophil counts. This was first reported in two Australian patients in 1973. These were two girls aged 14 and 16 years with lymphoblastic leukaemia and eosinophilia of 109 and 3.3 × 10^9/l respectively. They had a purpuric rash, and one had lung involvement.[1674]

Since then a total of 26 patients with this disease have been described. The mean age at diagnosis was 12 years. The youngest was aged 2 years. Eighty-one per cent were males. Median survival times were 18 months from diagnosis in children up to the age of ten, and 6 months in older individuals, but was not different from other patients with lymphocytic leukaemia. Eosinophilia preceded the leukaemia in half the patients, and in half, recurrence or an increase in eosinophil counts, preceded relapse of the disease. Cytogenetic studies have been reported on 14 patients. Three patients had 14q+ chromosomal abnormalities, with t(5,14),(q?,q32) in 2, including a 19-year-old man studied at the West Virginia University Medical Center, USA, from where a detailed review of the 26 patients was also provided. The q32 area of chromosome 14 is a common site for chromosomal rearrangements in patients with leukaemias and lymphomas, and this is also the site for the immunoglobulin heavy chain family of genes. It is not known whether eosinophilia is 'reactive', or part of the malignant clone in these patients, but the unusual morphology of the eosinophils, and the absence of a detectable eosinopoietic activity in serum, and in normal marrow cocultured with the malignant lymphoblasts, is consistent with the eosinophils being a component of the neoplastic process.[806] Some of the leukaemic lymphocytes possess helper T-cell markers, and some only markers of primitive lymphoid cells.

Nine of the cases which occurred in children under 13 and in five adolescents were reviewed in 1984, and an additional patient was reported. She was a 29-month-old girl in Chicago, who had acute lymphocytic leukaemia, with eosinophilia of 106×10^9/l. Treatment was started with steroids, vincristine, and L-asparaginase. Methotrexate and 6-mercaptopurine with cranial irradiation were also given. Eosinophilia disappeared 6 days from the onset of treatment, and she remained in remission for at least 10 months.[629] Nine of these 15 patients were boys, the same ratio as in HES. This disease can be compared with acute nonlymphocytic leukaemia where there is rearrangements of band q22 on chromosome 16. (See page 158). Although it is difficult to see a common genetic basis for the presence of abnormal eosinophils in these two diseases, these two chromosomal abnormalities should provide clues about the sites for the genes which regulate the synthesis of eosinophil granule constituents, and eosinophil differentiation.

Doubts about whether eosinophilia is part of the malignant process are not resolved, but measurements of the nucleotide content of the eosinophils in a Dutch patient with lymphoblastic leukaemia showed abnormal levels in both the tumour cells and the eosinophils.[413] Reports on 15 patients with lymphoblastic leukaemia associated with eosinophilia were reviewed in 1984.[1796]

In 1972 I showed that the injection of a rat T-cell lymphoma into PVG/C rats produced marked eosinophilia. This was steroid resistant and was unlikely to have been due to a graft-versus-host reaction, which induced a marked eosinopenia in the strain used. In this case it seemed probable that the circulating tumour cells were causing the retention of eosinophils in the blood, possibly by interfering with their normal emigration routes into the tissues.[1678]

Example of hypereosinophilia in patients with lymphoblastic leukaemia include:

1. a 2.5-year-old boy in London who developed a blood and CSF eosinophilia ten months after his disease presented. The appearance of the eosinophils in both sites preceded the appearance of leukaemic cells during subsequent relapses.[1360]

2. a four-year-old boy with an eosinophil count of 53×10^9/l, with lung, liver, and spleen involvement.[196]

3. a nine-year-old boy with eosinophilia of 2×10^9/l, with endomyocardial fibrosis, lymphadenopathy, and a macular rash.[180]

4. a 12-year-old boy with eosinophilia of 10.5×10^9/l, with lung and endomyocardial involvement, who died two months later.[1270]

5. a 13-year-old boy with eosinophilia of 67×10^9/l, and heart and lung involvement.[1387]

6. a 17-year-old boy with eosinophilia of 10×10^9/l, a purpuric rash, lymph node enlargement, and lung, heart, liver, and spleen involvement.[632]

7. a 27-year-old man with a lymphoblastic lymphoma, which was preceded by typical features of HES for one year. The lymphocytes had the phenotype of cortical thymocytes.[945]

Seven male patients, ages between 4 and 41, were described in 1980 from a number of European centres. In several patients the eosinophilia preceded the appearance of the tumour (or was present when the tumour was recognized), and the eosinophil counts usually fell during remissions. In five patients the blood eosinophils were hypogranular. Three of the tumours were of the C-ALL type, two were T-ALL, and one was a lymphoblastic lymphoma. One patient had several complications more commonly found in HES: eosinophilic endomyocardial disease and intravascular thrombi.[289]

11.1.4 *Other types of leukaemia*

Monocytic leukaemia has only rarely been associated with eosinophilia Four patients have been reported with plasma cell neoplasms, and hypereosinophilia, which were reviewed in 1984.[594]

11.2 Lymphomas

Malignant lymphomas, and tumours of Langerhans' cells (histiocytosis X) are the commonest types of malignancy which give rise to moderate eosinophilia. However, these tumours seldom produce as marked an eosinophilia as can occur in patients with carcinomas. Hodgkin's disease tissue, and the granulomas of histiocytosis X, can be densely infiltrated with eosinophils, even though the blood eosinophil count is only modestly raised. Eosinophil production has not been studied in these disorders, which may be greater than appears from the blood eosinophil counts.

11.2.1 *Hodgkin's disease*

Eosinophils are a common feature in tissues affected by Hodgkin's disease, and the number of tissue eosinophils reflects the Rye subtypes of the disease.[608] It is also a well-known cause of a moderate increase in blood eosinophil counts. A study on the possible significance of an increase in bone marrow eosinophils in Hodgkin's disease was reported from London in 1987.[1123] No clinical differences were seen between the 28 patients who had increased numbers of marrow eosinophils, and the 108 who did not. However, the same group showed that among 193 of 1260 (15 per cent) patients with Hodgkin's disease who had an increase in blood eosinophils at presentation, there was a survival advantage in 95 with disease of mixed cellularity and grade I nodular sclerosis, whether their disease was localized or widespread.[1843] This compares with a small series of 10 patients with the fibrotic type of Hodgkin's disease in Hungary, in whom over half of the cells in the tumour deposits were eosinophils, who only had a short survival.[1790]

Although Hodgkin's disease rarely induces a marked increase in blood eosinophils, 2 patients with hypereosinophilia were described in Australia, in 1966.[1758]. One was a 43-year-old man whose blood eosinophil counts rose to 48×10^9/l. The other was aged 34 years, and had abdominal Hodgkin's disease, and emboli to the lungs. The tumour was found to be infiltrated with eosinophils, and his blood eosinophil counts reaching 108 $\times 10^9$/l. Marked eosinophilia with Hodgkin's disease can also occur when the lungs are involved.[202] The highest blood eosinophil count yet seen in a patient with Hodgkin's disease is 160×10^9/l, which was reported in 1939.[1144]

It is not known if eosinophils affect the tumour cells or the surrounding tissues. They may play a more extensive role than appears from the number of intact eosinophils in affected tissues, as large amounts of EPO were detected by immunocytochemistry in the lymph nodes of 4 patients with nodular sclerosing disease, even though there were relatively few intact eosinophils.[1545] EPO was also found in the affected tissues of other patients with non-Hodgkin's lymphomas.[1547] Eosinophil MBP has also been found within affected lymph nodes of 13 of 18 patients with each of the principal histological types of Hodgkin's disease.[245]

11.2.2 *Non-Hodgkin's lymphomas*

Seven patients with non-Hodgkin's lymphomas and a marked increase in blood eosinophils were reviewed in 1984.[1429] Lymphosarcomas rarely cause eosinophilia. However, one example was seen in a four-year-old boy who presented with a lymphosarcoma which involved the lungs, lymphatic tissues, and cerebrospinal fluid. He had a blood eosinophil count of 25×10^9/l, and some of these cells had morphological abnormalities.[96].

In 1987, two patients were described who had pruritic skin lesions with a lymphocytic vasculitis and hypereosinophilia. Several years after presentation they developed peripheral T-lymphocyte malignancies, and died rapidly.[1337] These patients have some features in common with three patients with lymphomatoid papulosis whom we have seen in London.[1926] (See page 304).

Many non-Hodgkin's lyphomas contain eosinophils in the stroma of the malignant tissues, and this can be extensive in some. A review was published in 1987 of 28 cases of gastrointestinal tract T-cell lymphomas which contained massive numbers of eosinophils.[1608] Two were in the stomach, and 26 in the small intestine, and 8 were associated with coeliac disease. These tumours had several distinctive features on low and high power microscopy.

11.2.3 *Angioimmunoblastic lymphadenopathy*

This disease is probably a prelymphomatous state of immunoblastic sarcoma. It was reviewed in 1985.[1718] Although eosinophils with deposits of eosinophilic material are a characteristic feature of the lesions, only a third of affected people have an increase in blood eosinophils. Occasionally there may be a particularly high count, as seen in a man, aged 70, in Angers, France. His blood eosinophil count at presentation was 10×10^9/l, and reached 45×10^9/l, despite treatment with cytotoxic drugs.[623] The presence of an eosinophilic infiltrate in the affected tissues was a poor prognostic feature, according to a report in 1978 on 8 patients in Southampton, UK[886] and 30 in Lyon, France, who were followed prospectively for 42 months.[63]

11.2.4 *Sézary's syndrome and mycosis fungoides*

Very few patients with the cutaneous T-cell lymphomas (Sézary's syndrome and mycosis fungoides) have eosinophilia[1354] or an infiltrate of eosinophils into the tumours. This suggests that these tumours are seldom of the type which can produce eosinopoietic molecules.

11.2.5 *Lymphomatoid granulomatosis*

This premalignant or frankly malignant condition can be associated with peripheral blood eosinophilia.

11.3 Reticuloendotheliosis

The histiogenesis of the tumour cells involved in various clinical forms of reticuloendotheliosis was not known with certainty until it was recognized in 1983 that the malignant cell in most (if not all) of the malignancies classed as histiocytosis X belong to the Langerhans' cell lineage. They usually contain the characteristic Lx-bodies,[838], and are able to be stained with anti-Ia antibodies and the CD6 monoclonal antibodies.[1577, 593, 765]

As these granuloma cells can secrete IL-1,[64], which is a potent stimulus for vascular endothelial cell production of G-CSF and GM-CSF,[213] it is probably that the eosinophilic response in these diseases is the result of an indirect effect of granuloma cell products on endothelial cells, which cause the localization of eosinophils in the lesions, eosinophil activation, and occasionally increased eosinophil production in the marrow.

11.3.1 *Histiocytosis-X*

Histiocytosis-X is a general term used to cover the three diseases commonly referred to as Hand–Schuller–Christian disease, Letterer–Siwe disease, and eosinophilic granuloma. The relationships between the various clinical disorders in which granulomas affect the bone were reviewed in 1977.[2012] Eosinophilic granuloma, which comprises 60–80 per cent of the total cases of histiocytosis-X, is the least aggressive form of this disease. It may be (1) unifocal, unisystem, (2) multifocal, unisystem, or (3) multifocal, multisystem. Other classifications based on morphology of the lesions, or clinical criteria, have not proved useful.

Eosinophilic granuloma Eosinophilic granulomas, which were first described in 1940, are a well known cause of lytic lesions in the bones of children and young adults. They occur slightly more commonly in males, and are usually solitary in the skull, femur, or vertebral bodies[619] of children, and the ribs and other sites in adults. They can occur in soft tissues, including the thymus.[1625] Innumerable case reports of this condition have been published. In a typical example, published in 1987, a 37-year-old woman was reported who had a headache for three weeks. She was found to have a solitary eosinophilic granuloma in the temporoparietal region, which was cured by curettage.[391, 1384] The computed tomographic findings in vertebral lesions have been described in 1985.[1449]

It is now known that Langerhans' cells are the predominant cell type in these lesions,[2013] although many eosinophils can be found in them, and more rarely in the blood. Peanut agglutinin, which binds to Langerhans' cells, also binds to the granuloma cells, and this can be used to distinguish this disease from other granulomatous lesions.[732] The bony lesions may extend into adjacent soft tissues, and occasionally they originate in other sites. Computed tomographic scans are helpful for determining the extent of individual lesions. Although vertebral granulomas show increased density due to vertebral collapse, the lesions in other bones usually show decreased X-ray density, and can be highly characteristic.[1002] Biopsy with curettage is usually curative, but occasionally low doses of radiotherapy are given with success.[1922] All patients should be followed up for many years, as new lesions can develop as long as 12 years later.[1480]

As there are so many case reports of this condition this review will only describe some of particular interest:

1. An eosinophilic granuloma which was close to the foramen magnum, and produced torticollis in a five-year-old. It responded to a course of low dose radiotherapy.[110]. An eosinophilic granuloma affected the L4 vertebral body in another four-year-old girl.[307]

2. Eosinophilic granulomas affecting lymph nodes were described in two men aged 34 and 25 in 1977. Both had lymphadenopathy, with areas of necrosis, and many eosinophils in the lymphoid tissues. This may be a variant of the more common diseases in which eosinophilic granulomas develop in skeletal tissues, and it may also progress to a malignant histiocytosis in some patients.[1482]

3. A 48-year-old black patient in Nashville, USA with eosinophilic granuloma was described in 1987 who had painful deep draining sinuses, and nodules in both axillae, inguinal regions, and perianal areas. The diagnosis was made by lymph node biopsy. His disease responded to electron beam therapy. It was not stated whether the patient also had eosinophilia.[474]

4. An 11-year-old boy with eosinophilic granulomas which affected many sites and which was resistant to chemotherapy, was treated successfully by bone marrow transplantation in Sweden in 1987.[1493]

Hand–Schuller–Christian disease This syndrome, consisting of some or all of the classical triad of exophthalmos, diabetes insipidus, and focal bony lesions, occasionally shows a marked eosinophil infiltration into the tumour. Many different forms of treatment have been used, including etoposide in 1986.[802]

Letterer–Siwe disease Letterer-Siwe disease is seen in infants who present with lymphadenopathy, hepatosplenomegaly, and a bleeding diathesis, with bone and skin leions, which are usually fatal.

Familial reticuloendotheliosis with eosinophilia, Omenn's syndrome Among the 200 or more patients who have been found to have familial histiocytosis,[1675] there is a group of infants with skin lesions, hepatomegaly, variable splenomegaly and lymphadenopathy, fever and infections, and marked eosinophilia, now known as Omenn's syndrome. This is a rare autosomal recessive disease, first described in 1965, of which there are now about 20 reported cases. During the first or second month of life, these children begin to develop erythrodermia, chronic diarrhoea, severe infections, lymphadenopathy, hepatosplenomegaly, failure to thrive, and leukocytosis with marked eosinophilia. These babies have hypogammaglobulinaemia and low B cell counts, with increased levels of serum IgE, and reduced T-cell functions, associated with an absence of ecto 5'-nucleotidase in fresh, but not cultured lymphocytes.[631] A deficiency of IL-2 and interferon-gamma production is seen *in vitro*. Four patients, two of whom received bone marrow transplants, were reported in 1987 from Rome. Their blood eosinophil counts ranged between 0.4 and 11.1 × 10^9/l.[239]

It has been suggested that Omenn's syndrome is Letterer–Siwe disease in an immunodeficient individual. Lymph nodes biopsies show diffuse proliferation of histiocytes with eosinophil infiltration. The histiocytes are usually of the Langhans'-type with abundant cytoplasm, an eccentric round-to-oval nucleus with a nuclear groove, and no nucleolus.[139]

11.4 Neoplasms of vascular tissue

Each of the main types of vascular neoplasm has been associated (in small numbers of patients) with eosinophilia, involving an increase in both blood and tissue eosinophils. Examples of this include:

1. a patient with a histiocytoid haemangioma of the heart with an eosinophilia, who was reported from Taiwan in 1985. The eosinophilia disappeared after surgical removal of the tumour.[1017] The tumour cells

appeared metabolically active, suggesting that they might be secreting an eosinopoietic factor.

2. eight patients with epitheloid haemangiomas who were described in Fukuoka, Japan, in 1987.[1811] Although the lesions had some clinical similarities with Kimura's disease, they were smaller, and not in the preauricular region. They also contained irregulary hypertrophied vascular structures, and not lymphoid follicles, containing Langerhans' cells. For these reasons they were considered to be a distinct disorder.

11.4.1 *Angiolymphoid hyperplasia with eosinophilia (Wells' syndrome, eosinophilic granuloma of soft tissue, Kimura's disease)*

This tumour, which is often called Kimura's disease after the first author of a paper describing it in Japan in 1948,[965] is an uncommon and benign tumour affecting endothelial cells, lymphocytes, and eosinophils, in the head and neck region. A similar disease was described in London by Wells in 1969, which he called angiolymphoid hyperplasia with eosinophilia. Some earlier reports in the English literature were reviewed in 1982, and stress was given to the abnormalities of endothelial cells in this disease.[138] Not all patients have an increased number of eosinophils in the blood, although they are always found in the tissue lesions.

Some authors distinguish Kimura's disease from Wells' syndrome,[1015] as there are differences in sex incidence and histological appearances of the lesions. These have been compared in a paper from Japan in 1986[837] when it was suggested that the morphological differences could be due to the long interval (a mean of nine years) between onset and histology in the Japanese patients. There were 171 cases by 1978.[786] In Japan, 94 per cent are men, and mean age of onset is 32 years, and the lesions tend to be in deep tissues. In Europe, nearly all the patients are women, and the lesions are more superficial. In both regions, they are usually cured by simple excision. Case reports of the disease from Japan were published in 1986,[837] Hong Kong in 1984,[1015] London in 1987,[1904] and Memphis, USA in 1981,[625] which also provided good pictures of the gross appearances and histology of the lesions.

Histology shows varying degrees of infiltration with lymphocytes, histiocytes, mast cells, and eosinophils. Marked germinal centre formation may occur in Japanese patients. Fibrosis is common in Japanese, but rare in non-Japanese patients. The histopathological features in 116 cases referred to the Armed Forces Institute of Pathology, Washington, DC were reviewed in 1985.[1323] Orientals, blacks, and patients from the Middle East tend to have larger lesions (about 3 cm diameter) than other groups (about 1 cm diameter). Eosinophilia occurs in 17 per cent of Caucasians and 62 per cent of Orientals. Its behaviour is benign, and this is confirmed in the histology. Recurrences may develop, but spontaneous regression usually occurs. Treatment can include removal and irradiation.

The clinical and histopathological features of this benign disease in 12 patients studied at the Pittsburgh School of Medicine were published in 1980, with a review of the world literature then available; and the importance of differentiating it from an angiosarcoma was emphasized.[111] Two further patients with this disease were reported in detail in 1981, a 49-year-old woman and a 24-year-old man, and the histological appearances were provided.[106] Details of the histological appearances in Japanese patients were reported in 1986.[837] It was reported in 1984 that intralesional injections of triamcinolone were effective in treating a 12-year-old boy.[1271]

A characteristic feature of the lesions is the presence of 'flame figures' which contain eosinophil granules.[1709] Immunofluorescent studies using rabbit antibodies to MBP on skin biopsies from four patients with Wells' disease, were published in 1983, and showed MBP in the infiltrating eosinophils, and in the 'flame figures'. The localization of such large quantities of MBP in these lesions suggested that eosinophils may be involved in the pathogenesis of this disorder.[1391] A histopathological study from Stockholm, Sweden in 1986, showed that the flame figures consisted of eosinophil granules and not collagen bundles,[201] as suggested previously. Eosinophil-rich skin lesions with 'flame figures' have been seen in skin lesions from patients with a number of different diseases, besides Wells' syndrome. These include other skin diseases,[1951] vascular malformations,[1282] and renal diseases, including membranous glomerulonephritis, which disappeared after successful treatment of the skin lesion.[1665]

In a critical review which was published in 1982 of the relationship betwen Kimura's disease, and angiolymphoid hyperplasia with eosinophilia, Rosai, in Minneapolis, USA, argued that they were different diseases, and that the lesions were not always limited to the skin. He suggested that the lesions were due to a 'histiocytoid change' in endothelial cells, which then secreted substances that caused inflammatory cells to localize in the abnormal areas.[1514] Eosinophil chemotactic substances from the lesions of Kimura's disease, and the infiltrating T-cells have been described.[779] I suspect that the abnormal endothelial cells themselves are responsible for inducing the inflammatory changes, now that it is known that endothelial cells can secrete GM-CSF, and increase the survival and toxicity of eosinophils *in vitro*.[1522] These abnormal cells may release several other potent molecules into the blood. For example, large amounts of renin were secreted by the lesions in one hypertensive patient, which disappeared when the skin lesions were removed.[557]

In Toulouse, France, a patient has been described who had angiolymphoid hyperplasia with eosinophilia and a carcinoma of the lung. He was a 58-year-old man with these skin lesions affecting his neck, ears, and scalp. Cytotoxic drugs were effective in eliminating the skin lesions, and in temporarily reducing the size of the tumour.[477]

11.4.2 *Neoplasms of lymphatic vessels*

A number of tumours in which the malignant cells appear to be endothelial cells of lymphatic origin have been found to have marked eosinophilia in the blood or tissues. We have a record of this in an African patient with Kaposi's sarcoma (which is now known to be of lymphatic origin), and it can occur with lymphangiomas and lymphosarcomas.

11.5 Neoplasms of solid tissues

Solid tumours, especially those involving body surfaces, may contain many eosinophils and/or may give rise to a marked increase in blood eosinophils. The same types of tumour produce both types of eosinophil response, but peripheral blood eosinophilia is more common in patients with carcinomas of the lung, kidney, adrenal, thyroid, liver, gallbladder, pancreas, and breast, and in patients with peritoneal mesothelioma or liposarcoma.[1113] This could be of clinical importance, as patients with tumour-associated tissue eosinophilia without an increase in blood eosinophils may have a better prognosis than those without eosinophils in the tumour stroma. Conversely, an increased blood eosinophil count is often linked to the presence of metastases, and a poor prognosis.[1113]

It has been known since before the turn of the century that eosinophils can be a prominent component of solid neoplasms, and there are a large number of case reports describing this feature. One of the most widely quoted studies was carried out at the Mount Sinai Hospital, New York in 1946. Eighteen patients were described, and 15 further case reports were assessed. Most of the tumours were of epithelial, or connective tissue origin. It was concluded that eosinophilia usually indicated that the tumour had disseminated, and that there was a poor prognosis. Ninety per cent had metastases, and these were suspected in a further seven per cent.[843] By 1966 at least 29 patients had been reported with marked eosinophilia in association with solid tumours[137] since the first case report in 1893. This number had increased to 64 by 1977, when they were reviewed in a paper from Zurich, Switzerland.[1624] Although there was some evidence at that time that eosinophilia might be a poor prognostic sign in patients with solid tumours, this view has had to be modified as it may be a good sign in certain neoplasms.

The eosinophil response may involve the tumour itself, the draining lymph nodes, or the blood. In lymph nodes their presence may simply reflect the presence of tumour cells in areas where eosinophils are commonly found. This was supported by the finding that eosinophils were more often seen in the draining lymph nodes of adenocarcinomas of the large bowel than carcinomas of the breast, and the number of eosinophils in these nodes was not altered by the presence of lymphatic metastases.[814]

The incidence of eosinophilia in patients with a solid tumour has been assessed in several studies. It was 4.8 per cent in a group of 252 patients with solid neoplasms who were reported from Israel in 1986,[1617] 3 per cent of patients with cervical carcinoma in Malawi,[1114] and 2 per cent in an unselected series in London.[1113]

11.5.1 *Bone neoplasms*

The majority of eosinophil-rich lytic lesions in bones are eosinophilic granulomas, but there are also a number of primary bone neoplasms in which marked eosinophilia has been noted.

11.5.2 *Breast neoplasms*

An increase in blood eosinophil counts is extremely rare in patients with carcinomas of the breast. In 1983, a study on 419 patients with carcinoma of the breast suggested that when the blood eosinophil count was less than 0.055×10^9/l, that there was a greater risk of recurrence.[1349] This was not confirmed in a separate study on 83 patients reported in 1984.[1524]

In 1987, experiments were reported which showed that tumour-specific serum factors were involved in causing eosinophil infiltration into murine mammary tumours. Mice were implanted with the mammary carcinoma MC2, and after three weeks, although blood eosinophil counts only rose from 0.1 to 0.5×10^9/l, eosinophils began in infiltrate the tumour, with maximal numbers at five weeks. Unrelated tumours in the same animals were not infiltrated.[1815]. The nature of the factor(s) remains to be determined.

11.5.3 *Cardiac neoplasms*

A six-month-old baby boy was reported in 1965, who had an eosinophil count of 53.6×10^9/l, and an unresectable fibroma containing healthy-looking myocardial fibres in the right ventricle, giving rise to tricuspid stenosis.[770] A 59-year-old man with a malignant rhabdomyosarcoma infiltrating the right ventricular cavity was described in 1983, who developed an eosinophil count of 51×10^9/l. The tumour cells were of a large size, and contained NADH-positive striations.[1724] An adult was described in 1985[1017] with a histiocytoid haemangioma in the heart; this produced eosinophilia, which declined after the tumour was removed.

11.5.4 *Digestive system neoplasms*

Neoplasms affecting the gastrointestinal system may give rise to marked eosinophilia. In some patients blood eosinophilia precedes the clinical recognition of the tumour, and in others, the tumour is found to be heavily infiltrated, without producing marked blood eosinophilia. Some evidence has been presented that a marked infiltration into gastrointestinal tumours may indicate a better survival than normal.[1981]

Oesophageal neoplasms Only a handful of reports of oesophageal neoplasms with an eosinophilia, or eosinophil infiltrates into the tumour have been made. In 1980 there was a report of a patient who had marked eosinophilia due to a leiomyoma of the oesophagus, which caused superior vena cava obstruction.[795]

Stomach neoplasms Adenocarcinomas of the stomach are the commonest tumours of the digestive system associated with an increased blood eosinophil count.[1797] These tumours may also be infiltrated with eosinophils. The possible clinical importance of this was studied in Fukuoka, Japan in 1986.[856] Stromal eosinophilia was seen in 157 of 649 (24 per cent) resected tumours, and survival studies showed that in 59 with a marked infiltrate, 29 (57 per cent) were still alive at five years compared with 61 of 158 (39 per cent) patients with lesser numbers of eosinophils in the resected material.

Small intestinal neoplasms Neoplasms of the small intestine are rarely associated with eosinophilia. We have reported an unusual case of a patient with chronic strongylodiasis who developed a small intestinal lymphoma with eosinophilia,[337] and we raised the possibility that chronic parasitic infections could induce a malignant change at the site of parasite localization.

Caecal, colonic, and rectal neoplasms It has been known for many years that there may be a marked infiltrate of eosinophils in gastrointestinal carcinomas.[1981] In 1983, an analysis of 67 colorectal carcinomas in Cleveland, USA showed that although there was great variation in the numbers of eosinophils in sections of the tumours, varying from 0 to 233/mm^2, there was a positive correlation between the numbers of eosinophils and the survival time.[1448] In patients with a good prognosis, these eosinophils were more concentrated in the centre than the edges of the resected speciments.[1447]

In 1987 in Kiel, West Germany, a semi-quantitative assessment of the cells infiltrating 22 invasive adenocarcinomas of the large intestine also showed that although mononuclear cells were the most frequent infiltrating cells, there were sometimes large numbers of eosinophils in the tumour stroma. A moderate or marked infiltrate was seen in 9 of the tumours. The follow-up period was too short to tell whether this might correlate with prognosis.[815]

Eosinophils have been isolated from colonic tumours by enzymatic dissociation and countercurrent centrifugation, which gave 1.8×10^6 eosinophils/g mucosa.[146] This should enable studies to be done on their possible cytotoxic capacity against these neoplasms.

Peritoneal and retroperitoneal neoplasms Occasional reports of patients with slowly growing lesions in the peritoneal cavity who have marked eosinophilia have been published.[1015] We have noted an unusual progressive fibrotic reaction in the abdomen which had many features of a malignant condition, recurring after repeated surgery. See also page 187.

Liver and biliary tract neoplasms Neoplasms in these sites have given rise to marked eosinophilia on rare occasions. In 1986, a patient was reported with a sclerosing bile-duct carcinoma and hypereosinophilia.[1218]

Pancreatic neoplasms Pancreatic neoplasms are rarely associated with eosinophilia, except in the case of tumours which produce large amounts of lipases, which can also give rise to an unusual skin disorder resembling erythema nodosum.[1503] In 1981 a malignant islet cell tumour was described which produced persistent eosinophilia and non-bacterial thrombotic endocarditis.[1292]

Mouth neoplasms Tumours of the lip and tongue can be associated with marked eosinophilia. A large mandibular cyst associated with eosinophilia was reported from India in 1985.[730] Eosinophilia granulomas have also been seen in the soft tissues of the mouth.[677]

11.5.5 *Endocrine neoplasms*

Tumours of the thyroid[1215, 1831] and pituitary can occasionally produce marked eosinophilia.

11.5.6 *Nervous system neoplasms*

Only a few reports of tumours of the brain or spinal cord have described eosinophilia. In 1980, a cerebral histiocytic lymphoma was described which produced eosinophilia, and in 1981, a glioblastoma was reported which produced eosinophilic meningitis.[428]

In 1972 it was reported that a 62-year-old woman with a glioblastoma had blood eosinophil counts of up to 28.5×10^9/l.[353] The tumour was localized and not infiltrated with eosinophils. She only lived for two months, but during that time she developed cardiac failure and other features of eosinophilic heart disease. This case report is important (a) for showing that a localized malignant tumour can induce hypereosinophilia, and (b) that a localized tumour with eosinophilia can induce the development of a distant lesion: eosinophilic endomyocardial disease.

11.5.7 *Neoplasms in the ear, nose and throat regions*

Primary tumours in this region seldom produce an increase in blood eosinophil counts, although tumours of the nasopharynx[1113] and maxillary sinus[1560] are frequently infiltrated with eosinophils. The presence of eosinophils in the stroma of head and neck tumours appears to be a good prognostic indicator, according to a study of 82 tumours, reported from Chapel Hill, USA in 1987.[691]

Twenty-six per cent of nasopharyngeal carcinomas in a series of 422 reported from Kuala Lumpur, Malaysia in1987 contained stromal eosinophilia.[1098] Eosinophil accumulation was also seen in lymphatic metastases, but the clinical significance of these findings remains to be determined.

11.5.8 *Melanomas and squamous cell carcinomas of the skin*

The commonest primary neoplasms in the skin are vascular tumours and melanomas. In one series which was reported in 1977 of 132 patients with malignant melanomas in Houston, USA, 22 per cent had blood eosinophil counts greater than 0.3×10^9/l. This group responded slightly better to chemotherapy in the short term than the others, although their survival was not affected.[1175] In 1977, a 58-year-old man was reported to have developed an eosinophil count of 66.5×10^9/l, four years after he presented with a maglignant melanoma. The high count persisted for the last two months of his life.[1624]

In a study from Bari, Italy in 1986 it was found that 30 advanced and metastatic squamous cell carcinomas contained more inflammatory cells, including eosinophils, than 22 basal cell carcinomas.[330] Studies have been reported on the assessment of eosinophils in squamous cell carcinomas of the skin in several sites,[1109] and on the value of tissue eosinophilia in distinguishing keratoacanthomas from squamous cell carcinomas.[1112]

11.5.9 *Respiratory tract neoplasms*

Respiratory tract neoplasms are amongst the commonest causes of tumour-associated eosinophilia. Eosinophil-rich rumours are almost always large cell bronchial carcinomas. Eosinophils have not been reported in association with oat cell carcinomas, which more commonly produce paracrine effects. In a study which was reported in 1987 from New York on the occurrence of unexplained high blood counts in 105 patients with large cell carcinomas of the lung, there were 3 with hypereosinophilia, and it was suggested that these tumours were producing haemopoietic growth factors.[70] Three patients were reported from London in 1981,[1155] and 5 from Leeds, UK in 1986.[983] A possible role for eosinophils in determining the survival of patients with carcinomas of the lung has come from a study in 1979, showing that an eosinophil infiltrate improved the survival time.[994]

Malignant diseases involving the lung may produce both a peripheral blood and tissue eosinophilia. The commonest are respiratory metastases, but bronchial tumours themselves can cause both local accumulations and occasionally very high peripheral blood eosinophil counts. Bronchial adenomas have also been described with mucoid impaction and local eosinophil accumulation. Histological studies of lung tumours show that diffuse eosinophil infiltration occurs in as many as 50 per cent.[1249] In some cases eosinophilia is marked, and eosinophilotactic substances have been extracted from some of these tumours.[683] Marked eosinophilia can also occur both in Hodgkin's disease and in non-Hodgkin's lymphomas with lung involvement.[202]

11.5.10 *Urogenital neoplasms*

Amongst the many different forms of tumours which affect the urogenital tract, carcinomas of the cervix, bladder, and kidney are most commonly associated with eosinophilia.

Female genital tract neoplasms Carcinomas of the cervix may produce peripheral blood eosinophilia, but biopsies of the cervical tumour more commonly show a marked eosinophil infiltration into and around the tumour cells. Adenocarcinomas of the uterine body may occasionally be infiltrated with large numbers of eosinophils.

In 1937, a 47-year-old woman was described who had a carcinoma of the cervix with blood eosinophil counts of $10–22 \times 10^9$/l. Earlier work on the presence of eosinophils in tumours was reviewed, and it was suggested that they may have stimulated the bone marrow to produce excessive numbers of eosinophils.[1542]

In a study of 460 cases of cervical carcinoma, which was reported in 1981[1114] from Malawi, 13 (3 per cent) had a marked infiltrate of eosinophils into the tumour. They were all large cell non-keratinizing squamous carcinomas. No tumour necrosis or ulceration was seen. In 37 per cent there was a slight infiltrate of eosinophils. In London, 2 per cent of cervical squamous cell carcinomas had an equally marked eosinophil infiltrate.[1113] Six patients were reported from Ann Arbor, USA in 1982.[193] In 1985, 8 patients with tumour stromal eosinophilia were reported from Jacksonville, USA.[1987]

The presence of eosinophils in cervical neoplasms may be linked to an improved prognosis,[909, 1374] and conversely peripheral blood eosinophilia might be a poor prognostic feature. However, in five patients with cervical neoplasms containing many eosinophils and raised blood eosinophil counts who were treated surgically in Taipei, Taiwan, there was a fall in blood eosinophil counts in four patients, and these patients had no recurrences. In the one patient with metastases, blood eosinophil counts remained high, and she died two years later.[1966]

Male genital tract neoplasms Tumours of the male genital tract have only rarely been reported as producing eosinophilia.

Neoplasms of the kidneys, ureters, and bladder Renal tumours may occasionally produce marked eosinophilia.[137] Some bladder tumours have a marked infiltrate of eosinophils. A study in South Africa in 1978 found a marked eosinophil infiltrate in 16 of 151 tumours (11 per cent). Biopsies of adjacent normal tissue also contained an eosinophil infiltrate.[1783] In 1984, in a study of 1305 transitional-cell and squamous-cell carcinomas of the bladder, 36 (2.8 per cent) had a marked eosinophilic infiltrate within the tumour-cell islands and adjacent stroma. They were most numerous where the tumour was invading the muscularis.[1111] Further work on this series showed that they did not give rise to an increased number of eosinophils in the urine.[1110]

11.5.11 *Eosinophilia in animals with solid neoplasms*

A number of reports have been published of eosinophilia in dogs with tumours. One example was of a 2-year-old dog with a palatal fibrosarcoma. Eosinophilia was maximal at diagnosis (11.6×10^9/l). It fell after radiotherapy, then increased as the tumour metastasized.[363] Details of a dog with a mammary carcinoma and marked eosinophilia were published in 1986.[1107]

12. Musculo-skeletal diseases

Rheumatologists seldom see patients with eosinophilia, but when they do, eosinophilia is often strikingly high. The commonest musculo-skeletal diseases which produce eosinophilia are the fasciitis syndromes and rheumatoid arthritis. Patients with musculo-skeletal diseases can also develop eosinophilia due to drug reactions. Occasionally, large numbers of eosinophils are found in the joint fluid of patients with rheumatoid arthritis. The demonstration of increased ECP levels in joint fluid has raised the possibility that eosinophils could be involved in destructive processes within joints.

12.1 Bone and joint diseases

Primary bone diseases of developmental origin are seldom associated with eosinophilia, although this has been reported in patients with fibrous dysplasia of bone.

Eosinophilia is an unusual feature of joint diseases, including rheumatoid arthritis in which it has been most commonly described. Occasionally eosinophilia occurs as an isolated finding in patients with joint disease, and its significance is difficult to define. One example of this was seen in a woman with subchondral osteolysis of the femoral condyles.[860]

12.1.1 *Rheumatoid arthritis*

A slight increase in blood eosinophil counts is common in patients with rheumatoid arthritis, but some may have marked eosinophilia. This can persist for months or years, and in some patients can be life-long, raising the possibility that they have both rheumatoid arthritis and HES. As joint involvement is uncommon in HES, it seems unlikely that the joint disorder is secondary to an underlying eosinophilic process. In these rare cases it is more probable that the two diseases occur together, or that the arthritis has triggered the development of persistent eosinophilia. There are three settings in which eosinophilia occurs in patients with rheumatoid arthritis: in association with a vasculitis, in patients with associated respiratory disease, and in patients taking drugs known to produce eosinophilia, which is discussed under drug hypersensitivity reactions, page 306. Occasionally patients with juvenile or adult rheumatoid arthritis have been found to have serum anti-nuclear antibodies which bind to eosinophil but not neutrophil nuclei.[1517] None of these patients had eosinophilia.

Examples of rheumatoid arthritis with marked eosinophilia were published in the early 1970s.[1731, 1937] Five patients were described in 1971 with the classical features of rheumatoid disease, eosinophil counts of 0.7, 1.5, 2.6, 4.7, and 24 × 10^9/l, raised serum immunoglobulin levels, and relatively low serum complement levels.[1356] Another patient with rheumatoid arthritis and an extensive eosinophilic vasculitis was reported in 1979 from Sweden.[798] In 1980, a 58-year-old man was reported with an eosinophil infiltrate into the soft tissues around his joints and the synovium, which showed fibrinoid degeneration. Many degranulating eosinophils were also found in his skin nodules.[211] Two patients, who presented with active rheumatoid arthritis with nailfold vasculitis and hypereosinophilia were reported from Birmingham, UK in 1985. One, a woman aged 50, had an eosinophil count of 2.8 × 10^9/l at presentation, which persisted. The second patient had an eosinophil count of 1.5 × 10^9/l at presentation, but eosinophilia disappeared after successful treatment with penicillamine.[411] The features of rheumatoid arthritis with vasculitis, including observations on eosinophils in this disease, were reviewed in 1985.[1573] Some patients with rheumatoid arthritis and eosinophilia also have respiratory diseases, raising the possibility that the lungs, rather than the joints, are responsible for eosinophilia. This is most likely in patients with a high serum IgE level, as reported in 1978 in two patients, a man aged 57 and a woman aged 54, who had asthma, pulmonary infiltrates, high serum IgE levels, and cardiovascular involvement.[237] Other patients with respiratory diseases and rheumatoid arthritis who developed marked eosinophilia have been described in 1966,[1432] 1981,[357] and 1982.[368]

In 1985, serum ECP levels were assayed in 42 patients with rheumatoid arthritis in Uppsala, Sweden.[737] They had normal blood eosinophil counts, but the mean serum ECP level was 81 μg/l compared to 15 μg/l in normal people. Serum ECP levels fell after treatment with steroids, and the highest levels were seen in patients with early and active disease. Synovial fluid did not contain eosinophils, although there was a mean ECP concentration of 523 μg/l which did not correlate with serum ECP levels.

12.1.2 *Synovitis and joint fluid*

The finding of more than a small number of eosinophils in synovial fluid and in synovial biopsies is rare. Among the known causes are metastatic adenocarcinomas, parasitic diseases including ascariasis[1794] and guinea-worm infections,[501] radiation,[766] rheumatoid arthritis,[1937] HES,[211] and arthrography.[767] In one patient there was an associated hookworm infection, although no parasite was found in the synovial biopsy.[174] Occasionally, an eosinophilic synovitis can occur without any obvious disease associations.[1120]

A small number of patients have been described who had a strong allergic history.[981] In these patients, the joint involvement was mild, and although it recurred, it seldom lasted for more than a few weeks or months. The eosinophil count in their synovial fluid did not relate to their blood eosinophil counts. In some of them, an eosinophilic synovitis was identified by the presence of Charcot–Leyden crystals in the joint fluid.[1188] Thirteen patients were seen in Sherbrooke, Canada in 1986, and details of seven of these were reported.[215] They were aged 18–51 years, and had developed an acute, painless monoarthritis, following mild injury. The swelling resolved rapidly in most patients. They had a strong personal and family history of allergic diseases, and they all had dermatographism. The synovial fluid contained 5.7–19 $\times$ 10^9 white blood cells/l, and 2.4–9.7 $\times$ 10^9 eosinophils/l, although the blood eosinophil counts were normal. Some intracellular and extracellular Charcot–Leyden crystals were seen, and some of the eosinophils were partially degranulated.

Other reports of patients with an increased number of eosinophils in synovial fluid are:

1. a woman, discussed in 1980, who presented with a swelling of her elbow, a year after it had been injured. The fluid contained 83 per cent eosinophils and resolved without therapy.[1427]

2. an Iraqi child aged 10 with a history of atopy and an eosinophilic monoarthritis, described in 1983.[26]

3. a 15-year-old boy, described in 1987, with a three-month history of recurrent swelling of his knee joints, and a history of occasional asthma attacks for several years. The fluid was aspirated and found to contain 2.2 $\times$ 10^9/l eosinophils. He had a blood eosinophil count of 0.8 $\times$ 10^9/l. The synovitis resolved without treatment.[548]

4. a patient, who was described in France in 1987, who had delayed pressure urticaria, and joint effusions containing 9.5 $\times$ 10^9 eosino phils/l.[1217]

Raised levels of ECP have been found in joint fluid from patients with a variety of inflammatory arthritides, and these correlated with the amounts of lactoferrin present.[735] It is not known what effects, if any, eosinophil products may have within inflamed joints.

12.1.3 *Ankylosing spondylitis*

Although patients with ankylosing spondylitis do not have eosinophilia or histological signs of eosinophil accumulation in their affected joints, serum ECP levels have been found to be three times higher than normal in a group of 48 patients in Uppsala, Sweden. Treatment with sulphasalzine led to an improvement in nearly all the patients, with falls in serum ECP levels possibly due to a direct or indirect action of this drug on ECP secretion.[554]

12.2 Muscle diseases

Chronic inflammatory diseases affecting skeletal muscle seldom produce eosinophilia. It does not occur in giant cell arteritis or polymyalgia rheumatica. An acute inflammatory myopathy with an eosinophil-rich infiltrate is most commonly seen in patients with parasitic diseases such as trichinosis, but it can also occur in patients with actinomycosis,[76] dermatomyositis, and eosinophilic myositis.

12.2.1 *Eosinophilic myositis and polymyositis*

Several reports have been published of an eosinophilic myositis or polymyositis of unknown cause in man, with either widespread lesions in skeletal muscle, or a lump in one muscle group,[1979] which improve on treatment with steroids. Examples of this were reported in:

1. 1977, when three patient were described who had a systemic illness involving the heart, Raynaud's syndrome, splinter haemorrhages, a rash, anaemia, and eosinophilic polymyositis. Two of the patients had previous asthma and hay fever.[1039]

2. 1979, in a 43-year-old man with swelling of the leg muscles and a marked eosinophilic infiltrate into the muscle, but normal blood eosinophil counts.[1704]

3. 1980, when two patients were described: The first was a 47-year-old man with asthma, who had non-pitting oedema of the legs and eosinophilia of 1.96×10^9/l. This responded to treatment with indomethacin. The second was a 30-year-old woman who had tender leg muscles but no eosinophilia, whose symptoms responded to treatment with steroids.[1592]

4. 1981, in a 14-year-old boy, with a mass in the left side of the neck.[25]

5. 1983, in three men, who had peripheral blood eosinophilia and a myositis showing focal necrosis and degeneration with an inflammatory infiltrate containing histiocytes and eosinophils.[1641]

6. 1986, in a 40-year-old man who presented in Saudi Arabia with a swollen left calf muscle. He had pronounced cramps and weakness, but the muscles were not tender. The blood eosinophil count was 1.1×10^9/l, and the serum creatine phosphokinase level was raised to 872 IU/l. Biopsy showed 'focal degenerative changes with collection of eosinophils'.[538]

7. 1986, in a 40-year-old man who had eosinophilic myositis, with episodic weight gain of up to 11 per cent of his normal weight, hyperimmunoglobulin-E, and blood eosinophil counts as high as 41×10^9/l.[1732] His illness lasted for nine years, finally responding to alternate date steroid treatment. Some features of his illness, especially the weight gain and marked eosinophilia, are similar to those seen in patients with episodic angioedema (See page 299). Like them, he had none of the complications which are commonly seen in patients with HES.

Eosinophilic myositis is also a well recognized disease in dogs, sheep, and cattle, where it can present with muscle rupture, possibly as a result of weakening of the tissues by eosinophil granule components.[172] Bovine eosinophilic myositis affects up to 5 per cent of cattle in some parts of the USA. It is usually of unknown cause, although in about 7 per cent of cases, it is due to infection with *Sarcocystis spp*. This organism is a common incidental finding in skeletal and cardiac muscle in adult cattle and sheep, where it rarely gives rise to eosinophil infiltrates or muscle necrosis. The histological and parasitological findings in 53 bovine carcasses and 7 ovine carcasses with eosinophilic myositis in Colorado, USA were reported in 1986.[875] Sarcocystis is spread by cats and dogs which eat contaminated meat and excrete the sporocysts, which infect the livestock. Some cases of unexplained eosinophilia in man may be due to infection with this parasite, although this has not yet been described.

12.3 Fasciitis syndromes

Chronic inflammation in the vascular subcutaneous tissues, which is characteristic of eosinophilic fasciitis and the Spanish toxic allergic syndrome, can produce a very marked increase in blood eosinophil counts. The common denominator in these disorders may be an inflammatory response affecting certain blood vessels, and in both cases there is a dense deposit of fibrous tissue in the affected areas. Eosinophilic fasciitis was first defined by Shulman in 1974,[1619] so it is sometimes called Shulman's syndrome.

12.3.1 *Eosinophilic fasciitis*

Details of over 100 patients have been reported with this striking, but usually benign disease in adults and (less commonly) in children. The main features of the disease, which is a variant of systemic sclerosis, are pain, swelling, and tenderness of the distal part of the forearms and legs, and diffuse induration of the skin and subcutis. Movement of the hands and feet is limited. In several patients, the skin of the abdominal wall and face was involved. It can also produce the carpal tunnel syndrome.[888]

Most series of patients with eosinophilic fasciitis have been published in the USA,[1094] but a woman with the disease was also reported from Zambia. She had an eosinophil count of 2.4×10^9/l, and her symptoms improved after treatment with chloroquine, but not with aspirin or prednisolone.[34]. It has been reported in a child as young as 2 years 10 months.[1933]

In 1975, a report of six patients showed that blood eosinophil counts varied from 0.4 to 2.7×10^9/l, and they were above 1.2×10^9/l in four patients. Serum IgG levels were elevated in most of the patients. There was inflammation and thickening of the fascia between the subcutis and muscle, and the inflammatory lesions contained lymphocytes, plasma cells, and histiocytes, with some fibrin, but few eosinophils were found in the tissues.[1510] Initial descriptions of this condition in 1975 did not describe blood eosinophilia,[112, 1619] and in 1978 only 13 of 67 patients in a large series had transient eosinophilia.[576]

This disease is distinguished from systemic sclerosis by the absence of Raynaud's phenomenon and autoantibodies and by its responsiveness to steroid treatment; and from linear scleroderma, which can produce moderate eosinophilia in half of patients.[532] Nailfold capillary defects are also less common in eosinophilic fasciitis than in systemic sclerosis.[1527]

Eosinophilic fasciitis can be asymptomatic,[82] but later studies have also noted an overlap of eosinophilic fasciitis with systemic sclerosis,[692] especially as involvement of the oesophagus, liver, lymphatic tissues, lungs and heart has been noticed in an increasing number of patients.

The pathogenesis of eosinophilic fasciitis is not clear. In the acute stage, eosinophils are usually present in the affected tissues, but there are no reports yet of whether eosinophil granule constituents are secreted in the areas of injury, or whether they might cause some of the dermal injury, including oedema and fibrosis. The disease may have several causes. It has appeared in association with a number of diseases, including thyroid diseases and haematological disorders, including malignant diseases,[465, 858, 466] but their relationship remains unknown. In 1987 a 34-year-old man was given an HLA identical bone marrow transplant in an attempt to treat his eosinophilic fasciitis and myelodysplasia, but he died from an infection too soon for it to be clear whether the transplant would have been of long term benefit.[1750] In one patient, a graft-versus-host reaction appeared to have induced the development of eosinophilic fasciitis.[1832]

12.3.2 *The Spanish toxic oil syndrome*

From 1 May to 26 December 1981, 20,000 people in Spain were affected by a disease which produced a scleroderma-like syndrome known as the 'toxic oil syndrome'. There were 277 deaths.[1492] Marked eosinophilia was a characteristic feature of this extraordinary disease. In a study of 32 patients, blood eosinophil counts rose in 28 during the first month to a mean of 3.9×10^9/l (range $0.6–11.1 \times 10^9$/l).[35] Many of these eosinophils contained lipid bodies.[613] The diagnostic features were exposure to contaminated oil, the development of eosinophilia, chest X-ray abnormalities, and a variety of musculo-skeletal lesions.

This syndrome was probably the result of an allergic response to, or a direct toxic effect of one or more chemicals in cooking oils. Unfortunately, although considerable efforts have been made to discover the exact cause of the disease, and its sequelae have been described in detail,[709] the syndrome has not been reproduced in experimental animal models, so that its cause and the possible underlying nature of the inflammatory process have not been defined.

As several features of the disease such as thrombi, vascular leakage, and peripheral nerve injury are also seen in patients with other causes for hypereisonophilia, it has been suggested that some of the complications of the disease, including the peripheral nerve lesions,[1491] could have been caused by the release of granule proteins from eosinophils. Thrombi, a major problem in patients with the idiopathic hypereosinophilic syndrome, caused the deaths of 46 of 258 (18 per cent) affected people in one series, and it was suggested that eosinophilia which was present in 88 per cent of the patients for over six months could have been an important factor in producing the thrombi, as the highest blood eosinophil counts occurred at the time when thrombi were most prevalent: in the second and third months of the disease.[288]

12.4 Sjögren's syndrome

Sjögren's syndrome can produce a moderate increase in blood eosinophil counts. A case report of a 24-year-old man who had this disease, with 3.8×10^9/l eosinophils was described in 1984.[541] Eosinophils were also present in the skin, liver, and bone marrow.

13. Digestive system diseases

A wide variety of diseases of the gastrointestinal tract are associated with eosinophil infiltrates. These include parasitic infections, inflammatory bowel diseases, connective tissue diseases,[437] drug hypersensitivity reactions,[1161] and eosinophilic gastroenteritis,[294] but only in a proportion of these patients is there an increase in blood eosinophil counts.

The presence of many eosinophils in the lamina propria of the small and large intestines of patients with intestinal parasitic diseases has suggested that this is one of the major sites in which eosinophils act as effector cells in immunity to parasites and other potential disease-forming components of the bowel lumen. Although the intestine has been proposed as a possible site for the elimination of eosinophils in patients with blood eosinophilia, intestinal biopsies in man have not shown an increased number of eosinophils in patients with eosinophilia but without intestinal disease.[918] In rats aboard the Cosmos 1129 satellite, eosinophils were seen to accumulate in the lamina propria of the intestines, possibly as a result of the stress involved.[724] It is not known if a similar event occurs in human astronauts or in people in other stressful situations.

The finding which we reported in 1985 of large numbers of activated eosinophils in intestinal biopsies from patients with allergic gastroenteritis, with deposits of ECP and EDN/EPX, has suggested that eosinophils could be involved in the toxic reactions which cause damage to the bowel wall in this disease.[955] The peritoneal cavity can also contain many eosinophils in patients with the serous form of eosinophilic gastroenteritis, and they also appear to be activated.

13.1 Oesophageal diseases

Eosinophils have been described in the oesophagus in a number of disorders, including eosinophilic gastroenteritis,[585, 551, 1048] herpes simplex infection of the oesophagus, reflux oesophagitis, and achalasia,[1026] where it has been suggested that they damage the myoenteric plexus (Dahl 1987, personal communication).

An interest has developed since the early 1980s in the possibility that the presence of oesophageal intraepithelial eosinophils may be a useful histological feature for diagnosing reflux oesophagitis. Their occurrence in 10 patients with reflux oesophagitis was reviewed in 1985, when it was linked to the presence of oesophageal strictures in 3.[1048] This was supported by two studies on adults in 1984,[216] and children with the disease in 1985.[1618] However, in 1987, a report from New Haven, Connecticut, USA showed no differences in intraepithelial eosinophils in 73 adults with reflux oesophagitis, compared with 12 normal volunteers.[1798]

13.2 Diseases of the stomach and peptic ulcers

Eosinophils can be prominent in biopsy samples from patients with gastritis. Eosinophils are not a component of duodenal ulcers or most forms of duodenitis.

13.3 Eosinophilic gastroenteritis

Eosinophilic gastroenteritis has been recognized since 1937[901] to be an uncommon disease which can affect several parts of the intestines, producing eodema of the bowel wall, and a dense infiltrate of eosinophils. The gastric antrum[1838] and proximal small intestine are most commonly involved, but the oesophagus and large bowel can also be affected. The blood eosinophil count is raised in only 20 per cent of patients. Males have the disease twice as commonly as females, and it usually occurs in adults in their third decade, although 15 children with the disease had been described by 1977.[803] Further cases in children were reported in 1983.[345]

It has been divided into two forms: a polypoid form (which has sometimes been confusingly called inflammatory fibroid polyps or eosinophilic granuloma of the gastrointestinal tract (See page 186), and a diffuse type.[212] When the disease is localized it is sometimes difficult to distinguish from a tumour.

A review of the literature up to 1967 showed that 33 were of the polypoid type and 104 had diffuse disease.[1544] When the diffuse form of the disease affects the mucosa, it produces mălabsorption, protein loss, and anaemia. When the muscle layer is affected it can cause intestinal and biliary tract obstruction,[1528] and when the serosa is infiltrated with eosinophils, there is peritoneal involvement with ascites, which may contain many eosinophils. (See Fig. 13.1.) It is unlikely to be caused by a hypersensitivity reaction, as the serum IgE level is raised in only 20 per cent of patients, and proven food hypersensitivity reactions involving the gut in adults only rarely produce eosinophilia.[1585]

The disease can remit spontaneously, but relapses may also take place.[1685] It was first suggested in 1979, on the basis of the histological appearances of the small intestine of a 19-year-old man with eosinophilic gastroenteritis, that eosinophil products may injure the gut in eosinophilic gastroenteritis,[294] but this has yet to be shown directly. It is usually treated

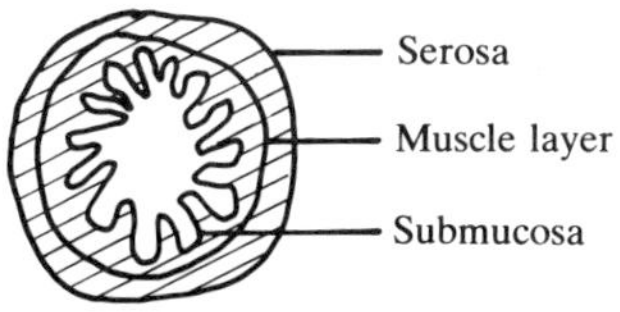

Fig. 13.1. Eosinophilic gastroenteritis. Involvement of each of the layers of the intestine produces different syndromes. Submuscosal lesions can be polyploid or diffuse. Redrawn from Spry (1984)[1685] with permission.

with 20–40 mg prednisolone for one to two weeks, but a tissue diagnosis is desirable before this is begun, as other disorders can produce a similar clinical picture.[1838] Surgery is only necessary if perforation or continued bleeding occurs.

The oesophagus can be involved in eosinophilic gastroenteritis. Seven cases had been reported up to 1985,[551] including a report in a 3-month-old infant boy in 1978.[585] They may have upper oesophageal strictures and/or polyploid lesions in the oesophagus.

The colon can occasionally be involved in eosinophilic gastroenteritis. Twenty patients were reported up to 1985,[1267] and a further case report was published in 1986.[1131]

The ultrasound appearances of antral thickening in a patient with eosinophilic gastroenteritis was reported in 1987, in a 15-year-old boy in Karachi, Pakistan.[936] The radiological appearances were discussed in 1981.[1158]

The pathology of eosinophilic gastroenteritis has been well described in a review of 120 patients in the UK made in 1978, which included 9 new patients.[883] Immunohistochemical studies on a resected stomach from a 50-year-old patient with eosinophilic gastroenteritis in 1985 showed many IgE stained mast cells in the areas rich in eosinophils, and it was suggested that mast cell degranulation may have contributed to the development of the lesions.[1350]

A 14-year-old girl with eosinophilic gastroenteritis who was described in 1985 was found to have large numbers of activated eosinophils in the lamina propria in duodenal biopsies, and their presence correlated with the degree of histological abnormality. She had 1.2–3.1 $\times$ 10^9/l blood eosinophils, which were activated. Unlike her brother, who also had eosinophilic gastroenteritis but no activated eosinophils, she had malabsorption. This suggests that degranulation of activated eosinophils in the gut could have caused her mucosal defects.[955]

13.3.1 *Eosinophilic ascites*

Eosinophilic ascites is a feature of eosinophilic gastroenteritis, when the serosal layer of the small intestine is involved. Adjacent lymph nodes are often enlarged, and the spleen may be incrased in size. By 1981, there had been 15 case reports of this condition.[757] For example:

1. a man aged 36 was described in 1967 who developed ascites with a blood eosinophil count of 2.1×10^9/l. There were 15 pints of ascites containing up to 98 per cent eosinophils. A pleural fluid collection contained 1.7×10^9/l eosinophils. The small bowel was thickened, and there was delayed transit time. He responded well to treatment with ACTH.[1544]

2. in 1970 two adults, a woman aged 25 and a man aged 57, were reported with these features and eosinophilic ascites.[979]

3. In 1979, a patient was described with widespread eosinophilic gastroenteritis involving the intestines, from the gastric antrum to the sigmoid colon, with eosinophilic ascites.[1062]

4. In 1979, a further example was given, and earlier reports were reviewed.[1184]

5. In 1985 a boy aged 9 years was described with eosinophilic ascites.[1795]

An eosinophilic ascites has also been described in patients undergoing peritoneal dialysis (see page 221), and a small number of other diseases, including granulomatous diseases. In two men aged 34 and 25 with widespread eosinophilic granulomas affecting lymph nodes, there were areas of necrosis and many infiltrating eosinophils, as reported in 1977.[1482] A patient with HES and endomyocardial disease had ascites which contained 86–90 per cent eosinophils, $3.2–10.4 \times 10^9$/l.[15] Spontaneous *E. coli* peritonitis, with large numbers of eosinophils in the peritoneal fluid was reported in one patient.[1525] This association is difficult to explain.

13.4 Inflammatory fibroid polyps

Granulomas, which are occasionally rich in eosinophils, can be found in the gastric antrum and occasionally in the wall of the small intestine. The pathogenesis of these diffuse or polypoid benign lesions is not clear. They have been referred to as eosinophilic granulomas of the gastrointestinal tract, but are probably best called inflammatory fibroid polyps.[884] A review of the pathology of 64 polyps was published in 1984.[1615] It is unusual for these patients to have an increase in blood eosinophils, even though the lesions can contain many eosinophils. Remnants of the herring parasite *Eustoma rotundum* have been seen in a few patients.[1012] The typical clinical features of this disease, which affected the ileum of a 55-year-old man, and produced an intersusception, was described in 1987.[387] It was treated successfully by resection.

13.5 Chronic eosinophilic pseudotumours in the abdominal cavity

A number of reports have been published of a puzzling disease or group of diseases, which produces progressing nonmalignant but chronic inflammatory lesions in the abdomen, with infiltrating eosinophils and blood eosinophilia. Examples include:

1. a patient who was reported from Houston, USA in 1980.[183] There were extensive necrotic eosinophil-rich lesions in the upper part of the stomach. These spread to the colon, diaphragm, and lung, and did not respond to steroid treatment.

2. a patient in Bilbao, Spain, who developed a retroperitoneal 'inflammatory fibrous histiocytoma' with eosinophilia.[1862]

3. a woman aged 23 years from the Antilles, who had a marked enterocolitis and eosinophilia, which did not improve with steroid treatment, reported in 1983.[1145] A colectomy was done, but the disease recurred in her rectum, producing tumour-like granulomas infiltrated with eosinophils, which caused her death seven years after presentation.

4. a 17-year-old Laotian woman who had a progressive disease with necrotic granulomas in lymphoid tissues, which induced a marked eosinophil infiltration and blood eosinophilia, with raised serum IgE.[338] The lesions regressed on steroid treatment, then recurred, and produced abdominal venous thrombi and small bowel necrosis, which were fatal.

5. I have also seen sections of the abdominal masses which developed in a young woman in the UK with an undiagnosed disease of this type. Her illness progressed slowly over several years, to produce large abdominal sclerosing lesions containing eosinophils, which finally produced a cuirass of chronic inflammatory tissue around the lower abdominal contents.

13.6 Enteritis and enterocolitis

13.6.1 *Coeliac disease*

Patients with coeliac disease do not have an increase in the number of blood eosinophils, although there is an increased number of eosinophils in their jejunal biopsies. In 1984, a report on 47 patients in Budapest, Hungary found that the number of eosinophils in the lamina propria was raised, and inversely related to villous height and the number of mast cells. The relative numbers of mast cells and eosinophils returned towards normal after gluten withdrawal.[1000]

13.6.2 *Cow's milk and soy protein allergy*

Cow's milk and soy protein allergy are important causes of intestinal disease in young children. This may take the form of rectal bleeding or chronic diarrhoea, with the small intestine or rectum affected, providing the two main forms of the disease: allergic gastroenteritis and allergic proctitis. Some patients have a similar disease called chronic nonspecific diarrhoea. In eight boys aged between one and five years, with chronic nonspecific diarrhoea and normal IgE levels, blood eosinophil counts were normal, but the number of eosinophils in duodenal biopsies was increased to $155/mm^2$ from a mean of $62/mm^2$ in seven normal subjects.[297]

Allergic gastroenteritis In 1986, details of 38 children aged less than two years with allergic gastroenteritis were analysed in Boston, USA.[689] They had vomiting, pain, some rectal bleeding, weight loss, an allergic history, anaemia, and increased serum IgE. The blood eosinophil count was raised in most patients up to $7.2 \times 10^9/l$, and was greater than one $\times 10^9/l$ in 21 patients. Mucosal abnormalities were present in biopsies from the gastric antrum, in the small intestine in 79 per cent, in the oesophagus in 60 per cent, and in the body of the stomach in 52 per cent. The inflammatory lesions, which contained scattered eosinophils, were usually diffuse and marked in the antrum and oesophagus, but generally focal and mild in the small intestine and stomach. Most of these children had multiple relapses, despite dietary elimination of possible allergens, but many recovered after steroids were given.

In severn children in the UK with diarrhoea due to cow's milk allergy, high serum IgE levels, and mean blood eosinophil counts of $0.87 \times 10^9/l$, there was a marked increase in the number of eosinophils in duodenal biopsies from a mean of $62/mm^2$ in controls to $368/mm^2$.[297] In a study from Lund, Sweden in 1982, serial serum ECP measurements were made after oral challenge of 18 patients with cow's milk intolerance.[1946] No consistent patterns emerged. In 7, serum ECP levels fell, whereas in 5 others it rose before falling again.

Allergic proctitis Allergy to milk and soy proteins in babies can give rise to a severe eosinophilic inflammatory reaction in the colon and rectum.[321, 874] Fifteen infants with this disorder were studied in Boston, USA in 1986.[689] Their disease began at less than six months of age, and all were under two years old when they presented with rectal bleeding alone or in combination with diarrhoea. Eight had increased blood eosinophil counts, reaching 1.9×10^9/l in one. In most cases there was a diffuse increase of eosinophils in the rectal lamina propria, together with a focal infiltration of the epithelium by eosinophils. They all recovered when the dietary antigens to which they had become sensitized were stopped.

13.7 Crohn's disease

A small body of evidence suggests that eosinophils are an important feature of the lesions of Crohn's disease. For example, in a study on 114 patients with Crohn's disease treated by 'curative' resection of the terminal ileum and part of the colon, there was a recurrent rate of 72 per cent within the first year. Ileal biopsies at this stage showed a marked inflammatory cell infiltrate in the lamina propria, containing numerous eosinophils, with fusion and blunting of the villi.[1534] These abnormal histological features were not always associated with symptoms.

In 1980, ultrastructural studies on surgical specimens from 13 patients with Crohn's disease showed that some eosinophils had become partially degranulated, with loss of many of the granule cores.[484, 488] When considered in relation to the degranulation of mast cells, and damage to vascular endothelium, antonomic nerves, and muscle cells in these sites, it was suggested that eosinophil constituents could be responsible, in part, for these changes.

13.8 Colonic diseases

Eosinophils may be a prominent component of the lesions in inflammatory bowel diseases.

13.8.1 *Ulcerative colitis*

Little is known about the properties or possible roles of eosinophils in ulcerative colitis, although they become more prominent in the blood and/or rectal mucosa as the disease progresses and becomes chronic. Genetic factors may be involved, as Indian patients in one series had blood eosinophilia at presentation,[155] whereas there was no increase in the number of tissue eosinophils in another series of Caucasian patients with a first severe attack of ulcerative colitis.[1935] Rectal biopsies have usually shown increased numbers of eosinophils just prior to[1100] or during relapses.

In 1966, during a trial of dietary treatment of ulcerative colitis, measurements were made of the number of blood and colonic eosinophils. Little relationship was found between them, although in some patients, blood counts rose during relapses, when the tissue eosinophil counts were highest.[1955] A report in 1987 failed to find a direct relationship between the number of eosinophils in rectal biopsies and the severity of ulcerative colitis, or an unfavourable response to treatment.[1558]

Eosinophilic enterocolitis has been described in dogs, cats, and in a captive orangutan which had diarrhoea with malbsorption, steatorrhoea, and blood eosinophilia of up to 7.2×10^9/l. The lamina propria of the small intestine and colon contained many eosinophils, and there was stunting of villi. The disease responded to treatment with oral prednisolone.[326] A dog with marked thickening of the colon, and mucosal ulcers with a marked eosinophilic infiltrate, has been described in Holland. The animal did not have an increase in marrow or blood eosinophils, but did have thrombi on the heart valves, with emboli in several organs.[1836]

13.9 Rectal diseases

Increased numbers of eosinophils in rectal biopsies are seen in a number of different disorders. These include parasitic infections, inflammatory bowel disease,[773] and allergic proctitis due to dietary allergens in children, where the eosinophil infiltrate is largely confined to the crypts.[689]

13.10 Liver and biliary tract diseases

Many different types of eosinophil-rich granulomas can produce an eosinophil infiltrate in the liver. Other major causes are parasitic infections, drug hypersensitivity reactions, and involvement in malignant diseases. Two reports of chronic active hepatitis with eosinophilia have been published.[1357, 761] Both patients improved with steroid treatment. Acute liver rejection with a marked eosinophil infiltrate following liver transplantation has also been noted in one patient.[1656] Patients with HES often show an infiltrate of eosinophils into the liver.

Sometimes, large number of eosinophils are found in gallbladders removed for cholecystitis. In one series of 625 resected gallbladders reported in 1972, 16 contained many eosinophils.[592] The infiltrate consisted almost entirely of eosinophils in three patients, all of whom were young women. The eosinophils were mainly subserosal, and in the muscle coats of the gallbladder. Other case reports have been published of patients with an eosinophilic infiltrate into the gallbladder,[1050] including patients with eosinophilic infiltrates into the cystic duct and lymph nodes,[241] and a patient with hepatic echinococcosis.[1531] Eosinophilia has also been noted in a patient with primary sclerosing cholangitis.[1269]

13.11 Pancreatic diseases

An acute pancreatitis can occasionally cause marked eosinophilia,[1252] and there are reports of three patients with an unusual combination of partial lipodystrophy, pancreatitis, and eosinophilia.[1654, 1367] Although alcohol-related pancreatitis is rarely found associated with eosinophilia, in 1985 a report from Toronto, Canada suggested that the pain of chronic pancreatitis related to alcohol could be due to toxic effects of eosinophils on nerves in pancreatic perineural areas.[946] This was based on the finding of a correlation between the number of eosinophils in these sites and pain severity in resected pancreatic tissues from 50 patients with chronic pancreatitis.

14. Diseases of the mouth

Eosinophils are not prominent in most of the diseases that affect the mouth and teeth, except for eosinophilic granuloma, which can affect the jaws and adjacent teeth. Eosinophils are probably not an important part of the protective mechanism of the mouth against infectious agents. The reason for this is not known, but it may be related to the different types of epithelial barrier which are found in each part of the gastrointestinal tract: eosinophils are commonest in sites where there is columnar epithelium.

There is an unusual type of chronic (traumatic) inflammatory ulcer of the oral cavity, which is often rich in eosinophils. Eighteen cases had been reported by 1981. The features have been the subject of reviews in 1983,[511] 1984,[1639] and 1986.[1992] It is a rare but benign disease of the oral cavity, usually affecting the tongue, and occurs in all age groups. It has been described under a number of different names, and is unrelated to histiocytosis X. It can last for several weeks, but may be treated conservatively with steroids. In 1987, a patient with this disease was reported to have multiple linear ulcers and fissures on the tongue in association with Waldenström's macroglobulinaemia.[2010]

15. Respiratory tract diseases

The respiratory tract, like the gastrointestinal tract, is one of the major sites for eosinophil localization in tissues in a wide variety of diseases. As in the gut, it has been suggested that this is because eosinophils are involved in the protective mechanisms of columnar epithelium. The capacity of eosinophils to secrete toxic basic proteins which can kill a variety of potential pathogens and damage the airways, and their ability to make molecules which affect the functions of smooth muscle and goblet cells, could also be important in these sites. The eosinophil EPO–H_2O_2–halide system can kill type II pneumocytes *in vitro*, and could produce tissue injury in patients with asthma and pulmonary eosinophilia.[24]

The special relationship between eosinophils and mast cells in the lung has been a subject of research for many years. A consensus view is now emerging that eosinophils are involved in inducing tissue mast cell degranulation. The earlier view, that they were involved in inhibiting mast-cell-mediated products, now seems rather unlikely.

The principal disorders in which eosinophils are involved in respiratory tract diseases are allergic and hypersensitivity disorders, but the presence of particularly large numbers of eosinophils in intrinsic asthma is an important fact which cannot be explained on the basis of an exogenous allergic stimulus producing eosinophil localization within the lung. It suggests that the factors involved in localizing eosinophils in the lung are produced locally within the lung itself. Eosinophils are only rarely found in normal lung tissue, and their presence in moderate or larger amounts is always associated with a disease process, either in the main bronchi or the peripheral lung tissues. It is unusual to find eosinophils in sputum, except when there is damage or loss of the respiratory epithelium. Eosinophils may be involved in stripping epithelial cells from bronchi, and there is experimental evidence to support this view.

Measurements of the amounts of eosinophil granule components in bronchial secretions in different diseases has now begun, but it is not yet clear whether this is useful in distinguishing between different lung diseases, or in following the effects of treatment.

Eosinophils are prominent in many disorders which affect the respiratory tract, and a number of classifications have been proposed. In 1952 it was recommended that a distinction should be made between patients with and without asthma.[369] In 1981, Schatz and colleagues suggested that classifications should be based on the aetiology of the respiratory disease,[1567] and I used this approach in my review of this topic in 1983[1684] which is also followed here with permission. It is also useful to subdivide these diseases on an anatomical basis into those which predominantly affect the bronchi, lungs, and pleura.

15.1 Sputum eosinophils

Sputum is readily available from most patients with respiratory tract disease. It is best to look for eosinophils in an unstained sample, viewed under a cover slip on a glass slide. If necessary, the sputum can be smeared, and stained with one of the Romanowsky stains. In patients with a history and signs of asthma, the presence of large numbers of eosinophils without many other inflammatory cells favours this diagnosis, aspirin-sensitive asthma, eosinophilic pheumonia, or bronchopulmonary aspergillosis. The presence of few eosinophils and many neutrophils favours a chest infection with or without one of the other causes of chest disease. Other components of the sputum which are worth looking for are Curschmann's spirals, Charcot–Leyden crystals, corpora amylacea, ciliated epithelial cells, and macrophages, including lipid ladened macrophages.

15.2 Bronchoalveolar lavage

The introduction of bronchoalveolar lavage (BAL) in the early 1970s has led to a greater knowledge of the nature of the cells and components which are secreted into the bronchial lumen and bronchoalveolar spaces in different disorders. Comparisons are usually made between the components in bronchial washings and in segmental washings. The largest yields of alveolar eosinophils have been from patients with eosinophilic pneumonia,[429, 715] but they are also prominent in BAL fluid from patients with allergic bronchopulmonary aspergillosis, asthma, and asbestosis.[1506]

Eosinophils were not found in BAL fluid from 18 non-smoking normal subjects in 1987.[525] Smokers have both a mild increase in blood eosinophil counts[922] and increased numbers of eosinophils in BAL fluid.

In 1984, a study at the NIH, Bethesda, USA showed that in patients with interstitial lung diseases, often more than 5 per cent of BAL cells were eosinophils,[409] The highest proportions of eosinophils were seen in patients with idiopathic pulmonary fibrosis (44 per cent of patients had greater than 5 per cent eosinophils), and they were also seen in fluid from some patients with sarcoidosis, hypersensitivity pneumonitis, collagen-vascular diseases, histiocytosis-X and chronic eosinophilic pneumonia.

The use of BAL to study the cellular and protein content of the bronchi in patients with asthma has been carried out in France, the USA, and in other countries since about 1980. It was found to be a safe procedure in patients with mild symptomatic asthma, both before[676] and after bronchial challenge.[1203]

15.3 Bronchial diseases

Asthma and hay-fever are the commonest cause of a raised blood eosinophil count in Western countries. The suggestion that eosinophils might be involved in the pathogenesis of several diseases affecting the bronchi and interstitial tissues of the lung has been a major stimulus for research into the association between eosinophils and respiratory diseases.

15.3.1 *Asthma*

The presence of eosinophils in the blood and sputa of patients with asthma has been known since 1889.[693] Later, histological studies showed that there were often many eosinophils in the bronchial submucosa of patients who died from asthmatic attacks, although this was not always the case.[1276, 667] The functions of eosinophils in these lesions were unknown, but their presence in the blood and sputum was taken to indicate that an allergic reaction was taking place in the lungs. This was useful in distinguishing patients with exacerbations of asthma from those who had acute respiratory infections, in whom blood eosinophil counts usually fell.

Later, as knowledge of the possible pathogenetic roles of mast cells in asthma developed, experiments were done with blood eosinophils to see whether they were able to detoxify products which were secreted from mast cells. The outcome of this work was interpreted in some centres as showing a beneficial role for eosinophils in asthma.

Knowledge of the toxicity of eosinophils themselves to human tissues has led to different experiments being done to see whether eosinophils could induce some of the pathophysiological features of asthma. Many of these ideas developed from studies at the Mayo Clinic which were reviewed in 1985[660] and 1986.[604] It seems probable that eosinophils may produce acute and chronic effects on the lungs in asthma, through their capacity:

(1) to secrete leukotriene C4, which can cause bronchial smooth muscle contraction,

(2) to secrete PAF-acether which produces bronchial hypersensitivity and vascular permeability;[1352]

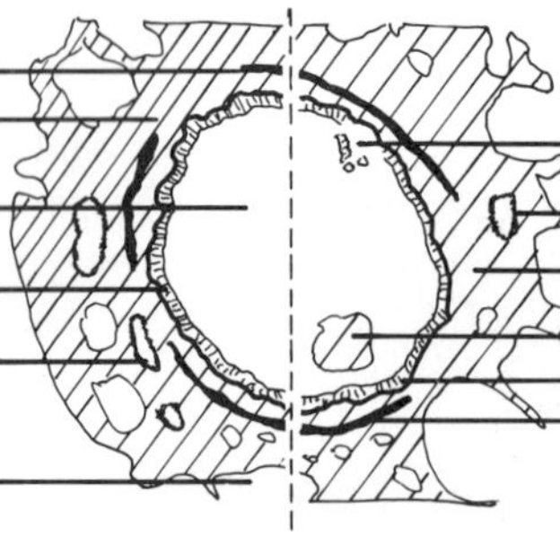

Fig. 15.1. Eosinophils and asthma. Eosinophils are associated with each of the major structural abnormalities seen in the bronchi of patients with asthma.

(3) to secrete toxic granule basic proteins, including MBP and EPO, which can induce mucosal cell desquamation, and injury to ciliated epithelial cells which help to reduce bronchial tone[574] and remove mucus and injured epithelial cells;

(4) to release reactive oxygen products, which can cause direct membrane damage to respiratory cells; and

(5) to stimulate mucus production from goblet cells. See Fig. 15.1.

Current clinical research is now designed to test these hypotheses. Experiments are beginning to show that in spontaneous or bronchial-challenge-induced asthma there are alterations in blood, sputum, and bronchoalveolar eosinophil structure, metabolism, activation, and functions. Eosinophils from patients with asthma have many of the properties required to mediate toxic-effector functions against normal tissues, although the overall importance of these findings in spontaneous attacks of asthma is still not known.

Antigen challenge of patients with mild asthma is beginning to show how these alterations in the properties of eosinophils come about. At the same time, it has become clear that eosinophils are probably more important in producing some of the features of the late asthmatic response after antigen challenge, than the acute changes which are linked more closely to the presence in the lungs of other inflammatory cells, such as mast cells, neutrophils, and macrophages. The efficacy of steroids in preventing late (nocturnal) asthmatic reactions following antigen challenge, and their variable effects in the acute response, confirms that the pathogenesis of the two events is different. As steroids are effective inhibitors of eosinophil degranulation *in vitro*, this finding supports an important role for eosinophils in late stage reactions. In animal models of late-phase asthma granulocyte depletion at the time of antigen challenge, prevented the late response and the increased bronchial reactivity.[1032]

The possibility that eosinophils may cause some of the serious features of asthma has led several pharmaceutical companies to search for drugs which may inhibit eosinophil activation and degranulation. In most of these studies, human or animal eosinophils have been stimulated *in vitro*, with and without test drugs. These are also several more ambitious projects in experimental animals, to study the systemic effects of drugs on eosinophil reactions in the lungs, peritoneum, and other sides (see below). The fruits of these experiments may well extend to other diseases where eosinophils are also thought to have deleterious effects.

The histopathology of asthma The pathology of fatal asthma has shown large numbers of eosinophils associated with areas of desquamation, bronchial plugging, and basement membrane thickening, which are the characteristic features of the late stage. Eosinophils are usually found around bronchial vessels, in the parenchyma of the lung, and under the submucosa. The most marked histopathological feature in light and electronmicrographs of bronchial biopsies from patients with asthma is damage to ciliated and other epithelial cells. This finding was reported in 1985, in a study of 24 endobronchial biopsy samples from different levels of the respiratory tract, in 8 patients with asthma who were studied by Laitinen and colleagues in Finland.[1021] Eosinophils were not seen in any of these samples.

The presence of MBP in histological sections of the lungs of patients with asthma was shown in a study which was reported in 1982 using fluorescein-labelled rabbit antibodies to MBP. After digestion of lung sections, the MBP was visualized in tissue eosinophils, as well as along the lining of bronchioles close to areas of damaged bronchial epithelium and mucus plugs. It was suggested that MBP was secreted into the lungs, and that it could have been responsible for the mucosal damage.[563]

Blood eosinophils in asthma Although eosinophilia has been thought to be a hallmark of intrinsic asthma,[1568] this is not always the case. For example, among 15 patients with extrinsic, and 12 with intrinsic, asthma not on steroids, who were studied in Holland, mean blood eosinophil counts were only 0.29 and $0.24 \times 10^9/l$ respectively.[221]. This shows that an increase in blood eosinophil counts is not a prerequisite for this disease, especially in its milder forms. But in patients with eosinophilia, there may be a link between blood eosinophil counts and bronchial responsiveness, as measured by the histamine PC20 method.[1760]

It has been taught for many years that alterations in the number of eosinophils in the blood and/or sputum can be useful for predicting steroid responsiveness, and monitoring steroid treatment. However, in a study in

1983 on acute exacerbations in 11 patients with chronic asthma, 3 had normal blood eosinophil counts. Measurements of the total number of eosinophils per day present in the sputum were more useful in predicting the response to steroids and monitoring their effects.[95]

The number of light density eosinophils in the blood may be a more useful measure of their involvement in asthma. This possibility arises from a study which was reported from the Mayo Clinic in 1985, showing that the proportions of light density eosinophils in the blood of normal people, patients with asthma, and patients with HES were 10 per cent, 35 per cent, and 95 per cent respectively.[611] A correlation between the log eosinophil count and the per cent light density eosinophils was seen among 22 patients studied. Further studies on the relationship of the number of light density eosinophils to disease activity and responses to treatment are awaited with interest.

It is possible that blood eosinophils from patients with extrinsic and intrinsic asthma are more activated than in normal people. This stems from the finding in 1986[1752] that when blood eosinophils from 26 patients with extrinsic asthma and 27 with intrinsic asthma were incubated with the calcium ionophore, they released significantly more LTC4 than normal subjects: 23.5 ± 14.8, 24.6 ± 20.6, and 8.3 ± 7.7 ng/10^6 cells, respectively. However, this was not seen in a previous study in 1984[1603] on 32 other patients.

Little is known about the properties of eosinophils in asthma, although it was shown that the content of arylsulphatase in the light density eosinophils of patients with asthma was normal.[921]

Serum eosinophil protein levels in asthma In 1977, work in Scandinavia showed that resting serum ECP levels were lower in patients with asthma than in normals or patients with eosinophilia due to other causes, although EDN/EPX levels were invariably raised.[1853] This was not due to a defect in eosinophils, as the ECP content of blood eosinophils in patients with asthma was normal.[382] No difference was seen in the diurnal variations in blood eosinophil counts or serum ECP levels in patients with asthma, compared with controls.[384] In 12 patients with asthma who were given an inhalation challenge, the serum ECP level rose at 1 hour, while blood eosinophil counts fell at 3 hours, only rising to higher levels at 24 hours. There was no relationship between the peak serum ECP levels and the severity of late reactions. As the EDN/EPX levels did not follow this pattern, it was suggested that serum ECP was being cleared at a different rate from EDN/EPX.[383]

Sputum eosinophils in asthma Large numbers of eosinophils in sputum are a feature of several diseases, especially eosinophilic pneumonia and aspirin-induced asthma. They are also increased in other forms of asthma and bronchial allergic responses. They are easily seen in phase-contrast preparations of fresh sputa, but it is also possible to carry out accurate differential counts on stained smears.[1858]. However, they are best assessed and quantified in timed samples. In 24 hour collections of sputa from a group of 11 patients with asthma, the mean number of cells was 8×10^7, and 26 per cent were eosinophils.[95]

Sputum eosinophil protein levels in asthma In a study on 15 patients admitted to hospital with asthma, the MBP content of the sputa was 0.3 to 92 μg/ml, geometric mean 7.1 μg/ml. Raised levels in sputa from a consecutive series of 100 patients with a variety of chest diseases showed that high sputum MBP levels were related to the presence of asthma and not other diseases. In a later study by the same group on 116 patients with a variety of respiratory diseases, including 10 patients in hospital with asthma, raised sputum MBP levels were again correlated with the presence of asthma.[460] As 10 μg MBP/ml was previously found to be capable of causing damage to human bronchial epithelium in tissue culture,[1247] it was suggested that the MBP in these patients was causing direct mucosal injury.[606]

The amount of CLC protein in sputa was raised in patients with asthma, but it was also high in other respiratory diseases, suggesting that this measurement does not have as high a discriminant value as sputum MBP assays.[460] LTC4 was not detected in the sputa of 17 patients with asthma, although it was detected in sputa from patients with cystic fibrosis.[1295]

Bronchoalveolar lavage in asthma By 1987, over 12 studies had been reported on the use of BAL to assess the number of inflammatory cells in the lower airways of patients with asthma. They all showed a similar picture: that in most patients eosinophils were increased in BAL fluid, but that they were only a small proportion of the recovered cells: less than 1 per cent[448, 579, 971] except in patients with aspirin-sensitive asthma,[676] when larger numbers were found.

Data on 171 patients who were studied in Montpelier, France were summarized in 1987. There were often no excess eosinophils in the lavage fluid in asymptomatic patients, and the mean number of eosinophils in 50 ml fluid in 93 symptomatic patients was only 7×10^5. No excess eosinophils were found in patients taking steroids.[675] In another study in 1987, it was found that only 0.6 ± 1.0 per cent of the cells in BAL fluid from 14 patients with mild asthma were eosinophils.[525] Even though they are present in small numbers, BAL eosinophils are metabolically active and can develop chemoluminescence *in vitro*[333] and synthesize LTC4 and 15-HETE.[1037]

Also in 1987, two studies were reported on MBP concentrations in BAL fluid from patients with mild asthma. In London, the amount of MBP correlated with the number of eosinophils in BAL fluid (Wardlaw, A. 1987, personal communication), whereas in Ontario, Canada MBP levels were not elevated.[971]

Bronchial challenge in asthma As a number of environmental antigens have been identified as causes of asthma, especially the house dust mite faecal particles, it has become possible to study the events which follow bronchial challenge. The response in the lungs has followed several patterns. In some patients there is an acute increase in bronchial resistance, which disappears after about 4 hours. In others there is a 'late phase' reaction, occurring between 4 and 12 hours after challenge. Some patients have both reactions. These two types of response are mediated by different mechanisms. Eosinophils may take part in both events, but they are believed to be especially important in the late phase reactions by secreting LTC4 and toxic granule basic proteins.[220] No consistent alteration takes place in blood eosinophil counts during the late-phase reaction following antigen challenge of patients with asthma. This reaction is not usually associated with a leukocytosis, or fever, although the patient may feel hot, and sweat excessively. About half of the patients developed eosinophilia in a study in 1986.[1386] In a study from Scandinavia in 1979, the blood eosinophil count fell slightly at 3 hours, and then increased at 24 hours.[383] However, in a report from London in 1985, 11 patients with late phase reactions to inhaled allergens had raised blood eosinophil counts at 24 hours, whereas this did not occur in 6 with single reactions, or after methacholine challenge. The initial blood eosinophil counts were related to the methacholine reactivity in the 11 patients.[481]

In 15 patients with asthma who were studied at the Mayo Clinic and reported in 1985, plasma MBP levels correlated with the number of blood eosinophils.[611] An eosinophil chemotactic activity was reported to be present in the sera, and to correspond to the times of bronchospasm in 10 patients with seasonal asthma who developed biphasic, or late-phase responses after bronchial challenge.[1204]

In 1985, de Monchy and colleagues in Holland reported on the results of bronchoalveolar lavage, which was done 6 hours after antigen challenge in 6 patients with asthma due to house dust antigens. The number of eosinophils was greater than in control subjects, or in patients who only had early reactions.[416] Twelve atopic patients were studied in Iowa City, USA, in 1986.[1205] Lavage eosinophils, which were increased in number at 4 and 24 hours, were also found to have lost their central cores. Taken together, these studies supported the view that eosinophils are particularly involved in the late asthmatic reactions to inhaled antigens. This was confirmed in a study from Chile which was published in 1987, in which bronchoalveolar cell numbers were assessed in the late-phase asthmatic reactions induced by antigen challenge in 6 patients.[449]

The results of a similar study in Padua, Italy in patients challenged with toluene diisocyanate which was causing occupational asthma, showed similar increases in the number of bronchoalveolar eosinophils in 6 late responders, but not in 6 early responders or 6 normal subjects. As there was also an increase in neutrophils, it was suggested that late asthmatic reactions and the associated increase in airway responsiveness could be induced by both cell types during airway inflammation.[527] In a study in 1987 on 44 patients with asthma due to plicatic acid from red cedars, BAL with bronchial biopsies after bronchial challenge showed many eosinophils in lavage fluid, but little neutrophil infiltrate.[1022] Although eosinophils were seen infiltrating the bronchial epithelium and submucosa, no relationship was seen between the number of eosinophils and sloughing of bronchial epithelial cells, albumin leakage, or airflow obstruction. It was suggested that macrophages were responsible for the sloughing. A small increase in blood eosinophil counts was seen at 24 hours.

A useful assessment of the effects of bronchial challenge on the human bronchial mucosa, and BAL cells was reported from Iowa City in 1987.[1206] The local effects on the lower bronchi were assessed in 11 asthmatic patients with a history of late reactions and six controls. An immediate pallor was followed by reactive hyperaemia, oedema, and bronchial narrowing. The challege site and a control site were relavaged at 48 or 96 hours. Eosinophils were a significant component of the BAL fluid at both times, whereas neutrophil counts rose initially, then returned to normal at 96 hours. Eosinophils were also found to be degranulated at both times, and macrophages had ingested intact eosinophil granules.

In a study reported from Holland in 1985, in which BAL was done 6 hours after antigen challenge in 6 patients with late phase reactions due to house dust antigens, the ECP/albumin ratio in the lavage fluid was greater than in control subjects, or in patients who only had early reactions.[416]

Asthma and parasitic infections An interest has been taken for many years in the occurrence of asthma in populations having many parasitic infections. The importance of this is that eosinophils induced by one disease could affect the other,[1803] either by altering the severity of the asthma[18] or by influencing the capacity of the individual to resist parasitic diseases. Although these possibilities have not been investigated adequately, it seems likely that any effects are probably minor.[721]

This was supported by a study from Papua, New Guinea in 1985, where it was found that the incidence of hookworm infections in asthmatic and control patients was equal, 75 per cent.[464] However, a study in this region in 1980 had shown that patients with asthma had significantly less parasite eggs in their stools than parasitized patients without asthma.[1612]

Intrinsic asthma In patients with intrinsic asthma, who are often of a older age group than those with extrinsic asthma, blood eosinophil counts are often higher. This has not been explained, and it is not known whether this is linked in any way to morbidity and mortality in this patient group.

Aspirin-induced asthma The syndrome of asthma, drug intolerance, and nasal polyps (AIA) has been known for many years.[2] It is caused by a number of drugs, including aspirin and other non-steroidal, antipyretic analgesic drugs, and some food colourants. The clinical details of this triad have been described in a number of papers from the West, and recently from Osaka, Japan. There were 18 patients: 6 males and 12 females. The mean age of onset for rhinitis was 25, and for asthma 32 years. Thirteen had nasal polyps, 8 had urticaria, and 15 sinusitis. Fourteen of 16 patients had a blood eosinophilia, but no relationship with skin test results or IgE levels was found.[1301] This syndrome may result from an effect of these cyclo-oxygenase pathway inhibitors causing an over production of SRS-A and altered prostaglandin synthesis. This would cause bronchoconstriction.

15.3.2 *The Churg–Strauss syndrome*

The classic post mortem study of patients with asthma who developed a disease with granulomas containing necrotizing vasculitic lesions with many eosinophils affecting many different tissues, and high blood eosinophil counts, was carried out by Churg and Strauss in 1951.[323] This disease, which is named after them, may present with granulomatous pulmonary eosinophilia, and there may be considerable difficulty in diagnosing it, if tissue is not available for biopsy. It was previously known under a variety of different names, which are sometimes used today, and I suspect that many of the earlier descriptions of patients with eosinophilia, respiratory tract disease, and involvement of the pleura, pericardium, peritoneum, kidneys, gut etc. (many of whom were diagnosed as having polyarteritis nodosa) would be classified today as having the Churg–Strauss syndrome. A possible example of this is ‘polyserositis’, which was described in 8 patients in 1941. Six of the patients in this report developed pleural effusions; 3 had ascites containing many eosinophils, and 2 developed constrictive pericarditis, which was confirmed at post mortem.[754] Occasionally a disease similar to the Churg–Strauss syndrome can occur without the presence of a vasculitis. Two patients of this kind were reported in 1986.[1833]

The aetiology of the syndrome is unknown, but it may be exacerbated by an excessive eosinophil inflammatory response to allergens, as was reported in 6 patients who developed systemic vasculitis with eosinophilia after allergic hyposensitization therapy. In these patients, eosinophilia continued after the treatment had been stopped.[1402]

Clinical features of the Churg–Strauss syndrome Characteristic clinical features of this disease are a family history of asthma or a recent presentation with asthma,[728] and marked peripheral blood eosinophilia. In a group of 43 patients reported from Paris in 1987, the average blood eosinophil count was $8.2 \pm 6.2 \times 10^9/l$.[728] Granulomas can occur in many different tissues including the pericardium, heart, gastrointestinal tract, skin, and peripheral nerves where they produce a mononeuritis multiplex. The eosinophil count can fluctuate, and may occasionally be normal.[1030] A patient with the Churg–Strauss syndrome has been described with an eosinophil-rich vasculitis affecting the sural nerve,[1303] In previous patients, nerve damage has not been reported with eosinophil infiltrates, although this probably occurs frequently. Asthma is one of the principal features of the disease, and this was emphasized in a paper describing 10 patients in Lille, France in 1984. In 3, BAL fluid contained many eosinophils.[1274]

Cardiac complications of the Churg–Strauss syndrome The cardiac complications of the Churg–Strauss syndrome are particularly dangerous, as they can give rise to arrhythmias, and sudden death. This probably accounts for the high mortality of the disease. Long term effects of the disease are also suspected: Among three patients with this disease who were seen at the Brompton Hospital, London, two had pericardial involvement, and one progressed to a dilated cardiomyopathy.[410] A special interest was taken in this disease at the Hammersmith Hospital, London. Our work there showed deposition of the activated form of ECP and ECN/EPX in two patients at post mortem. These deposits and activated eosinophils were found within the heart of a patient who died with an arrythmia, and in the spleen and other tissues of both patients. The close apposition of the eosinophil granule proteins to damaged cardiac myocytes suggested that they could have caused the myocyte necrosis.[1737] (Plate 12)

Treatment of the Churg–Strauss syndrome Immediate treatment with large doses of corticosteroids can be life-saving,[320] but even with steroids, immunosuppressive drugs, and plasma exchange, the mortality rate is 16 per cent.[728] The use of alternate day steroids to treat the Churg–Strauss syndrome is not recommended during the active phase of the disease. For example, in an account of a patient with widespread mononeuritis multiplex, 100 mg prednisolone on alternate days failed to control the disease.[643] Pulse methylprednisolone has been effective in one patient whose disease was resistent to prednisolone.[1122]

15.3.3 *Respiratory hypersensitivity*

Inhaled antigens can give rise to many different types of respiratory tract damage. Reversible bronchial obstruction may develop, or extensive damage, giving rise to fibrous tissue formation. Eosinophils are probably involved in both types of response, and are prominent in the peripheral airways of patients with fibrosing alveolitis. Many organic and chemical dusts can give rise to hypersensitivity pneumonitis, which was first recognized in maple bark strippers, and in farmers working with mouldy hay. In 1986, an association was found with exposure to the neoprene rubber thermoinjection process, which produced eosinophilia in 10 of 18 people.[1771] It can develop when cocaine is inhaled. A genetic component may provide increased susceptibility to these diseases, which are due to both antibody and cell-mediated reactions to the inhaled antigens in the lungs.[33]

Extrinsic allergic alveolitis In some patients with moderate or severe respiratory tract involvement, often with X-ray changes and defects in respiratory gas exchange, rather than obstruction, eosinophils can be a prominent feature of disease.

Hayfever Hayfever is the commonest cause of a moderately raised blood eosinophil count in Western countries. This causes difficulty in defining the 'normal' blood eosinophil count, as patients with mild disease may not report that they have it. A longitudinal study on 16 children with hayfever and 16 with hayfever and asthma was reported in 1986 from Aarhus, Denmark.[785] The main findings were that the blood eosinophil counts increased in both groups during the pollen season, and it was greatest in those with asthma. Asthma sufferers also had the greatest alteration in exercise-induced bronchoconstriction, suggesting that the two may have been related.

In patients with chronic hayfever and allergic rhinitis who develop polyps, eosinophils are often a prominent component of the nasal washings and the mucosa of the polyps. It is possible to obtain them in nasal washings, and their properties may then be studied.

15.3.4 *Acute and chronic bronchitis*

Bronchitis is seldom associated with eosinophilia. Although eosinophils are found in the sputa of patients with chronic bronchitis, their numbers are much less than is seen in asthma.[1655] The presence of large numbers of eosinophils in the sputa of these patients suggests that the epithelium may have been colonized with fungi, especially *Aspergillus spp*.

15.4 Lung diseases

Eosinophils are important components of a wide range of parenchymal lung diseases. They range from granulomatous and vasculitis disorders to the large group of patients classified as having pulmonary eosinophilia. Their causes are usually unknown, and they present a challenge for diagnosis and treatment in many instances. In patients with a parasitic, fungal, or bacterial hypersensitivity reaction, pulmonary eosinophilia probably develops as a reaction to antigens released from these organisms. However, there is little evidence for an allergic cause of the lung disease in patients with cryptogenic pulmonary eosinophilia.

In many of these patients, chest radiographs may show pulmonary infiltrates, which can be characteristic of the disorder (eosinophilic pneumonia), and more marked than was suspected from the clinical features. Investigations often prove to be difficult to interpret. No consensus view has developed concerning the diagnostic groupings and pathological descriptions of these lung disorders, which makes them difficult to review.

15.4.1 *Pulmonary eosinophilia*

Pulmonary eosinophilic syndromes are characterized by the presence of an interstitial inflammatory reaction in the lung, containing large numbers of eosinophils. The blood eosinophil count is often raised as well. Some classifications of pulmonary eosinophilia have as their basis the occurrence of asthma in some patients.[369, 1804] The principal difficulty with this approach is that asthma can occur (albeit rarely in some diseases) in every clinical syndrome associated with pulmonary eosinophilia. I have argued[1684] that it is better to separate pulmonary eosinophilic syndromes of extrinsic or known cause (secondary pulmonary eosinophilic syndromes) from diseases of unknown pathogenesis (cryptogenic pulmonary eosinophilic syndromes). The second group consists of three main subtypes:

(a) acute;

(b) chronic disorders, which may repond well to steroids and are usually easy to manage; and

(c) more severe syndromes, which are chronic and are usually difficult to treat. The more serious disorders include the chronic eosinophilic pneumonias, and some vasculitic and granulomatous diseases of the lung, such as Wegener's granulomatosis.

Löffler's syndrome The classical description of patients with a fleeting infiltrate and moderate eosinophilia was made in 1932 by Löffler in

Switzerland.[1091] Two of the five patients who had recurrent infiltrates developed blood eosinophil counts of only 7 per cent and 9 per cent. Symptoms were mild in all of the patients. Löffler's syndrome is now seldom seen or described in publications and was probably due to ascaris and other parasitic infections in childhood.

PIE syndromes Patients with eosinophilic inflammatory reactions in the lung, similar to eosinophilic pneumonia but of less severity, have been designated as having the pulmonary infiltrates with eosinophilia (PIE) syndrome. They show similar clinical features to those described below.

Chronic eosinophilic pneumonia Chronic eosinophilic pneumonia, which became widely known following a pathological study in 1969,[281] is the most severe form of cryptogenic pulmonary eosinophilia. It requires hospital treatment and careful follow-up. The principle difficulties are in distinguishing it from infective lesions, emboli, and malignant diseases involving the lung. About 50 per cent of these patients have preceding adult-onset asthma, but most are not atopic. Patients usually experience fever, night sweats, weight loss, cough and dyspnoea, which becomes progressively worse over several days or weeks.

Twenty-seven patients with cryptogenic pulmonary eosinophilia were described in 1973, among a group of 43 patients with pulmonary eosinophilia of different causes, who were seen during a two-year period at the Brompton Hospital, London. Interestingly, 2 of the patients later developed polyarteritis nodosa.[1170] In 1976 a detailed description was published of a further 15 patients in London. Ten were women (mean age 35 years) and five were men (mean age 42 years). Eight had had previous attacks of asthma. The mean blood eosinophil counts were $4.3 \times 10^9/l$, range $0.8–12.8 \times 10^9/l$. The principle clinical features were anaemia, weight loss, and fever, in addition to their respiratory symptoms. Four had splenomegaly, and 3 hepatomegaly. One also had hilar node enlargement. In each case, there was a dramatic resolution after treatment with steroids. Some patients had minor elevations in serum IgE. The pathology of the lung lesions was described in lung biopsies from 3 of the patients.[1805]

In 1977 4 women with this disease were reported from Salt Lake City, USA, and their features were correlated to give a picture of this disease as seen in all 27 patients whose details had been published up to this time.[41] They were nearly all women, with breathlessness, weight loss, fever, eosinophilia, and peripheral alveolar infiltrate in chest radiographs.

Details of a further 8 patients with chronic eosinophilic pneumonia were described in 1978. Four were allergic to penicillin.[1382] Although the pathogenesis of cryptogenic pulmonary eosinophilia presenting as eosinophilic pneumonia is unknown, in one series about half the patients had intrinsic asthma which began within five years of diagnosis.[1562] Other series have shown a lower incidence of preceding asthma.[1382] However, patients often have a history of atopy in relatives, drug hypersensitivity, or allergic rhinitis. A strong genetic element in the disease was suggested in a report from the UK of cryptogenic pulmonary eosinophilia in identical twin sisters, at the ages of 25 and 29 years.[113] Both responded well to treatment with steroids. Six patients with chronic eosinophilic pneumonia were reported from Chapel Hill, USA in 1986.[854] Two had atypical features with diffuse abnormalities on chest radiographs. They developed the adult respiratory distress syndrome, which responded slowly to treatment with steroids.

About two-thirds of these patients have raised blood eosinophil counts which can be over 5×10^9/l,[281] and are generally higher in this group of patients than in those with pulmonary eosinophilia of known cause.[1170] However, in 13 per cent of histologically confirmed cases, a raised blood eosinophil count was intermittent or absent.[591] Pulmonary function tests can show airway obstruction in addition to restricted volumes and reduced diffusing capacity.[1245]

Chest radiographs show areas of patchy consolidation, which are usually peripheral, with dense and ill-defined areas that lack lobar, or segmented distribution. They may be unilateral or bilateral, and the latter give the appearance of a 'photographic negative' of pulmonary oedema.[281] In 1977 16 patients in a large series of 24 with pulmonary eosinophilia had these charasteristic 'ground glass' abnormalities, which related to areas where positive lung biopsies were obtained. Details on 81 other patients with pulmonary eosinophilia were assessed in this comprehensive paper.[615] Opacities may recur in the same site on several occasions.

These radiological features, in association with eosinophilia (or occasionally without) are sufficiently distinct for a diagnosis of chronic eosinophilic pneumonia to be made without a lung biopsy. However, in some patients with an atypical illness, bronchoscopy with BAL (looking for large numbers of eosinophils, and/or trans-bronchial lung biopsy may be required to establish the diagnosis.

BAL has been used to diagnose[715] and to follow the effectiveness of steroid treatment of eosinophilic pneumonia.[429] In 1987, large amounts of prostaglandin E2 were found with many eosinophils in BAL fluid from two patients with eosinophilic pneumonia, which fell after steroid treatment.[1302] In a study on four patients with eosinophilic pneumonia seen in Israel, blood eosinophil counts were $0.78–1.8 \times 10^9$/l, and BAL showed that eosinophils made up 23–76 per cent of the cells recovered in the fluid.[715]

In BAL of three patients with eosinophilic pneumonia, one with polyarteritis nodosa, and one with a drug hypersensitivity pneumonitis who were studied in Lille, France in 1986, light density and degranulated eosinophils were noted to have an increased capacity to generate chemoluminescence after stimulation with alveolar macrophage supernatants. They also possessed IgE on their surface.[1451]

By 1981, there had been over 60 published case reports of the histological appearances of chronic eosinophilic pneumonia.[591] The focal areas of infiltration contain eosinophils, mononuclear cells, and occasional plasma cells. Granulomas with giant cells and Charcot–Leyden crystals also occurred.[1078] Bronchiolitis obliterans and vasculitis were sometimes noted, and eosinophils in the lesions were frequently degranulated. Deposits of IgG and IgA have been seen by immunofluorescence.

Electronmicroscopy and tissue immunofluorescence studies for MBP showed extensive eosinophil degranulation in one patient,[1463] while deposits of MBP and free granules within the pulmonary microvasculature in the lesions of another patient with chronic eosinophilic pneumonia were reported from Galveston, Texas, USA in 1987.[695] MBP was found in the lung and pleural fluid of a patient studied at the Mayo Clinic in 1986.[712] Intracytoplasmic inclusions in other patients have been interpreted as Birbeck granules, but these were probably phagolysosomes.[1463] As there was also exfoliation of alveolar lining cells, with clustering of eosinophil granules against a denuded basement membrane, it was suggested that these eosinophils may have contributed to the damage which occurred in the respiratory parenchyma.

Over 80 per cent of the 31 reported patients responded to steroid treatment. This resulted in a rapid resolution of clinical and radiological features. Oblique or vertical lines may persist in chest radiographs, and cavitation can develop in rare instances. This disease is a chronic one, and lesions can recur in previously affected parts of the lung after steroid treatment has been stopped. For this reason a long follow-up period is important. As spontaneous remissions occur in less than 10 per cent, almost all patients require some form of treatment. Corticosteroids usually produce such a dramatic response, that this can be used to confirm the diagnosis. As little as 10 mg prednisolone on alternate days may be effective.

Treatment is usually continued for several weeks after clinical and radiological resolution is complete. Unfortunately, 30 per cent of patients in whom steroids have been stopped, relapse and require further treatment. Some patients may require long-term corticosteroid therapy. One group of patients had to be treated for a mean of four years to control relapses, and some patients needed treatment for eight years.[1382] Inhaled steroid derivatives should not be used to treat chronic eosinophilic pneumonia. Although clinical and radiological appearances may resolve rapidly, lung function tests appear to be slower to improve, and these are useful to monitor relapses. Blood eosinophil counts, red cell sedimentation rates, and chest radiographs can also be helpful to detect relapses at an early stage.

15.4.2 *Pulmonary fibrosis*

Studies on BAL cells in patients with cryptogenic pulmonary fibrosis usually show an increased number of eosinophils,[1968] although this is not so in all series.[1616]

However, when large numbers of eosinophils are present, patients have more severe disease and a worse prognosis. This was first shown at the Brompton Hospital, London, where serial BAL was also shown to help in management.[1806] The initial observation was confirmed in 1987 in a group of 27 patients who were studied in Iowa, USA[1399] and in Denver, Colorado, USA.[1892] Increased numbers of eosinophils have also been seen in BAL fluid from patients with the CREST syndrome and interstitial fibrosis.[1388]

The reasons why eosinophilia in BAL may have a poor prognostic value in pulmonary fibrosis compared with other diseases such as eosinophilic pneumonia and histiocytosis X, where the eosinophil infiltrate is usually greater, may be related to the different sites in which eosinophils localize in the lungs in these diseases,[1076] and to the capacity of eosinophils to induce a fibrotic reaction, under certain circumstances.

A guinea pig model of interstitial lung disease has been described, in which guinea pigs were given aerosols of polymyxin B for four weeks. They developed an eosinophilic alveolitis, but no fibrosis. In this model, it was found that alveolar eosinophils but not blood eosinophils were able to kill fetal lung fibroblasts spontaneously.[1726]

15.4.3 *Wegener's granulomatosis*

Wegener's granulomatosis is occasionally associated with eosinophilia, although the necrotic lesions in the lungs and kidneys seldom contain eosinophils. A wide range of pulmonary eosinophilic syndromes can be associated with vasculitic and granulomatous reactions in the lungs. Although apparently distinct syndromes have been defined, the illness in individual patients often does not correspond with them. This difficulty is seen in occasional patients who present with chronic eosinophilic pneumonia, but who then develop a systemic vasculitis. For this reason these disorders are best described as a spectrum of diseases.[545] A general description and a modern attempt to provide a rational classification of these diseases was put forward by A. Churg in 1983.[322]

Earlier work stressed the importance of pulmonary involvement in polyarteritis nodosa. For example, in the widely quoted study of Rose and Spencer in 1957,[1516] of 111 patients with polyarteritis, 14 had lung involvement, 10 of whom also had peripheral blood eosinophilia. However, these patients had many features which suggest today that they had Wegener's granulomatosis, in which the characteristic histological features are necrotizing vasculitis and eosinophil accumulation. At present, polyarteritis involving the lungs is rarely diagnosed, probably because of the distinctions which are now being made between the various types of vasculitis. Granulomatous disorders which produce pulmonary eosinophilic syndromes are much more common.[1844, 828]

The proportion of patients with Wegener's granulomatosis who develop eosinophilia varies from 60 per cent in some series to none in others.[546] A preceding history of pulmonary infection can be used to distinguish this type of granulomatous disease from the Churg–Strauss syndrome. Lesions are usually better defined than in other diseases with pulmonary eosinophilia, and cavitation can occur leaving areas of scarring. Extrapulmonary lesions are an important feature, and involve the upper respiratory tract, kidneys, eyes, brain, skin, and other sites. In these patients the pulmonary lesions can recur at an early stage during relapses, and chest radiographs are useful to monitor the progress of the disease. Cyclophosphamide appears to be of particular benefit in Wegener's granulomatosis, and patients are usually also treated with high doses of corticosteroids initially.

15.4.4 *Lymphomatoid granulomatosis*

Lymphomatoid granulomatosis is a somewhat similar disease to Wegener's granulomatosis, but it is much less common than other granulomatous diseases of the lung with eosinophilia.[1079] This disease, which is often fatal, is characterized by lesions containing a mixture of inflammatory cells infiltrating blood vessels and tissues, without necrotizing vasculitis. Cavitating lung nodules appear, and lesions also occur in the skin and kidneys. The upper respiratory tract is seldom affected. Patients may show leukopenia, unlike other forms of granulomatous and vasculitis disorders affecting the lung. Early treatment with cyclophosphamides and corticosteroids may reduce the high mortality.

15.4.5 *Eosinophilic granuloma of the lung*

Another rare cause of eosinophilia and pulmonary disease is eosinophilic granuloma of the lung. This was first described in 1951, and over 200 patients have been reported since then. It was also discussed in 1986.[2017] It occurs in 20 per cent of patients who have the histiocytosis X group of diseases.

Patients usually present with bilateral reticulonodular lesions, which may be found in chest radiographs carried out to investigate nonspecific respiratory symptoms. Pneumothorax is an important complication, and 10 per cent of the patients have hemoptysis: 6 of 74 patients in one series.[1068] In these patients, granulomas with eosinophil infiltrates may also develop at sites outside the lung, including the skeletal system, brain, and other systems. Patients with localized disease respond well to treatment with corticosteroids and cytotoxic drugs, but diffuse disease can be rapidly fatal.

The lesions are small nodules which centre on small airways and develop into fibrotic areas.[341] Electronmicroscopic studies on the abnormal histiocytic cells in lung washings and lung biopsies show characteristic cytoplasmic rod-shaped bodies (X-bodies).[1014] When these are found in lung washings, and used in conjunction with the staining of Langerhans'-type cells with CD6 monoclonal antibodies, it is possible to make a firm diagnosis.

Experimental work on the induction of granulomas in the lungs of rabbits has suggested that prostaglandin E2 and other cyclo-oxygenase products may be important in the development of eosinophil-rich granulomas after the inhalation of toxic substances.[746]

15.4.6 *Obstructive lung diseases and pulmonaryt emphysema*

The chronic effects of obstructive lung disease, which give rise to pulmonary emphysema, are rarely associated with an increased number of eosinophils in the blood or tissues.

15.4.7 *Sarcoidosis*

Sarcoidosis is characterized by macrophage and lymphocyte infiltrates into tissues, and eosinophils are rarely a prominent part of the disease pathology.

15.4.8 *Adult respiratory distress syndrome*

Studies in Uppsala, Sweden have implicated eosinophils in the adult respiratory distress syndrome (ARDS). This conclusion was based on the finding of high ECP levels in serum[736] and BAL fluid, which correlated with the severity of the lung disease. The study was carried out on 12 patients with ARDS, 15 patients undergoing major surgery, and 17 having minor surgery.[1228] BAL was done just after anaesthetic induction. Patients having major surgery also had BAL one hour after surgery was completed. Patients with major surgery had higher levels of BAL fluid ECP after surgery, increasing from 25 to 50 μg/l, but blood ECP levels did not increase. Eight patients with severe ARDS had mean lavage fluid ECP levels of 200 μg/l. The highest level was 272 μg/l in a patient who subsequently died. In 4 less severely affected patients, lavage fluid contained 75 μg/l. Serum ECP levels were only slightly elevated in most ARDS patients, but the highest serum level was 107 μg/l, in a fatal case. As very few eosinophils were found in the blood, it was suggested that eosinophils were trapped in the lungs, where they degranulated and may have caused tissue injury. Neutrophil lactoferrin and myeloperoxidase were also increased in the lavage fluid,[739] suggesting that neutrophils were affected in much the same way as eosinophils.

15.5 Pleural diseases

Several of the parenchymal diseases of the lung which are associated with eosinophilia, can also affect the pleura. Reactive eosinophilic pleuritis[73] is a disease of unknown cause which can give rise to a spontaneous pneumothorax. The pleural biopsy shows sheets of histiocytes mixed with eosinophils in the pleural tissues.

15.5.1 *Pleural effusions*

Eosinophils have been noted in pleural effusions since 1894. Particular note is taken of the presence of eosinophils in pleural fluid when they comprise 10 per cent or more of the cells in the effusion. Five to 8 per cent of pleural effusions are of this type. Eosinophilic pleural effusions have been seen in a wide variety of diseases, especially following introduction of air into the chest, trauma,[389] infections including tuberculosis,[1210] and more rarely in patients with a malignancy, benign asbestos lesions, pulmonary infarction, sarcoidosis,[480] and rheumatological diseases including systemic sclerosis.[456] In a series of 30 patients reported in 1979, trauma was involved in 11, and an allergy in 8, but no cause was seen in 11.[1854] This report commented on the large numbers of lymphocytes in these effusions, and the benign course of the effusions in most patients. In 1974, a study on 78 patients with an eosinophilic pleural effusion showed that 48 had tuberculosis, and 6 a tumour. No definite diagnosis was made in 16, even after pleural biopsies had been taken.[993] In 1981, a study from Finland found that tuberculosis was no longer an important cause of an eosinophilic pleural effusion.[1401] Occasionally, an eosinophilic pleural effusion develops in patients with viral respiratory diseases.[836] An historical review of 343 published patients was done in 1985, and showed no clear association with any single disease, although the presence of an eosinophilic effusion reduced the likelihood of a malignant disease or pulmonary tuberculosis compared to other benign diseases.[17] A negative correlation between an eosinophilic pleural effusion and malignant disease was also found in a study of 334 patients in Sweden in 1985,[1159] and in 36 patients studied in Israel in 1985.[1959] In about 10 per cent of eosinophilic pleural effusions no cause can be detected, although some of these may be due to asbestos, as half of known asbestos-associated pleural effusions are eosinophilic. These idiopathic cases usually resolve spontaneously, and empirical treatment for other diseases such as tuberculosis is probably unwarranted in most instances.

16. Diseases of the ear, nose, and throat

16.1 Diseases of the ear

The external ear may be involved in a number of diseases which affect other parts of the skin, including Kimura's disease and angiolymphoid hyperplasia with eosinophilia. Eosinophils have been seen in the exudate from the ear in a proportion of patients with chronically discharging ears (17 per cent in one series of 84 patients),[1306] but the reasons for this are not known.

In otitis media, eosinophils are occasionally found in cytological preparations, but they are seldom present in any large numbers, except in patients with aspergillus infections.

16.2 Diseases of the nose

Eosinophils are not found normally in the nose, although large numbers can be found in patients with allergic nasal diseases. Early reports described eosinophils in the nose of normal children under six months of age, but this was not confirmed in a groups of 22 children aged two days to 12 months, who were studied in San Francisco, California, USA in 1985.[335] Although patients may occasionally have focal lesions in the nose rich in eosinophils due to such rare disorders as nasal tumours and the Churg–Strauss syndrome, the majority of patients with nasal symptoms and eosinophil accumulation in the nose or in the blood have allergic rhinitis, with or without nasal polyps. An important form of rhinitis which does not appear to have an allergic cause (NARES) can also present with many eosinophils in nasal washings. Occasionally, patients with allergic bronchopulmonary aspergillosis can also present with allergic rhinitis.[707]

16.2.1 *Rhinitis*

Rhinitis is usually divided into allergic and non-allergic types. Allergic rhinitis may be perennial or seasonal. A general review was published in 1984.[1381] The nasal smear contained eosinophils in 71 per cent of one group of 770 patients with allergic rhinitis studied in Helsinki, Finland in 1984.[171] Nasal eosinophilia is more common in those with perennial allergic rhinitis than in seasonal allergic rhinitis. Nasal eosinophil levels are related to blood eosinophil counts, but as there may be a significant difference in the numbers of eosinophils recovered from each nostril, the association is not close. Non-allergic rhinitis has been described both in adults and children.[1529] It has many different causes, including drug reactions, aspirin sensitivity, vasomotor rhinitis, and NARES. NARES is associated with more than 5 per cent eosinophils in nasal smears. (Occasionally a 25 per cent lower limit is used to make this diagnosis). In a study from Providence, Rhode Island, USA in 1985 on 78 patients with non-allergic rhinitis who had negative skin tests, 61 per cent had vasomotor rhinitis, 33 per cent NARES, and 6 per cent sinusitis. Among the 25 patients with NARES, 3 had mean blood eosinophil counts of 0.95×10^9/l. These are sometimes classified separately as BENAR (blood eosinophilia non-allergic rhinitis) syndrome. There is some evidence that patients with non-allergic rhinitis and an increased number of eosinophils in nasal secretion respond best to medication.[1248]

16.2.2 *Nasal polyps*

Nasal polyps in patients with chronic rhinitis are often rich in eosinophils and nasal secretions from these patients usually contain large numbers of these cells.[600] The proportion of polyps which contain eosinophils varies from 26 per cent in Japan, to 94 per cent in several parts of Europe.[811, 231] The incidence of atopy in patients with eosinophilic polyps is one in four, and about half have asthma. Polyps in children with cystic fibrosis contain few eosinophils.[1666]

A study on nasal polyps from 77 patients in Tokyo showed that 43 (56 per cent) contained eosinophil infiltrates. Thirty per cent were atopic. IgG-immune complexes were found in five of the six polyps studied,[1298] and IgE has also been detected in nasal polyps.[600] Polyps also occur in patients with aspirin sensitivity, who may have marked blood eosinophilia. The incidence of nasal polyps in patients with aspirin-induced asthma ranges from 60–100 per cent.[1301] In a study on 22 nasal polyps, it was found eosinophils were responsible for the formation of large amounts of 15-HETE in this site, but their role(s) within and on the surface of polyps remains unknown.[1649]

16.2.3 *Paranasal sinus diseases*

Aspergillus infections of the sinuses have been noted to be able to cause a marked eosinophil-rich infiltrate in this site.[920] In 1987, the clinical features of allergic fungal sinusitis due to *Curvularia lunata* were described.[1127]

16.3 Pharyngeal and laryngeal diseases

The pharynx and larynx may contain many eosinophilia in rare individuals with tumours, granulomatous diseases, or rheumatoid arthritis. In 1985, three patients were described in Norwich, UK, with an eosinophil-rich fibrotic reaction in the submucosa of the upper respiratory tract, and subepiglottic region of the larynx.[1496] Their illnesses may have been related to primary eosinophilic granuloma of the larnyx, which was described in three patients in 1981.[603]

17. Diseases of the nervous system

Eosinophils are not normally found within the nervous system, and their presence there is always evidence for a disease process. Much of the interest in the relationship between eosinophils and the nervous system has centred on the capacity of ECP and EDN/EPX to cause demyelination in experimental animals. However, there is no direct evidence that ECP or EDN/EPX injures the brain in man, and high levels of ECP in the cerebrospinal fluid do not seem to cause demyelination. However, it is possible that one or more of the eosinophil effector mechanisms may accentuate lesions in the meninges and within the brain in inflammatory disorders where they are prominent, and further work in this area will be of interest. The peripheral nervous system is commonly affected in patients with hypereosinophilia, but it is not known whether eosinophil constituents affect nerve conduction.

17.1 Central nervous system diseases

Few primary diseases of the central nervous system result in eosinophil accumulation within the brain, and it is very seldom that they give rise to peripheral blood eosinophilia. The common forms of cerebrovascular diseases do not give rise to eosinophil infiltrates.

17.1.1 *Diseases affecting meninges, and eosinophils in the cerebrospinal fluid*

The finding of eosinophils in the cerebrospinal fluid (CSF) is uncommon,[1007] except in countries where eosinophilic meningitis due to *Angiostrongylus cantonensis* is prevalent, which gives rise to the highest CSF eosinophil counts. This was reviewed by Kuberski in Honolulu in 1981.[1008] A number of other parasitic diseases produce an increase in CSF eosinophils,[167] including echinococcosis, cysticercosis, and toxoplasmosis. It can also occur in other infectious diseases, including (rarely) tuberculous meningitis, coxackie B meningitis,[313] chronic lymphocytic choriomeningitis, and Rocky Mountain spotted fever.[367] The other main causes are neoplastic diseases, including lymphocytic leukaemia,[967, 1360, 995] Hodgkin's disease,[1716, 295, 1375, 809, 260] myeloproliferative disorders,[861] pneumococcal meningitis,[302] as well as following myelography, surgical operations on the brain,[872] and the presence of shunts in children treated for hydrocephalus.[1808] Other causes are meningeal carcinomatosis,[352] cerebral eosinophilic granulomas,[1638] and drug hyersensitivity reactions such as gentamycin hypersensitivity, which induced a blood and CSF eosinophilia in a patients with a ventricular shunt,[1216] and ibuprofen, which produced an aseptic meningitis.[1462] Only one report has described a minor increase in CSF eosinophils in a patient with HES.[1900] The meninges can be infiltrated with eosinophils in some patients with central nervous system involvement in eosinophilic leukaemia.

In one series of patients with meningitis, measurements of ECP in the cerebrospinal fluid showed that patients with the highest levels had the slowest recovery.[740]

In 1985, ultrastructural studies were carried out on subdural haematomas from five patients in whom eosinophils were seen in the outer membranes of the haematomas. They appeared to be degranulated, and free granules with altered matrix were found outside the cells. Eosinophils might release constituents which could contribute to the increase in fluidity of chronic subdural haematomas causing further leakage of blood into the capsule of the haematoma.[1965]

17.2 Peripheral nerve diseases

There are no specific disorders in which the peripheral nerves or cranial nerves are involved by eosinophils, although cranial nerve lesions and peripheral damage are common in patients with hypereosinophilia. The pathology of these lesions has not been investigated, but it is possible that the damage is vascular in origin, probably due to occlusion of central and perineural blood vessels. In 1986 four patients were described from Stanford, Connecticut, USA who had multiple peripheral nerve lesions in association with eosinophilia. They also had chronic sinusitis and asthma, and responded to steroids, with relapses. Biopsies failed to show any vasculitis lesions, although these could have been localized and difficult to detect. Whether these patients fall into the HES clinical spectrum remains to be seen. It was postulated that eosinophil granule components might have caused the nerve lesions.[461]

17.3 Schizophrenia

Although there is no clinical evidence to suggest that eosinophils are involved in schizophrenia, a study from Uppsala, Sweden in 1982, showed raised serum levels of ECP in several patients.[743] As these correlated with raised serum lactoferrin levels, it was suggested that these changes might accompany an alteration in inflammatory reactions which have been noted previously in schizophrenia.

18. Eye diseases

The principal eye diseases associated with eosinophils are parasitic and allergic diseases.

18.1 Conjunctival diseases

The presence of eosinophils in tarsal conjunctival scrapings is a feature of a number of hypersensitivity disorders such as vernal conjunctivitis, seasonal allergic (hay fever) conjunctivitis, atopic conjunctivitis, and other non-specific allergic diseases. In some patients with these diseases it may be difficult to demonstrate the eosinophils in tear fluid or scrapings, although they are present in conjunctival biopsies.[1] Occasionally only eosinophil granules may be seen.[602] Other causes of an eosinophil-rich conjunctivitis are filarial infections and the Churg–Strauss syndrome.[1613]

18.1.1 *Vernal conjunctivitis*

In vernal conjunctivitis, which often starts in childhood and is associated with itching and mucus secretion, eosinophils can be a prominent cell type in the affected tarsal conjunctiva. In ten patients with vernal conjunctivitis, biopsies showed the presence of many eosinophils in the epithelium and the substantia propria. As similar features were seen in 38 per cent of the biopsies of the tarsal conjunctiva from 15 patients who wore hard or soft contact lenses, and who had developed a similar clinical picture of giant papillary conjunctivitis, it was suggested that the two diseases were related.[30, 31] Both MBP and CLC protein were detected in significant amounts in the tears from five of seven patients with vernal conjunctivitis.[1809]

18.1.2 *Seasonal and perennial allergic (hay fever) conjunctivitis*

Allergic conjunctivitis is an IgE-mediated acute allergic reaction in the conjunctiva, due to air-borne allergens, especially pollens. It gives rise to relatively mild symptoms, but these can last for several months, and a large number of people are affected each year. It responds well to treatment with antihistamine and 2 per cent disodium cromoglycate. The conjunctival fluid usually contains eosinophils and raised levels of IgE. In one study on 25 patients with seasonal allergic conjunctivitis and 14 with perennial allergic conjunctivitis, eosinophils were found in carefully prepared samples of tear fluid in 25 per cent and 43 per cent respectively.

Seventy-eight per cent of the patients with perennial allergic conjunctivitis had higher levels of IgE antibodies in their tears than in sera, suggesting that house dust mite antigens were responsible for their disease.[392]

The rabbit and guinea pig conjunctival sacs have been used for many years as sites in which to test for immediate hypersensitivity reactions to drugs and chemicals. This assay may detect the presence of mast cells sensitization with IgE. It was also proposed that antigen caused them to release histamine, which attracted blood eosinophils into the conjunctival epithelium.[1953]

18.2 Corneal diseases

The significance of finding eosinophils in the human cornea had been reviewed in 1986.[1080] They have been seen in failed corneal transplants, and smaller numbers were seen in a wide variety of other corneal diseases.

18.3 Retinal diseases

One of the best known causes of an eosinophilic lesion in the retina is *Toxocara canis* infection, which can produce a diffuse unilateral subacute neuroretinitis,[1333] in addition to focal lesions, which may mimic retinoblastomas.

18.4 Diseases of the orbit

Several reports have been published of eosinophilic granulomas affecting the orbital frontal bones and the lateral orbital wall.[553]

19. Urological diseases

Eosinophils are prominent in the urological system in several parasitic diseases, in a variety of granulomatous and allergic diseases, and in patients undergoing renal or peritoneal dialysis. (See Fig. 19.1.) The presence of eosinophils in the urine can be of diagnostic value in a number of diseases.

19.1 Kidney and ureteral diseases

Drug-induced interstitial nephritis and acute tubular necrosis can both produce an eosinophil-rich infiltrate into the kidneys, and eosinophiluria. In a study reported in 1987, on 81 patients, 28 of whom had a hypersensitivity reaction to non-steroidal inflammatory drugs or antibiotics, both types of renal lesions were detected by renal biopsy.[1025] Eosinophil-rich allergic reactions to drugs can also produce glomerular lesions.[49] See page 309.

19.2 Renal dialysis and eosinophils

Patients with renal failure often have a small increase in blood eosinophil counts, and their serum ECP levels are usually raised.[738] In a study from Denmark in 1987, 13 per cent of 99 patients about to start maintenance haemodialysis had mean counts of 0.8×10^9/l, range $0.4–2.7 \times 10^9$/l, and many of them were male.[601] Renal haemodialysis can produce a rapid fall in blood eosinophil counts. This was well documented in 1980, in 8 patients whose blood eosinophil counts fell to 80 per cent of the initial levels. They gradually returned towards normal by three hours.[125] Haemodialysis also decreased the density of white blood cells, possibly as a result of the formation of C5a by the dialysis membrane.[1071]

It has been known for over 20 years that treatment of end-stage renal failure by either peritoneal dialysis or haemodialysis can induce a marked increase in the number of eosinophils in the peritoneal fluid and occasionally in the blood.

As eosinophils are rarely seen in the peritoneal fluid from patients with bacterial peritonitis, a search for eosinophils in cloudy peritoneal fluid can be a useful and rapid way to distinguish these two types of peritonitis.[1673]

Peritoneal fluid from patients having ambulatory dialysis can also be a

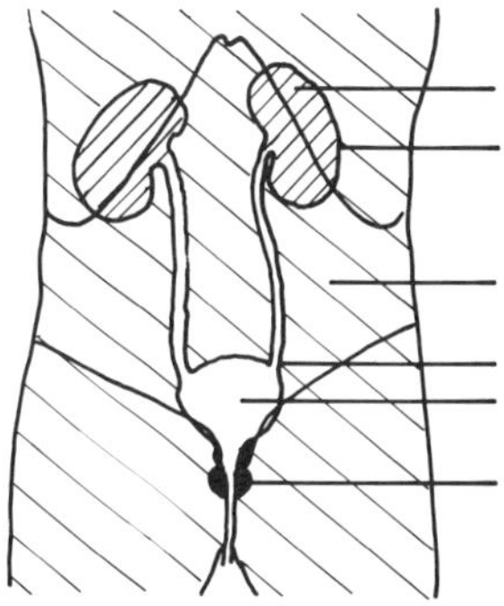

Fig. 19.1. Eosinophils in urological diseases.

source of eosinophils which have traversed into tissues, useful for structural and functional studies. In one report from Washington DC in 1986, 0.3–288 × 10^8 eosinophils were obtained from each bag.[583]

19.2.1 *Peritoneal dialysis and eosinophils*

Many reports have been published of eosinophilia in patients undergoing maintenance peritoneal dialysis. In 1981 three patients were reported from Newcastle-upon-Tyne, UK,[688] and ten were described in the USA.[826] Eight more were reported in 1982.[1673] Twenty-nine patients with this complication were reviewed in 1985, and previous cases were reviewed.[304] The typical clinical features of these patients were that two weeks to four months after implantation of the peritoneal catheter, they developed a cloudy peritoneal fluid, without having fever, abdominal pain, nausea, vomiting, or rebound tenderness, which are characteristic of a peritoneal infection. They did not have a skin rash or itching. The fluid contained as many as 1.9 × 10^9 white blood cells/l, and up to 95 per cent were eosinophils. Some patients also developed blood eosinophilia. In most patients the fluid became clear again after several days or weeks, without the use of antibiotics. Quantitative counts of peritoneal fluid eosinophils and blood eosinophils, and the time course of disappearance of peritoneal eosinophilia was assessed in 61 patients in Pittsburgh, USA, in 1984,[1423] and it was found that the counts fell from initial high levels, and continued to fall at six months.

The cause(s) of this eosinophilic response has been the subject of considerable interest. One possibility was that they had become sensitized to impurities released from the tubing, bags, or fluids used for the dialysis. Ethylene oxide was considered to be a possible sensitizing agent,[708] as it can be eluted from dialysis tubing.[1378] Plasticizers in dialysis bags were also considered.[1265] An explanation of this kind was supported by a study in

1986 which showed that the frequency of tubing changes was linked to the incidence of eosinophilia.[90]

The possibility that eosinophils in the peritoneal fluid appear as a result of the entry of air into the peritoneal cavity was tested in two patients on continuous ambulatory peritoneal dialysis (CAPD) in 1985. The number of eosinophils increased from a mean of 1.5 to 50 × 10^9/l in one patient, and from 0 to 60 × 10^9/l in the other, during the week following air injection, showing that this could be a factor in the appearance of eosinophils in peritoneal fluid.[394] In 1987 the same group reported that peritoneal fluid eosinophilia was produced in four of five patients on CAPD by the injection of 100–500 ml air into the peritoneum. With the larger amounts of air, eosinophilia persisted for five weeks.[395]

19.2.2 *Haemodialysis and eosinophils*

Nephrologists have known for many years that patients with end stage renal failure on haemodialysis can develop eosinophilia. As the highest counts were usually seen in patients who had been on dialysis the longest, and as a raised serum IgE level was more common in haemodialysis patients with eosinophilia than those without,[1288, 1875] it was natural to suppose that an allergic reaction to a component in the dialysis fluid was responsible. However, alterations in the rinsing procedure did not affect the development of the reactions in a study reported in 1984.[1875]

Among a group of 240 patients undergoing haemodialysis in Lisbon, Portugal, 14 per cent had blood eosinophil counts greater than 0.4 × 10^9/l. The mean eosinophil count was 0.613, and the range 0.410–1.780 × 10^9/l. Thirty-one per cent of the HBsAg positive patients who were on coil dialysis had eosinophilia. No difference was seen in the incidence of eosinophilia between patients on coil and on capillary dialysis machines, nor was there any relationship to their parathyroid status.[1436]

In studies from Uppsala, Sweden reported in 1982[742] and 1984,[388] it was found that blood eosinophil and neutrophil counts fell during the first ten minutes of haemodialysis, although they subsequently returned to normal levels. During the first two hours of dialysis, the serum ECP level also rose. It was then seen that when fresh blood containing eosinophils was passed through a dialyser, the ECP level rose steadily, so that at two hours it was 76 times higher than at the start, and the eosinophil count had fallen to 67 per cent of the initial level. This effect on eosinophils was most marked when cuprophane membranes were used. It was suggested that during haemodialysis, the contact of eosinophils with the dialysis membrane caused them to release their constituents into the blood. These would not attach to the membrane, as experiments showed that only 10 per cent of added ECP bound to dialysis membranes. This possibility was supported by a study from Italy in 1985, which suggested that MBP was released from eosinophils, and that this neutralized some of the heparin anticoagulation which their patients were receiving.[1556] Dialysis membranes can cause complement activation with aggregation and stimulation of neutrophil degranulation in the lungs. Whether eosinophils could also be affected by complement activation products in this way is not known.

Microangiopathic changes in the skin of patients undergoing haemodialysis were reported in 1987, from a group of 63 patients with end stage renal failure in Japan. Marked basement thickening of epidermal capillaries was seen, and it was suggested that this was due to inflammatory reactions induced by uraemic toxins. As some of these patients had eosinophilia, it was thought possible that eosinophils could have been involved in the production of these vascular changes.[835]

19.3 Eosinophilic cystitis

Eosinophil cystitis, which was originally defined in 1960 as 'eosinophilic granuloma of the bladder', is a rare disease. Only 39 cases were reported by 1982,[1087] although by 1987 there were a total of 50 case reports. It is more common in men than women, and there may be a history of allergy or previous trauma to the bladder. These patients had episodes of haematuria, frequency of urination with dysuria, and syprapubic pain. At cystoscopy there were raised erythematous mucosal lesions which often looked like polyps, or even tumours. In the acute stages of the disease, the mucosa, submucosa, and muscularis of the bladder wall was found to be infiltrated with many eosinophils and mast cells, with muscle necrosis and surrounding oedema.

Later, chronic inflammation lead to fibrosis, especially of the superficial layer, and this required urinary diversion and cystectomy in some patients.[1623] About one-third had eosinophilia. One patient with eosinophilic cystitis also had Glanzmann's thrombasthenia.[195]

Light microscopy and EM studies on biopsies from the bladder of a 63-year-old woman with eosinophilic cystitis showed giant cells ingesting eosinophils and free granules.[44] An assay for ECP in urine was developed in 1986, and it was recommended as a useful technique for indentifying patients with eosinophilic cystitis,[595] but this was not confirmed in a study the following year.[1121]

Eosinophilic cystitis can cause obstruction of the ureteral orifices with eosinophil-rich inflammatory tissue.[1219] This may necessitate surgical resection and reimplantation of the ureters, and/or repeated hydrostatic dilatation.[1308] Rarely, the ureters only are affected by a similar process,[775] or an eosinophilic granuloma.[1814]

An 'allergen provocation test' with tomatoes in a 35-year-old woman with eosinophilic cystitis showed an eosinophil-rich infiltrate into the bladder, and it was suggested that this or similar allergens could be the cause of this disease in some patients.[1551]

Eosinophilic cystitis can also occur in children, when it appears to have a more benign course than in adults.[1727]

19.4 Eosinophils in the urine

Eosinophils can occur in the urinary sediment with other inflammatory cells in a wide variety of diseases, as reviewed in 1987.[359] In a study from Chicago, Illinois, USA in 1985, eosinophils were found in the urine of 65 of 470 patients whose urine was specifically examined. Infections in the upper and lower urinary tract was responsible in 29 (45 per cent), and 9 patients had acute interstitial nephritis.[360] About 60 per cent of patients with interstitial nephritis have eosinophiluria,[321, 1728] but the incidence can be even higher. Eosinophiluria was found in 10 of 11 patients with drug-induced acute interstitial nephritis, reported in 1986.[1284] Other diseases where they have been seen include rapidly progressive glomerulonephritis, acute prostatitis, and occasionally acute cystitis and postinfections glomerulonephritis. A patient with systemic atheroembolism, renal damage, and eosinophiluria was described in 1986.[2018]

19.5 Prostatic diseases

Eosinophils are prominent in the prostate gland in several types of granulomatour prostatitis, including:

(1) allergic eosinophilic prostatitis, in which eosinophil-rich granulomas are found in patients with asthma or other allergic diseases;

(2) non-specific granulomatous prostatitis; and

(3) post-transurethral resection prostatitis.

Seven patients at the Johns Hopkins Hospital, Baltimore, Maryland, USA with eosinophil-rich granulomatous prostatitis, were described in 1984.[522] Three had nonspecific granulomas, and four had post-transurethral resection granulomas. Two other cases of non-allergic eosinophilic prostatitis were described in 1984.[1978, 1481]

19.6 Renal allograft rejection

In renal transplant patients, an increase in blood eosinophil counts is invariably associated with an acute rejection episode 1–4 days later, but it is not related to the extent of the cellular infiltrate into the graft.[1036] In one patient, eosinophil counts returned to normal four days after the removal of a rejecting graft.[1596] Eosinophils are usually present within rejecting renal allografts, where they may play a role in the rejection process itself, by causing further tissue injury. This possibility was discussed in 1986 following an analysis of acute rejection episodes in 112 patients with renal allografts, which showed that an increased percentage of eosinophils in the blood and in renal biopsies was linked to a poor outcome from rejection episodes.[1901]

20. Female genital tract diseases and pregnancy

It has been known for many years that eosinophils are prominent in the endometrium of rodents undergoing oestrus. Experimental studies have looked for oestrogen receptors on rodent eosinophils, and an effect of eosinophils on the endometrium. This work has been based on the hypothesis that eosinophils may release a number of molecules, including leukotrienes, during oestrus which would affect the permeability of uterine blood vessels. However, in man, eosinophils do not appear to have oestrogen receptors, and only small numbers are found in the endometrium. The presence of large numbers of eosinophils in the human genital tract is always abnormal. The principal disorder of the genital tract in which eosinophils are prominent is carcinoma of the cervix as described on page 174. No studies have been done using monoclonal antibodies to look for secreted eosinophil products in the uterus in different diseases. There may be a role for MBP in pregnancy, although there is no evidence that eosinophils are involved in gestation.

20.1 The uterus and uterine diseases

The number of eosinophils in the human uterus varies during the menstrual cycle, so that they are least during the luteal phase, when implantation may occur.[286] They are mainly localized, with larger numbers of neutrophils in the endocervix, and lower uterine segments. Peroxidases, which are produced by granulocytes in these sites, may have a protective role against bacterial infections.[1445] A marked cervical eosinophil-rich infiltrate of unknown cause was reported in 1977 in a baby who died at birth with dysplastic kidneys and hypoplastic lungs.[377]

An extensive literature is available, much of it from Tchernitchin's group in Chile, on the occurrence of eosinophils in the rodent uterus. This was reviewed in 1986.[656] Their main conclusions were that oestrogens induced eosinophils to localize and degranulate in the wall of the uterus, where they contributed to the large amounts of uterine peroxidase which is present in late oestrus. It is not known whether these eosinophils induce a vascular permeability increase that occurs at this time, or whether they have a role in protecting the rodent uterus from infection.

20.2 Pregnancy

Although there is either no change in blood eosinophil counts during pregnancy or a slight fall,[1424] plasma and serum MBP levels (but not ECP, EDN/EPX, or CLC protein levels) have been found to increase to about 7.5 μg/ml at 20 weeks, when it levels off, only returning to previous levels at term.[1128] MBP has been detected in the placenta, in anchoring villi, placental X-cells, and giant cells,[1882] and this may be the source of the serum MBP in pregnancy. Pregnancy-associated MBP appears to be identical with eosinophil-derived MBP.[1129] As there was a relationship between increased plasma MBP levels late in the third trimester and at the onset of spontaneous labour, it was suggested that plasma MBP levels could be useful in predicting when this was about to occur.[1881] An increase in plasma MBP has also been noted in the pregnant gorilla, cynomologus monkey, and rhesus monkey, and MBP was also found in primate placental X cells.[1880]

21. Cardiovascular diseases

Eosinophils have an important relationship with a number of heart diseases. Eosinophils may cause endomyocardial fibrosis, both in patients with a marked and persistent eosinophilia, and in tropical endomyocardial fibrosis. A range of inflammatory heart muscle disease also occurs in which eosinophils are often found, including cardiac rejection, drug reactions affecting the heart, and the Churg–Strauss syndrome. Cardiac involvement in systemic diseases producing eosinophilia is usually a serious prognostic sign, and many of these patients develop arrhythmias or heart failure. It is therefore important to examine the heart carefully in all patients who have eosinophilia. Any abnormalities which are detected at the bedside, or following electrocardiograms (ECGs) and chest radiographs should be followed up with further studies, providing treatment is not delayed, as many of these disorders can progress rapidly.

21.1 Diseases of the heart and pericardium

21.1.1 *Pericardial diseases and pericardial effusion*

An unusual eosinophilic disease of unknown cause can give rise to constrictive pericarditis. In a study from Hawaii, USA reported in 1984, three patients were described with constrictive pericarditis, in whom eosinophils were found in the resected tissue. In one of them there was a blood eosinophil count of 2.2×10^9/l. They were treated successfully by pericardectomy.[1867] I have also seen two women, aged 45 and 65 years with this disease, and both needed pericardectomies. Granulomas were not found in the pericardium, and there was no evidence for a systemic illness to account for their pericardial lesions and eosinophilia, although one had a history of asthma. Details of the first patient were published in 1978.[358] The second patient had a similar history, although her eosinophilia persisted despite continuous treatment with steroids for over 10 years. Few reports describe the discovery of large numbers of eosinophils in pericardial fluid, but they have been noted in patients with asthma, malignant lymphomas, Hodgkin's disease, and drug reactions. A 28-year-old woman was described in 1964 who had pulmonary eosinophilia and pericarditis, in whom the pericardial fluid contained 11.3×10^9 white cells/l, 96 per cent of which were eosinophils.[733] Four previous case reports of eosinophils in pericardial fluid were discussed in a case report in 1983 of a woman with asthma, and blood eosinophil counts of $6.2 \times 10^9/l$, who developed a pericardial effusion, containing 540 ml, and 80 per cent eosinophils.[885]

21.1.2 *Cardiac allograft rejection*

Rejection of the transplanted human heart is usually associated with an increased inflammatory infiltrate. In a study on 18 transplants reported in 1987 from the John Hopkins Hospital, Baltimore, Maryland, USA, more eosinophils were seen in biopsies showing myocyte necrosis than in pre-rejection biopsies, but they were not useful as a predictor of rejection episodes.[792]

21.1.3 *Coronary heart disease*

As coronary artery occlusions induce blood neutrophils to localize in areas of ischaemia and necrosis, with some extension of the areas of myocardial injury,[1690] it is important to consider whether eosinophils can also be localized in the areas of myocardial ischaemia. This is of potential importance as eosinophils can produce large amounts of reactive oxygen species, and secrete their cardiotoxic proteins. Raised levels of serum ECP were reported in 1979 in a group of Swedish patients admitted to hospital with a myocardial infarction, even though none of them had eosinophilia. This report suggested that eosinophils might be involved in the inflammatory response to myocardial injury, although they are seldom seen in histological sections of myocardium. This study also showed that treatment of normal individuals with 0.5 mg methylprednisolone did not alter serum ECP levels, although it caused blood eosinophil counts to fall, suggesting that the rise in serum ECP following myocardial infarction was not a steroid-induced effect.[741] Eosinophils may also affect the long-term outcome of a myocardial infarction, as a study from Nashville, Tennessee, USA in 1985 found that cardiac rupture following myocardial infarction seemed to be related to the presence of an increased number of eosinophils in the area of myocardial damage.[74]

21.1.4 *Myocardial diseases*

Eosinophil infiltrates can also be found in the heart in a wide variety of inflammatory disorders, which we have reviewed in 1985.[1700] They include eosinophilic and tropical endomyocardial fibrosis, which are reviewed in the next chapter, drug hypersensitivity reactions[170] (see page 309), cardiac transplantation, and a poorly defined disorder called necrotizing eosinophilic myocarditis.[793] Focal areas of vasculitis and granulomatous reactions, as seen in the Churg–Strauss syndrome, can also give rise to large numbers of eosinophils in areas of myocardial injury. Parasitic diseases such as trichinosis can also induce areas of myocardial injury rich in eosinophils.[40] Congestive cardiomyopathy is the end result of a wide range of different types of myocardial injury. We raised the possibility that some patients may have a disease process involving cardiotoxic eosinophil constituents in a small study in which we found that serum ECP levels were higher than normal.[1698]

21.2 Vascular diseases

Eosinophils are often found with mast cells in the adventitia of veins in the lung, intestine, and other sites, but the presence of eosinophils in the vessel wall itself is uncommon, except in vasculitis disorders. The occurrence of thromboemboli complications in patients with persistent eosinophilia, especially HES, is an important clinical observation, suggesting that eosinophils could produce effects on the endothelium or platelets. Although there is limited work in this area, it has been shown that ECP can:

(a) produce changes in the intrinsic coagulation system;

(b) reduce thromboxane production by isolated endothelial cells; and

(c) occasionally stimulate platelet aggregation.[398]

The relative importance of these processes in thromboembolic complications of hypereosinophilia are not known, and it is also not clear whether therapy to prevent platelet aggregation is beneficial in patients with persistent hypereosinophilia.

21.2.1 *Atherosclerosis*

Eosinophils are not a component of atherosclerotic lesions. However, patients who develop the 'multiple cholesterol emboli syndrome' with visceral infarction due to the release of cholesterol-rich plaques, for example during arterial catheterization, may have marked eosinophilia with thrombocytopenia and hypocomplementaemia. Biopsies may be needed to distinguish this syndrome from vasculitic diseases.[1984] Eosinophilia occurs in 80 per cent of reported patients with atheroembolic renal disease, according to a literature review made in 1987. Eosinophilia is often mild, and may last only a few days.[914]

21.3 Vasculitis

A large number of diseases have a vasculitic element which can contain many eosinophils. A useful review of these diseases was published in

1985,[1504] and the difficulties in providing distinct categories of arteritis were discussed in 1986.[303]

Polyarteritis nodosa is the best known example of a systemic vasculitis without granulomatous inflammation, and many textbooks on general medicine state that it is an important cause of marked eosinophilia. This stemmed from early reports[1464] and difficulties at that time in distinguishing polyarteritis nodosa from the Churg–Strauss syndrome which does give rise to marked eosinophilia. However, both diseases are closely related, and in the classification of patients with vasculitis put forward by Dr Anthony Fauci in 1983,[543] they were combined under the general term 'polyarteritis nodosa group of systemic necrotizing vasculitis'.

Although hypereosinophilia is not a characteristic of classical polyarteritis nodosa,[545] these patients often have mild or transient eosinophilia.[1581, 1246] A moderate increase in blood eosinophil counts is also common in patients with microscopic polyarteritis with crescentic and necrotizing glomerulonephritis. This was discussed in a study on polyarteritis nodosa and necrotizing glomerulonephritis in 1987.[370]

Serum antibodies which stain the cytoplasm of circulating neutrophils have been detected in patients with necrotizing vasculitis. These were found in two patients who also had eosinophilia. One was a 17-year-old boy with the Churg–Strauss syndrome, cardiac involvement, and blood eosinophil counts of 18×10^9/l, and the second was a 55-year-old man with pulmonary eosinophilia and a blood eosinophil count of 4×10^9/l.[1891]

Wegener's granulomatosis, first described in the 1930s, is a systemic disease which gives rise to necrotizing granulomas in the upper and lower respiratory tract, glomerular lesions, and injury to the skin, joints, and peripheral nerves. It mainly affects the respiratory tract, and is discussed on page 209.

An unusual type of temporal arteritis can be found in young adults, and there is a case report of this disease in a young adult with eosinophilia of 28–48 per cent of $9.9–13.9 \times 10^9$/l total white blood cells.[187]

Spontaneous dissection of the left anterior descending coronary artery, which was reviewed in 1982,[1505] has been described in 54 people who developed chest pain or died suddenly. A striking feature is an eosinophil-rich inflammatory reaction in the adventitia, with dissection in the outer third of the vessel. The coronary sinus can be involved in a similar disease process as described in a 44-year-old woman in Sydney, Australia in 1980.[206]

22. Endomyocardial fibrosis

22.1 History

Eosinophilic endomyocardial fibrosis (E-EMF) (see Plate 7) was probably first seen in 1893 in a 31-year-old woman who had a tumour in the neck, with a blood eosinophil count of 57.6×10^9/l. At post mortem the right ventricular endocardium was found to be covered with a greyish-white mural thrombus.[1485] In 1936 Professor W. Löffler published detailed clinical descriptions of two patients in Basle, Switzerland, who had E-EMF, although at that time it was called endocarditis parietalis fibroplastica, or Löffler's endomyocardial fibrosis. His first patient was a woman of 45 who died one year after presentation with severe right and left sided eosinophilic endomyocardial disease. The second was a 37-year-old man who died after 21 months with similar complications. In one patient the heart disease was associated with a severe illness, whereas the second patient presented with heart failure without a systemic illness. Another difference was that eosinophilia increased in one patient whereas it disappeared shortly before death in the other.[1092] An English translation of Löffler's seminal paper was published in 1948,[1059] and the disease was reviewed in a German paper published that year.[158]

A second form of this disease, called tropical endomyocardial fibrosis (T-EMF) as it is mainly confined to tropical regions, has been known since 1946.[145] For several years these diseases were considered to be distinct, although the possibility that there was a disease spectrum ranging from 'tropical' endomyocardial fibrosis to 'Löffler's' endomyocardial fibrosis was suggested by Davies and Ball as early as 1955.[406] Histological studies in the 1970s demonstrated that they were pathologically indistinguishable, despite the different clinical settings in which they were found. In the first of these studies in 1970, detailed post mortems were carried out on three men aged 25, 26 and 35 who died with HES. The findings supported the possibility that tropical endomyocaridal fibrosis might be a later stage or an inactive form of E-EMF.[1500]

In the second, a comparative pathological and clinical review of 90 patients with E-EMF was carried out in 1973. Eosinophilia was of unknown cause in 50 per cent, reactive in 25 per cent (polyarteritis, asthma, drug sensitivity, Hodgkin's disease, and carcinomas), and due to eosinophilic leukaemia (or HES) in 25 per cent. Among 30 hearts examined, 10 were in the acute necrotic stage, with an illness lasting a

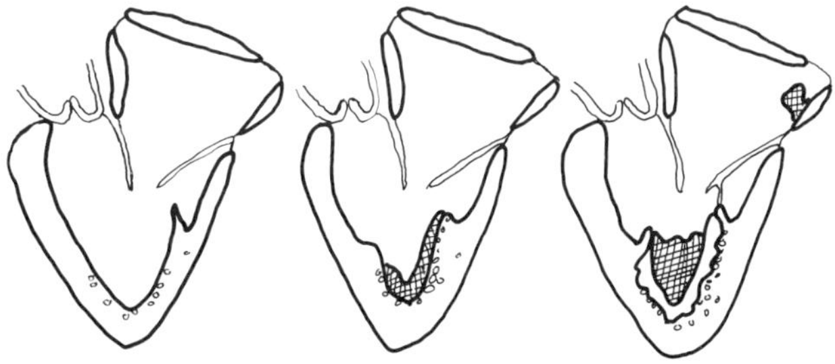

Fig. 22.1. Three stages in the development of eosinophilic endomyocardial fibrosis. Modified from Spry *et al.* (1983),[1693] with permission.

mean of 5.5 weeks, 8 were in the later thrombotic stage, with an illness of 10 months, and 12 were in the fibrotic stage, with an illness lasting 24.5 months. (See Fig. 22.1.) Samples from 16 patients in the thrombotic and fibrotic stages of E-EMF were compared with 32 specimens from patients with T-EMF, and no significant pathological differences were found. It was concluded that T-EMF and E-EMF had a similar pathogenesis, such as a toxic effect of eosinophils on the myocardium.[209] This review is based on my related article[1689] (with permission).

By 1972 the frequent occurrence (20 per cent or more) of E-EMF in patients with 'eosinophilic leukaemia' (two rare disorders occurring together with high frequency) led to the suggestion that there might be an intimate cause–effect relationship between the two disorders, similar to that of the cardio-pulmonary lesions in the metastatic carcinoid syndrome:

> Forceful cardiac contractions might cause excessive destruction of eosinophils, and a continued high concentration of their chemicals and hydrolytic enzymes within the heart. This in turn may cause endocardial inflammation and injury. In prolonged eosinophilia, regardless of etiology, this sort of change is likely to occur more frequently, and to be more severe. It would appear that the endocardial lesion is the result of the eosinophilia . . . [1962]

It is now thought likely that eosinophils are involved in the development of the endocardial lesions in both forms of the disease. This association has been most clearly demonstrated in E-EMF, and there is strong circumstantial evidence that a similar but more slowly progressive disease occurs in the tropical form of the disease. However, the predilection of the endocardium for this type of damage has not been explained, but it does raise the possibility that regional differences in disease susceptibility within the heart may account for a number of other focal or diffuse cardiac diseases of unknown cause. It also shows how an inflammatory response can give rise to distant effects on other otherwise normal tissues, especially when the inflammatory process is prolonged.

Twenty-six patients with E-EMF were described during the period 1936–57, and reviewed by Weiss-Carmine. Several patients had arteritic lesions, and thrombo-emboli were also noted to be an important feature of the disease.[1903] Another review was published in 1955.[804]

A second major review of E-EMF was carried out in 1963 with details of 14 further patients, including 3 more of their own, by Brink and Weber (1963). This paper suggested that high blood neutrophil counts might be associated with endomycardial fibrosis, although this has not been substantiated subsequently.[207]

During the past decade, the development of effective invasive techniques for studying the heart have enabled clinicians to diagnose both diseases at an earlier stage than was previously possible. The advent of 2-D echocardiography, endocardial biopsy, and surgical treatment has also enabled clinical and experimental studies to be carried out on the nature and pathogenesis of EMF.

We reviewed the clinical features and pathophysiology of E-EMF in 1983,[1318] 1985,[1319] and 1987.[1691, 1689]

By 1980, over 100 patients with E-EMF had been described.[1893] Because an underlying eosinophilic disorder, often HES, tended to dominate the clinical picture, the heart disease was usually described in less detail. However, the general awareness that cardiac complications were the main presentation in at least half of the patients with HES, and that over 80 per cent would finally develop heart disease,[1683] stimulated detailed cardiological studies on these patients.

Two series of patients with HES who have a high incidence of E-EMF have been studied over more than a decade in the USA,[1366] and by us in the UK.[1694]

Although EMF, with or without eosinophilia, was initially only known in Uganda[404] and Nigeria, there have been detailed reports from a number of other countries, including South India in 1983[402, 310] and 1986,[104] Ivory Coast in 1985,[163] Venezuela in 1983,[1457] Brazil in 1984,[284] Japan in 1985,[1743] Thailand in 1984,[1719] Spain in 1982,[1828] the Middle East in 1985,[549] and France in 1983.[471] In French speaking regions, no attempt was made to distinguish the tropical forms of the disease from the eosinophilic form. In other countries, they are usually described separately.

In 1979, an analysis of the cardiological features of E-EMF was reported from the NIH, Bethesda, Maryland, USA.[1366] This paper reviewed 65 previous case reports, in which 57 per cent had histological features of E-EMF, combined with descriptions of a further 26 patients. M-mode echocardiograms were thought to show an increased left ventricular wall thickness and raised left ventrical mass in 18 of the 22 patients (82 per cent). It was suggested that this was an early feature of cardiac involvement in HES, and might be helpful in following the progression of the disease. In 7 of 8 patients, who did not show a good response to treatment with prednisolone, with or without hydroxyurea, there appeared to be a progression of echocardiographic abnormalities, whereas in 8 of 10 patients adequently treated, this did not occur. Although this was one of the first detailed descriptions of the disease, using a combination of echocardiography and ventricular angiocardiograms, cardiac biopsies were not done in any of the 26 patients. Three of the 26 patients died: one following busulphan treatment, one with a possible arrhythmia, and one with the Budd–Chiari syndrome. Although only one patient had emboli, because of the likely presence of thrombi in the left ventricle of some patients, it was recommended that anticoagulation should be carried out. Several patients had angiographic evidence for coronary artery disease, but this was not a clinical problem in any of these patients.

The cardiological features of E-EMF seen in outpatients range from apparent normality in patients at the first stage, to gross heart failure in patients in the late fibrotic stage of the disease. In 1974, a review of the cardiovascular complications which occurred in the NIH patients with HES and eosinophilic leukaemia showed that they were the same, and that the endocardial lesions were indistinguishable from those seen in T-EMF.[1499] A further report from the same centre was made in 1983.[755]

The awareness of the high incidence of eosinophilic heart disease in patients with persistent eosinophilia has made many clinicians more alert to the earlier signs of cardiac involvement; asymptomatic murmurs, micro-embolic disease, especially splinter haemorrhages, minor strokes, and non-specific ECG abnormalities.[262] Today, eosinophilic heart disease can be recognized when it gives rise to a number of different abnormalities, besides a restrictive cardiomyopathy. In the series of 14 patients, published in 1985 by Take and colleagues in Japan,[1743] 5 patients had acute carditis, 3 had electrical disturbances, 3 had ventricular dilatation, and 3 had a restrictive cardiomyopathy.

22.2 Eosinophilic endomyocardial fibrosis

The clinical features of the underlying eosinophilic disorders may mask or affect the clinical presentation of the heart disease, which is usually diagnosed at a late stage in the development of the cardiac pathology, although methods are now available for recognizing this at an early stage.

22.2.1 *Eosinophilic diseases with endomyocardial fibrosis*

By definition, E-EMF always occurs in patients with eosinophilia. It can occur in patients with any of the principal causes of chronic eosinophilia.

For example, a 52-year-old man was described in 1959 who had tuberculosis treated with isoniazid and PAS. He developed an eosinophil count of $14 \times 10^9/l$, and died later with E-EMF. Other early work, describing patients with infections, eosinophilia, and endomyocardial disease were also reviewed in this report. These included patients with syphilis, malaria, tonsillitis, amoebiasis, dengue fever, and allergic reactions to parasites, including *Loa loa*.[1486] In Western countries the commonest disease association is HES, but it also includes parasitic diseases, chronic drug reactions, and tumour-induced eosinophilia.

E-EMF complicating HES can occur in infancy and childhood. Examples include:

1. a girl aged five years, who died within a month of presenting with HES. At post mortem, there were thrombi in the left ventricle and right atrium, and emboli in a pulmonary artery, but there was no endomyocardial fibrosis, probably because the illness was of such short duration.[1479]

2. a child aged seven years, who developed HES. She died after a 10 month illness, and was found to have bilateral E-EMF, with peripheral emboli originating from the left ventricle.[982]

3. a 9-year-old boy who died after a 10 month illness due to HES, and showed the features of E-EMF at post mortem.[1324]

4. a boy aged 12, who was found to have an eosinophil count of $170 \times 10^9/l$. Three years after the onset of his illness, he died with congestive cardiac failure, due to bilateral E-EMF.[1075]

E-EMF is an important complication of eosinophilic leukaemia. A review in 1961 showed that among 9 patients with acute eosinophilic leukaemia with blast cells, 5 had cardiovascular abnormalities. Seven of the 11 patients who only had mature blood eosinophils (which might today be called HES) also had heart involvement. This is a total of 12 cases of heart disease in 20 patients (60 per cent).[156] In 1978 E-EMF was described in a patient with Phi positive chronic myeloid leukaemia and a hypoplastic right ventricle.[1651]

Although it is unusual for patients in Western countries with E-EMF to have a parasitic infection, in 1972 a 40-year-old woman was described who died with E-EMF and eosinophilia of '60–70 per cent', and who was found to have a 10 metre long *Taenia saginata* worm in her intestines.[50] Patients with E-EMF and fascioliasis have also been reported from France in 1975,[386] and 1978.[1434]

Patients with a drug-induced hypersensitivity disease may develop E-EMF. In 1946 a 41-year-old man was described who had been treated with neoarsphenamine for syphilis, and developed eosinophilia of $2.5 \times 10^9/l$, with heart failure which was found to be due to E-EMF.[492] In 1959, E-EMF was described as a complication of eosinophilia due to streptomycin hypersensitivity.[624]

Vasculitic diseases with eosinophilia are also known to be able to lead to the development of E-EMF, including the Churg–Strauss syndrome.[1029]

E-EMF has been seen in patients with lymphocytic-leukaemia-associated hypereosinophilia.[180, 629]

An unusual clinical story of a woman with chronic eosinophilic pneumonia who developed hypereosinophilia and E-EMF, was given in a clinico-pathological conference in 1980. When she was 31, she developed pulmonary infiltrates with an eosinophil count of $6.4 \times 10^9/l$. This improved on treatment with prednisolone, 13 mg per day. At age 35, after the steroids had been stopped and eosinophilia had recurred, she developed chest pain and went into severe heart failure with an enlarged heart and a pericardial effusion. A right ventricular biopsy showed E-EMF in the acute necrotic stage. Treatment with steroids, warfarin, and digoxin resulted in an improvement. The discussion by Dr Sheldon Wolff centred on the differential diagnosis of this unusual combination of clinical problems. It illustrated the wide range of eosinophilic disorders in which E-EMF can occur.[2014]

22.2.2 *Clinical features*

Over a hundred case reports of patients with E-EMF have been published. As the majority of patients with E-EMF have HES, the most extensive studies have been carried out in this group of patients, and most is known about the clinical features of the disease in this setting. About half the patients presented with late-stage disease, and half developed it during the subsequent several years. The age, and sex incidence of the patients reflect that of HES: a mean age of 37 years and predominantly male. In the late stage of the disease it has many features in common with other forms of restrictive cardiomyopathy, and it can be confused with pericardial constriction. This difficulty in distinguishing constrictive pericarditis and E-EMF was well illustrated by a case report from the Johns Hopkins Hospital in 1952. The correct diagnosis was only made when surgery was carried out to remove what was thought to be a constricting pericardium.[1176] Löffler himself described the ways in which E-EMF is now known to affect cardiac function: 'endocardial thickening prevents normal diastolic relaxation of the ventricles, and thrombotic masses decrease the capacity of the ventricles'.[1093] Unlike T-EMF, ascites is uncommon, and oedema of the face and upper extremities is not often seen, even when the patients are in gross heart failure with persistently high right atrial pressures and pulmonary oedema. The main features at the bedside are signs of chronic heart failure, with wasting, oedema, and heart murmurs which are most marked in patients with mitral incompetence.

E-EMF is invariably associated with a systemic disorder giving rise to eosinophilia. This ranges from a malignant process which may remain hidden for several months or years, and HES, to rare cases of eosinophilic leukaemia. In some patients with acute eosinophilic leukaemia, blood disease may progress so rapidly that they do not have time to develop cardiac disease before they die.

22.2.3 *Investigations of E-EMF*

The investigations of E-EMF can be considered under two headings: outpatient investigations, and inpatient invasive studies designed to determine the extent of the lesions and the potential value of surgery. The cardiac silhouette is generally normal in patients with the early or later stages of E-EMF, until heart failure supervenes. In occasional patients calcification can be seen in lateral chest radiographs, although this is much more common in T-EMF. Marked calcification was reported in one patient.[1057] When pulmonary oedema occurs, this has no special features. Pleural effusions and pericardial effusions are sometimes seen.

Electrocardiography in E-EMF Electrocardiograms (ECGs) are normal until the later thrombotic and fibrotic stage of the disease has developed, when there are repolarization changes, characteristic of endocardial lesions. Following the development of heart failure, a number of other abnormalities in the ECG can develop, but none of these are diagnostic. Holter monitoring has generally not been of great help, except in defining the types of arrythmias that often develop sporadically in patients who have the late stage of the disease, and who may be improved by anti-arrythmic therapy. However, as arrythmias usually respond to successful cardiac surgery (valve replacement with or without endocardectomy), arrythmias seem to be more related to heart failure than to involvement of conducting systems or other sites by the fibrotic process.[336]

Conduction defects have been reported on several occasions.[910] Arrythmias were a problem in a 48-year-old man with E-EMF who had conduction defects, a wandering atrial pacemaker, and intermittent 2:1 dissociation which required treatment with a pacemaker.[1652] Another example was in a 79-year-old man who developed complete heart block.[1467] This study also reviewed 65 other cases of E-EMF, and found that 19 (29 per cent) had conduction disturbances. An HIS bundle electrogram has been carried out on a patient with E-EMF. Right atrial pacing showed increased P1-A interval from 25 ms to 100 ms, followed by Mobitz type 1 block. This suggested that there was a conduction delay in the atrium and AV node, possibly due to fibrous tissue. Details of the catherization and angiocardiography findings in this patient were also published.[705] It may be very difficult to place a transvenous pacing electrode into the right ventricle, due to the presence of thrombus and fibrosis in the cavity,[1583] and an open procedure may be preferable.

Ventricular fibrillation has been documented in a few patients.

Echocardiography in E-EMF Echocardiography is the most useful technique for defining the structural changes within the heart and the abnormalities in the ventricular wall which are characteristic of endomyocardial fibrosis. M-mode echocardiograms are most useful in defining the mitral valve defect that occurs in the late stage of the disease. M-mode echocardiography findings were described in 1977 in 10 patients with HES studied at NIH, Bethesda, Maryland, USA. Symmetrical thickening of the left ventricle of greater than 11 mm, with increased left ventricular mass (greater than 275 g) was reported in all the patients. These observations have not been confirmed in other series of patients with E-EMF, and they remain puzzling.[191]

2-D echocardiography, which can be combined with colour-coded enhancement of the images, has provided clear evidence during life of the sites of involvement of the heart in endocardial fibrosis the abnormalities in the septal wall, and the presence of thrombi within the heart. It has become the technique of choice in first-line investigations of patients suspected of having endomyocardial disease.[182, 1509] Unfortunately, only patients in the late stage of the disease show abnormalities which can be considered characteristic of this disorder. These include enhanced echos from the endocardium in either ventricle, the septum, and the base of the posterior papillary muscle.

In 1980 the findings were published of 2-D echocardiography in 21 patients at NIH.[1366] In 9 patients who had clinical evidence of mitral regurgitation, the 2-D echo features were correlated with the gross features seen at operation or at post mortem. In 6 patients who had peripheral emboli, the presence of thrombus or thickening of the posterobasal wall of the left ventricle was detected, and it was suggested that this was the site of origin of these emboli.[703] Three patients with HES were described from Philadelphia, USA in 1983 with cardiac dilatation on echocardiography.[434] Mural thrombi have also been clearly shown by echocardiography[1009] and computed tomography.[1377] In 1987, pulsed Doppler echocardiography showed the marked contribution of right atrial systole to pulmonary flow in a woman with HES and a large right ventricular thrombus.[1446]

A detailed report on echocardiographic studies on E-EMF was reported from Hungary in 1982,[1058] and this led to the correct diagnosis in 6 of 8 patients.[69]

In London, M-mode and echocardiography were done on 9 patients with E-EMF, among our series of patients with HES looked after at Hammersmith Hospital. The value of this series, which was also published in 1982, was that all the patients had undergone full cardiological investigations, and the extent and staging of their heart disease was known. Amplitude processed 2-D echocardiography appeared to be more sensitive than conventional 2-D echocardiography in detecting areas of increased relative echointensity. M-mode echocardiography only showed non-specific abnormalities, but was particularly useful in assessing the functional defects in myocardial function and mitral valve disease. It was also clear from this study that echocardiography was not as sensitive as endocardial biopsy in detecting the earlier stages of the disease. This limitation may be important if echocardiography is to be used to monitor the effects of treatment on the progression of endocardial fibrosis, as it may not be able to detect structurally small but functionally significant deteriorations in cardiac performance.[397]

Cardiac catheterization in E-EMF Before the introduction of echocardiography, E-EMF was often mistaken for constrictive pericarditis and cardiac catheterization with pressure studies was then the only technique for providing a definitive diagnosis of the disease prior to operation. One of the first patients in whom this was done was reported in 1956.[327]

Intracardiac pressure studies are used today to help in the assessment of pulmonary hypertension and the work of each side of the heart, and to assist in functional studies on the possible effectiveness of steroids and other drugs in preventing the progression of the disease to the later thrombotic and fibrotic stages. Angiocardiography, which is usually carried out at the same time, is also helpful in defining the extent of the lesions and the effects of these lesions on ventricular function. Angiocardiography is particularly good at demonstrating intracavity thrombi.

We published the results of detailed cardiovascular assessments of 11 patients with E-EMF who were studied at Hammersmith Hospital between 1975 and 1981.[401]

The characteristic lesions of endocardial fibrosis have been described in many patients with E-EMF. Good examples of this are given for two patients reported from St Thomas' Hospital, London in 1976,[152] and for a 45-year-old man described in the USA in 1977. The latter patient died 14 months after the onset of heart failure due to biventricular E-EMF, complicating HES. He underwent a variety of cardiac investigations, including catherization with pressure studies and cardiac biopsy, and although his blood eosinophil counts were reduced with hydroxyurea and vincristine, his disease appeared to progress.[734] An earlier report in 1974 of right-sided catheterization showed almost complete obliteration of the ventricle.[179]

Pressure studies during left ventricular catheterization of a woman in 1987 with eosinophilia of 6.068 × 10^9/l showed a 90 mmHg subaortic gradient, while the catheter was pulled back from the apex to the aortic root. This was interpreted as evidence for an obstructive cardiomyopathy, but was more likely due to thrombus which was also demonstrated in the cavity.[1214]

Cardiac biopsy of E-EMF has been carried out since 1972. Histological studies on these biopsies and post mortem material have defined the three stages of the disease. Cardiac biopsy has become one of the principle methods for diagnosing E-EMF in its early stages. This technique has the theoretical advantage that it samples the endocardium, which is the principal site of the lesion being studied.[1456] Occasionally, the endocardium is so thickened by fibrous tissue that it may not be possible to obtain a biopsy. As the fibrotic areas are surrounded by softened areas of acute inflammation, the myocardium may be perforated. Pericardial haematomata have also resulted from cardiac biopsy.

Endocardial biopsy in the diagnosis of endomyocardial fibrosis has been used in London since 1976, when the findings in two patients were reported,[152] and in the USA since 1980.[616, 1278] The experiences at NIH were reviewed in 1982.[544]

Right ventricular biopsy is most commonly carried out, because the lesions of E-EMF are always bilateral. If the tropical form of the disease is suspected, it may be also necessary to carry out left ventricular biopsy, because the lesions can occasionally be restricted to the left side of the heart.

In the earlier stages of the disease, biopsy of the septal wall can usually provide diagnostic material. Generally, four to seven biopsies are taken. In the late stage of the disease fibrotic lesions may not be easily sampled, and the catheter may move to unaffected endocardium from which normal samples may be obtained. This means that careful placement of the bioptome is essential.

Histopathology of E-EMF The histological appearances of E-EMF show involvement of the endocardium, underlying areas of the myocardium, small vessels, and interstitial tissues in the granulation tissue layer of the heart. These lesions are confined to the inflow tract and part of the outflow tract of the heart, where a rolled edge is often seen in post mortem samples. Occasionally, thrombi can be found attached to the mitral or tricuspid valve leaflets, and less commonly to the walls of the atria. Results of histological studies of E-EMF, using both light and electronmicroscopy, were reported from the UK in 1981[87] and 1982,[1314] Denmark in 1977,[86] and Japan in 1985.[1588, 1264]

Electronmicroscopy of eosinophilic heart disease has shown the presence of degranulated cells within the myocardium.

22.2.4 *Treatment of E-EMF*

The treatment of E-EMF depends on the stage at which it is diagnosed. In the early acute necrotic stage, the aim is to prevent progression of the disease. In the later thrombotic phase, the goal is to prevent emboli and further disease progression. In the final stage it becomes necessary to treat heart failure and to consider the use of surgery. As yet there is no medical treatment which will prevent the progression of E-EMF, although we have preliminary evidence that prednisolone 5–15 mg/d slowed the progression of the disease. The insensitivity of echocardiography in following the progression of the disease, except in the later stages, is clearly a difficulty here, and cardiac biopsy has not been carried out routinely in treated and untreated patients to determine which form of therapy might be most effective.

The recognition that endocardial thrombi were clinically important,[1753] and that thromboembolic complications were the most common cause of death in patients with E-EMF[1694] has led to the general use of anticoagulation in this disorder. However, there is no convincing evidence that this has resulted in a reduction in vascular occlusive episodes. Indeed, we have looked after several patients who developed large emboli after anticoagulation was begun.

Heparin may not be as effective as warfarin in controlling the formation of clots in patients with HES. This was seen in a patient who had mitral and tricuspid valve replacement with Bjork–Shiley prostheses for E-EMF, and was then treated with subcutaneous heparin eight hourly, instead of warfarin. One month later he was admitted to hospital with a thrombosed mitral valve and peripheral emboli. The mitral valve was replaced with a porcine graft. When the coagulation response to heparin was assessed, he was found to need over twice the expected amount of heparin, and it was recommended that the activated clotting time should be carefully assessed in these patients in view of their increased thrombotic tendency.[751]

Anti-platelet drugs including aspirin and dipyridamole have also been used, but again, their efficacy in this condition has not been proven. Anticoagulation should be continued for life after cardiac surgery for E-EMF.[1533]

Medical treatment which improves the underlying eosinophilic disorder in patients with HES, in turn may prevent the progression of heart disease in these patients, but no long-term reports have yet been provided of the use of different forms of medical treatment, such as chronic steroid treatment, cytotoxic drugs, or other medication. Steroids may benefit patients by inhibiting eosinophil granule secretion, and as a result, the amount of granule toxin present within the heart. This was shown to have occurred in a 51-year-old woman with the acute necrotic stage of E-EMF, complicating asthma, and a radiculopathy, who was treated with prednisolone 60 mg/day for several days, followed by tapering lower doses. Cardiac biopsies were done before this, and two months later, when the acute changes had resolved.[963]

Surgery At one time the apparently bad prognosis of the underlying eosinophilic disorder discouraged surgeons from attempting a surgical approach to E-EMF. However, the outlook of the majority of eosinophilic disorders has improved so much that surgery has become a worthwhile form of treatment in most patients with severe endomyocardial fibrosis.

No consensus view has yet emerged about the stage at which surgery should be carried out, whether the mitral valve should be preserved,[1950] the type of valve that should be used, or the possible danger of an increased thrombotic tendency affecting the new valve. Prior to 1980, early work in Switzerland and the USA had led some surgeons to suspect that valve replacement would not benefit these patients due to the high incidence of thromboembolic complications. Indeed, occasional patients have been described who developed prosthetic valve endocarditis. Three of the patients in the series at NIH, Bethesda, Maryland, USA who developed heart failure complicating HES had atrioventricular valve replacements. One patient had recurrent thrombotic involvement of the valves despite anticoagulation, and after these had been replaced with pig allografts, the patient died with *Staphylococcus aureus* endocarditis. The other two patients, one of whom also had removal of a left ventricular thrombus, did much better post-operatively, although there was little improvement in pulmonary hypertension. This report emphasized the serious feature of the hypercoaguable state in this disease; the importance of carrying out valve replacement early before irreversible changes have occurred in the lungs and other organs as a result of the heart failure; and the possible value of steroids.[756] This danger was seen in a 45-year-old Finnish woman with asthma and eosinophilia of $9.4 \times 10^9/l$ who developed intracardiac thrombi. Removal of the thrombus and replacement of the mitral valve with a Bjork–Shiley tilting disc valve only prolonged the life of the patient for 14 months, as she died after the prosthesis had become blocked with thrombus, despite treatment with anticoagulants.[839] A patient with HES in India was reported to have died from a pulmonary embolus from the right ventricle in 1985.[1469] Removal of a large intracavity thrombus can be successfully carried out, as described in 1982 in a patient with an underlying malignant eosinophilic disorder.[589]

Each centre has its own approach as to how surgery should be carried out. The principle points to emphasize are that the restricting fibrotic tissue can be removed successfully, and that it does not recur at the sites of surgery. The lesions may be more difficult to see at operation than in angiograms, and the extent of fibrous tissue removal should be decided pre-operatively. A plane of cleavage can be found in some patients, but in others a ragged surface will be left, but this does not cause any special postoperative problems. The valves should be replaced with the best known material on which thrombi will not form, in view of the high risk in these patients.

When mitral valve incompetence suddenly occurs in a patient with left ventricular disease, the effects are much more serious than when a similar process occurs on the right side of the heart, and surgery then becomes urgent. Surgery for E-EMF was first carried out in 1972 in London, and this patient still remains well in 1987.

By 1985, there had been reports of the use of surgery in 41 patients with E-EMF.

Four of these patients were operated on in Budapest, Hungary between 1979 and 1984. Two required thrombectomy, two had bilateral valve replacements, and two died. Although eosinophilia persisted in the two survivors, there was no evidence for recurrence of the endocardial disease, and the patients were much proved.[69, 68]

In 1980, we published details of the first two patients at Hammersmith Hospital with severe E-EMF who underwent open heart surgery. One patient, with predominant right ventricular disease, was treated by right ventricular endocardectomy with tricuspid and mitral xenograft valve replacement. (See Plate 9) In the second patient, it was only necessary to replace the mitral valve. Both patients showed marked clinical improvement post-operatively, which was documented by cardiac catheterization and angiography. Our review of the results of surgery on 22 other patients with endocardial fibrosis, some of whom had eosinophilia, showed equally encouraging results overall. In none of these patients was there any evidence for recurrence of the endocardial lesions or progression of the heart damage for periods of up to seven years.[399]

Three patients with HES and E-EMF were reported from St Thomas' Hospital, London in 1976. One of them, a 47-year-old man, underwent mitral annuloplasty and coronary bypass surgery, and remains well 13 years later.[152]

Probably the first patient to have surgery for E-EMF in the USA was a 16-year-old boy with HES and heart failure who had a Hancock mitral valve replacement on 1 April 1976. However, his disease, including the heart failure, progressed, and he died 19 months later.[1826] Mitral valve surgery was successful in a 23-year-old black woman with blood eosinophil counts reaching $8.75 \times 10^9/l$, who had E-EMF causing mitral regurgitation. This responded well to mitral valve surgery.[15] A further account of the successful use of surgery for endomyocardial fibrosis was reported from Houston, Texas in 1981,[706] but there has been no comprehensive survey of the North American experience of surgery for EMF.

In 1985 it was proposed that it might be easiest to destroy the thickened endocardium by laser photoablation, using the focused beam of a carbon dioxide laser or argon laser light delivered through a 200-micron optical fibre,[852] but this has not been described to date.

22.2.5 *The pathogenesis of E-EMF*

The first suggestions that E-EMF and T-EMF might have a common pathogenesis were made in the Ivory Coast in 1956[636] and in Nigeria in 1970, where it was proposed that 'the eosinophil leucocytes in susceptible persons, by some unknown mechanism, caused endo- and myocardial damage'.[208] Subsequent papers have emphasized this possibility, describing the way in which eosinophils might be damaged as they hit the wall of the ventricle, where they could release toxic substances, or binding to thrombotic material on the endocardium and damaging underlying contractile tissues.

We first became interested in these possibilities in 1975, and our subsequent experimental studies have confirmed that eosinophils have a marked propensity to damage myocardial cells through a unique series of interactions with cardiac cells.

Why the lesions are localized to the endocardium in this disease is still unknown. The two main possibilities are that the thrombus layer on the endocardium concentrates the cells and the toxic proteins, so that the underlying tissue receives the largest amounts of toxic granule constituents. The second possibility is that endocardial cells have a metabolic or structural difference from other parts of the heart and other tissues, which makes them susceptible to eosinophil-mediated damage. The peculiar blood supply to the cells in this region indicates that they might differ from other parts of the heart in their response to inflammatory cells, but this has yet to be documented.

Human studies In 1976, we reported that a distinctive feature of these patients, which was linked to the development of E-EMF, was the presence of vacuoles and a decreased number of specific granules in many blood eosinophils. This was documented in four patients who had more than 1×10^9 eosinophils/l which were vacuolated and contained reduced numbers of crystalloid granules. A higher proportion than normal of these patients' eosinophils had FcγR for rabbit IgG-coated erythrocytes, and could phagocytose erythrocytes coated with rabbit IgG or human C3b, suggesting that a large proportion of the blood eosinophils were activated or stimulated in these patients.[1696]

As eosinophils had been shown to be able to damage some antibody-coated parasites *in vitro*, a study was done at NIH in 1978 to see whether eosinophils could kill antibody-coated heart cells *in vitro*. Blood eosinophils were isolated from 10 patients with HES, and their cytotoxic capacity was assessed against antibody-coated human or chicken red blood cells, Chang cells, and Girardi human heart cells during an 18 hour assay. As only 15 per cent of the Chang or Girardi heart cells had been killed, and only 33 per cent and 43 per cent of human and chicken red blood cells respectively were lysed, it was concluded that eosinophils were unlikely to damage the heart in this way.[1367] A direct effect of eosinophils or their products on the heart seemed more likely, as seen in post mortems showing eosinophils microabscess in the heart.[1385]

At that time our principle reason for believing that E-EMF was caused by eosinophils was that it was described in each of the diseases which produce eosinophilia. The only common pathogenic feature of these different diseases was the presence of a marked increased in blood eosinophils.[1317, 2015, 1692, 1688]

Few patients with eosinophilic leukaemia develop E-EMF because they usually die from leukaemic complications soon after diagnosis. However, a patient has been described who had marked blood eosinophilia with blast cells in the circulation, and who developed endomyocardial fibrosis.[1095]

Several case reports of carcinoma-of-the-lung-induced E-EMF have been published, in which the onset of the heart disease could be correlated with the eosinophilia. We reviewed these reports in 1985, and added details of a patient of our own in 1985.[1701]

One of the first papers to describe this association was reported from London in 1975. The patient was a 51-year-old man with a large cell carcinoma of the lung, who was studied over a two year period before he died in heart failure, and was found to have biventricular E-EMF at post mortem. He also had alcohol-induced flushing attacks, violent headaches, and eosinophil counts which rose as the tumour mass increased, and fell after excision of the main tumour mass and subsequent radiotherapy. It was suggested that E-EMF was the result of an allergic response to the tumour, involving eosinophils.[117]

In 1978, a patient was studied in detail in Boston, Massachusetts, USA.[871] In this case report, the association between degranulated eosinophils in the blood and the development of heart disease was particularly well documented, supporting the view that eosinophil granule products might be involved in the development of the heart disease.

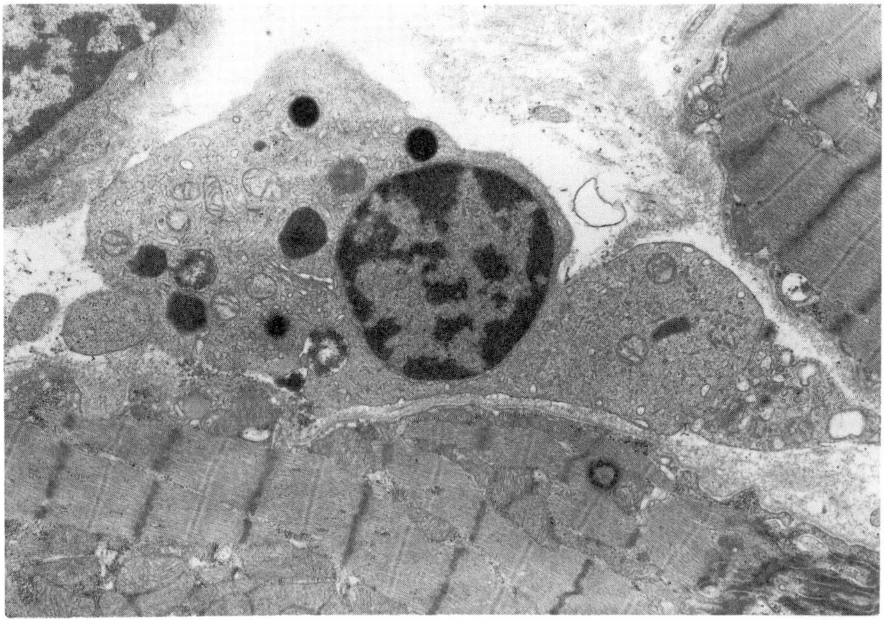

Fig. 22.2. Electronmicrograph of an eosinophil adjacent to a cardiac myocyte. The eosinophil granules have undergone changes in electron density, and electron-dense material appears to be discharged from one of the granules close to the surface of the heart cell. This was obtained from a left ventricular cardiac biopsy in a 68-year-old Japanese man with HES. Eosinophils in the heart muscles were also activated. From Nakayama *et al.* (1985),[1264] with permission.

Other reports of a similar disease process were published in the USA in 1982[1647] and 1983.[1961]

One of the most striking demonstrations of the interaction between eosinophils and the heart is in an ultrastructural study from Japan, where degranulating eosinophils were seen adjacent to a cardiac myocyte, in a cardiac biopsy from a patient with eosinophilic endomyocardial disease.[1264] (See Fig. 22.2.) A monoclonal antibody which only binds to activate eosinophils[1742] can be used to look for the presence of these cells in the blood, but no formal study has yet been carried out to see whether the number of activated cells in the circulation can be used to define or monitor patients most likely to develop E-EMF.

A growing body of evidence suggests the possibility that eosinophils may stimulate the coagulation system, not only by effects on the clotting sequence,[1148, 381, 1849] but also by affecting endothelial cells and platelets.[1049] Patients with marked eosinophilia and E-EMF appear to be forming thrombi continually, as judged by high serum levels of platelet factor 4, β-thromboglobulin, and fibrinogen.[398] The possible importance of this mechanism in the induction of E-EMF has been outlined in an echocardiographic study in which thrombi were considered to precede and/or augment the fibrotic process, leading to atrioventricular valve dysfunction. It was suggested that scar formation in the ventricles in patients with E-EMF was the result of the organisation and incorporation of thrombus into the ventricular cavity wall,[703] although this has not been seen in other studies.

In 1987, we reported the results of an immunopathological study on cardiac tissues taken at necropsy or cardiac biopsy from 18 patients with E-EMF, to look for the presence of the toxic eosinophil granule proteins within the heart. Serial sections were stained for MBP by indirect immunofluorescence, and for ECP, EDN/EPX, and activated eosinophils with alkaline-phosphatase-linked monoclonal antibodies. Activated eosinophils and secreted eosinophil granule proteins were mainly detected within the necrotic and later stage thrombotic lesions, in areas of acute tissue damage in the endocardium, and in the walls of small blood vessels. These findings suggested that eosinophil granule proteins could be causing the cardiac muscle damage and vascular injury which leads to the development of endomyocardial fibrosis.[1733] Several diseases which give rise to persistent eosinophilia are not commonly associated with eosinophilic heart disease. These include bronchial asthma, cryptogenic eosinophilic pneumonia,[41] hayfever, and other allergic disorders. This implies that there may be a protective factor(s) in the blood of these individuals, or that the stimuli which cause eosinophil degranulation in these diseases are different, and only affect eosinophils which are distant from the heart.

Experimental studies Direct evidence that eosinophil granule proteins were involved in the killing of heart cells has come from our studies on isolated rat heart cells which were killed in a dose-dependent manner by secretion products from human blood eosinophils.[1736] These produced an alteration in the plasma membrane of isolated myocytes, which stimulated increased oxygen uptake to provide additional ATP. A second mechanism was shown to involve a direct toxic effect of eosinophil granule proteins on cardiac mitochondrial enzymes. 2-oxoglutarate dehydrogenase was inhibited in a stochiometric fashion, and pyruvate dehydrogenase was also inhibited. These were sufficiently potent and irreversible effects for it to be clear that heart cells would die if these proteins could traverse the plasma membrane, and reach mitochondrial constituents. See also page 118.

Confirmation for the effects of eosinophil cationic proteins on cell membranes was seen in a study in which they induced pores to form in the surface of lipid bilayers.[1986]

Two of the most toxic cationic proteins in eosinophil granules, ECP and EDN/EPX, both have ribonuclease activity, and have probably evolved from a common gene.[661] Whether ribonucleases have a predilection for the endocardium has not yet been studied, but this could explain the unusual distribution of cardiac necrosis and fibrosis in this condition. Other possibilities which have been considered are the special blood supply to this part of the heart, or physical effects of the blood stream within the cavity of the heart affecting the inflow tract and apex of the ventricles.

Future work on endocardial fibrosis will be concentrating on the nature of the eosinophilic disorders themselves which give rise to this disorder; the nature of the stimuli which induce eosinophil secretion within the heart; and the factors within the endocardium which localize the lesions to these unusual anatomical sites. It is hoped that when more is known about these, effective forms of therapy, and prevention of E-EMF may become available, and it may be possible to distinguish patients in the tropics at risk of developing T-EMF.

22.3 Tropical endomyocardial fibrosis

Tropical endomyocardial fibrosis (T-EMF) was first described in 1946 in African troops serving in the Middle East by Bedford and Konstam.[145] They summarized their finding of 40 African troops, mainly from West Africa, who had unexplained heart failure. Some of the patients had eosinophilia, and many had parasitic infections. Post mortem examination of 17 showed 'an obvious and extensive subendocardial fibrosis, with fibrous areas resembling shallow infarcts in the ventricles, adherent to which was organized antemortem clots'. (See Plate 8) The disease was rediscovered by J. N. P. Davies in 1948 in Uganda. It occurs in regions five degrees north and south of the Equator in Africa, India, and South America. Sporadic cases occur in other parts of the world. Most patients in the UK have lived in the tropics for several years before the disease presents.[210] In parts of Nigeria 21 per cent of acquired heart disease is due to this disease,[43] and it is equally common in parts of South India. It has many features in common with eosinophilic endomyocardial fibrosis, and the diseases are pathologically indistinguishable. However, the different clinical backgrounds of the patients with each type of heart disease was the reason why the two disorders were treated separately for many years. The pathogenesis of both disorders is probably linked to marked blood eosinophilia and eosinophil granule deposition within the endocardium in the early stages of the heart disease. In the case of the tropical form of the disease, evidence to support this has been difficult to obtain. Few patients are seen in the early stages of the disease, and so no cardiac biopsies have been done at a time when the lesions are developing. The tropical form of the disease may progress slowly, so that the heart has time to hypertrophy, and most patients only present when they develop heart failure. In 1982, a workshop on endomyocardial fibrosis was held in London, with contributions from Africa, India, South America, and Europe. The clinical features of the various forms of the disease in each of these parts of the world was presented, with work on pathology, pathogenesis, and treatment.[1320]

22.3.1 *Clinical features of T-EMF*

T-EMF occurs in a younger age group than the eosinophilic forms of the disease. Children are affected as well as teenagers. Occasionally the disease is seen in older people. It occurs equally in males and females.[1597] In some patients the disease is unilateral, affecting only the right ventricle in 15 per cent of cases, and only the left ventricle in 5 per cent of cases.

These patients usually come from poor, malnourished communities, and presumably have a high parasite/worm burden, although no comparison has been done of this in relation to unaffected people living in the same region. A marked association with filarial infections has been noted in Nigeria,[855] but this is unlikely to be an important cause of the disease in patients with EMF in South America. On the other hand in Kerala, South India, where filariasis is hyperendemic, this may be the major parasite inducing eosinophilia, hypergammaglobulinaemia, and subsequent endocardial damage.[1861]

The classical clinical appearances of patients in the late stage of T-EMF include an oedematous face and eyelids, ascites, relatively few heart murmurs, but a markedly enlarged heart, and no ankle oedema.[405] The patients looks malnourished and chronically ill, but the heart failure appears to be remarkably well-compensated for in many cases. Goodwin has noted that marked right ventricular disease with almost complete obliteration of the ventricular cavity in T-EMF, is seldom seen in E-EMF.[697]

Thrombotic and embolic lesions are uncommon, and retinal abnormalities, which are common in HES, have not been reported in T-EMF.

T-EMF is seldom associated with gross heart murmurs even in the late stage of the disease, in contrast with E-EMF, where a murmur is almost invariably present. Amongst a group of five patients in Ibadan, Nigeria, with clubbing of the fingers and cyanosis, the cardiac murmurs most often noted were an opening snap, and a mid-disastolic murmur at the apex.[535] The classic features of a restrictive cardiomyopathy are present in most patients in the late state of the disease. Occasionally patients may have a markedly dilated left and/or right ventricle, particularly in the tropics, and in rare cases it may be difficult to distinguish endocardial fibrosis from constrictive pericarditis. The differential diagnosis includes Ebstein's anomaly.[29] Atrial fibrillation, myocardial calcification, and pericardial effusions are more common in endomyocardial fibrosis than in Ebstein's anomaly.[102] A comparison of the ECG findings in 18 patients with Ebstein's anomaly, and 20 with right ventricular T-EMF was published from South India in 1982.[863] Other important differential diagnoses are rheumatic heart disease, cardiac tumours, ventricular thrombi, and congenital heart diseases presenting in later life.

22.3.2 *Investigations in T-EMF*

Now that surgery has become available for T-EMF, investigations need to be as thorough as in the eosinophilic form of the disease. In tropical countries chest radiographs and echocardiograms are most useful, but cardiac catheterization is usually carried out prior to surgery. Investigations for associated disorders such as parasitic infections are obviously important in patients in the tropics, and these should be treated before surgery is done.

The cardiac silhouette is usually markedly increased, with or without pulmonary infiltrates, and occasionally marked calcification can be seen.[1258] ECGs show axis deviation, repolarization changes, and rhythm abnormalities in proportion to the degree of heart failure.

Echocardiography in T-EMF Echocardiography is the most useful single investigation of T-EMF, and several groups have now reported their findings.

M-mode echos provide measurements of the degree of mitral valve involvement, and the abnormalities in the septal wall. These are helpful prior to cardiac surgery, but cannot be used for diagnostic purposes, as they may be found in other cardiac disorders. Several echocardiographic studies on EMF have been published.[265] M-mode echocardiographic findings have been well described in one group of 21 patients.[635]

Two-dimensional echos provide a clearer picture of the left and right ventricles and the extent of endocardial fibrosis. In our studies in Kerala, South India, we found that it was helpful to use colour coded 2-D echocardiography to define the sites of fibrosis.[1860] Abnormalities in the movement of the ventricle can help to distinguish ischaemic and dilated ventricular muscle diseases from T-EMF, in which ventricular contractility is often well maintained, and infundibular contractility is enhanced. This was seen in a 2-D echocardiography study in Venezuela, which also demonstrated the value of this technique in distinguishing T-EMF from Chagas' heart disease which is common in that region. Preservation of the left ventricular apical systolic inward motion in T-EMF contrasted with other diseases which caused apical abnormalities.[14]

Cardiac catheterization in T-EMF Cardiac catheterization is rarely carried out in T-EMF, except in patients who are to undergo surgery. The procedure is not without danger, especially in patients with severe and long-standing heart disease with rhythm abnormalities. It is rarely carried out for diagnostic purposes, although this may occasionally be necessary when 2-D echocardiograms are difficult to interpret.

In South India, the results of cardiac catheterization of patients with T-EMF were described in 1983.[310] The appearance of minimal involvement of the right ventricle in patients with predominant left ventricle disease have been reported.[1559] Selective coronary angiography was done in 24 patients with T-EMF in the study carried out in the Sree Chitra Tirunal Institute for Medical Sciences and Technology, Kerala, South India. Eight had right ventricular disease, 2 left ventricular disease, and 14 biventricular disease. Abnormalities included a vascular blush, localized ventricular filling from the region of the blush, and tortuosity of the coronary arteries, lending support to the suggestion that mural thrombi could be important in the development of the endomyocardial lesions.[103] Post mortem coronary angiograms have been reported from Japan.[840] In four cases studied in China in 1983, massive enlargement of the right atrium was noted.[1088]

The outline of the left and right ventricles is clearly shown to be abnormal in classical angiocardiographic studies.

Cardiac biopsies have been carried out on a small number of patients with T-EMF, since this procedure was first reported in 1971.[1662] The procedure can be especially difficult in patients with gross heart failure, because heavy deposits of fibrous tissue can resist the jaws of the bioptome.

Histopathology of T-EMF The gross appearances of T-EMF have been well described and reviewed: The thickened endocardium may end in a thick-rolled edge in the outflow tract, and granulation tissue often extends from the thickened endocardium into the underlying myocardium.[1313] The post mortem and histological appearances of T-EMF are indistinguishable from those seen in the late fibrotic stage of the eosinophilic form of the disease.[1501]

The post mortem histological features of T-EMF have been reviewed in studies from Uganda[1598] and South India.[912] The immunohistochemical features in some patients in South India have also been published.[911]

Only a few ultrastructural studies on T-EMF have been published. The appearances in two patients who were studied in France were reported in 1977. One showed the classical appearances of pure fibrosis, which was acellular and associated with degenerative changes in the heart muscle cell; the other consisted of young fibrous tissue with numerous fibroblasts secreting a copious fibrillary substance which may have been the precursor of collagen fibres.[719] In 1984, the ultrastructural features of the lesions were described in seven patients in South India. The eosinophils showed alterations in their granule morphology, which were similar to those seen in patients with E-EMF.[1005]

Extra-cardiac lesions in T-EMF Although there is little clinical evidence for involvement of skeletal muscle in the process which leads to T-EMF, in 17 of 20 consecutive angiographically proven cases of EMF in South India, there was evidence for myopathic changes in electromyograms of skeletal muscle, which was more pronounced than in a control group of patients with heart failure due to other causes. However, light-microscopic study of the quadriceps muscles in 8 of these patients showed no abnormality.[72]

Renal involvement, although well known in HES, has rarely been noted in T-EMF. Glomerular lesions included capillary wall thickening, basement membrane duplication, mesangial expansion and interposition, intraluminal fibrin, and dense subendothelial deposits. These changes were thought to result from the deposition and organization of immune complexes.[393]

Feminization, which is not seen in patients with E-EMF in temperate climates, has been described in patients in Nigeria with T-EMF. This was related to low serum testosterone levels.[185] Interestingly, the same group also found raised serum immunoreactive prolyl hydroxylase protein levels, galactosyl-hydroxylysyl glucosyl transferase activity, and type III procollagen aminopropeptide levels in the sera of some of these patients.[186]

22.3.3 *Treatment of T-EMF*

At present the treatment of T-EMF is largely limited to the late fibrotic stage, when surgery is the only effective treatment for patients who may have been in heart failure for several months or years. Preparation for surgery is clearly important, and bedrest combined with carefully regulated diuretic treatment is usually required. A problem with diuretics is that the cardiac output depends to some extent on a high filling pressure, so treatment should be given carefully and over several weeks, in order to prevent a sudden fall in cardiac output.

Surgery By 1985, there had been reports of the use of surgery in 94 patients with T-EMF,[69] and many more surgical operations have been carried out successfully since then. Surgery for endomyocardial fibrosis is now carried out in each of the major areas of the world in which this disease occurs, and the success rate has been much higher than might have been expected a decade ago. This is largely because the underlying myocardium remains intact in the majority of patients, and the relief of incompetent valves, and removal of restricting fibrotic tissue can return the cardiac output to near normal.

The main issues to consider before surgery is carried out, are whether the procedure should involve valve repair or replacement, endocardectomy, and/or thrombus removal. A small number of patients with dilated hearts and poorly functioning left ventricular muscle may not benefit from any of these procedures,[1792] emphasizing the importance of considering surgery before the cardiac disease has led to irreversible myocardial injury. Occasionally, it may be possible to remove localized areas of fibrosis from the left ventricle, leaving the mitral valve intact.[1259]

In 1971, Dubost's group in Paris began to use open heart surgery to treat endomyocardial fibrosis. His patients came from the Gabon, a French colony with a high incidence of filariasis, especially loiasis. The importance of this pioneering work was not immediately recognized outside France, although it is now clear that Dubost's, and Carpentier's group have operated on more patients with this disease than any other groups outside the tropics.[1450, 637] The techniques and results of cardiac surgical treatment in five patients with T-EMF treated in Paris were reviewed by Dubost and his colleagues in 1976 and 1977. The operations included endocardectomy on the left and/or right side, and valve replacements, with Starr or Bjork prostheses or heterografts. Survivals ranged from 2 to 56 months or more.[469, 470]

Between 1975 and 1985 4 women with T-EMF in Budapest, Hungary, had endocardectomy, and 2 had thrombectomy successfully performed, among a group of 11 patients with endomyocardial fibrosis. One had bilateral valve replacement. The outcome was successful in all 4 patients.[69]

The indications for surgery for T-EMF in French-speaking areas in the tropics have been defined,[163] and the extensive work in Abidjan, Ivory Coast have been reported. Results in 55 operated patients were given in 1985.[1199] Twenty patients were reported in an earlier paper from the same centre.[1200] The value of mitral valve repair in 4 patients was also described by this group.[1201] Difficulties in diagnosing localized left ventricular disease affecting the mitral valve has also illustrated in a report of 6 patients in the same centre.[1202]

The indications and results of cardiac surgery were reported from South India in 1983: from Kerala[1827] and Tamil Nadu.[311] In Kerala, 17 of 25 patients with T-EMF were followed up for a mean of over 13 months after endocardectomy and atrioventricular valve replacement. Although there was no change in right ventricular shape after endocardectomy, left ventricular shape was restored to near normal. This study, like earlier reports, stressed that the benefits were mainly a result of the correction of mitral regurgitant lesions, and an improvement in ventricular compli-

Plates

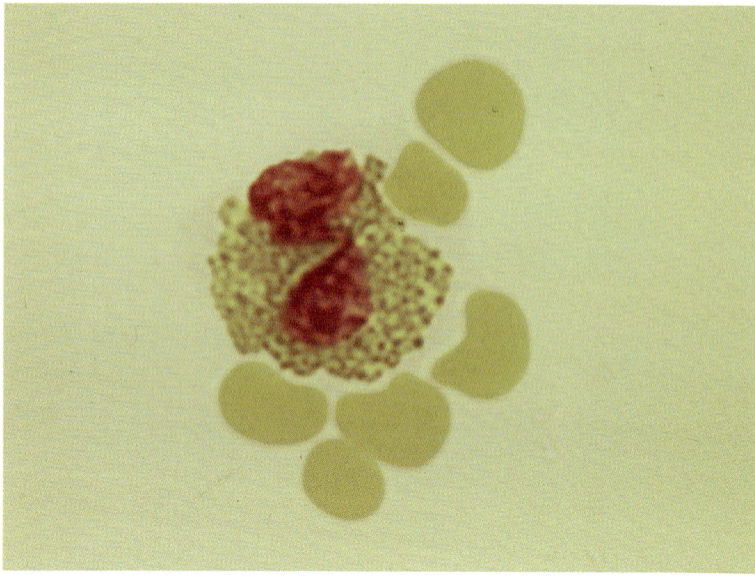

1. A normal blood eosinophil forming a rosette with complement coated sheep red blood cells. It shows the light microscopy appearances of normal eosinophils (see p. 37), and the presence of complement receptors on the cell membrane (see p. 81). Cytocentrifuge preparation. Giemsa's stain (× 500).

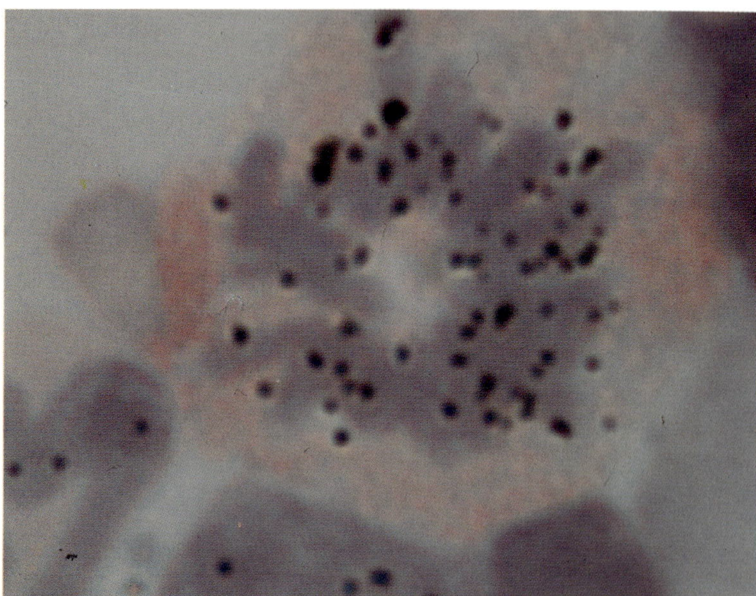

2. Autoradiograph of a rat bone marrow eosinophil metaphase following the injection of ^{3}H-thymidine. This shows the presence of the isotope as black grains over the chromosomes, one hour after the injection. The percentage of labelled eosinophil metaphases was used to measure their cell cycle time (see p. 14). Cytocentrifuge preparation. Haematoxylin, and Biebrich scarlet (× 1200).

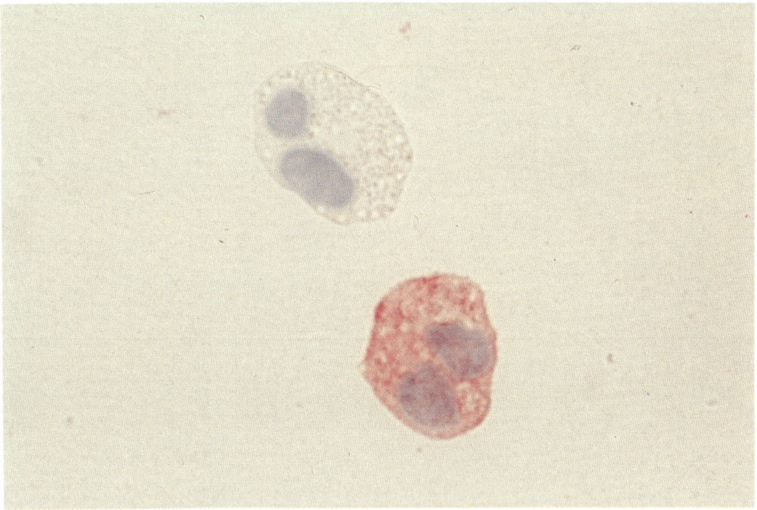

3. Two human blood eosinophils, one of which is stained red as it contains the activated form of ECP, and EDN/EPX, as shown by the binding of monoclonal antibody EG2. The localization of this antibody was demonstrated with alkaline phosphatase immunocytochemistry with fast red dye. These were normal eosinophils, which had been incubated with eosinophil activating factor. The reaction was stopped when some of the eosinophils had become activated (see p. 103). Cytocentrifuge preparation. Haematoxylin, and alkaline phosphatase/fast red stain (× 800).

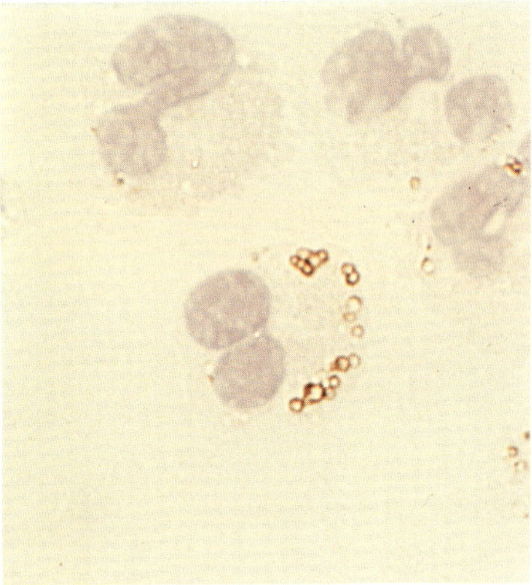

4(a). Blood eosinophils from a patient with HES showing the presence of the activated form of ECP, and EDN/EPX, using monoclonal antibody EG2. The binding of the monoclonal antibody to these proteins was detected by peroxidase immunocytochemistry with diaminobenzidine. The secreted forms of these proteins were present in the blood cells of patients with HES, unlike normal blood eosinophils (see p. 283). Cytocentrifuge preparation. Haematoxylin, and peroxidase stain (× 800).

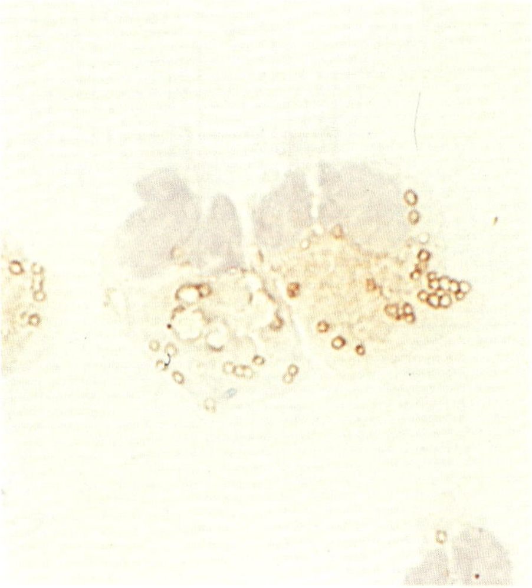

(b). Eosinophils from the blood of a patient with HES, stained for ECP, using monoclonal antibody EG1, and peroxidase immunocytochemistry with diaminobenzidine. This antibody binds to ECP in the granules, cf. 4(a), and ECP in the vacuoles (see p. 283). Cytocentrifuge preparation. Haematoxylin, and peroxidase stain (× 800).

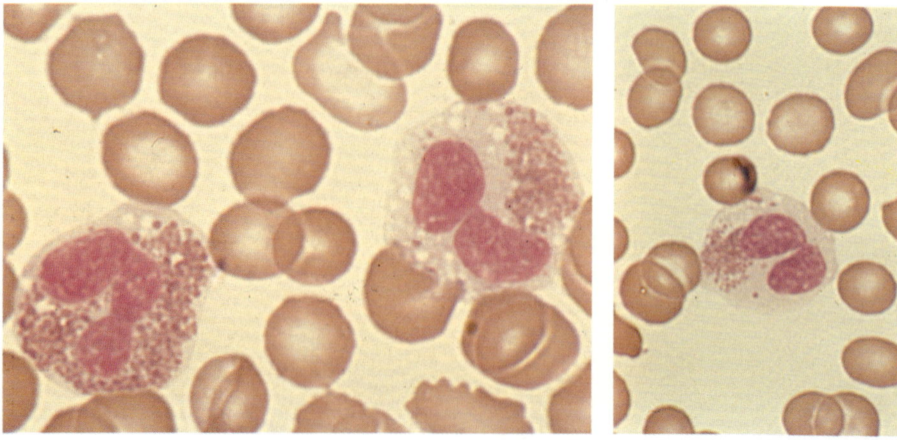

(a) **(b)**

5(a). Blood eosinophils from a patient with HES and endomyocardial fibrosis. Two eosinophils are shown. One contains two vacuoles. The other is partially degranulated, and contains many vacuoles. Degranulated eosinophils in the blood of patients with hypereosinophilia have been linked to the development of endomyocardial fibrosis (see p. 280). Giemsa's stain (× 900).

(b). A markedly degranulated eosinophil in the blood of a patient with HES (see p. 280). (Giemsa's stain × 600.)

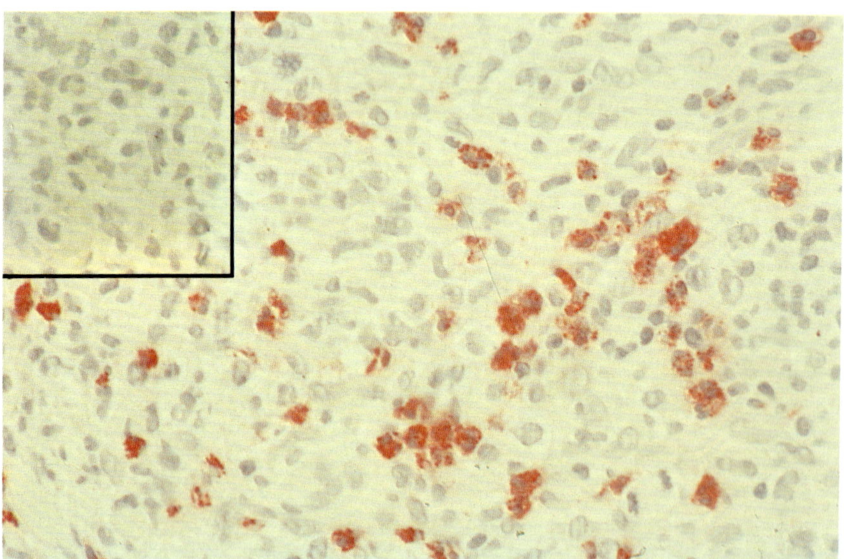

6. Eosinophils infiltrating a T-lymphocytic lymphoma in the skin, stained with monoclonal antibody EG2, which binds to the secreted forms of ECP and EDN/EPX. The binding of this antibody was shown by alkaline phosphatase immunocytochemistry with fast red dye. The majority of eosinophils were activated. Haematoxylin counterstain. A control section treated with an unrelated antibody and stained in the same way is in the *top left corner* for comparison (see p. 103) (× 400).

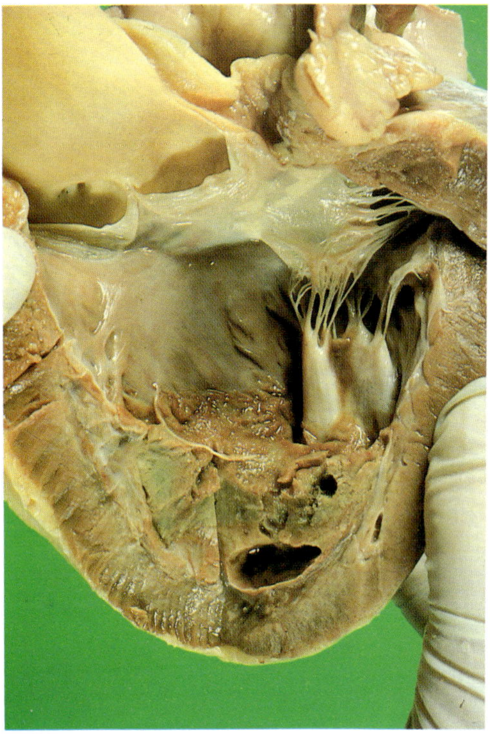

7. The heart of a patient with HES, who died with eosinophilic endomyocardial fibrosis in the acute thrombotic stage. The longitudinal section through the heart showed the presence of thrombus affecting the posterior papillary muscle, some liquefaction in the base of the thrombus, and hypertrophy of the ventricular muscle. The outflow tract was uninvolved (see p. 232).

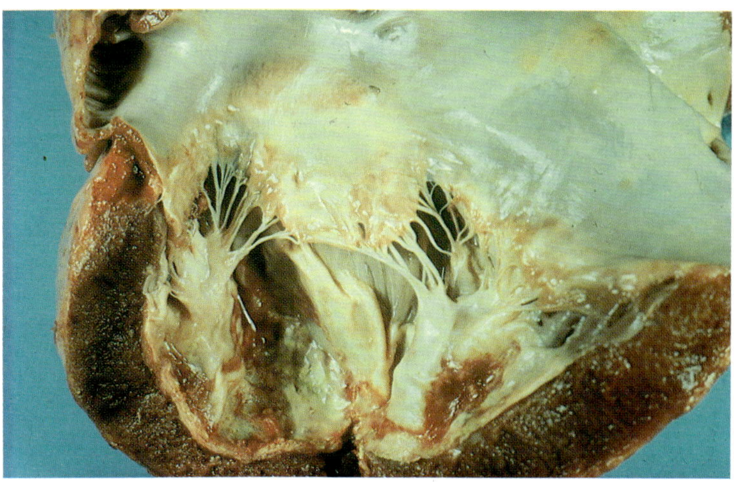

8. The heart from a patient with tropical endomyocardial fibrosis. The endomyocardium of the left ventricle was markedly thickened by fibrous tissue, and the myocardium was hypertrophied. Some thrombus was present on the endocardium. This is the late fibrotic stage of the disease, which is also seen in patients with eosinophilic endomyocardial fibrosis (see p. 249).

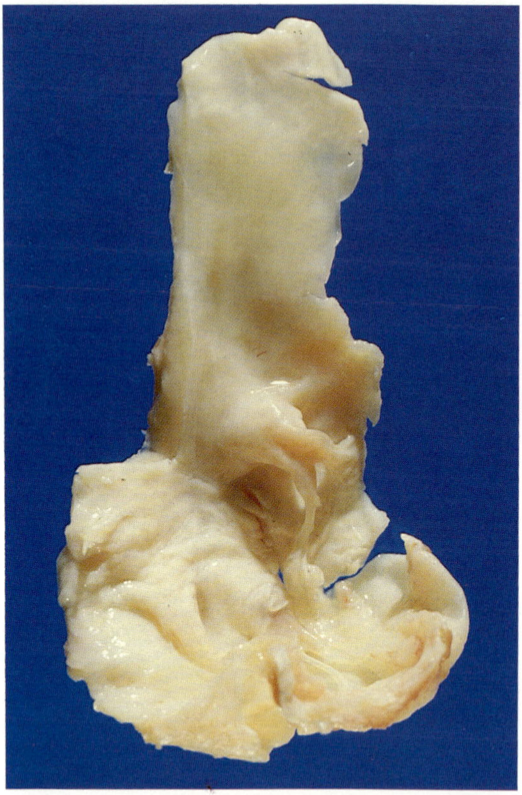

9. Resected fibrotic endocardium from the right ventricle and tricuspid region of a patient with eosinophilic endomyocardial fibrosis. This shows the amount of scar tissue which can be removed at operation from the cavity of the heart, to overcome the restriction on diastolic relaxation, and contraction of the underlying muscle (see p. 244). (Reproduced by permission of Mr Ralph Sapsford.)

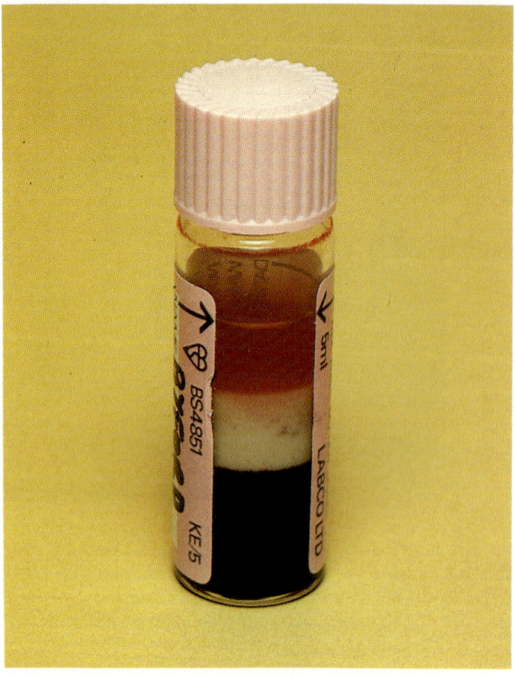

10. Blood count bottle from a patient who presented with nonspecific aches and pains, and a blood eosinophil count of 247 × 10^9/L. These form the large pale buffy coat layer, occupying as much space as the plasma. The patient responded to treatment with steroids, and is asymptomatic fiv.e years later, although the eosinophilia persists (see p. 278).

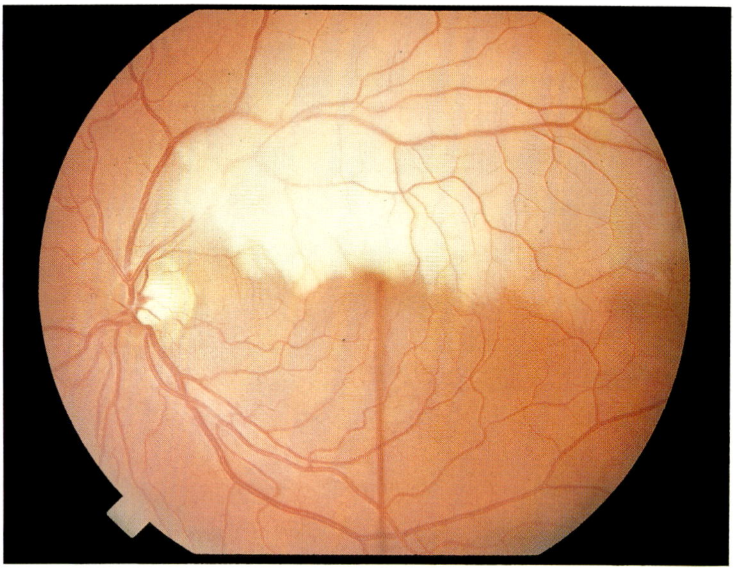

11. The right retina of a patient with HES who presented with sudden loss of vision in the upper nasal quadrant due to occlusion of the retinal artery in this region. There was no response to treatment with anticoagulants. This is a common complication in patients with HES (see p. 275). (Reproduced by permission of Mr James Govan.)

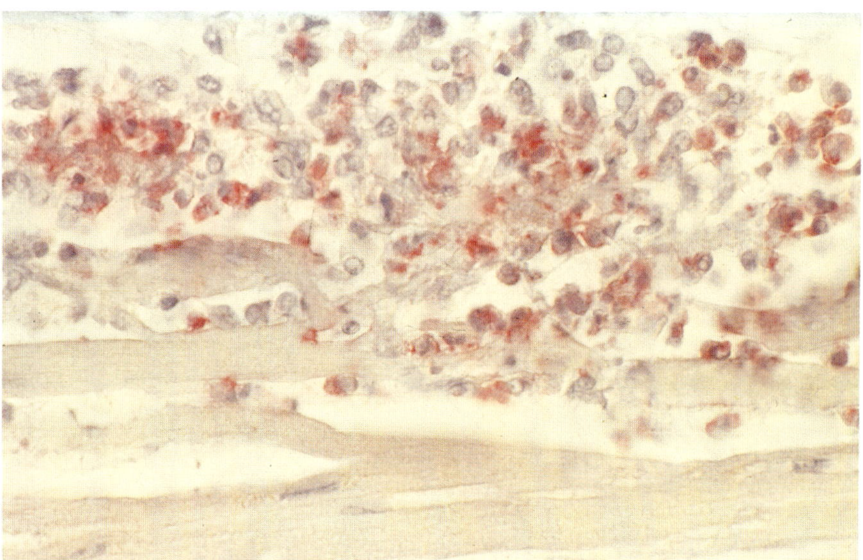

12. An area of acute necrosis, and eosinophil infiltration in the myocardium of a patient with the Churg–Strauss syndrome. The section was stained with monoclonal antibody EG2, which binds to the secreted forms of ECP and EDN/EPX. The majority of eosinophils were activated, and many were on the surface of cardiac myocytes. This suggested that they may have been releasing their toxic constituents, and damaged adjacent heart cells (see p. 203). Alkaline phosphatase immunocytochemistry with fast red dye, and haematoxylin (× 200).

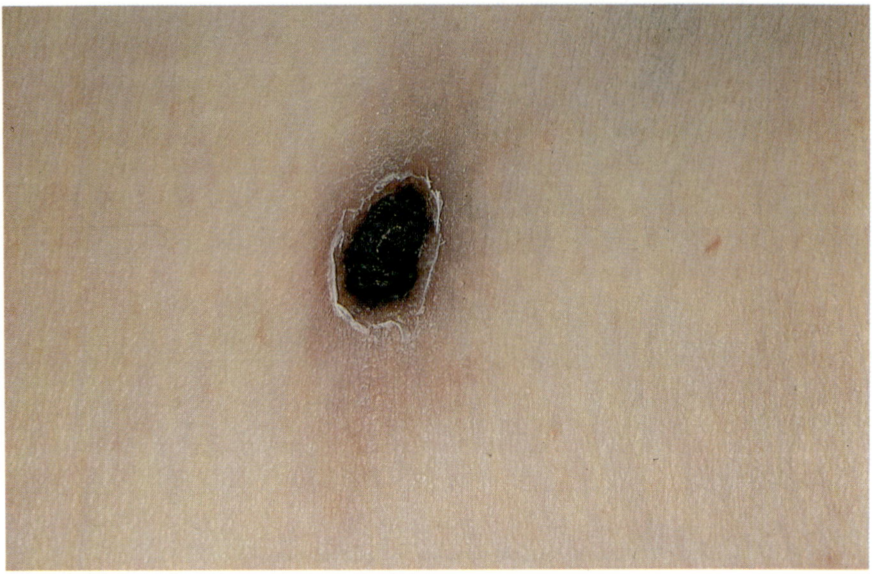

13. A necrotic, and ulcerating skin lesion on the lower arm of a man with lymphomatoid papulosis, and hypereosinophilia. This patient was one of three in whom it was thought that T-lymphocytes had become malignant, and may have secreted eosinopoietic factors (see p. 304). The lesion is 1.5 cm diameter. (Reproduced by permission of Dr Robin Russell Jones.)

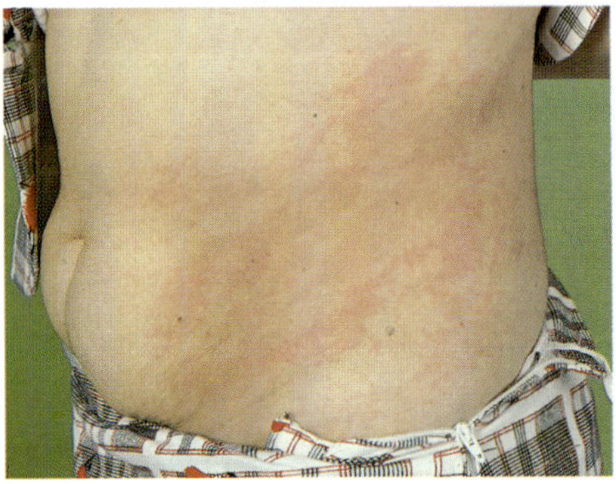

14(a). An area of eczematous eruption on the lateral abdominal wall of a woman with episodic angioedema, and hypereosinophilia. The lesions were worse during the period of maximal weight gain, and increase in blood eosinophil counts (see p. 299).

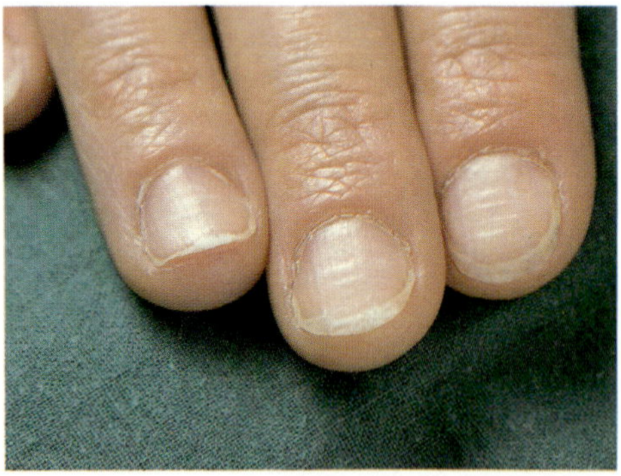

(b). Fingernails in the woman whose skin is shown in (a). The ridges corresponded to the monthly episode of angioedema, and eosinophilia (see p. 299).

ance.[104] Successful surgical correction of T-EMF has been carried out in India in a child only 12 years old.[878]

In Recife, Brazil, 30 patients with T-EMF were submitted to endocardial decortication and atrioventricular valve replacement between 1977 and 1981, and the benefits of cardiac surgery were considerable.[1238]

As T-EMF is rarely seen in the USA, there have been no large series of surgically treated patients, although I know of one who had an unsuccessful cardiac transplant in 1983. Similarly, in other parts of the world, only occasional reports have been published. One of these was from Tehran, Iran in 1979, of successful decortication of the right ventricle, mitral valve repair, and tricuspid valve replacement.[1606]

22.3.4 *Pathogenesis of T-EMF*

Many different pathogenetic mechanisms have been proposed for T-EMF, but there is still no generally accepted explanation for why it is largely limited to regions close to the equator, and to the poorer people living in these areas. As it may occasionally develop in Western visitors to these places,[210, 719] it is likely that environmental factor(s) are involved. There is little evidence for a familial susceptibility, although the disease has been seen in more than one member of a family in Kerala (Vijayarhagavan 1985, personal communication).

The unusual geographical distribution of T-EMF, especially its high incidence in Rwandan immigrants to Uganda compared to the local population, led to the suggestion that genetic factors might be important in addition to environmental factors such as diseases causing eosinophilia. However, as a comprehensive epidemiological study on the prevalence and natural history of T-EMF is not available, it has not been possible to determine the relative importance of genetic and other factors.[832]

In Nigeria, where T-EMF is a disease of the rain-forest belt, several prospective studies are under way to look at these questions.[533] The finding of raised IgM levels with normal IgG and IgA levels in some patients in Nigeria, strengthens the case that an unusual response to an infectious disease may underlie this disease.[279, 864]

Circumstantial evidence has been available for many years that an inflammatory reaction might be the initiating event in the development of T-EMF. In 1965, Parry and Abrahams noted in Nigeria that in some patients who developed T-EMF, a constitutional illness could precede clinical cardiac disease. In patients who were judged to be at the earlier stage of the disease, there were often inflammatory cells and necrosis in the endocardium.[1370] Shaper in Uganda in 1972 detected antibodies to heart muscle antigens in some patients, but there was a closer association of this disorder with malaria antibody levels.[1599] He suggested that some unknown mechanism induced both the heart damage and eosinophilia which is often associated with the disease.[1597]

Eosinophils and T-EMF The suggestion that eosinophils could be responsible for the endocardial lesions in T-EMF stems from the clear evidence that they are involved in causing the eosinophilic form of the disease. Several reports in Western countries have described patients who had marked eosinophilia, which disappeared several years before they were shown to have endomyocardial fibrosis.[1868] Unfortunately, T-EMF is seldom diagnosed at an early stage, and there are few reports of accurate eosinophil counts in this disease. However, 12 of the first 24 patients with T-EMF who were reported by Davies in 1948 had eosinophilia.[403] In a detailed study in 1967 on 16 patients with T-EMF in Uganda, although absolute eosinophil counts were not reported, 6 had eosinophil differential counts of up to 64 per cent.[350] In 1977, mean blood eosinophil counts in 15 patients with T-EMF in Uganda were $1.13 \times 10^9/l$, compared with $0.72 \times 10^9/l$ in a control group, but the range of counts was similar, and the differences were not significant.[1376]

Amongst the group of 77 patients who were studied in 1967 in Nigeria, 33 (43 per cent) had eosinophil counts greater than $1.0 \times 10^9/l$.[855] Several surveys are continuing in West Africa and India, where there is some evidence that patients with eosinophilia may later develop T-EMF. In Venezuela, a small prospective study was carried out on 14 patients with eosinophilia for a mean of 14.5 months, but echocardiography and clinical studies showed no abnormality.[14] It may be more important to assess the numbers of degranulated eosinophils, rather than total eosinophil counts, as 2 patients with T-EMF in the Venezualan study were noted to have degranulated blood eosinophils.[14]

In a study on 10 patients with T-EMF in Nigeria, serum ECP levels were not statistically different from 15 controls. This may have been because they were in the late stage of the disease.[1813]

An alternative view is still held, which stems from early work in Uganda showing connective tissue swelling in the endocardium and inner myocardium in post mortem.[351] This view proposes that the cardiac injury is primarily the result of an immediate hypersensitivity reaction, in which eosinophils only play a secondary role.[39] These issues were discussed by Falashe in 1985.[534]

A strong possibility has been present for many years that some patients with filariasis may go on to develop EMF. Amongst a group of 77 patients who were studied in 1967 in Nigeria, 70 (91 per cent) had loiasis. This study was one of the first to suggest that there might be an association between filariasis, eosinophilia, and the development of T-EMF in this area.[855] It was suggested in India that obstruction of heart lymphatics in lymphatic filariasis could produce T-EMF,[1478] but there is no supporting evidence for this.

The possibility that filariasis and eosinophilia may lead to the development of T-EMF was examined in a prospective study on 1956 patients aged less than 20 in northern Nigeria, which was reported in 1981. Forty-four patients (2.2 per cent) had eosinophil counts greater than 3×10^9/l. Twenty-two patients had filariasis (loiasis), with mean eosinophil counts of 1.48×10^9/l, and all responded to treatment with diethylcarbamazine. Thirteen patients had heart disease at presentation, and 8 were found to have T-EMF, even though their eosinophil counts had returned to normal with treatment.

Angiocardiograms were done in six patients. One patient died, and was shown to have T-EMF at post mortem. This study adds further evidence to the possibility that chronic eosinophila due to filarial infections can lead (over several months or years) to the development of endomyocardial fibrosis. This sequence of events was documented in a six-year-old boy in this series.[38] Full details of his illness were published later: He was admitted to hospital with acute filariasis, and despite effective treatment and disappearance of eosinophilia, he died 2 years later with predominant right-sided T-EMF.[39]

By 1981, 25 Europeans resident in the tropics had been reported to have developed T-EMF. Nineteen had marked eosinophilia, and 15 had micro-filiaria in their blood. Disappearance of eosinophilia at the late stage of the heart disease has also been noted in some of these patients.[39]

22.4 Animal models of endomyocardial fibrosis

There is some hope that an animal model of EMF could be produced. For example, in male Sprague–Dawley rats, endomyocardial fibrosis which mostly affected the left ventricle was observed 1–14 weeks after a course of treatment with the carcinogen N-nitrosomorpholine.[1169] Endomyocardial lesions were also seen in mice which were given a lethal infection of *Plasmodium berghei*.[503]

22.5 Comparisons of E-EMF and T-EMF

In 1983, Olsen in London reviewed the concept which unites T-EMF and E-EMF.[1316] He felt that the evidence linking these apparently separate diseases together with a common pathogenesis (eosinophil-mediated cardiac injury) means that endomyocardial fibrosis should now be classified as a specific heart muscle disease, rather than a cardiomyopathy, which by definition is of unknown aetiology.[1315]

In the same year, we reported the results of a comparative study of T-EMF and E-EMF in patients with HES, in London, to try to explain the different clinical features of the two disorders. Forty-seven patients with T-EMF were studied in South India, and 8 in Brazil. Their clinical features

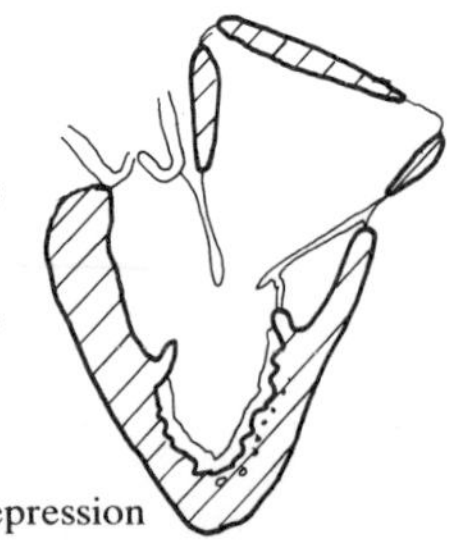

Fig. 22.3. A comparison of EMF in temperate and tropical regions. Although differences are seen in the clinical settings in which these diseases occur, the pathogenesis of the heart damage is probably identical. Adapted from Davies *et al.* (1983),[402] with permission.

were compared with 11 patients with E-EMF studied in London. See Fig. 22.3. The patients in Britain were older than the patients in the tropics, and the male predominance in the UK was not found in the other patient group. In Britain, half of the patients presented in the acute necrotic stage of the disease, whereas patients in the tropics only presented in the late stage. This was linked to the association of endomyocardial fibrosis in London with HES, which has a mean age incidence of 37, whereas in the tropics, the patients were from poor malnourished communities, with heavy parasite loads, especially filariasis. Another important difference was that isolated right or left ventricular disease was found in a quarter of the patients in the tropics, whereas this did not occur in patients in London. In order to account for these differences, it was suggested that the rate at which the heart disease developed in these different regions was determined by the underlying disorder producing eosinophilia. In temperate climates, the systemic effects of toxic eosinophil granule proteins was thought most likely to produce bilateral rapidly progressive disease, whereas in the tropics, the eosinophilic disorder might be more chronic, and the effects could be limited to one or the other side of the heart, depending on where eosinophil degranulation was induced to occur.[402]

23. Diseases of the blood

Although any disease which affects the bone marrow may affect eosinophil production, this is seldom commented on, and primary disorders which principally or exclusively affect eosinophils are relatively rare.

23.1 Inherited diseases affecting eosinophils

A few inherited blood disorders such as Omenn's syndrome (see p. 166), and other immunodeficiency diseases can be associated with a marked increase in blood eosinophil counts. Other inherited disorders can produce defects in eosinophils. For example, they occur in eosinophils from patients with gangliosidase deficiencies. This was shown in 1985 in blood and bone marrow samples from four patients with GMI gangliosidosis type I. The cells contained poorly stained and unevenly spaced granules, many of which were larger than normal and had abnormal ulatrastructural appearance.[647]

Several of the major immunodeficiency diseases which are noted mainly for their effect on neutrophils also affect eosinophils. These include chronic granulomatous disease, the inherited Pelger–Huët anomaly, and the Chediak–Higashi syndrome. See also page 295.

23.1.1 *Eosinophil peroxidase deficiency*

The only genetic disorder confined to eosinophils is peroxidase (EPO) deficiency, which has been noted sporadically. Genetic defects in neutrophil myeloperoxidase are common. The gene for this tetrameric protein was cloned in 1987,[881] and it was found that the deficiency was due to the inheritance of abnormal myeloperoxidase gene(s) which did not undergo correct post-translational processing. A patient with deficiency of the neutrophil cationic proteins defensin and gelatinase, has been reported,[1147] but genetic abnormalities in the eosinophil basic proteins, ECP, EDN/EPX, and MBP, have not yet been noted.

EPO deficiency occurs either as a complete or partial deficiency. Interestingly, members of the cat family and some other animals have blood eosinophils which do not stain for peroxidase.[1810] See page 123.

In 1968, two children aged 3 and 7 were found by Presentey to have blood eosinophils which had hypersegmented nuclei, decreased numbers of granules, and complete absence of staining for EPO and phospholipids. Myeloperoxidase was unaffected.[1437] This appeared to be a new inherited enzyme deficiency, [1439] which was due to an autosomal recessive defect.[1440]

He then made a detailed assessment of the staining characteristics of EPO-deficient eosinophils from two families, which showed that as Sudan black staining phospholipids were also reduced, phospholipids were probably associated with EPO in eosinophil granules.[1438] By 1976, he had extended his studies to more families, and was able to show that this anomaly was not associated with clinical problems.[897] In a six year study of 63 465 Jews resident close to Rehovet and in Galilee, Israel, he reported in 1982 that there were 74 with complete absence of EPO, and phospholipid deficiency in blood eosinophil granules. These people were mainly Yemenite Jews. It was shown to be an autosomal recessive trait, and 14 individuals had a family member who was affected. Partial loss of peroxidase staining was seen in 14 people. None of the EPO-deficient people had a related clinical disorder, and they were able to produce eosinophilia normally. This deficiency could be used as a genetic marker in affected populations.[1444]

Although complete EPO deficiency is very rare in Caucasians, twins with this defect were reported from Lille, France, in 1987.[1060] As yet no functional studies have been reported using EPO-deficient eosinophils. It is not known, for example, if they can kill parasites *in vitro*, or degranulate normally, and whether they have a normal complement of the other basic proteins. Ultrastructural studies have showed enlargement of the cores of the granules, and thinning of the matrix region, where EPO and phospholipids are usually found.[1441, 1060]

Partial EPO-deficiency is seen less commonly, but the use of automated flow cytochemistry, which uses peroxidase staining, has brought some cases to light. In 1980, partial deficiency of myeloperoxidase, with complete absence of EPO, was detected using an automated Hemalog D machine. The patient was a 48-year-old man with intellectual deterioration due to ceroid lipofuscinosis: Kuf's disease.

Electronmicroscopy studies showed that many eosinophil granules did not stain for peroxidase. The peroxidase deficiency did not explain the neurological disorder, as other patients with complete EPO deficiency have not had cerebral disease.[200] However, partial deficiency of EPO in a 4-year-old Turkish boy with mental retardation was also noted in Holland using a Technicon H-6010 automated-flow cytochemical analyser. The residual peroxidase activity was almost completely cyanide resistant,[805] like the peroxidase in normal blood eosinophils.[1226]

23.1.2 *Other inherited blood diseases affecting eosinophils*

The Chediak–Higashi syndrome affects many species besides man. The eosinophils are structurally abnormal with giant cytoplasmic granules.

These probably arise from the fusion of pre-existing granules.[531] In the X-linked form of chronic granulomatous disease, there is an abnormality in a gene which codes for a transmembrane protein, which anchors cytochrome b558 to the plasma membrane. The nature of the defects in the other genetic forms of the disease have not yet been defined.[1147] In 1986, a report on the eight patients seen at NIH, Bethesda, Maryland showed that they all had a minor increase in blood eosinophil counts. Eosinophils in four patients had a small capacity to form formazan from nitrobluetetrazolium salts, and it was suggested that this could produce a false positive result in this test for the disease.[1498] An autosomal dominant trait in which eosinophils and basophils contained unusual cytoplasmic crystalline inclusions was described in 1978. This did not appear to have caused any clinical problems.[1793] In 1981, a familial trait in eosinophils, which contained more than five cores per granule, was also reported.[1361]

The Pelger–Huët anomaly can occur as an inherited or an acquired abnormality in eosinophils. An example of the inherited form was described in 1987 in a three-year-old boy, who had blood eosinophil granules which were reduced in number and contained crystalloids of many different shapes.[1332]

The acquired form of Pelger–Huët may be more common, as it occurs in patients with myeloproliferative diseases,[1153] and it can be limited to the eosinophil series. The fourth example of this defect in eosinophils from a patient with myelofibrosis was described in Italy in 1980.[588]

23.2 Fanconi's anaemia

Abnormalities of eosinophil development have been seen in occasional patients with Fanconi's anaemia. Abnormal crystalloids were seen within eosinophil granules in one patient. In another patient there were nuclear pockets, and eosinophil granules contained globular material, with some autophocytic vacuoles in the cytoplasm.[120]

23.3 Cyclical haematopoiesis and eosinophils

Several patients have been described with cyclical alterations in the number of eosinophils in the bone marrow and blood.[16, 513] This appears to be part of a disturbance of haematopoisis which affects some or all of the blood cells, and produces maturation arrest for a period at the myelocyte or myeloblast stages of differentiation. The most significant alteration is in blood neutrophil counts, which fall periodically. About 20 per cent of these patients have moderate eosinophilia.[1028]

23.4 Acquired platelet dysfunction with eosinophilia

The syndrome of acquired platelet dysfunction with eosinophilia, which is mainly seen in children in tropical countries, has been known for over a decade.[1223] Although its pathogenesis is unknown, it has been linked to the presence of intestinal nematode infections.[1010] Most publications on this syndrome have come from Singapore, Thailand,[1729] and India. I have seen several patients with the syndrome in Kerala, South India. There is also a report of a patient in the USA,[140] and another in the UK: This was a girl aged 8.5 years, who returned from a visit to Malaysia with multiple painless bruises. Her blood eosinophil count was 1.66 × 10.9/l. Her bleeding time was 20 minutes, and her platelets did not aggregate with collagen. Immune complexes were also found in her serum. The disease could be either due to a defect in the platelets, making them unable to release ADP after stimulation with collegen, or a 'storage pool' effect of immune complexes on blood platelets.[1255] Seven adults aged 19–21 years were reported from Singapore in 1984.[1767] The defect can be partially corrected by platelet transfusions.[769]

24. The idiopathic hypereosinophilic syndrome (HES): Clinical features

The idiopathic hypereosinophilic syndrome (HES) is a term used to cover a variety of eosinophilic diseases, in which the cause is unknown, but which share a number of unusual features. (See Fig. 24.1.) The term was introduced by Hardy and Anderson in 1968,[753] who used it to cover both malignant and non-malignant diseases affecting the eosinophil series. The first patient with HES was probably reported in the USA in 1912.[1711] The first case report of HES in the UK (from Durham) was published in 1922. This was a man who had an eosinophil count of $23.8 \times 10^9/l$. The eosinophils had more lobes than normal, and the cytoplasm contained vacuoles and smaller numbers of granules than normal. These cells were able to form crystals (possibly Charcot–Leyden crystals) after they had been incubated at 37°. The crystals were soluble in hot water, 2 per cent acetic acid, and sodium hydroxide. It was thought that this patient had an eosinophilic leukaemia but, in retrospect, it is possible that he had HES.[1172]

In 1938 a detailed clinical description was made of a 35-year-old man who died with HES, complicated by heart disease and cerebral thrombo-embolic disease. Eighteen earlier reports were reviewed: 14 of the patients were male, and 5 female. They were aged between 6 and 54. Eleven had died, and 6 had post mortems. Four had heart failure, 2 cerebral haemorrhages, and 5 had thrombi in the heart.[1458] This was not a complete review, as it did not include the patients already described by Löffler in 1936 in German.

By 1969 there were at least 48 reported cases of 'eosinophilic leukaemia', and details of 5 were reported by Benvenisti and Ultmann.[157] In 1971 3 patients with HES were reported from St Thomas' Hospital, London, 2 of whom died from endomyocardial fibrosis.[1607] In 1975, the sydrome was redefined by Wolff and his colleagues at the NIH, Bethesda, Maryland, USA.[325] They argued that a clear distinction of eosinophilic leukaemia was now possible, and they restricted HES to patients with a non-malignant but persistent eosinophilia of more than $1.5 \times 10^9/l$ with evidence for

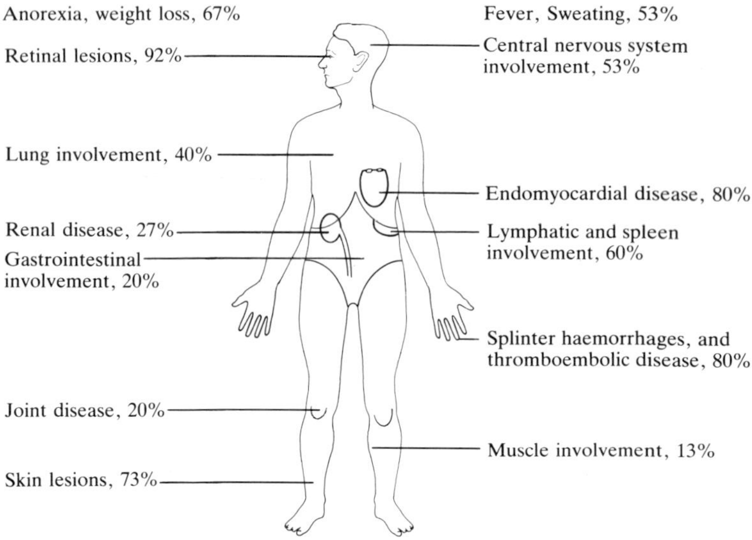

Fig. 24.1. The principal complications of the idiopathic hypereosinophilic syndrome (HES).

organ damage, such as endomyocardial fibrosis, skin lesions, and respiratory tract involvement. This was reviewed in 1980.[438]

The diagnosis is made by the exclusion of other distinct diseases, such as parasitic infections, which can give rise to a similar clinical picture. Even after a diagnosis of HES has been made, it is important to bear in mind that any of these diseases, such as tumours, parasitic diseases, and hypersensitivity disorders may only become apparent later. The main reason for classifying patients as having HES is that they share a number of serious complications, many of which are probably caused by toxic effects of eosinophils on normal tissues. Although HES appears to occur world-wide, and there are over 100 reports of patients with the disease, only two centres have described their clinical experience with more than 10 patients with HES. Most haematologists in large hospitals have had experience of treating these patients, but they are also seen in other clinical departments, especially departments of cardiology, dermatology, and neurology, because of the wide range of organs affected in this group of diseases.

The problems involved in distinguishing eosinophilic leukaemia from nonmalignant (leukaemoid) diseases with marked eosinophilia were carefully studied by Bousser in 1957.[198] As these diseases were rare, questionnaires were sent to well known haematology centres in France and abroad, to obtain their experience of diagnosing and treating patients with high blood eosinophil counts of unknown cause. As a result, it was clear that there were two distinct diseases. In one group of patients, death was usually the result of heart failure. These patients also had pulmonary infiltrates and central nervous system disease. This illness was clearly different from eosinophilic leukaemia which affected a smaller number of patients. As there seemed to be no overlap between the two diseases, he proposed that the main treatment for patients who did not have the malignant form of the disease should be steroids and anticoagulants. He stressed the importance of continually searching for possible causes of eosinophilia (allergic and parasitic diseases for example), as specific treatment would be curative. A small number of patients with HES also developed a malignant bone marrow disorder, several years after they presented with HES.[1345]

In 1969, a group was set up at the National Institutes of Health (NIH), Bethesda, Maryland, USA by Dr Sheldon Wolff to study patients with unusual vasculitic diseases. As a result of this interest, patients began to be referred who had hypereosinophilia, which they defined as a blood eosinophil count greater than 1.5×10^9/l. Many of them did not have a vasculitis, which was surprising, as polyarteritis nodosa was considered at that time to be one of the main causes of marked eosinophilia. However, they all had a number of serious clinical complications which fell into a single syndrome, which they called 'the hypereosinophilic syndrome'. This was the first time that a significant number of these patients had been studied. Their results have formed the basis for all the subsequent work which has been carried out on this syndrome.[325]

They showed that the blood eosinophil counts were almost always greater than 1.5×10^9/l, and (by definition) no cause for eosinophilia could be found. In addition, a majority of the patients had evidence for tissue damage. Their first report described the clinical and haematological features of 14 patients, all of whom were male; and a comprehensive review of the English language literature brought to light 57 other patients with the same syndrome, 91 per cent of whom were also male. As the mean survival time of the earlier patients was only nine months, and as many deaths appeared to have been due to myelotoxic side-effects of cytotoxic drug therapy, treatment was more expectant in their own patients. In patients with evidence of active tissue injury, steroids were given first, followed by busulphan, chlorambucil, and 6–mercaptopurine in patients who remained ill. No attempt was made to bring eosinophil counts into the normal range: treatment was based on the extent and severity of ongoing tissue damage. This approach resulted in a marked improvement in survival.

The NIH series of 50 patients was reviewed in 1982.[544]

It is likely that HES embraces a number of different diseases. Although most of the patients initially studied at NIH did not have a malignant disease (many have been followed up for more than 15 years), several had circulating myeloblasts and raised serum B12 levels, with low folate levels, basophilia, and low alkaline phosphatase scores, suggesting that their illnesses were related to chronic myeloid leukaemia.[325]

24.1 Disease processes underlying HES

It is still not known whether HES is an intrinsic bone marrow defect in which eosinophils or their precursors themselves are at fault, or whether a factor or regulatory mechanism affecting eosinophil production is abnormal. In 1982, it was reported that a 26-year-old woman with HES, pulmonary lesions, E–EMF, and a blood eosinophil count of $54 \times 10^9/l$ had given birth to a healthy boy with a blood eosinophil count of $55 \times 10^9/l$.[278] At one month it was still $61 \times 10^9/l$, but it then began to fall, so that it was $13 \times 10^9/l$ at four months, and in the normal range of eight months. It was suggested that maternal eosinophilia had induced the eosinophilic response in the baby, but no special studies were done on this possibility. If this reaction were due to an eosinopoietic factor from the mother, its effect must have persisted for a remarkably long time. The activity of injected CSFs on eosinopoiesis are lost within three days.

No genetic studies have been reported on whether eosinophils in patients with HES are derived from a single clone, and no patient with HES has yet received a bone marrow transplant which might help to clarify this question. No reliable animal model of the disease has been found. A number of patients with HES have a preceding parasitic or allergic illness in which eosinophilia probably occurred. In these patients, it is tempting to suggest that this was the initial stimulus which led to persistent eosinophilia. Two patients with eosinophilic leukaemia, who were studied in South Africa, also had schistosomiasis. This finding suggested to these authors that chronic stimulation of eosinophil proliferation might have been followed by a structural change in an adjacent part of chromosome 12, where eosinophil proliferation may be regulated, possibly involving the c-Ki ras 2 gene, which is present at 12p12.1.[943] It is hoped that studies will develop along these lines into the genetic basis of eosinophil proliferation in normal and malignant diseases. See pages 25–6, and 155–6.

24.2 Variants of HES

There are four clinical variants of HES which show some overlap.

1. Some patients with HES have asthmatic symptoms, or a hypersensitivity, or allergic disorders. They may have raised serum IgE levels,

suggesting that the disease has an allergic basis. The symptoms and signs of disease in these patients usually respond within a few days to treatment with steroids, and patients' blood eosinophil counts can return to normal while they are taking steroids.

2. A second group of patients with HES have a disease which gives rise to few symptoms or signs, despite the presence of a persistently raised blood eosinophil count. Treatment is not needed, and the disease may be of little inconvenience to the patient.

3. In a third group of patients, who form the majority of patients with HES, there are one or more less serious complications of the disease which require treatment. This may range from coughing attacks and skin lesions, to endomyocardial fibrosis. Treatment is again symptomatic, and in periods of relative quiescence of symptoms, the patients often feel well. Blood eosinophil counts are consistently raised, on or off treatment. They have a life-long illness, and their lesions can progress.

4. Patients in the fourth group present with the more serious complications of the disease, such as heart failure and vascular occlusions, including strokes or diffuse central nervous system involvement. These patients often have the highest blood eosinophil counts, and their blood eosinophils are often hypogranular. Eosinophil production in these individuals appears to be poorly regulated compared to other patients with HES. For this reason cytotoxic drug treatment, in addition to steroids, may be required to suppress their bone marrow, and to help patients to recover from acute episodes of their illness, which generally recur at intervals of several weeks or months.

24.3 Animal models of HES

It would be of great value if animal models of HES could be developed. This may well be possible, now that methods have been devised for producing marked eosinophilia in rodents by treating them with cyclophosphamide, followed by an allergic or parasitic eosinopoietic stimulus. We came across this possibility in 1980, when six LOU strain rats were infected with *T. spiralis* two larvae/g, two days after a heat wave. They developed eosinophil counts of up to 32×10^9/l. Antemortem thrombus was present within both ventricles, with extensive eosinophil infiltration into lymphoid tissues and lungs, and one rat had cirrhosis.[1699] It would be worth seeing whether recombinant GM-CSF or IL-5 could be used to develop a model of HES in rodents.

A spontaneous hypereosinophilic disorder has been well-defined in cats. Six were described in 1981,[783] and in 1985, three cats which had the disease for 4 months, 1.5 years, and 3.5 years, were found at necropsy to have many mature eosinophils in lymphatic tissues, the liver and the subendocardium, but without endomyocardial fibrosis.[1173] Two dogs with a similar disease were described in 1983.[702]

24.4 Patients affected

HES is a sporadic disease which does not appear to have a strong genetic element in its pathogenesis, as there are no reports of the disease occurring in more than one member of a family. The remarkable sex incidence of HES (and a number of other eosinophilic disorders) has yet to be explained. Nine males with the disease are reported for each female affected.

The mean age of onset of HES is 37 years, and few cases have been reported in childhood or old age. The youngest child with the disease was aged 5.5 years at presentation.[325] A review of previously published cases of hypereosinophilia of unknown cause in children was published in 1987. There were only 18, which emphasizes the rarity of HES under the age of 15. Five of the children died with a leukaemic process, and the others probably had HES.[27]

Examples of HES in children under 13 years of age include:

1. a five-year-old girl described in 1973, who died 25 days after she presented with abdominal pain, vomiting, and fever. Her blood eosinophil counts rose from 78 to 126 × 10^9/l. She also had cardiac, central nervous system, renal, liver, and spleen involvement.[1479]

2. a seven-year-old boy reported in 1950, who presented with an eosinophil count of 10 × 10^9/l, and had skin, heart, lymphatic, and joint involvement. Although the marrow was said to contain 53 per cent blast forms, he was alive 12 years later after treatment with only adrenocorticotrophic hormone (ACTH), making it probable that he had HES, not eosinophilic leukaemia as originally proposed.[458]

3. a seven-year-old boy described in 1942, who had an eosinophil count of 79 × 10^9/l, with cardiac, respiratory, joint, and thrombotic complications. He died 11 weeks after presentation with coronary artery thromboses.[512]

4. an eight-year-old boy described in 1956, who presented with respiratory, cardiac, and abdominal symptoms. His liver and spleen were

enlarged, and his blood eosinophil count was 79 × 10^9/l. Treatment with ACTH reduced the size of these organs, and the eosinophil count was lowered to 7.7 × 10^9/l. However, the eosinophil count rose again, and he died six months later, after the marrow eosinophils had become increasingly immature. Thrombus and fibrosis were found in the heart, and eosinophilic infiltrates in tissues. Vascular changes were also noted in the spleen and kidneys.[514]

5. a 10-year-old boy discussed in 1956 who developed an illness which affected his skin, cornea, heart, kidneys, joints, and muscles. His liver and spleen were enlarged. The eosinophil count rose to 10.5 × 10^9/l. He also had a marked increase in serum immunoglobulins. Surprisingly, treatment with ACTH increased the eosinophil count, although the immunoglobulin levels fell. This disease appears to be different in many ways from classical HES.[514]

6. a six-year-old girl described in 1984 who had an eosinophil count of 4.8 × 10^9/l, with heart, skin, kidney, lung, and liver disease, while taking anti-tuberculous drugs. She died three and a half years later. The possibility of rifampicin-induced hypersensitivity was a possibility in the aetiology of her eosinophilia, especially as she had circulating immune complexes and a glomerulonephritis, but the illness was diagnosed as HES.[582]

7. a nine-year-old boy described in 1985 with blood eosinophil count of 64 × 10^9/l, and heart, central nervous system, skin, respiratory, and lymphatic involvement. He died six months later with endomyocardial fibrosis.[791]

8. a seven-year-old girl described in 1958 who had an eosinophil count of 18 × 10^9/l, with heart, central nervous system, skin, respiratory, and lymphatic involvement. She died after 10 months, with severe heart lesions and peripheral emboli.[982]

9. a nine-year-old boy described in 1985 who had a blood eosinophil count of 64 × 10^9/l, with heart, central nervous system, skin, respiratory, and lymphatic involvement. He died six months later with endomyocardial fibrosis.[791]

10. two Indian children aged three and five years described in 1983, who had abdominal pain and a cough respectively. Although their blood eosinophil counts were between 4 and 9 × 10^9/l, no clinical complications developed during follow-up periods of over 18 months.[1602]

11. a preterm boy described in 1981 who died aged four days with a perforation of the terminal ileum, which was infiltrated with eosinophils, as were his kidneys, lymph nodes, bone marrow, portal tracts of liver, gall bladder, and bile duct.[1254]

24.4.1 *Demography*

All races appear to be affected, although no accurate statistics are available. Besides the patients described above, there are also reports of HES from Scotland,[151] Eire,[1461] France,[1024, 509, 526] Italy,[334] and Austria.[1571] Most of the patients described in the USA and England were white, although several were blacks.[530, 325, 2016, 1900] Although reports of HES were initially confined to temperate climates and it may be very difficult to distinguish it from chronic parasitic diseases, there are now several reports of HES from India.[1841, 1602, 1469]

24.5 Presentation

HES may present in a number of different ways. Sometimes the raised blood eosinophil count is found accidentally. In the NIH series this occurred in 12 per cent of patients.[544] However, in others, a serious illness leads to urgent hospital admission, and the diagnosis soon becomes clear. Most patients fall between these two extremes, and present with thrombotic complications, coughing, weight loss, or general malaise. The frequency of symptoms and signs in the NIH series[544] was tiredness in 26 per cent, cough in 24 per cent, breathlessness in 16 per cent, muscle pains or angioedema in 14 per cent, a rash or fever in 12 per cent, and retinal lesions in 10 per cent.

24.6 Nonspecific symptoms

Sweating is a common feature of HES, and some patients also have a low-grade fever. Although eosinophils were thought at one time to be able to produce endogenous leukocyte pyrogen,[1207] which is now known as IL–I, this now seems to be unlikely, although no formal study has been done on this using eosinophils from patients with HES and a fever.

Twelve per cent of the NIH series of patients presented with fever. It is seldom due to an infection, and the large amount of sweating in some patients is out of proportion to the rise in body temperature. Few patients have weight loss unless the disease is active and they have lost their appetite. They seldom develop a catabolic state, as seen in some patients with malignant diseases.

Some patients with marked eosinophilia have been found to have alcohol-related symptoms, such as flushing attacks, redness of the face, weakness, nausea, and diarrhoea[1046]. I have one patient with HES who had these symptoms with lymphoma-induced hypereosinophilia. It has also been reported in a patient with eosinophilic leukaemia in 1984,[1351] and in a patient with bronchial carcinoma-induced hypereosinophilia.[117]

24.7 Cardiovascular complications

Cardiovascular complications are amongst the most serious features of HES. The principal ones are eosinophilic endomyocardial fibrosis (see Chapter 24), and thromboemboli. Arterial calcification has also been noted in three patients with HES.[1286, 646]

24.8 Thromboembolic complications

Eosinophils are able to affect the coagulation system by actions on endothelial cells, platelets, and clotting factors. IL–I has been found to be a potent inducer of tissue-factor like procoagulant activity, and this maybe an important event in intravascular coagulation produced by immunological and inflammatory diseases.[164] For this reason it is not surprising that small vessel and large vessel thrombotic occlusions are an important feature of HES, and may well cause the death of patients if they are not recognized and treated. Extensive cardiac ventricular intracavity thrombi and emboli can develop in some patients with HES. A striking example of this was described in 1977 in a 30-year-old Japanese man who presented with thrombophlebitis and an eosinophil count of 109.7×10^9/l. He was treated with prednisolone and busulphan until his death three years later, when he had also developed eosinophilic heart disease. At post mortem the heart was found to contain a large mural thrombus below the mitral valve, overlying fibrous endocardium. Thromboemboli were also seen in other organs: the spleen, kidneys, liver, and brain.[846] A Swedish patient with similar cerebral, renal, and pulmonary infarcts, and thrombotic endocarditis, was reported in 1979.[847]

The principal small vessels which are known to be involved include small vessels in the nail beds of the fingers, where they produce 'splinter haemorrhages',[1460] and retinal vessels, which were occluded in 10 of 12 patients in our series.[296]

Large vessel occlusions probably occur mainly as a result of emboli leaving the wall of the left ventricle. These have been noted most commonly in femoral arteries and the lower aorta, but can also occlude coronary arteries, or give rise to minor strokes and major thrombi in the central nervous system.

Other forms of arterial disease can also affect the large vessels of patients with HES. Two patients with arterial calcification were described in 1971.[1286] There is also a report of the development of thromboangiitis obliterans requiring amputation of the legs in a 47-year-old man with HES.[556] This patient also had an occluded temporal artery, with eosinophils infiltrating the vessel wall. It was suggested that these vascular lesions had occurred as a result of eosinophil-dependent damage to the vessel wall, but the patient was also a smoker.

24.9 Respiratory tract complications

One of the main presenting features of HES is an intractable nocturnal cough which wakes the patient and forces him to cough repeatedly for several minutes. A small amount of sputum may be produced. These coughing attacks can occur during the day, and may be very disabling. Chest radiographs are normal before and during these attacks. In one patient, I was able to show that large numbers of blood eosinophils were being sequestered in the lungs during an attack.

Pulmonary infiltrates are often seen in patients with HES. These have to be distinguished from heart failure, embolic lesions, infective episodes, and tumour deposits, which can also give rise to eosinophilia.[521] When lung infiltrates in patients with HES are biopsied, they usually show an interstitial infiltrate of mononuclear cells and eosinophils.[493] In a report in 1984 on a patient with progressive infiltrates, the eosinophils were found surrounding and infiltrating small pulmonary arterioles.[797]

In 1982, details were given of a patient with HES and endomyocardial fibrosis with heart failure, who had respiratory failure due to respiratory infiltrates. His lung lesions cleared within two weeks of treatment with steroids.[93]

24.10 Digestive system complications

Many patients with HES complain of indigestion and discomfort in the abdomen, but it is uncommon for them to have diarrhoea, gastrointestinal bleeding, or other serious problems affecting the gut. When they do occur, a careful search should be made for the site of the abnormality, and the nature of the organ involvement can vary considerably. Detailed inpatient investigation may be required. Unusual complications include small bowel obstruction,[1652] and jaundice due to pancreatic involvement.[526]

Several patients with HES have been described, who had painful ulcers in their mucous membranes. Two patients with oral and genital ulcers were reported from the Mayo Clinic in 1982.[1054] This preceded other more serious complications of HES, such as heart disease. We are also looking after a patient with HES and lichen planus, which is producing severe pain in the mouth and pharynx, and has been refractory to a wide variety of drugs.

Diarrhoea occurs in about 20 per cent of patients with HES, and the bowel wall may be infiltrated with eosinophils.[325, 1694] In one of our patients who had repeated attacks of gastrointestinal bleeding, this was eventually shown to be due to a vascular malformation in the ileum. In another patient, persistent diarrhoea was the presenting feature for an eosinophilic disorder which was subsequently shown to be eosinophilic leukaemia.

The liver can be enlarged in patients with HES, and biopsies often show the presence of many periportal eosinophils. One patient with the Budd–Chiari syndrome complicating HES was reported from Creteil, France, in 1985.[509]

24.11 Skin complications

A wide variety of skin lesions have been noted in patients with HES. These were reviewed in 1979, when the findings in eight patients at NIH were described.[937] They were usually mild, with erythematous pruritic papuls and nodules, or urticaria, and angioedema, and had a variable response to treatment with steroids. It was reported in 1984 that an intensly pruritic erythematous rash in a patient with HES responded to oral sodium cromoglycate (200mg, four times daily). Topical steroids had no effect.[1952]

Many patients have itching of the legs, and scratch marks are common. Some patients show marked dermatographism, but this does not appear to correlate with any features of the illness, and a few patients may have urticaria within two minutes of applying pressure to the skin for 30 seconds, a condition not seen in other types of pressure urticaria.[908] Eczematous skin lesions can occur in HES, but they have no diagnostic features.

Papules and macules are common in patients with HES.[937] An unusual skin disorder was seen in a man of 24 with HES who had pruritic papules involving many parts of his skin. He also had an enlarged liver, and an eosinophil count of 2.7×10^9/l. Treatment with prednisolone gave some benefit, but dapsone was more effective. On the basis of the results in this patient, and a review of three others, it was suggsted that dapsone might be helpful in other patients with similar skin complications.[1279] The term 'hypereosinophilic dermatitis' was used to describe this skin abnormality.

In other patients, localized abnormalities occur in the skin, which may ulcerate. We have looked after one patient with severe ulcerating lesions, which appeared several weeks before she died. They were associated with thrombi in dermal arterioles.[1694] Similar lesions were described in a patient with HES in Puerto Rico in 1982.[1550] We have also noted three patients with HES, who were later found to have lymphomatoid papulosis.[1926] In these patients we suggested that the T-cell abnormality which gave rise to the skin disorder could also induced eosinophilia. See page 304.

24.12 Nervous system involvement

The central nervous system is often involved in patients with HES, and individual peripheral nerves can also be affected. Many patients have psychological problems, although no formal studies of this have been carried out. Several of the major neurological complications of HES were defined in a detailed study in the UK in 1971.[627] Four patients were described who had optic ataxia and paralysis of visual fixation (Balint's Syndrome). Post mortem studies in one patient showed brain infarcts, with subintimal fibrous tissue in the left posterior cerebral artery. These were also present in a 59-year-old man, who had cerebral infarcts and emboli, but without arteritis. These central nervous system complications only seem to occur in the most seriously affected patients, who seldom live for more than one or two years after they have developed. It is not known whether they are the result of microemboli, local thrombosis in cerebral vessels, or a more subtle effect of the disease on the brain tissues.

The ways in which HES causes neurological problems is still not known, although a number of post mortems have been carried out on these patients. No reports have been published of demyelination or loss of Purkinje cells, which occurs when ECP or EDN/EPX are injected into the cerebrospinal fluid of experimental animals. As high levels of these proteins have been detected in the cerebrospinal fluid in a variety of eosinophilic disorders, it is probable that these effects of the eosinophil basic proteins in animals are unimportant in human neurological complications of HES. However, this area needs further work, and its importance may only come to light when experimental studies have been done using isolated nerve cells and purified eosinophil constituents.

24.12.1 *Central nervous system complications*

Patients with HES may have diffuse central nervous system disease, or focal lesions, or combinations of these. The commonest abnormality is an alteration in their capacity to think rationally. This has been difficult to define, but I have noticed it especially during periods when my patients have had progressive disease. Neurological disease affecting the NIH group of patients with HES was assessed in 52 patients, and reported in 1985. Thirty-four (65 per cent) had neurological abnormalities, including encephalopathy, peripheral neuropathy, and focal lesions. Seven patients had more than one of these abnormalities.

In the NIH series, five patients were described who had a distinctive encephalopathy, characterized by changes in behaviour, confusion, loss of memory, and ataxia. They had upper motor neuron signs, with increased muscle tone, deep tendon reflexes, and a positive Babinski sign. Two had epileptic fits.[1233] The nature of the alteration in brain function is not known. In our series of patients, four of whom had post mortems, no lesions were found in the brain, and this was also the case in a post mortem of another patient with HES and confusion, reported from Texas, USA in 1985.[1900]

Major complications of HES are repeated minor or major strokes which can cause the patient's death. These are usually multifocal, and can involve any of the major centres of the brain. They probably involve occlusions of vessels by emboli from the left ventricle,[1383] and possibly by local thrombus formation. At the NIH, six patients had focal central nervous system disease, which was transient. Five others with these features also had heart disease, suggesting that they may have had thromboemboli, and two had recurrent attacks.[1233]

24.12.2 *Eye diseases*

Although only one patient with retinal haemorrhage was reported amongst a group of 52 patients with HES at the NIH,[1233] we have found retinal abnormalities in many of our patients with HES (see Plate 11). This was documented in 10 of our patients in whom lesions were visible, either by direct examination or by fluorescent retinal angiography.[296] Defects were the result of vascular occlusions affecting the retinal and choroidal vessels. One patient developed showers of splinter haemorrhages, and had coincidental retinal lesions. Other case reports of patients with HES and retinal vascular lesions were reported from Louvain, Belgium in 1980,[1073] and from Creteil, France in 1982.[540]

24.12.3 *Peripheral nerve diseases*

Several types of peripheral nervous system disease may develop in patients with HES.[151, 717] These include mononeuritis multiplex, symmetrical sensorimotor neuropathy, multifocal neuropathy, and radiculopathy. In some patients it may be difficult to distinguish nerve involvement in HES from other causes of a neuropathy and eosinophilia, especially vasculitic and granulomatous disease. This is well shown in a study on three patients with a peripheral neuropathy reported from Palo Alto, California, USA in 1983,[462] and in these patients the presence of allergies, asthma, and granulomas mitigated against a diagnosis of HES.

Mononeuritis multiplex is common in patients with HES, involving the peroneal nerve and other long nerves supplying the legs, and arms. They may cause considerable pain and discomfort, but tend to resolve over several weeks, sometimes leaving no residual abnormality. An example of this was in a 16-year-old man in Kuwait, who also had respiratory and cardiac involvement which were eventually fatal.[507] Another patient was described in 1985.[1233]

A sensorimotor neuropathy was described in 1982,[544] and 23 patients among 52 with HES at NIH had various forms of sensorimotor loss. Three other had a radiculopathy.[1233] Seven of these patients, three of whom had clinical evidence of peripheral nerve injury, underwent nerve conduction studies, elctromyograms, and sural nerve biopsies. These showed axonal neuropathy, axonal loss, and some demyelination. It was suggested that these changes could have been produced by EDN/EPX.[1928] A patient with HES and a purely motor neuropathy was described in 1986. This patient also had bilateral facial palsies and focal central nervous system lesions.[1162]

Multifocal neuropathy in HES has been described in 1975,[325] 1983,[462] and 1985.[717]

24.13 Musculoskeletal complications

Many patients with HES have aches and pains which are often poorly localized. Muscle biopsies have shown no specific abnormalities. Bony deposits of primitive eosinophils are a feature of eosinophilic leukaemia, but it has only been reported in one patient with HES, who also had hypercalcaemia.[646]

Joint involvement is also unusual, but there are a number of patients with a disease similar to rheumatoid arthritis who have a marked and persistent eosinophilia for many years. We are looking after a woman with this association who has had HES and rheumatoid arthritis for 24 years. A 58-year-old man with eosinophilia of 4.5×10^9/l was described in 1967 who developed swollen, tender, and stiff joints. His skin became doughy and erythematous. The erythrocyte sedimentation rate was 68 mm/h. Although he was treated with steroids, his eosinophil counts increased, splenic infarcts occurred, and he died in heart failure. However, as blast cells eventually appeared in his blood, and these were also found infiltrating into the heart, he may have had eosinophilic leukaemia.[1404]

Skeletal muscle wasting associated with eosinophil infiltrates may develop in a few patients with the hypereosinophilic syndrome,[1652] although muscle biopsies usually show no specific abnormalities.

24.14 Renal complications and hypertension

About 10 per cent of patients with HES have renal complications, but less than this have hypertension. One of the first was reported in 1965.[1293] Some reports have been published of renal interstitial eosinophil infiltrates, and vascular damage to renal arteries, shown by intimal proliferation and medial injury.[1351] These vascular changes have also been seen in other sites.[308]

Renal impairment with glomerulonephritis has been described in a small number of patients with HES and eosinophilic endomyocardial fibrosis.[1661] In two cases which were reported in 1969, the renal damge may have been due to bacterial endocarditis. A post mortem on a 25-year-old man who died 1.75 years after onset of his illness showed thickened glomerular basement membrane, with fibrinoid necrosis of arterioles, but he was also found to have vegetations on the aortic and mitral valves. A second man, aged 35, with eosinophilic heart disease complicated by bacterial endocarditis and myocardial abscesses, had renal disease during life. Similar glomerular lesions were found at post mortem.[1502]

Several patients with HES have had hypertension and impaired renal function. This has been shown to be associated with arteriolar thickening in renal biopsies, and it has been suggested that eosinophils might be involved in damaging blood vessels in these areas. The hypertension responds to therapy, but the renal impairment does not appear to improve. No patient with HES has progressed to end-stage renal failure.

24.15 Breast involvement

A single report of breast involvement was reported in 1985.[1772] This was a 56-year-old woman with HES who developed swollen, painful, red breasts, in which the ducts were heavily infiltrated with eosinophils, and contained areas of necrosis, but no fibrosis. The skin was indurated, and the breasts were stony hard. This lesion resolved following treatment with steroids.

25. The idiopathic hypereosinophilic syndrome (HES): Investigations

The clinical investigation of HES involves an assessment of the nature and mechanisms of the complications which are usually the presenting features of the illness, and a careful search for the underlying causes which may only become apparent several months or years after the patient becomes ill. As this disease is usually life-long, it is suggested that patients be admitted to hospital for several days for a careful assessment of each of the major organ systems which might be involved at the time, or subsequently, and in order for a careful long-term plan of management to be organized. These patients should be reviewed at one of the major centres where there is a special interest in the disease, although their subsequent care can be carried out in the outpatient departments of most district hospitals. As many organ systems can be involved, patients may need to be seen by different specialists for this initial workup.

This chapter will outline the special investigations which have proved to be useful in discovering the nature of the underlying abnormalities in the eosinophil series in this disorder. Details of cardiological studies are given on pages 238–42.

25.1 Blood eosinophils in HES

An unusually high blood eosinophil count in patients with HES is the first investigation which points to this diagnosis. (See Plate 10). Nearly every patient with HES has eosinophilia throughout the rest of his life, with counts remaining remarkably constant in the majority of patients. In a few patients with the aggressive forms of the disease, the counts may rise to higher levels, but these can return toward their previous levels after treatment, and they may then persist at this level for several years before relapses occur. The majority of patients with HES have eosinophil counts between 2 and 20 × 10^9/l. The highest count I have seen recorded in HES is 220 × 10^9/l.[1009] There is no direct relationship between the eosinophil count and the severity of the clinical complications. Some of the highest blood eosinophil counts have been found in patients with the more benign forms of the disease. Serial blood eosinophil counts have only been published in a relatively small number of patients, but the management of these patients is greatly helped by graphing their blood counts on log paper over a prolonged period. This is important if minor fluctuations in the counts are not to be overinterpreted as signs of alterations in the underlying disease process.

A wide range of special studies have been carried out on blood eosinophils from patients with HES, and many of the papers published on the properties of eosinophils are describing HES eosinophils. Comparisons of their properties with eosinophils from other disorders are still limited, but it is likely that differences will be found. Some of these may be linked to the increased rate of production of eosinophils in HES, but others may be due to the underlying abnormality in the eosinophil series, which probably occurs in some patients with HES.

25.1.1 *Eosinophil density*

In a study reported from the Mayo Clinic in 1987, blood eosinophils from 10 normal people had a mean peak density in Percoll of 1.088 g/ml, and only 10 ± 7 per cent (mean ± SD) had a density less than 1.082, which was defined as the cut off point to distinguish normal density from light density eosinophls. In four patients with HES, the mean peak density was much lower: 1.075, and 97 per cent of the eosinophils were of light density. The density of blood eosinophils correlated with their MBP content.[1389] Current research in several centres is looking at how normal eosinophils could become lighter in density. The first successful *in vitro* technique, reported in 1987,[1522] involved the use of prolonged culture with endothelial cells or their products. (See also page 35.)

25.1.2 *Morphology of blood eosinophils in HES*

It has been known for many years that blood eosinophils in patients with marked eosinophilia may be structurally abnormal, and these were often thought to be leukaemic. For example in 1919, a patient with 'eosinophilic leukaemia' in New York, was seen to have many blood eosinophils with fewer eosinophilic granules than normal. This important observation was recorded in a colour plate.[1600] Similar findings were reported in 1960.[308]

Light microscopy of HES blood eosinophils In blood smears, eosinophils from patients with HES show a range of abnormalities, which include hypersegmentation of the nucleus, cytoplasmic vacuoles, a decrease in the number of specific granules, and granules of smaller size than normal. Measurements of the proportions of cells in the blood which show these abnormalities may be of clinical value in distinguishing HES from other causes of eosinophilia. The presence of many degranulated eosinophils in a blood smear can be striking. When there are more than $1 \times 10^9/l$, it is likely that the patient has HES and eosinophilic endomyocardial fibrosis. (See Plate 5.)

Hypersegmented blood eosinophils with decreased numbers of granules and vacuoles are not confined to patients with HES. For example, eosinophil peroxidase deficiency can occur with these abnormalities in blood eosinophils,[1437] and I have seen them in a patient with severe tropical (filarial) eosinophilia.

Histochemical and immunocytochemical studies on HES blood eosinophils have shown several qualititative differences from normal eosinophils, but they have not been studied sufficiently to know whether these can be used in diagnosis. The alterations were well illustrated in a detailed study in 1964 on the morphological and histochemical characteristics of blood and bone marrow eosinophils from a 38-year-old man with 'eosinophilic leukaemia', which would be diagnosed today as HES. Abnormalities in the neutrophil series were also seen.[3]

Ultrastructural studies on HES blood eosinophils Blood eosinophil ultrastructure in patients with HES shows several features consistent with the possibility that they are activated and secreting their granule contents.

Scanning electronmicroscopic studies on human blood eosinophils from patients with HES have shown no surface features to distinguish them from eosinophils or neutrophils in normal individuals. As yet, no studies have been done to see if activated eosinophils develop ridges and projections which are found in other stimulated cells. The first detailed morphometric study on HES blood eosinophils was carried out in 1986 on peripheral blood eosinophils from a woman aged 41 with HES and a blood eosinophil count of $202 \times 10^9/l$. The principal findings were that the eosinophils were larger in size than normal, with a 34 per cent increase in volume; and 19 per cent had three or more nuclear lobes. Mitochondria were more numerous, and 50 per cent larger than normal. The volume of the specific granules was 35 per cent smaller than normal, and there were slightly less of them than normal. These findings suggested that in this patient blood eosinophils were metabolically more active than normal, and that the granules were undergoing dissolution or secretion.[1659]

A detailed ultrastructural study was carried out in Seattle, Washington, USA, in 1987, on five patients with HES. The mean diameter of the crystalloid granules was reduced to 82 per cent of normal, and there were only 27 per cent of the normal number of granules. Lipid bodies were prominent in the cytoplasm; and in two patients, some eosinophils were found to contain Charcot–Leyden crystals.[780]

The ultrastructural appearances of blood eosinophils in patients seen at the Mayo Clinic are given in two reports. In the first, published in 1976, there were unusual electron-dense inclusions in the cells.[1661] The appearances of the cells in three other patients were reported in 1987. Over 90 per cent of the eosinophilis were of light density: less than 1.082 g/ml. The total number of granules were the same as in normal people, although the granules were of smaller mean area than normal: 0.14 μm^2, compared to 0.26 μm^2. The eosinophils were of the same size, with the same number of lipid bodies, and equal proportions of eosinophils with reversed staining were seen.[1389] The reasons for this are not known, but it was suggested in 1975 that the hypogranular eosinophils could be less mature than normal.[455]

Freeze-fracture studies of HES blood eosinophils have shown the presence of membrane structures similar to those seen in blood neutrophils.[780]

25.1.3 *HES blood eosinophil cell membrane components*

The plasma membrane of blood eosinophils from patients with HES has been studied using a variety of different techniques. In 1976 we showed that HES blood eosinophils had more FcγR and complement receptors than normal.[1738] In one patient with HES it was found that the cell surface charge was low, similar to that of stimulated normal blood eosinophils.[127]

We have raised monoclonal antibodies to HES blood eosinophil membrane constituents.[1734] These recognized a number of structures which were also present on neutrophils, but which were occasionally found in greater amounts on the surface of HES blood eosinophils, than on normal eosinophils. The nature of the membrane antigens which they bound to, has still be be defined, but they appear to be components of the membrane which are involved in activating the cells to secrete.

25.1.4 *Constituents in HES blood eosinophils*

Many of the studies which have described the purification of eosinophil constituents have used blood eosinophils from patients with HES, as they are the easiest to obtain. However, in some patients with HES, there is less ECP and MBP in blood eosinophils than normal. In the past, this led to difficulties in measuring the absolute quantities of the different basic proteins in human eosinophils. The reasons why there are less of these proteins in these patients' cells is not known, but could be due to either reduced synthesis in the marrow, or to preferential secretion from the blood cells. A study in 1983 on blood eosinophils from six patients with HES showed that they contained 6.3–63.5 more MBP than ECP. This may have been related to the amount of degranulation that has occurred, as this ratio was smallest when the cells contained the highest concentration of ECP.[9]

Blood eosinophils from patients with HES have a lower and a more variable content of MBP than normal.[7] The MBP content of blood eosinophils with a density less than 1.082, in four patients with HES was 3670 ± 368 ng/10^6 cells, compared to 8619 ± 1445 ng/10^6 cells in normal subjects.[1389] The content of ECP in blood eosinophils from patients with HES is usually less than normal.[1944] There are no reports on the eosinophil content of EDN/EPX or EPO in HES blood eosinophils. Cytochemical electronmicroscopy has shown that acid phosphatase was unmasked in eosinophil granules from one patient with HES.[127] Blood eosinophils from patients with HES have over twice the capacity to secrete LTC4 in response to stimulation with A23187 as eosinophils from normal blood: 69 ng compared with 38 ng/10^6 eosinophils.[1915] One case report has described PAF-acether production by blood eosinophils from a 32-year-old woman in Brazil, who had HES with cerebral and retinal vascular occlusions, and endomyocardial fibrosis. These produced 4×10^{-10}M PAF-acether per 1×10^6 eosinophils, and it was suggested that this could have contributed to the development of her thrombotic lesions.[299] HES eosinophils produce large amounts of PAF-acether in response to the calcium ionophore A23187.[898]

25.1.5 *Metabolism of HES blood eosinophils*

Many metabolic studies on human eosinophils have been carried out using blood eosinophils from patients with HES. An example of this was the study done by Mickenberg and colleagues in 1971. They isolated blood eosinophils from a 45-year-old man with HES, eosinophilic endomyocardial fibrosis, and multiple embolic episodes. The cells' capacity to kill bacteria and to metabolize glucose after a phagocytic stimulus was compared with blood eosinophils from other patients with eosinophilia. After incubation of the patient's eosinophils with bacteria, more of the organisms were killed at two hours than when control eosinophils were used. The patient's eosinophils had a higher oxidative capacity for 1-^{14}C-glucose than controls, either resting, or after phagocytosing particles *in vitro*.[1207]

Similar studies were done in 1981 on nine patients with HES, with blood eosinophil counts between 2.1 and 7.2×10^9/l, by Bass and colleagues. They showed that the patients' blood eosinophils had a higher uptake of deoxyglucose than normal, both resting and after stimulation with zymosan activated serum, than normal blood eosinophils.[127] The amount of superoxide produced by purified eosinophils from a patient with HES was shown to be related to the degree to which the cells were stimulated.[1418]

25.1.6 *Motility and chemotaxis of HES blood eosinophils*

Histamine diphosphate induced purified blood eosinophils from four patients with HES and from one other patient, to migrate up a concentration gradient, but random motility was not increased. At high concentrations of histamime, migration was inhibited.[328] In a paper published from Lille, France in 1987, it was found that light density blood eosinophil from four patients with HES migrated less well towards LTB4 than normal density eosinophils from the same patients. The sera from five patients with HES was found to be as effective as LTB4 in inducing eosinophils from other patients without HES, to migrate into polycarbonate filters. i.e., the sera contained chemotactic activity. This activity was found in 600 kDa and 240 kDa fractions. Preincubation of normal density HES eosinophils with this active sera reduced their capacity to migrate towards LTC4 and fMLP. From these results, it was suggested that the sera of these patients with HES contained two (deactivating) components which might inhibit the capacity of their blood eosinophils to leave the circulation, and that this could explain their high blood eosinophil counts.[700] Unfortunately some data was missing from this report, and it did not address the question of why HES blood eosinophils should be able to migrate *in vitro*, if they had already been deactivated *in vivo*.

25.1.7 *Activated blood eosinophils in HES*

The monoclonal antibody EG2, which distinguishes activated from nonactivated blood eosinophils,[1742] has shown that a variable proportion of eosinophils in the blood of patients with HES are activated (Plate 4). So far, no study has been carried out to see whether this can be clinically useful in determining the degree of activation, or severity of complications in these patients.

25.1.8 *Secretion from HES blood eosinophils*

The capacity of HES blood eosinophils to secrete their granule contents in response to stimuli, such as complement-coated particles, is very variable in different patients. The reason for this is not clear. However, in any one patient, the secretory response to a set stimulus is reproducible, and this has enabled studies to be carried out on the effects of drugs on eosinophil secretion.

In 1987, blood eosinophils from five patients with HES were isolated, to study the amounts of EPO which were secreted following stimulation with opsonized zymosan and the calcium ionophore A23187. Under optimal conditions, 23 per cent of the EPO was secreted following stimulation with A23187, which was seen to induce vesiculation of granule contents, and fusion of adjacent granules in electronmicrographs. Opsonized zymosan also induced vesiculation, with granule fusion and secretion into the endocytic vacuoles, but only 13 per cent of the EPO was secreted.[780]

25.1.9 *Cyotoxic capacity of HES blood eosinophils*

The capacity of HES blood eosinophils to kill a variety of targets has been assessed: They have been shown to be able to kill a number of antibody- and complement-coated parasites, and nucleated cells.[1367]

25.1.10 *The half-life of injected blood eosinophils*

Isolated blood eosinophils have been labelled with ^{51}Cr or ^{111}In, and reinjected into patients with HES. This has shown that they have the unusual capacity to marginate in the circulation for 1–2 hours, and then to re-emerge with a subsequent prolonged half-life compared to blood neutrophils or eosinophils in patients with parasitic diseases,[385] and I have similar unpublished data on five other patients injected with ^{111}In-labelled blood eosinophils.

25.2 Serum and plasma constituents in HES

Plasma MBP levels in four patients with HES were 2.928 ± 1.567 μg/ml compared to 0.307 ± 0.038 μg/ml in 10 normal subjects.[1389] In one patient with HES, large amounts of ECP were found complexed to α-2 macroglobulin.[1398]

Several patients with HES have been noted to have high serum B12 levels.[910, 575, 1461, 1024] In the large study from the NIH, Bethesda, Maryland, USA, in 1981, it was the commonest additional abnormality in 32 patients with HES.[573] In 1984, serum cobalamin (vitamin B12) and unsaturated B12 binding capacity were measured in 16 patients with HES.[2002] They were markedly elevated, and this was principally due to an increase in R binders (transcobalamins I and III). The cell source of this additional B12-binding capacity is not known. A proportion may have come from neutrophils, which normally contain over four times as much unsaturated B12 binding proteins as normal eosinophils. In a study in 1984 on partially purified eosinophils from a patient with HES, transcobalamin 1 was detected at 10 ng/10^8 eosinophils: half the amount found in normal neutrophils.[22]

Although Strath and Sanderson in 1986 detected an eosinopoietic activity in the sera of mice infected with *Mesocestoides corti*,[1714] they have had no success in developing a reliable assay system using human sera. However in 1987, the serum from six patients with hypereosinophilia who were studied in Hamburg, West Germany induced additional production of eosinophils in 12-day liquid cultures of normal bone marrow.[954]

25.3 Bone marrow features of HES

In patients with HES, up to 80 per cent of the dividing cells in the bone marrow may be of the eosinophil lineage. No morpholigical features distinguish these dividing eosinophils from eosinophils in normal bone marrow, but other studies with these cells have shown that there are important abnormalities in up to ten per cent of these patients. The quantity of reticulin and fibrous tissue in the bone marrow is often increased. In the majority of patients the red cell series is well-preserved.

One patient has been reported with polycythaemia and HES.[1842] Platelet production is normal or increased, although the blood platelet count can be low, due to platelet consumption. Neutrophil production is usually not affected, but some patients have unusually basophilic granules in a proportion of their neutrophils. A normal neutrophilia can develop in patients with HES who developed a bacterial infection.[124]

Thirty-two patients with HES who presented at NIH between 1968 and 1979, had bone marrow and other haematological studies done. Later, a numerical score was given to each of their clinical and haematological features depending on its severity. It was proposed that the treatment of other patients should be based on the size of their 'score' in relation to the NIH data.[573] I disagree with this approach. Patients with HES should be given expert medical advice on treatment and they should not be managed by inexperienced physicians on the basis of an arbitrary score chart drawn up in one referral centre until this has been verified elsewhere.

A small number of patients with HES have a marked increase in fibrous tissue in the marrow. Examples of this include:

(1) a patient reported as having 'eosinophilic leukaemia' in 1969;[157]

(2) a 57-year-old man with refractory heart failure, and an eosinophil count of 12.4×10^9/l in 1972.[572]

(3) a 54-year-old man with blood eosinophil counts of up to 13×10^9/l in 1972.[638]

(4) three patients in Copenhagen, Denmark in whom it was suggested that eosinophils could be producing a factor, such as platelet-derived growth factor, which could induce the fibrotic reaction.

(5) four patients who were reviewed in 1974 in a report which also described a 16-year-old black patient who died in a blast cell crisis, and was found to have endocardial disease.[710]

25.3.1 *Bone marrow culture in HES*

In 1981, we measured the number of eosinophil colonies which could be grown from the bone marrow and blood of four patients with HES. The total number of colonies which grew from the marrows of two of the patients were not different from normal, but the proportion which were eosinophilic was increased. No eosinopoietic effect of the patients' lymphocyte conditioned medium was found.[774] In 1982, 13 patients with HES at NIH, were assessed for the number of CFU-Eo which grew from bone marrow and blood. In seven, normal numbers were found. In five, increased numbers developed, and in three of these, bone marrow cells produced excess CSF. One patient produced a smaller number of colonies than normal. None of them showed the *in vitro* growth characteristics of leukaemic cells.[176] This study demonstrated that there may be heterogeneity in HES, depending on whether there is a defect in eosinophil progenitor cells, or in the cells which produce CSFs.

25.3.2 *Cytogenetic studies in HES*

A wide range of chromosomal abnormalities have been described in patients with persistent eosinophilia. Some of these patients have an eosinophilic leukaemia, either of the acute or chronic form. Whether any of these patients should be included under the general term of HES is questionable. My own feeling is that once a cause has been found for hypereosinophilia, the illness should be placed in a separate category from HES. The cytogenetic defects in eosinophilic leukaemia are described in pages 155–7.

25.4 Immunological investigations in HES

The commonest immunological abnormality in patients with HES is a raised immunoglobulin level in serum. This is nearly always polyclonal, mainly affecting IgM, IgG, and/or IgE. Defects in lymphocytes have been less consistent.

The clinical significance of a polyclonal increase in serum immunoglobulins in patients with HES is not known, as it does not appear to be related to any particular clinical complication. Occasionally, as reported in 1976, in a 56-year-old London man, a paraprotein can be present.[152]

Although many tests of T-lymphocyte numbers and functions have been carried out in patients with HES, no consistent abnormality has been detected.[1369]

It was reported in 1983 that blood mononuclear cells from a 54-year-old man with HES who had eosinophilic heart disease (but no thromboembolic episodes) produced three or four times more procoagulant activity than normal monocytes on stimulation with endotoxin *in vitro*. As this abnormality returned to normal during treatment, it was suggested that this might be a cause of thromboembolic complications which are common in patients with HES.[1373]

25.5 Coagulation studies in HES

We have carried out coagulation studies in nine patients with HES, and compared them with normal subjects. There were marked elevations in the levels of β-thromboglobulin, platelet factor 4, fibrinogen, factor VIII C:Ag, and R:Ag. In one patient, eosinophil supernatants produced platelet aggregation *in vitro*. As many of these patients had a low platelet count with increased numbers of bone marrow megakaryocytes, it was probable that there was continuing spontaneous coagulation even when there was no clinical evidence of thrombotic lesions.[398] It would be interesting to study patients with eosinophilia of other causes, to see whether eosinophils induce these coagulation abnormalities. Abnormalities in fibrinolysis, and increased procoagulant activity secretion from monocytes in patients with HES would also be worth studying.

26. The idiopathic hypereosinophilic syndrome (HES): Course of the disease, and treatment

The management of HES has to take into account the life-long nature of the disease, its propensity to relapse and remit, the prevention and treatment of complications as they occur, and the avoidance of harmful side effects of powerful drug therapies which may be employed.

A number of charts of the course of the disease in individuals with HES have been published; see, for example, some of our patients' charts in Reference 1694. Studies on the survival rate of patients with the disease have shown a progressive improvement since the early sixties, when therapy was based on current treatments for leukaemia. The realization that a leukaemic disease process was not present in the majority of patients with HES has altered this approach, and now very few patients die from complications of their treatment. A breakdown of patients into the 4 groups described on pages 266–67 can be helpful. Patients

(1) with allergic features are given steroids intermittently in relation to symptoms;

(2) with disease of mild severity are treated with low doses of steroids and antiplatelet drugs;

(3) with moderately severe disease are treated with moderate doses of steroids, intermittent courses of hydroxyurea, and anticoagulants; and

(4) with severe progressive disease are treated with high doses of steroids, continuous hydroxyurea, or another cytotoxic drug, with intermittent injections of vincristine and anticoagulants.

Treatment can enable most patients to lead normal lives, and hospital admissions can be kept to a minimum. Many patients are surviving for more than 10 years after diagnosis. Two patients, who were reported in 1971, survived for 11 and 17 years after the onset of their illness.[1487]

On the other hand, other patients, especially those who develop the thromboembolic complications involving the central nervous system may die within a few days or months. All patients are at risk from developing endomycardial disease and major vascular occlusions.

26.1 Treatment of HES

Radiotherapy was one of the first treatments to be given to patients with HES. This was reported in 1912 in two patients. One had an eosinophil count of 7 × 10^9/l, and was in heart failure. A transient increase in the eosinophil count occurred immediately following each treatment, but no long-term reduction was seen.[75] A second patient with persistent eosinophilia of 4.5 × 10^9/l was given an unspecified amount of irradiation. The blood eosinophil count increased to 8.1, and then fell to 3.2 × 10^9/l the following day.[1034] Despite these intriguing findings, no formal study of the effects of irradiation on patients' eosinophil counts has been published subsequently.

Splenectomy was first used by Giffin in 1919 to treat a patient with a persistently high blood eosinophil count at the Mayo clinic. The patient was a 31-year-old man, who had eosinophil counts of up to 16 × 10^9/l. He died four years later from obliterative endocarditis, pericarditis, and cirrhosis.[642] In 1922 splenectomy in a patient with HES led to an increase in blood eosinophil counts.[1172] In 1971 splenic irradiation was used in a patient with HES, without obvious benefit.[1286]

The use of modern drugs to treat HES began with corticotropin, and then steroids in the late 1950s. Corticotropin (ACTH) was first used in 1953 to treat a 61-year-old woman with hypereosinophilia, producing a fall in her blood eosinophil count.[1523] The development of antineoplastic drugs in the 1960s was soon followed by the use of these compounds to treat HES, but the outcome was generally bad, as patients died from infections due to agranulocytosis. Bone marrow transplantation has not been attempted in this condition, although it is possible that it could cure some patients in whom the disease is confined to the marrow. The difficulty has been to decide whether the disease would recur in the transplanted marrow.

26.1.1 *Steroids in HES*

In 1978, a review of the value of drug treatment in 24 patients seen at the NIH showed that some responded to steroids, and others to cytotoxic drugs. Among these 24 patients, 15 were given steroids. Five improved, 5 showed little change, and 5 did not improve. The 5 unreponsive patients were also given hydroxyurea, and 4 responded favourably. Six patients did not need to be treated with steroids or cytotoxic drugs. Ninety-six per cent of the patients survived for over 3 years, and 77 per cent for over 10 years.[1368] This series was extended, so that 32 patients had been seen by 1980, when their treatment was reviewed again.[1575] Six had no specific therapy. Twenty-six were given steroids, 9 of whom responded. Seventeen were treated with cytotoxic drugs, of whom 9 responded, but 4 had progressive disease despite these treatments. Additional details were published in 1981.[573, 1574]

Most patients with HES receive steroids at some time during the course of their illness, to treat the less serious complications, such as coughing attacks, malaise with sweating, and uncomfortable skin lesions. Doses of prednisolone between 7.5 mg and 20 mg/day are usually given, and the lowest dose which is effective is maintained for several weeks. Alternate day therapy is used in some centres, but it has not been particularly useful in my hands. Few patients have suffered from the serious complications of steroid therapy, although some have developed mild diabetes, hypertension, or a cushingoid appearance. A patient was described in 1982 who developed disseminated tuberculosis,[540] and I know of one other (Bain, B. 1988, Personal communication).

It was suggested in 1978 that steroids may be particularly effective in treating patients with HES who have a history of asthma and pulmonary infiltrates. This was put forward as a result of the successful treatment of two patients, a man aged 57, and a woman aged 54, who had asthma with pulmonary infiltrates, high serum IgE levels, cardiovascular involvement, and rheumatoid arthritis. One of these patients had a mononeuropathy, and the other purpura.[237] In the NIH series of 32 patients, 14 of 17 with splenomegaly at presentation did not respond to steroids, but 3 of 9 who did not have splenomegaly responded well.[1574]

Steroids may improve patients' symptoms by their capacity to inhibit eosinophil production, and the release of mature eosinophils from the marrow. This effect has been studied in rats. Injection of 5 mg cortisol into the peritoneum of normal rats 66 hours after injection of ^{3}H–thymidine reduced blood eosinophil counts, but the percentage of labelled blood eosinophils was not lowered, suggesting that eosinopoiesis was not altered by single doses of steroids. However, when several doses were given over a three-day period the emergence of labelled eosinophils from the marrow was inhibited.[36] Steroids also reduce the secretion of eosinophil granule components, which may cause some of the complications of HES.

Oral steroids usually produce a fall in blood eosinophil counts during the first few hours or days after starting therapy, but they then usually return to their pretreatment levels. This can be a useful way of distinguishing steroid-sensitive allergic diseases from HES. However, as mentioned above, in asthma-associated HES, steroid treatment can return the patient's symptoms and blood counts to normal within a few days.[27]

No studies have been reported on the possible benefits of high-dose pulse therapy with steroids on rapidly progressive disease, although it has been used occasionally.

Troleandomycin 250 mg/day, which has steroid sparing effect in asthma,[1869] was used successfully in a 26-year-old woman with HES, after she failed to respond to steroids, and hydroxyurea.[493]

26.1.2 *Antineoplastic drugs in HES*

Many different antineoplastic drugs have been given to patients with HES, but the ones which are most commonly used today, are those which are effective in chronic myeloid leukaemia. The point at which to change from steroids alone to steroids with cytotoxic drugs should be jüdged on the clinical state of the patient, and not on a wish to produce a 'remission', or to lower high blood eosinophil counts in the absence of signs of continuing tissue damage. Treatment should also be based on the principle that HES is usually a non-malignant and life-long disease, so that the long-term acceptability of each treatment and its side effects are of great importance.

Doses of hydroxyurea between 1 and 2 grams per day appear to be effective in patients with more severe forms of the illness, and blood eosinophil counts may return to near normal with a combination of steroids and hydroxyurea.[93]

Vincristine has been particularly effective in patients with hyper-eosinophilia

(a) who do not respond to steroids and hydroxyurea; or

(b) who have serious complications which would benefit from a reduction in eosinophil production; or

(c) who have thrombocytopenia. Vincristine is also effective in patients with eosinophilic leukaemia and its variants.

One useful regime in adults with the most active forms of the disease is to give 1.5 grams of hydroxyurea and 10–15 mg prednisolone per day, with 1.5 mg of vincristine intravenously at two week intervals. One of our patients has remained well and at work on this treatment for five years, marrying and having two healthy children. Several case reports have described its use in HES.[1839, 334] Intravenous cytarabine and oral 6-thioguanine was given successfully to a patient with HES in 1982.[489]

26.1.3 *Anticoagulation and antiplatelet drugs*

As many patients with HES have thrombotic and embolic complications, and as endomyocardial lesions are commonly coated with thrombus, many patients are treated with oral anticoagulants. However, there is no proof that these prevent thromboembolic disease in these patients, and several patients in our care have had major embolic episodes after anticoagulation has been introduced. Most patients are treated with warfarin, and the dosage is carefully regulated with blood tests every two weeks. As this treatment is likely to be continued for the rest of their lives, care should be taken in deciding which patients might benefit.

The antiplatelet drugs, aspirin and dipyridamole, are also often prescribed for these patients on the basis that platelet aggregation could be an important feature; and in view of the low risk of side effects from these drugs, they are commonly given. Again, there is no controlled study to show that they are effective.

26.1.4 *Leukapheresis and plasma exchange in HES*

Leukapheresis in patients with extremely high blood eosinophil counts is effective in lowering the viscosity of the blood, but there is no evidence at present that this is of therapeutic benefit in patients with eosinophilia,[1421] despite a report from Boston, USA in 1974 that it could have helped a patient with a drug-induced hypereosinophilic state. This was a 25-year-old woman who had a hypersensitivity reaction to sulphisalazole. She developed myositis, myocarditis, and a vasculitis, with eosinophilia of 10×10^9/l. On two separate days, 22 and 9.6×10^{10} cells were removed, and she improved during the subsequent two weeks.[506] However, the fall in blood eosinophil counts was probably mainly due to stopping the sulphonamide. A therapeutic leukapheresis was also done in 1979 in an 18-year-old New Zealand boy with HES and retinal disease.[178]

Surprisingly, plasma exchange produces a larger and more consistent fall in blood eosinophil counts than leukapheresis. This may be because some plasma components are involved in retaining eosinophils in the circulation. Davies and I reported in 1982 a comparison of the effects of plasma exchange, and leukapheresis on blood eosinophil counts in four patients with HES.[400] In three patients there was a larger percentage fall in eosinophil counts following plasma exchange (90 per cent, 83 per cent, and 35 per cent) than following leukapheresis (38 per cent, 27 per cent, and 35 per cent). Serial plasma exchanges continued to be as effective on three consecutive days. These findings suggested that there might be a plasma factor retaining eosinophils within the circulation, and that removing it allowed eosinophils to become marginated. This might not always be beneficial, and it is not recommended that plasma exchange should be used as a treatment for the hypereosinophilic syndrome until more is known about its effects. However none of our patients had adverse effects.

26.1.5 *Bone marrow transplantation in HES*

If HES were due to a defect in dividing eosinophil precursors in the bone marrow, then marrow ablation followed by marrow transplantation could be curative. However as HES may have a number of different causes, and there is no way of distinguishing between them at present, there has been a natural reluctance to consider this therapeutic option, except in patients who appear to have a clonal (malignant) eosinophilic disease. Two patients have received transplants in 1987, and 1988. One died three months later with cytomegalovirus infection, in France, and the other remains well in the UK 2 months post-transplant (Powles, R. 1988. Personal communication).

27. Diseases in neonates and infants

In normal infants less than 28 days old, the eosinophil count is less than $0.70 \times 10^9/l$,[515] although occasionally counts of $1–2 \times 10^9/l$ have been found in otherwise normal babies.[1898] In a study on cord blood samples, which were collected from 242 babies of five different ethnic groups living in London, there was no difference in eosinophil counts between the groups. This suggested that raised blood eosinophil counts, which were previously reported in Indian and African infants, may have had environmental causes.[301]

The discovery of eosinophilia in neonates and in infants is not often described, although it may be quite common: 22 per cent in one series.[1038] Cord blood contains more eosinophils and more progenitor cells than adult peripheral blood, and is a good source of GM-CSF,[1989] so neonates appear to have a well developed capacity to produce high blood eosinophil counts. In one series of 21 neonates receiving surgical treatment in Milwaukee, Wisconsin, USA in 1979, 14 (67 per cent), had blood eosinophil counts greater than $0.740 \times 10^9/l$.[959]

27.1 Premature infants

A number of preterm but otherwise normal infants have been reported to develop marked eosinophilia soon after birth. The reasons for this are not known. Twenty of 38 premature infants who were described in a report from the University of Arizona, USA in 1979, developed eosinophilia greater than $1.0 \times 10^9/l$, which began 19 days after birth, and lasted for two weeks. It was suggested that eosinophilia was linked to the development of an anabolic state.[641] In 1982, a prospective study of 45 premature infants found that preterm babies had the highest blood eosinophil counts, especially when they had been subjected to invasive procedures.[166] A second prospective study in 1983 in Johannesburg, South Africa on six premature babies who developed mean blood eosinophil counts of $2.7 \times 10^9/l$ three weeks after birth, and four comparable babies who did not have eosinophilia, suggested that eosinophilia was part of a biphasic granulopoietic response in infants.[1521]

27.2 Familial and genetic diseases

Relatively few newborn children with familial or genetic diseases have been described with eosinophilia. A syndrome of 'hereditary' or 'familial eosinophilia' has been previously noted, in which several members of a family, including children, were found to have a raised blood eosinophil count.[1155] As it has not been reported for the past 20 years, it may not exist today.

In a study on eight people with Down's syndrome in Australia, the morphology of bone marrow and blood eosinophils was normal, except for an increase in the percentage of marrow eosinophils with three or more nuclear lobes. As this is the reverse of the findings in neutrophils, it is likely that the mechanisms which regulate nuclear lobation in neutrophils and eosinophils are different.[62]

Intrauterine blood transfusions, with exchange transfusions, can produce a hypersensitivity reaction, with a rash, eosinophilia, thrombocytopoenia, and lymphopoenia. This was described in 21 of 35 (60 per cent) neonates in San Francisco, California, USA in 1982.[319] It did not appear to be a graft-versus-host reaction, as it did not occur when intrauterine transfusions alone were used, and its cause remains to be determined.

27.3 Eosinophilic diseases in infants

Malignant diseases are an important cause of marked eosinophilia in infants. The malignant process may involve the eosinophil series, as in eosinophilic leukaemia, or act indirectly. Examples include:

1. eosinophilic leukaemia in a one-year-old girl who died three months after presentation with widespread tissue infiltration with eosinophils and thrombi.[424] I have details of a similar case in a neonate in London.

2. two infants with lymphoblastic leukaemia and marked eosinophilia.[1936, 629]

Occasionally marked eosinophilia of unknown causes can occur in infants. One example was of an 18-month-old child who had eosinophilia reaching 47.6×10^9/l. A lymphocyte-derived factor may have been involved, as conditioned medium from the child's blood cells induced marrow cells to make more eosinophil colonies in agar than normal.[108] In 1987 it was reported that a boy aged 5.5 months had developed marked eosinophilia, skin lesions, a hemiparesis, and hepatosplenomegaly. His blood eosinophil counts rose to 115×10^9/l. He was treated with steroids and hydroxyurea, and eosinophilia disappeared 15 months after presentation.[1958] Clearly, this illness had much in common with HES in older children and adults, but I do believe that HES should not be diagnosed unless eosinophilia persists.

Pertussoid eosinophilic pneumonia is a disease of unknown cause which produces a severe, bilateral, eosinophil-rich infiltrative inflammatory response in the lungs of infants. Twenty-three cases were reviewed in 1977.[1296] High immunoglobulin levels suggest that it might be an infectious disease, but no pathogen has yet been isolated from the lungs in this disease. It appears to have a good prognosis.

28. Skin diseases

The normal skin contains very few eosinophils, but they are found in large numbers infiltrating from venules into lesions as different as atopic eczema, bullous pemphigoid, lymphomatoid papulosis, drug reactions, and insect bites. In these diseases, many eosinophils in the skin show ultrastructural evidence for secretion of their granule contents,[2006] and the amount of deposited eosinophil granule material can be extensive. This leaves little doubt that eosinophils are an integral part of the pathogenic processes in these lesions. However, the ways in which this occurs, and the different clinical manifestations of these disorders, suggest that there is no single disease mechanism which eosinophils serve in the skin. These may include alterations in permeability leading to oedema,[1055] the stimulation of fibrous tissue deposition, and the formation of bulli, itching, and chronic inflammatory injury. See Fig. 28.1.

Research on the relationship between eosinophils, and skin diseases is just beginning. The presence of eosinophils in scleroderma, Well's syndrome, recurrent angioedema, and filarial dermatitis has begun to be described and explained. This is obviously an important area for research on the properties of eosinophils in disease, in view of the accessibility of the skin for experimental studies, and the large background of research on the pathogenesis of skin disorders. Little related work has been done on animals, although the characterization of ectoparasite-induced eosinophil responses in guinea pigs and other animals has been studied in Yale University, USA since the late 1970s.

Several diseases give rise to marked eosinophilic infiltrates into the fatty tissues of the skin, producing the histological appearance of 'eosinophilic panniculitis'. This term is not particularly helpful when considering the possible roles of eosinophils in skin diseases, as there is no suggestion that eosinophils interact with fat cells. A description of 18 patients seen at the Mayo Clinic, USA with this histological appearance was made in 1986. The diseases encompassed by this term included erythema nodosum, immune vasculitis, eosinophilic dermatitis, Well's syndrome, injection granulomas, and lymphomas affecting the skin.[1940]

28.1 Dermatitis

Eosinophil-rich inflammatory diseases of the skin associated with itching occur in several well-defined skin disorders. The numbers of eosinophils

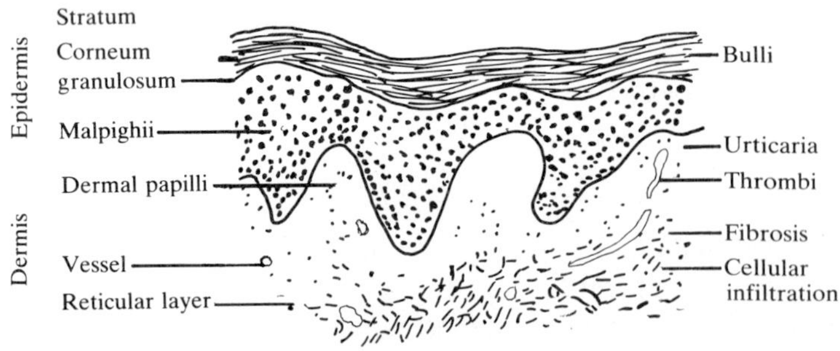

Fig. 28.1. Eosinophilic diseases involving the skin, and the effects they may produce there.

in the lesions varies considerably from patient to patient, and there is no unifying concept about how eosinophils are involved in these disorders; some unusual skin disorders of this type remain to be classified. For example, a 66-year-old man has been described with papules, pruritus, and urticarial lesions on his thigh and trunk, with eosinophilia of up to 1.6 $\times$ 10^9/l, and raised serum IgE, which responded to a short course of treatment with ketotifen. Differences with Kimura's and Well's syndrome were outlined.[1570]

28.1.1 *Atopic dermatitis*

Eosinophils are clearly involved in atopic dermatitis, as large amounts of secreted MBP were see in the skin of 18 patients studied at the Mayo Clinic. The distribution of the MBP followed a fibrillar pattern, similar to that seen in the lichenified lesions of untreated onchocerciasis. As few intact eosinophils were seen in the skin, the extent of eosinophil involvement in atopic dermatitis has probably been underestimated in the past. It was suggested that MBP deposition occurred as a consequence of an IgE-mediated late-phase reaction, and that they contributed to the tissue damage present.[1052]

As eosinophils are involved in the development of late-phase asthmatic responses, and as skin test reaction in patients with atopic dermatitis are often delayed, an experimental study was carried out to examine the possible role of eosinophils in atopic dermatitis. Fifteen patients with atopic dermatitis, 10 atopic patients with asthma and rhinitis without atopic dermatitis, and 10 non-atopic subjects were studied to see whether epicutaneous patch tests with aqueous allergen preparations and intracutaneous tests would give different inflammatory reactions in skin than normals. Eosinophils first appeared in the dermis at 2–6 hours, and in the epidermis at 24 hours. Dermal eosinophils were activated (stained with antibody EG2), whereas epidermal eosinophils were non-activated, and often lay adjacent to Langerhans' cells. Eosinophils might influence the late responses in the skin, possibly by affecting the capacity of Langerhans' cells to present antigens in the skin of atopic patients.[222]

28.1.2 *Urticaria*

Many different forms of urticaria occur which are often distinguished by their mode of induction, and by the type of cellular reaction which develops. Chronic urticaria in children, which is often associated with eosinophilia, is usually of unknown cause.[760] Intact eosinophils are only found in urticaria in which there is an acute inflammatory response, such as delayed pressure urticaria.[376] Typical of the types of eosinophil-rich urticarial skin lesions, which are difficult to define, is a report of a 68-year-old man with widespread itching papular eruptions, following an episode of facial oedema. He had raised blood eosinophil count and IgE, and skin biopsies showed a diffuse perivascular infiltrate of eosinophils. It responded to treatment with steroids.[1834]

In 14 patients with urticarial vasculitis, we noted the presence of activated eosinophils in biopsies from 7 with dense perivascular infiltrates,[1532] and secreted ECP was seen in the dermis of 12.[1742] Deposits of MBP had also been seen in the skin of patients with chronic urticaria in 1983,[1392] and in the skin lesions of 10 patients with pressure urticaria. The extent and intensity of anti-MBP staining was not related to the number of intact eosinophils in the tissues. Deposits were seen in both spontaneous and induced lesions. It was suggested that eosinophil mediators, particularly MBP, were involved in the development of oedema in the skin.[1393]

MBP, ECP, and EDN/EPX have been shown to produce a dose-related wheal-and-flare reaction after intradermal injection into human skin, and MBP has also been found in the late phase of the immediate wheal-and-flare reaction (Leiferman, Haugen, and Gleich 1987, personal communication).

Itching papular eruptions preceded by angioedema have been described in a 68-year-old man who developed a blood eosinophil count of up to 9 $\times$ 10^9/l. Several forms of treatment were ineffective, until he was given PUVA therapy. After a three-month course, his symptoms and eosinophilia disappeared, and no abnormalities were found during the next two years.[1835]

28.2 Episodic angioedema with eosinophilia

The syndrome of episodic angioedema associated with eosinophilia was described at the Mayo Clinic in 1984. (See Plate 14). Four patients were reported, who had recurrent attacks of angioedema with weight gain of up to 18 per cent, urticaria, fever, and blood eosinophil counts of up to

$95 \times 10^9/l$. They were aged 4, 7, 16, and 28 years. Three were male, and one female. Steroid treatment appeared to help the patients over each episode. MBP was found in skin biopsies, and high serum MBP levels were measured. Blood eosinophils had ultrastructural features of degranulation. Only one patient had raised serum IgE levels. It was suggested that eosinophils induced the oedema and weight gain, through an effect of their granule proteins and LTC4 on blood vessels and adjacent mast cells. Although these patients had features of HES, it was suggested that they had a distinct disorder, as follow-up for 5–37 years had shown no signs of visceral organ involvement.[672, 673]

A related disease, in which recurrent oedema was restricted to the face, was described in 1985 in two patients who had eosinophilia. One had a high level of serum MBP. In both patients, skin biopsy samples showed a nonspecific mononuclear cell infiltrate, with deposits of extracellular MBP.[1664]

Other patients with episodic angioedema with eosinophilia have been described. (See also page 180). They include:

1. a two-and-a-half-year-old girl in Boston who had monthly attacks of angioneurotic oedema, in which she gained up to 20 per cent of her total body weight, with malaise and fever, preceded two days earlier by pruritic papules. She had pulmonary infiltrates on one occasion, which resolved 10 days later. The blood eosinophil count was $17.2 \times 10^9/l$ in an attack, and $6.8 \times 10^9/l$ on recovery. A slight increase in serum IgE (154 IU) and IgM (2.1 g/l) were found. MBP was found in a skin biopsy, and a few scattered eosinophils were also seen there. Thirty-two per cent of her CD4 positive blood lymphocytes expressed HLA–DR antigens. Steroid treatment resolved the oedema in four days, and eosinophil counts were transiently reduced, but they returned to high levels, reaching $58 \times 10^9/l$ at their highest.[919]

2. the only child reported from the NIH series of patients with HES in 1975, who was a ten-year-old boy who had attacks of fever, angioneurotic oedema, malaise, and eosinophilia which responded to steroid treatment.[325]

3. a 64-year-old man reported from Creteil, France in 1987, who had eight years of cyclical fever, itching, diffuse muscle pains, and angioedema lasting 5–7 days, which recurred with regular 28 day cycles. Blood eosinophil counts rose to $30 \times 10^9/l$ during these episodes from baseline levels of $1.5–2 \times 10^9/l$. No MBP deposition was seen in biopsies of stomach, skin, or muscle. As there was no evidence for cardiac injury

or other serious complications of HES, it was suggested that the disease was the result of a cyclical stimulation of eosinophil progenitor cell proliferation.[261]

4. a 65-year-old man described in 1985 in the UK, who presented with episodic facial angioedema and associated eosinophilia up to 14×10^9/l. Marrow cultures grew an increased number of eosinophil colonies, and T-suppressor cell counts in his blood were increased.[407]

5. a 12-year-old boy described in 1986 in Australia, who had episodic facial and peripheral angioedema for seven years, and associated eosinophilia up to 48×10^9/l. No excess eosinophil colonies grew from his bone marrow, and no excess CSF production was detected.[796]

In one of the patients with episodic angioedema and eosinophilia of 13×10^9/l who was studied at the Mayo Clinic, 90 per cent of the blood eosinophils were of density less than 1.082, and they contained only 37 per cent of the MBP found in normal eosinophils: 3197 compared to 8619 ng/10^6 eosinophils. In this patient, plasma MBP levels were 7.8 times higher than in normal plasma: 2408 compared to 307 ng/ml.[1389]

These descriptions appear to be distinct from earlier reports of patients with eosinophilia with a vasculitis, angioedema, and hypocomplementaemia. A six-year-old girl with the latter disease was reported from Beirut, Lebanon in 1977.[630] Biopsies of her skin and muscle showed many eosinophils in the walls of blood vessels, which also contained deposits of immunoglobulins and C3. Her illness responded to steroid treatment.

In 25 patients with cancers treated with recombinant IL-2-activated autologus peripheral blood cells, 16 gained more than 10 per cent of their initial weight, and 20 had pulmonary oedema. Although no mention was made in the publication of this study,[1518] or in other early reports of patients treated with IL-2, a marked eosinophilia of up to 20×10^9/l can develop, and 24 of their patients had greater than 5 per cent circulating eosinophils.

Side effects of treatment of patients with IL-2, including eosinophilia, fluid accumulation, and respiratory difficulties, may be due to stimulation of eosinophil proliferation and secretion by T-cell factors which have been produced in response to the IL-2. This possibility was based on the finding that eosinophils secrete LTC4 and PAF, and can damage endothelial cells *in vitro*. Some of the anti-tumour effect of IL-2 might be mediated via eosinophils.[1001] However, steroids, which inhibit eosinophil functions, did not prevent the oedema caused by IL-2 treatment. (See also page 20).

Another syndrome, which may have a common pathogenesis with

episodic angioedema with eosinophilia, comprises oedema, hypergammaglobulinaemia M, eosinophilia, and tiredness. Several patients have been described,[1160] and although the disease persists, they seem to have an excellent prognosis.

28.3 Skin eruptions in pregnancy and in infancy

Eosinophils are one of the main cell types found in the nonspecific pleomorphic skin lesions which are sometimes seen in pregnancy. They occur with histiocytes and lymphocytes in the dermis and epidermis,[1241] but their pathogenesis is unknown.

Skin diseases in infants which can give rise to a marked eosinophil-rich exudate include erythema toxicum neonatorum, and acropustulosis, which was described in a baby in 1982.[1119]

28.4 Scleroderma syndromes

The scleroderma syndromes are divided into several subgroups. Localized forms of skin thickening can occur, which may be extended on the arms and legs. In some patients there is more generalized disease, systemic sclerosis. Eosinophilia can occur in any of these, but marked blood eosinophilia is most commonly seen in eosinophilic fasciitis. Eosinophils are usually not a prominent part of the lesions themselves, and eosinophilic fasciitis might be better called fasciitis with eosinophilia. Eosinophilic fasciitis is reviewed in pages 181–2.

28.5 Bullous skin diseases

Several different bullous diseases of the skin can be associated with the presence of eosinophils both in the blood, and in the skin lesions. The most striking example of this is bullous pemphigoid. In 1968, the term 'eosinophilic spongiosisis' was introduced for the histological appearance of many eosinophils in the skin, with patchy areas of swelling of the connective tissue. It was thought at first that these features were confined to patients with pemphigus, but it has been shown subsequently that this can also occur in bullous pemphigoid, bullous impetigo, pruriginous erythematous exanthema, and melanoerythroderma. In one 68-year-old woman with the latter diagnosis, who was reported in 1986, her blood eosinophil count was about 5×10^9/l, the serum IgE level was raised, and she had eosinophilic spongiosis, with deposits of IgG in the epithelium.[482]

28.5.1 *Bullous pemphigoid*

It has been known for nearly 100 years that this disease can occur with large numbers of eosinophils in the inflammatory lesions and blood.[238] The lesions are probably due to binding of antibodies to the basement membrane, where complement is activated. This induces eosinophils to release toxic molecules directly onto the basement membrane zone, to produce a loss of dermo-epidermal adherence, which causes blister formation.[1548] In 1982 it was shown that eosinophils in the lesions had ultrastructural features to suggest that they could be degranulating, and damaging the basement membrane.[487] Eosinophil granule proteins have been found in the bullous fluid of some of these patients, and eosinophil peroxidase has been found along the basement membrane.[468] Eosinophil activating factors, which might be involved in triggering eosinophil degranulation, have also been extracted from blister fluid.[1840]

Treatment is difficult. In 1987 a 48-year-old man with bullous pemphigoid lesions containing many eosinophils responded to treatment with tetracycline. Drugs which can inhibit the binding of tRNA to mRNA, and so block protein synthesis, could be effective in this disease by inhibiting the toxic properties of granulocytes, including eosinophils.[1781]

28.5.2 *Dermatitis herpetiformis and linear IgA disease*

Eosinophils were prominent in the skin of 6 of 26 patients (23 per cent) with dermatitis herpetiformis reported from London in 1983.[181] In linear IgA disease there is a continuous and homogeneous band of IgA along the basement membrane of the skin, and the formation of subepidermal bullae. It is closely linked to dermatitis herpetiformis, although it does not occur in patients with intestinal diseases. Eosinophils can be prominent in or below the bullae. They were seen in this site in 7 of 30 patients studied in London who were reported in 1983.[181]

28.6 Incontinentia pigmenti

This rare inherited disease is named after the characteristic areas of increased skin pigmentation, which occurs in whorls, stripes, and other angular shapes. These are present at birth, or first appear in the newborn period, and in 60 per cent of children they are associated with neurectodermal defects. The lesions begin with an inflammatory (vesiculobullous) phase, which may be extensive. The patients are usually afebrile, and they may have a marked increase in eosinophils in the lesions and blood. The inflammatory phase may evolve through a verrucous phase, to the pigmented stage, which fades with age. In Sendai, Japan, an eosinophil chemotactic factor was defined, with LTB4, in the eosinophil-rich lesions.[1745]

28.7 Eosinophilic pustular folliculitis

Eosinophilic pustular folliculitis (Ofuji's disease) was first described in 1970 in three young Japanese patients who had marked eosinophil infiltrates into areas of pruritic follicular papulopustular eruptions, and high blood eosinophil counts.[1297] Since then other patients have been reported from Japan,[1744] North America in 1985,[1118] the USA in 1986,[865, 453, 346] including three patients with AIDS,[1657] Italy in 1985,[1289] and France in 1986.[1859]

This is a rare disease, in which there are recurrent sterile papulopustules and plaques which increase in size. They are commonest in hair-bearing areas, although the palms and soles can also be involved. Microscopy shows subcorneal and intrafollicular abscesses containing many eosinophils or neutrophils, with spongiosis of the outer root sheath, and a dense infiltrate of eosinophils around dermal vessels. Occasionally, tinea infections can mimic this disease.[1016] It also occurs in dogs,[1582] and in both it is a chronic disease, with a variable response to steroids. Dapsone was effective in one patient.[1705]

28.8 Psoriasis

Eosinophils can be a prominent component of the skin lesion in some patients with psoriasis,[1706] and there may be an increase in blood eosinophil counts, especially in patients with psoriatic arthropathy.

28.9 Erythema nodosum

Occasionally, erythema nodosum can be associated with an eosinophilic panniculitis and marked eosinophilia.[1940]

28.10 Lymphomatoid papulosis

A small number of patients with lymphomatoid papulosis have large numbers of eosinophils in their skin lesions,[1240] in addition to atypical lymphocytes. Occasionally the lesions may contain more histiocytes than lymphocytes, and it has been suggested that these may be a separate form of the disease.[1181] In 1988 we reported three patients who had lymphomatoid papulosis and the hypereosinophilic syndrome.[1926] (See Plate 13.) As the dermal lymphocytes had some of the phenotypic features of helper cells, we suggested that the eosinophilia could have been due to the secretion of an eosinopoietic cytokine, such as IL-5, from these atypical T-cells.

28.11 Erythema annulare

Increased numbers of eosinophils have been found in the skin lesions of patients with granuloma annulare. They were present in 18 of 45 biopsies (40 per cent) in a study reported in 1985.[1631] They are also found in other cutaneous granulomas, such as necrobiosis lipoidica, and reactions to insect bites.

29. Immunological diseases

Diseases of the immune system are often associated with eosinophilia, especially the hypersensitivity group of disorders, and immunodeficiency diseases. This is not surprising in view of the importance of T-cell regulation of eosinophil production, and the capacity of lymphokines to affect the properties of eosinophils.

29.1 Autoimmune diseases

Although eosinophil infiltration into affected tissues has been observed in experimental animals injected with autologous endocrine tissues, a blood eosinophilia with eosinophils in the affected organ seldom occurs in autoimmune diseases. However, Addison's disease can rarely present with eosinophilia. I reported my studies on one patient in 1976.[1679] Some clinical and experimental evidence suggests that eosinophils could be involved in the development of certain types of diabetes mellitus. In 1978, an eosinophil infiltrate was found in the pancreas of a premature baby born to a diabetic mother.[116] An eosinophil infiltration into the islets of Langerhans has been noted in guinea pigs, in which diabetes was induced by immunization with pancreatic tissues. In 1987 it was found that BB rats, which develop diabetes spontaneously, developed eosinophilia at the onset of diabetes.[1020]

29.2 Drug hypersensitivity reactions

The normal immune response to allergens often includes eosinophils, and it is likely that they play an important role in protecting lymphoid tissues against potentially toxic or harmful products which enter the body through afferent lymphatics. This mechanism may occasionally lead to a detrimental host response such as occurs during drug hypersensitivity reaction.

Eosinophils can be found both in immediate hypersensitivity, and in chronic or delayed hypersensitivity responses. In each case, the blood eosinophil count is usually raised as well as there being large numbers of eosinophils in the lesions themselves. In hypersensitivity diseases, blood eosinophil counts are seldom as high as can be seen in patients with HES, although this can occur in drug hypersensitivity reactions. Drug reactions are an important cause of eosinophilia. This review is based on my earlier article[1681] with permission. The finding of a raised blood eosinophil count in patients taking drugs can be useful as an early warning of potentially dangerous hypersensitivity reactions, which could lead to permanent tissue injury, or even death. The eosinophilia forms part of an immediate hypersensitivity reaction, or delayed cell-mediated response to the drug or its breakdown products. Most of the diagnostic tests which are used to decide whether a drug is responsible for an adverse reaction are based on these two possible mechanisms.

It is not known why these reactions occur in some patients, except that they can be dose-related, and it is not clear why eosinophils are involved in some hypersensitivity reactions and not others. No work has been done on how eosinophils could be involved in drug reactions, either as effector cells of the immune response, or as protective cells against the damaging effects of drugs and their metabolites. Most reactions end when the drug treatment is stopped, but steroid treatment can be valuable, accelerating recovery from cell-mediated reactions. Very rarely, drug-induced eosinophilia may progress to a chronic persistent eosinophilia.

In the majority of patients it is not difficult to recognize this complication of drug treatment. Problems mainly arise when the drug history is incomplete, or when several drugs are being used to treat a disease which may itself give rise to eosinophilia. Then special investigations are worthwhile to determine the aetiology of the eosinophilia, especially when drug treatment ought to be continued. No common chemical or pharmacological feature in these agents accounts for the development of the eosinophilia. In treated patients the incidence of eosinophilia is probably less than 0.1 per cent except for a few treatments, such as sodium aurothiomalate therapy, which can produce eosinophilia in 20–50 per cent of treated patients.[491] The prevalence of drug-induced eosinophilia is, however, relatively common in hospitals, largely because drugs are so widely prescribed there. See Fig. 29.1.

29.2.1 *Clinical features of drug hypersensitivity diseases*

Allergic and hypersensitivity reactions to drugs can occur without any alterations in blood eosinophil counts, and acute anaphylactic reactions are usually not accompanied by eosinophilia. Drug-induced eosinophilia may not be related to the occurrence of toxic side-effects in patients taking D-penicillamine.[1648] Drug-induced hypersensitivity reactions with eosinophilia usually only develop after several weeks or months of treatment, but it may recur rapidly when the drug is taken again. This suggests that an immune response has developed. Sometimes it can be difficult to

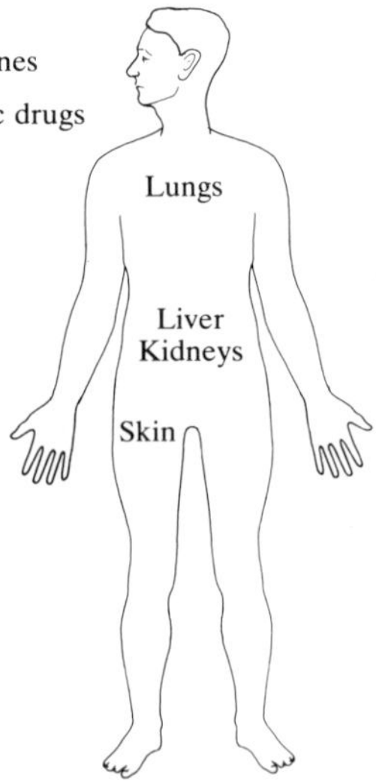

Lungs	Liver	Kidneys	Skin
Sulphonamides	Phenothiazines	Antibiotics	Antobiotics
Nitrofurantion	Antidiabetic drugs	Sulphonamides	Antifungal agents
Methotrexate	Allopurinol	Cimetidine	Anti-neoplastic drugs
Anti-neoplastic drugs	Aspirin	Non-steroidal anti-inflammatory agents	Anticoagulants
Non-steroidal anti-inflammatory agents		Allopurinol	Allopurinol
Anti-tuberculosis drugs		Phenytoin	
Anti-diabetic drugs		Phenylbutazone	

Fig. 29.1. The major target organs affected by eosinophils and other inflammatory reactions in patients suffering from drug-induced hypersensitivity reactions.

recognize that eosinophilia is drug-related, especially when it is overshadowed by other complications. Failure to do so may be responsible for the development of progressive lesions which may be fatal. Useful clinical features which suggest that eosinophilia is due to drug treatment are fever, skin rashes, lymphadenopathy, splenomegaly, pulmonary infiltrates, and (more rarely) hepatic, renal or cardio-toxicity. However, in a review of drug fever which was published in 1987, fever was infrequently associated with eosinophilia.[1126]

Eosinophilia that accompanies drug reactions ranges from just above normal to very high levels, but the majority of affected patients have counts between 1 and 10 × 10^9/l. Eosinophilia may take several weeks to return to normal after the drug has been stopped.

Fever with eosinophilia may be the only clinical manifestation of a drug reaction, and this is well described for hypersensitivity to the penicillin, barbiturate, and hydantoin groups of compounds. In 1987, details were given of a 15-year-old boy who developed a hypersensitivity reaction to phenytoin, with a blood eosinophil count of 2.1 × 10^9/l. A review of 17 similar patients aged 2 to 21 years with hypersensitivity reactions to phenytoin showed that eosinophilia occurred in 76 per cent.[1435]

Reactions affecting the skin Skin reactions with eosinophilia are common in patients taking antibiotics, antifungal agents, and allopurinol.[234, 1027]

Fatal angioedema due to bleomycin was reported in 1984.[958] The varied skin lesions which have been described under the general term of eosinophilic panniculitis are often due to a drug reaction, although this can be difficult to prove.[1940] Carbamazepine-induced erythema multiforme with eosinophilia has been described in a patient in 1984.[1187]

Reactions affecting the lung and heart Pulmonary hypersensitivity reactions can develop with eosinophilia in patients taking nitrofurantoin,[1131] suphonamides,[1807, 293, 1825] penicillin, mephenesin and azathioprine,[1601] methotrexate,[1924] bleomycin,[1988] chlorpropamide,[153] tolbutamide, and carbamazepine,[1708] and naproxen.[578] Occasionally the reaction can progress to fibrosis.[1519]

Several drugs which are used to treat pulmonary tuberculosis can cause damage to the lungs with eosinophilia. These include paraaminosalicylic acid,[1635] isoniazid, rifampicin, and capreomycin sulphate (16 of 38 patients in one series).[1335]

Eosinophilic myocarditis is an important complication of some types of drug-induced hypersensitivity reactions. Twenty-four patients with this reaction were reviewed in New York in 1982.[555] Twenty had died suddenly, and it was recommended that a careful search for this dangerous reaction should be made in patients with drug-induced eosinophilia. Pericardial lesions can also develop. Sodium cromoglycate produced an allergic response in a 46-year-old woman who presented with pericardial symptoms and signs, and a blood eosinophil count of 12.5×10^9/l, which resolved when this drug was stopped.[1642]

Reactions affecting the kidneys Both glomerular and tubular injury can occur during eosinophilic hypersensitivity reactions to drugs.[49] Glomerular lesions may develop during treatment with penicillins, amphotericin B, sulphonamides, and phenylbutazone.[1061]

Interstitial nephritis, in which there is an eosinophil infiltrate into areas of renal damage, can complicate treatment with a wide variety of drugs. It was reviewed in 1980.[1083] Offending drugs include penicillins, including methicillin, and ampicillin (4 of 7 patients in one series),[105] cimetidine, non-steroidal anti-inflammatory drugs, and allopurinol.[1183, 748]

The interstitial lesions may be due to the production of antitubular basement membrane antibodies.[190] Although peripheral blood eosinophilia is not always found in drug-induced interstitial nephritis, when it occurs, it can be marked, and persist for weeks after stopping treatment. Phenytoin can cause marked eosinophil infiltration into the kidneys,[1611, 1171] as can cephalosporin[1856] and sulphasalazine.[314]

Rarely, drugs can cause an eosinophilic reaction in the bladder, as described in a patient taking an anti-allergy drug in Japan.[1261]

Reactions affecting the liver Many drugs are able to produce a granulomatous hepatitis, in which eosinophils are a prominent feature. In a series from Charleston, USA published in 1981, they accounted for 29 per cent of granulomas in liver biopsies.[1182] Drug reactions only rarely produce extensive hepatic injury with eosinophil infiltration and peripheral blood eosinophilia. Phenothiazines are probably the commonest type of drug causing liver injury and eosinophilia, with jaundice of an obstructive type. A patient with carbamazepine-induced acute cholangitis and hypereosinophilia was described in 1987.[1031] Other drugs which have been reported to induce liver injury include tolbutamide, chlorpropamide,[1999] and allopurinol.[1636] Eosinophilic hepatitis has also been seen in patients with juvenile rheumatoid arthritis treated with aspirin: six in one series,[1489] and acute rheumatic fever treated with high doses of aspirin: 10 of 11 in a series from South Africa.[645]

29.2.2 *Drugs which induce hypersensitivity reactions*

Many different types of drug can induce eosinophilia.[1957] Especially important causes of eosinophilia are antibiotics and fungicides; drugs acting on the central nervous system such as phenytoin;[763] anticoagulants such as phenindione and chlorophenindione, anti-inflammatory and anti-neoplastic drugs, including dacarbazine,[1372] and oral hypoglycaemic agents. These adverse reactions usually become apparent one to three months after treatment has started;[1090] Even small inorganic substances such as potassium iodide have been shown to produce eosinophilic hypersensitivity reactions as high as 63×10^9/l.[857] Radiographic contrast media, which may release small quantities of free iodine, can also produce eosinophilia and mild urticaria (21 of 101 patients undergoing intravenous urography in a series in Boston, USA[1865]), but this is rarely of clinical importance.[1425]

29.2.3 *Susceptibility to drug hypersensitivity reactions*

Although as many as 10 per cent of patients in hospital have adverse reaction to drugs, and approximately 11 per cent of these are hypersensitivity reactions,[830] and although skin rashes may develop in 5–7 per cent of patients receiving ampicillin and amoxicillin,[1431] the prevalence of hypersensitivity reactions with eosinophilia is probably less than 1 per cent. For example, although penicillin and cephalosporin and their related derivatives are highly immunogenic in man and are well known for their capacity to produce eosinophilia,[109, 430] allergic reactions develop in only about 1 per cent of treated patients.[817]

Renal failure is an important predisposing factor in the development of drug-hypersensitivity reactions. The reasons for this are not known, but may involve slow elimination of immunogenic metabolites. The incidence and severity of reactions to allopurinol is also increased in acute and chronic renal failure.[300] However, in many patients with renal failure who develop eosinophilia, it may be difficult to incriminate the drug responsible for the reaction. We have seen eight patients with renal failure who developed eosinophilia of unknown cause, and who were receiving several different drugs. In each case resolution of the eosinophilia occurred as renal function improved, suggesting that the response was in some way associated with the excretion of a sensitizing agent. In one of these patients tartrazine was suspected to be the cause of the eosinophilia, and the eosinophilia closely followed renal function.[205] Tartrazine may be a common cause of eosinophilia in patients with renal failure. It is a yellow dye which can also give a red or green colour, and it is widely used in foodstuffs and medications. The incidence of hypersensitivity reactions to drugs is also increased in patients with liver failure,[1999] probably for the same reasons. However, eosinophilia does not seem to develop as frequently as in renal failure.

The main genetic factor known to predispose a patient to drug-induced eosinophilia is slow acetylator status, which is important in patients taking drugs which are altered by this pathway, such as the sulphonamides. For this reason, some reactions are dose-related, and slow elimination through the liver or kidneys then becomes more important. Patients with atopy, or a family history of allergic diseases do not appear to have a higher risk of developing drug hypersensitivity reactions, although there is the possibility that they may be more severe when they do occur. A previous history of drug reactions or allergic diseases is often held to increase the likelihood of hypersensitivity reactions developing to other drugs,[829] but this has not been substantiated in the case of penicillin sensitivity.[817] Patients with asthma also rarely develop hypersensitivity reactions to drugs. But when it occurs in them it may be particularly severe. It should be noted that there is a rare syndrome of asthma, nasal polyps and eosinophilia which is regularly aggravated by aspirin ingestion.[644] (See page 214.)

29.2.4 *Mechanisms of drug hypersensitivity reactions*

Drugs produce hypersensitivity reactions by binding to proteins, forming larger immunogenic hapten–protein conjugates. This usually leads to the production of antibodies which can form immune complexes with the drug. Large amounts of circulating complexes can injure blood vessels, producing the clinical features of serum sickness (type III reactions). IgE antibodies may be produced. These are present on the surface of mast cells, and combine with the drug to give acute type I reactions including urticaria, angioedema, and anaphylactic reactions. However, the most important mechanism in drug-induced eosinophilic hypersensitivity reactions is T-lymphocyte dependent: the cell-mediated (type IV) reaction. Histologically, the main features of drug-induced lesions are a monunuclear cell, and eosinophil-rich inflammatory reaction in all three layers of the walls of small arteries, arterioles, and venules, without the presence of a necrotizing vasculitis or fibrinoid necrosis.[1251]

IgG-mediated reactions Many drugs give rise to small amounts of IgG antibodies but generally these have no clinical significance. Eosinophilic hypersensitivity reactions to nitrofurantoin often occur in patients with higher IgG antibodies to the drug than in control patients, but as some patients with the highest IgG antibody levels do not have reactions, it is likely that other factors are also involved. In the majority of patients who develop allergic reactions to the penicillin group of drugs there is no correlation with IgG or IgM antibody levels.[2004] However, in a few patients, immune complexes can develop, causing serum sickness accompanied by eosinophilia and complement activation. This has been described in a patient given cephalothin.[199]

IgE-mediated and mast-cell-mediated reactions IgE-mediated (anaphylactic) responses to drugs have often been incriminated in the development of drug-induced eosinophilia. Penicillin allergy is the best known. Here bivalent penicilloyl-haptens cross-link IgE antibodies on the surface of mast cells, and induce the secretion of mast cell mediators. In other drug reactions the involvement of IgE has been conjectural, and largely based on increased total IgE levels in serum, such as in patients with allergic reactions and eosinophilia after treatment of rheumatoid arthritis with gold salts.[408] Among 50 patients who received sodium aurothiomalate, 20 developed eosinophilia. Of these, 35 per cent had raised IgE levels, whereas only 11 per cent among the other patients showed increased levels. Unfortunately, specific IgE antibodies to gold salts or their metabolic products have yet to be defined, and the possible importance of eosinophilia as a useful indicator of an adverse reaction to gold salts was not confirmed in two other studies.[876, 935]

As mast cells degranulate during acute allergic reactions to drugs, a number of diagnostic tests for drug hypersensitivity have been developed using basophil degranulation *in vitro*. These are technically difficult, as basophils can degranulate nonspecifically; so they are now seldom done, except in specialized laboratories. Another test which has now been largely abandoned is serial measurements of blood cell accumulation in skin abrasions, to which glass coverslips or chambers containing the drug have been applied ('skin windows'). It is not clear what type of response this measures, and it is difficult to interpret.

Cell mediated (type IV) reactions Most drugs probably produce eosinophilia by stimulating T-lymphocyte responses *in vivo*. This is studied by incubating patient's blood lymphocytes with the suspect drug, and measuring the degree of lymphocyte proliferation by the uptake of ^{3}H-thymidine. This mitogenic response has been widely used in attempts to find the drug responsible for hypersensitivity reactions, and there are a number of reports where a positive response has been detected using lymphocytes from patients with drug-induced eosinophilia.[1484] Positive results with this type of test have also been reported in patients with hypersensitivity reactions and eosinophilia, which developed during treatment with antituberculous drugs and nitrofurantoin.[89] Five of seven patients with eosinophilia due to carbamazepine had lymphocytes which showed a positive mitogenic response. In the other two patients, a positive response was seen only in samples taken several months later, possibly due to a depression of lymphocyte responsiveness by the illness itself. These patients also produced positive patch tests for the drug, suggesting that delayed (type IV) hypersensitivity had developed.[818] The value of the mitogenic response in diagnosis has, however, been questioned. For example, in a group of patients with asthma who developed hypersensitivity reactions to sodium cromoglycate (cromolyn sodium), there was no difference in lymphocyte responsiveness to the drug compared with other unaffected asthmatic patients. However, by measuring lymphocyte-derived migration inhibitory factor, which is secreted during delayed hypersensitivity reactions, it was possible to discriminate between the two groups.[1605] Other drugs, in which mitogenic responses have been correlated with hypersensitivity reactions and eosinophilia, include phenytoin[1611] and allopurinol.[1146] Evidence that lymphocytes are involved directly in these responses also comes from studies on circulating lymphocytes, which may show a number of morphological abnormalities, for example in patients with phenytoin hypersensitivity.[1702]

These findings fit in well with experimental work in animals on the role of T-lymphocytes in the induction of eosinopoiesis. Basten and Beeson[136] showed that eosinophilia did not occur in rats injected with *T. spiralis* larvae unless they possessed normal T-lymphocyte populations. A similar conclusion was reached in regard to basophilopoiesis in studies in rats infected with *T. spiralis*. Congenitally T–lymphocyte-deficient rats did not show either basophilia, or eosinophilia when infected.[1300] However, it is not known whether the same lymphocyte subpopulation induces both eosinophilia, and delayed (type IV) reactions, or whether one response influences the development of the other.

In further experimental studies, the importance of inflammatory lesions in the induction of eosinophilia was clearly demonstrated.[1872] In the absence of an inflammatory reaction, stimuli which would normally produce eosinophilia appeared to be ineffective. How far this was due to a nonspecific effect of the inflammatory reaction on the immune response, or a direct effect of these reactions on eosinopoiesis was not clear. However, it may be useful to consider whether a drug-induced hypersensitivity reaction has an underlying inflammatory reaction if there is an associated eosinophilia.

29.2.5 *The roles of eosinophils in drug reactions*

Although tissue eosinophils are a prominent component of tissue lesions in patients with hypersensitivity reactions, it is not known what part they play there, and they are not involved in acute anaphylactic reactions.[669] They may be involved in the production of chronic tissue injury in drug hypersensitivity reactions, but as they are rarely associated with endomyocardial fibrosis, their effects are probably localized.

Blood eosinophils in these patients may contain many vacuoles,[347] and degranulated eosinophils have been seen in the blood[1443] and in drug-induced tissue lesions. Tissue eosinophils containing vacuoles have been seen in 'skin window' preparations in a group of 45 allergic patients. The maximum number of vacuolated eosinophils (42 per cent) was seen four hours after the drug was applied to the skin.[451] However, it is not clear whether eosinophils contribute in any way to the clinical or pathological consequences of these reactions.

29.3 Graft-versus-host disease

Mild eosinophilia is common in chronic graft-versus-host (GvH) disease, but occasionally the blood eosinophil count can be strikingly high. Blood eosinophil counts did not correlate with increases in IgE levels in 14 patients with GvH disease.[1494] In one patient reported in 1986, eosinophilia due to GvH disease after a bone marrow transplant was also accompanied by polymyositis.[1812]

29.4 Immunological deficiency syndromes

Immunological deficiency syndromes in childhood and later life, and several acquired immunodeficiency syndromes can all be associated with a marked increase in eosinophil counts. At first sight this seems surprising in view of the role of T-cells in eosinophil production. However, in these disorders it is likely that there is an imbalance in the regulation of the production of lymphokines, which leads to an over production of lymphokines with eosinopoietic activity from other cells, such as endothelial cells.

Children with severe defects in cell-mediated and humoral immunity, such as the severe combined immune deficiency syndrome, may have marked eosinophilia.[896] See also Omenn's syndrome, page 166.

A number of children with hypogammaglobulinaemia and *Pneumocystis carinii* pneumonia have been found to have eosinophilia. In a five-month-old child with this syndrome and a blood eosinophil count of $14.2 \times 10^9/l$, who was reported in 1987, the eosinophilia disappeared after he was treated with intravenous gammaglobulin.[1380]

29.5 Absence of eosinophils

Occasionally, blood films may have less than three eosinophils per 200 white blood cells, although eosinophils are present in the bone marrow. As I have found that germ-free rats and mice have very few blood eosinophils, this may be a reflection of the absence of stimuli, which might otherwise increase the eosinophil count, rather than an abnormality in these individuals. In hospital practice, low eosinophil counts are also sometimes seen, but it is very rare for this to occur in serial blood samples. This was studied in 1987 in 24 300 patients admitted to hospital in Pittsburgh, Pennsylvania, USA. Only 24 had blood eosinophil counts of less than $0.010 \times 10^9/l$, and in each case this was linked to current steroid treatment, or the presence of a serious underlying disease.[1003]

A small number of patients with a variety of immunodeficiency syndromes, which are often associated with a thymoma or asthma, have no eosinophils in their marrow, blood, or peripheral tissues, as judged by staining with eosin and other similar stains. During the 1950s and 1960s, there were several single case reports of this association.[696, 1474, 587, 1870] The syndrome was reviewed in 1968 by Good and colleagues, who had made several of the earlier descriptions of these patients.[877] In 1977 five patients with this syndrome were discussed in a short review,[2011] and an additional patient was mentioned in a review in 1977.[147] Other reports of patients with no eosinophils are:

1. a 52-year-old man in Uppsala in 1977, who had a wide range of recurrent and persistent infections, including chest infections, tuberculosis, multiple warts, recurrent gastroenteritis, a persistent salmonella infection, and scabies. He also had a haemolytic anaemia, selective IgA deficiency, asthma, and an absence of eosinophils and basophils in his marrow and blood. A small number of mast cells were found in tissues. The plasma was found to induce white cells from normal individuals to degranulate, suggesting that newly formed cells were unable to reach maturity in this patient.[899]

2. a woman in the USA in 1981, with episodic urticaria and rhinitis who had no circulating eosinophils or serum MBP.[596] She had 0.4 per cent basophils, and normal immunoglobulins. In 1984 it was reported that she had an eosinophil-specific serum inhibitor of CFU-Eo growth.[1262]

3. a 59-year-old woman in Brussels, Belgium in 1982, who had no eosinophils in her blood or marrow for at least eight years after she had recovered from an episode of drug-induced agranulocytosis.[1765] The lack of eosinophils was thought to be due to a defect in the marrow environment for eosinopoiesis, as she had normal numbers of CFU-Eo, and could make Eo-CSA, and she did not have an antibody preventing the growth of immature eosinophils.

4. a man aged 55 years reported in London in 1983, who had a spindle cell thymoma, with hypogammaglobulinaemia. Two years after he had a thymectomy, blood and marrow eosinophils disappeared, and eosinophils were noted to be absent in skin allergen patch test sites. As there was a marked increase in his blood T-lymphocyte suppressor activity, it was possible that suppressor cells were inhibiting T-lymphocytes which would normally stimulate eosinophil production.[1221] This report also suggested an alternative mechanism for his lack of eosinophils. The defective T-cells might be the ones which would normally supply the 'helper' functions for eosinopoieis.[1220]

5. a 52-year-old woman described in 1984 with asthma, diabetes, and seasonal rhinitis, with a history of drug allergy, who had a mild leucocytosis but no blood eosinophils. Her serum IgG inhibited CFU-Eo growth specifically, and it was suggested that the eosinopenia was due to an autoimmune process.[1262]

6. a second patient with reported from Uppsala in 1988, who had no blood or marrow eosinophils or basophils, although there was a low level of serum ECP.[900] The cause of the eosinopenia in this patient was not determined.

29.6 Hypergammaglobulinaemia E and infection syndrome

The syndrome of recurrent pyogenic infections and high serum IgE levels is occasionally associated with marked eosinophilia. Two boys with recurrent infections, very high serum IgE levels, poor secondary antibody responses, and reduced delayed hypersensitivity reactions with marked eosinophilia were described in 1972.[227] In 1975 serum IgE levels of over

20,000 IU/ml, and increased numbers of IgE-staining B-cells were noted in a patient who had blood eosinophil counts of 4 to 18 × 10^9/l.[1379]

In 1976 eleven other patients with this syndrome were reported from Minneapolis, USA. They all had recurrent staphylococcal abscesses involving the skin and the respiratory tract, chronic eczematous dermatitis, and high levels of serum IgE. In ten patients the peripheral blood eosinophil count was 10 per cent or more of the total white blood cell count.[379] A patient was reported from Denmark in 1980,[144] and 16 patients who were seen at NIH, Bethesda, USA were reviewed in 1983.[457] Six had blood eosinophil counts above 1 × 10^9/l, and eosinophils were also present in abscess fluid and sputum.

Appendix A

Research groups working on eosinophils and eosinophilic diseases, 1988

Many scientific and clinical centres have an interest in the study of eosinophils and eosinophilic diseases. The following list includes the major centres which have published several English language papers on eosinophils, from 1985–1988.

Australia

Division of Human Immunology, Institute of Medical and Veterinary Science, Box 14 Rundle Mall Post Office, Adelaide, South Australia 5000. Dr Mathew Vadas. Genetic factors and eosinophil production. Colony stimulating factors, and eosinopoiesis. Eosinophil activation.

The Walter and Eliza Hall Institute of Medical Research, Post Office, Royal Melbourne Hospital, Melbourne, Victoria 3050, Australia. Dr Donald Metcalf. Eosinophil CSFs.

Chile

Laboratory of Experimental Endocrinology, University of Chile Medical School, Casilla 21104, Correro 21, Santiago, Chile. Dr Andrei Tchernitchin. The relationship between oestrogens and eosinophils in the rodent uterus.

France

Centre d'Immunologie et Biologie Parasitaire, Institut Pasteur, 1 Rue du Professeur Calmette, 59019 Lille, Cedex, France. Dr Monique Capron. Eosinophil-dependent killing of parasites. IgE receptors on human eosinophils. The properties of light-density and activated eosinophils.

Italy

Clinica Malattia Infettive, Universita La Sapienza, Rome, Italy. Dr C. DeSimone. Eosinophil activation and cytotoxicity.

Japan

Clinical Research Centre for Rheumato-Allergology, National Sagamihara Hospital, Kanagawa, Japan. Dr H. Saito. Eosinophil malignancies. Eosinophil cell lines.

Department of Pathology, Kumamoto University Medical School, Japan. Dr M. Hirashima. Eosinophil chemotactic factors.

Department of Medicine and Clinical Immunology, Dokkyo University School of Medicine, Mibu, Tochigi-Ken 231–02, Japan. Dr Sohei Makino. Eosinophils in asthma. Eosinophil heterogeneity.

Sweden

Research Dept. 2. E. Blocket Floor EB–14, University of Lund, Lund Hospital, S–221 85 Lund, Sweden. Dr Inge Olsson. Purification and characterization of ECP. Biosynthesis of eosinophil granule proteins.

University Hospital, Department of Clinical Chemistry, S–751 85 Uppsala, Sweden. Dr Per Venge. Separation and properties of ECP. Characterization of EDN/EPX. Eosinophils and coagulation. Eosinophils and lymphocyte proliferation. The involvement of eosinophils in asthma and other diseases.

UK

Immunology Division, Cambridge University Department of Pathology, Tennis Court Road, Cambridge CB2 1QP, UK. Dr Anthony Butterworth. Eosinophil-parasite interactions, especially eosinophil killing of schistosomula. Eosinophil activating factors.

Beecham's Group Research, Biosciences Research Centre, Great Burgh Yew Tree Bottom Road, Epsom, Surrey KT18 5XQ, UK. Dr Harry Smith. Effects of drugs on rodent eosinophils.

Department of Allergy and Clinical Immunology, The Cardiothoracic Institute, Brompton Hospital, Fulham Road, London SW3 6HP, UK Dr Barry Kay. Eosinophil chemotactic factors. The properties of eosinophils in the blood and BAL of patients with asthma. Eosinophil leukotriene production.

National Institute for Medical Research, Mill Hill, London NW7 1AA, UK. Dr Colin Sanderson. Liquid culture of murine and human eosinophils. T-cell clones making eosinopoietic factors. Murine and human eosinophil differentiation factor (IL–5).

Department of Immunology, St George's Hospital Medical School, Cranmer Terrace, London SW17 ORE, UK. Dr Christopher Spry. The clinical features of HES and other diseases with eosinophilia. Preparation of monoclonal antibodies to eosinophil granule and secreted components, and eosinophil membrane antigens. Mechanisms of eosinophil secretion. The pathogenesis of eosinophilic endomyocardial fibrosis, and tropical endomyocardial fibrosis.

Agricultural Research Council, Poultry Research Centre, Roslin, Midlothian EH25 9PS, UK. Dr M. H. Maxwell. Avian eosinophils.

USA

Building 31, National Institutes of Allergy and Infectious Diseases, National Institutes of Health, Bethesda, Maryland, 20205, USA. Dr Anthony Fauci. The idiopathic hypereosinophilic syndrome. The properties of eosinophils in patients with hypereosinophilia.

Laboratory of Parasitic Diseases, National Institutes of Allergy and Infectious Diseases, National Institutes of Health, Bethesda, Maryland 20205, USA. Dr Eric Ottesen. Eosinophil interactions with filaria and other parasites.

Harvard–Thorndyke Laboratory, Department of Medicine, Beth Israel Hospital, 330 Brookline Avenue, Boston, Massachusetts 02215, USA. Dr Peter Weller and Dr Stephen Ackerman. Characterization of the components in human eosinophil granules and cell membrane. The biochemistry of the Charcot–Leyden crystal protein, lysophospholipase. Eosinophil–complement interactions. Lipid metabolism in eosinophils.

The Seeley G. Mudd Building, Room 604, 250 Longwood Avenue, Boston, Massachusetts 02115, USA. Dr K. Frank Austen and Dr John David. Eosinophil chemotactic factors. Eosinophil–mast-cell interactions. The constituents in eosinophils. The production of leukotriene C4 and other lipid mediators. Extended culture of human eosinophils. Eosinophil activating factors. Properties of activated eosinophils.

Division of Allergy, New England Medical Centre Hospital, Tufts University School of Medicine, Boston, Massachusetts 02142, USA. Dr Stephanie Pincus. Guinea pig and human eosinophils biochemistry, and responses to parasitic infections.

Department of Microbiology, Vanderbilt University School of Medicine, Nashville, Tennessee, USA. Dr Daniel Colley. Murine eosinophils. Eosinophil-parasite interactions. Eosinophil activation. T-cell involvement in eosinophil functions *in vivo*.

Research Laboratory for Allergic Diseases, Mayo Clinic and Foundation, Rochester, Minnesota 55905, USA, Dr Gerald Gleich. The isolation and biochemistry of eosinophil granule components, especially MBP. Study of the roles of eosinophils in diseases. Clinical disorders in which eosinophils may have a pathogenetic role, especially asthma and allergic diseases. MBP in pregnancy.

School of Medicine, University of California Medical Centre, San Francisco, California 94143, USA. Dr Edward Goetzl. Eosinophil-derived lipid mediators of inflammatory reactions. Eosinophil chemotactic factors.

University of Washington, Seattle, Washington 98195, USA. Dr Seymour Klebanoff. Eosinophil peroxidase. The interaction of EPO with mast cells and parasites. Eosinophil ultrastructure and secretion.

Appendix B

The scientific literature of eosinophils

Over 400 papers on eosinophils and eosinophilic diseases are published each year. Only one third of the literature on eosinophils is in journals which are readily available in most medical schools; one third is in less commonly taken journals; and a third is in literature which is difficult to retrieve.

The principal journals in which papers on eosinophils have appeared during the period 1977–87, and which are indexed in Medline in decreasing order of frequency of publication are: the *Journal of Immunology*, *Blood*, the *Journal of Allergy and Clinical Immunology*, the *New England Journal of Medicine*, the *American Journal of Tropical Medicine and Hygiene*, *Annals of Internal Medicine*, *Lancet*, *Annals of Allergy*, *Clinical and Experimental Immunology*, *Immunology*, *International Archives of Allergy and Applied Immunology*, the *American Journal of Medicine*, *Archives of Dermatology*, and the *Journal of Experimental Medicine*.

The National Library of Medicine's Medline MEZZ database has indexed 8759 articles, 6283 in English, on eosinophils and eosinophilic diseases under the Medical Subject Headings 'eosinophils' and 'eosinophilia', since it began in 1966. Of these, 3825 were published from 1977 up to the time that this book was completed on 15 January 1988. 1977 was chosen as the starting date for this review, as this was the year in which Beeson and Bass published their comprehensive book on 'The Eosinophil'[147]. A free text search of the MEZZ database for the same period led to the selection of a further 300 references, providing a core material of 4125 references, many of which also had abstracts. These were downloaded, and read into a Cardbox-Plus reference database on my own microcomputer. Over 1000 photocopies were obtained of selected articles which could not be read in my Medical School libraries, or at the library of the Royal Society of Medicine, London. As the work of extracting information from these references, and preparing the book proceeded, 1173 earlier references and related material was added to the database, so that my database finally contained 5298 references on eosinophils and eosinophilic diseases. Over one-third of these references are discussed in this book. A copy of the complete database can be obtained from the author.

The order of the chapters and headings on eosinophils in disease and individual diseases broadly follows the listings in the Medline Medical Subjects Headings Tree Structure, to make it easier to search for subsequent references from the Medline databases.

As this book was designed to be a source and synthesis of information on human eosinophils, and of diseases affecting eosinophils in man, animal studies were only included where they related to human eosinophils, except for Chapter 7, which centres on eosinophils in normal animals.

Books and reports of meetings

Few books have been written on eosinophils. The most comprehensive on 'The Eosinophil', was published in 1977 by Paul Beeson and David Bass.[147] It described eosinophil production, their structure, biochemistry, and occurrence in a wide range of clinical disorders, and reviewed 1485 references in a scholarly and critical fashion. This book was the first to bring together clinical information about diseases in which eosinophils were either common, less common, or rare. It also gave a detailed and balanced account of experimental studies on eosinophils in animals and man. It remains an indispensable source of information on literature dealing with eosinophils in disease.

In 1979, on the centenary of the discovery of the eosinophil by Paul Ehrlich, a meeting was organized at Brook Lodge, Michigan, USA. The proceedings were published, with chapters from different groups in several parts of the world. It is one of the most useful reviews of the properties of eosinophils and their constitutents.[1134]

The proceedings of a small meeting at the Royal Society of Tropical Medicine and Hygiene in London in 1980 was published as a supplement to *Transactions*.[226]

In 1981, the 'First International Workshop on the Eosinophil' was held in Fukuoka, Japan, and the presentations were published in 1983.[1982] This meeting was one of the first occasions in which eosinophil activation was discussed in detail by several groups.

Review articles in books and journals

Many of these articles are useful for obtaining an overview of various aspects of eosinophil cell biology and their occurrence in disease. It is difficult to learn about these, as multi-author books are not indexed in reference databases, and many reviews are provided in the introduction and discussion sections of more detailed papers. The following articles provide a detailed assessment of the literature, as well as useful sources for further reading.

Published in 1914–76

1914: Schwarz, E. Die Lehre von der allgemeinen und ortlichen '*Eosinophilie*'. 2758 references.[1580]

1975: Chusid, M. J. Dale, D. C. West, B. C. and Wolff, S. M. *The hypereosinophilic syndrome: analysis of fourteen cases with review of the literature.* 94 references.[325]

Published in 1977

Butterworth, A. E. *The eosinophil and its role in immunity to helminth infection.* 239 references.[248]

Gleich, G. J. *The eosinophil: structure and biochemical composition.* 30 references.[651]

Gleich, G. J. *The eosinophil: new aspects of structure and function.* 26 references.[652]

Kay, A. B. *Eosinophil leucocytes: recruitment, localization and function in immediate-type hypersensitivity.* 30 references.[925]

Published in 1978

Konig, W. (*Structure and function of the eosinophils leucocytes*). 56 references.[997]

Spry, C. J. *Eosinophils as effector cells in disease.* 51 references.[1680]

Zucker-Franklin, D. *Eosinophil function related to cutaneous disorders.* 45 references.[2006]

Published in 1979

Kay, A. B. *The role of the eosinophil.* 53 references.[926]

Olsen, E. G. and Spry, C. J. *The pathogenesis of Löffler's endomyocardial disease and its relationship to endomyocardial fibrosis.* 138 references.[1317]

Olsson, I. and Venge, P. *The role of the eosinophil granulocyte in the inflammatory reaction.* 81 references.[1330]

Schiffmann, E. and Gallin, J. I. *Biochemistry of phagocyte chemotaxis.* 300 references.[1569]

Sullivan, T. J. *The role of eosinophils in inflammatory reactions.* 156 references.[1725]

Weller, P. F. and Goetzl, E. J. *The regulatory and effector roles of eosinophils.* 210 references.[1912]

Published in 1980

Slater, J. M. and Swarm, O. J. *Eosinophilic granuloma of bone.* 227 references.[1643]

Spry, C. J. *Eosinophilia and allergic reactions to drugs.* 67 references.[1681]

Valone, F. H. *Modulation of human neutrophil and eosinophil polymor-*

phonuclear leukocyte chemotaxis: an analytical review. 149 references.[1830]

Weller, P. F. and Goetzl, E. J. *The human eosinophil: roles in host defense and tissue injury.* 179 references.[1913]

Published in 1981

Butterworth, A. E. and David, J. R. *Eosinophil function.* 7 references.[252]

Root, R. K. and Cohen, M. S. *The microbicidal mechanisms of human neutrophils and eosinophils.* 313 references.[1513]

Schatz, M., Wasserman, S., and Patterson, R. *Eosinophils and immunologic lung disease.* 76 references.[1567]

Smith, J. A. *Molecular and cellular properties of eosinophils.* (*A review.*) 137 references.[1650]

Tavassoli, M. *Eosinophil, eosinophilia, and eosinophilic disorders.* 350 references.[1759]

Zucker-Franklin, D. *Eosinophils.* 55 references.[2008]

Published in 1982

Ackerman, S. J., Durack, D. T., and Gleich, G. J. *Eosinophil effector mechanisms in health and disease.* 117 references.[4]

Bass, D. A. *Eosinophil behavior during host defense reactions.* 168 references.[124]

Dessein, A. J. and David, J. R. *The eosinophil in parasitic diseases.* 234 references.[440]

Hudson, G. and Maxwell, M. H. *Eosinophil leucocytes. Granules and cell functions.* 269 references.[824]

Kay, A. B. *Complement receptor enhancement by chemotactic factors.* 20 references.[927]

Spry, C. J. *The hypereosinophilic syndrome: clinical features, laboratory findings and treatment.* 123 references.[1683]

Spry, C. J. and Kumaraswami, V. *Tropical eosinophilia.* 100 references.[1695]

Published in 1983

Cohen, S. G. and Ottesen, E. A. *The eosinophil, eosinophilia, and eosinophil-related disorders.* 429 references.[339]

Engle, W. A., and Schreiner, R. L., and Baehner, R. L. *Neonatal white blood cell disorders.* 89 references.[515]

Favara, B. E., McCarthy, R. C., and Mierau, G. W. *Histiocytosis X.* 68 references.[547]

Gleich, G. J. Ackerman, S. J. and Loegering, D. A. *Procurement and purification of eosinophils.* 118 references.[655]

Gleich, G. J., Loegering, D. A., Frigas, E., and Filley, W. V. *The eosinophil granule major basic protein: biological activities and relationship to bronchial asthma.* 20 references.[662]

Klebanoff, S. J., Henderson, W. R. Jr, Jong, E. C., Jorg, A. and Locksley, R. M. *Role of peroxidase in eosinophil function.* 82 references.[976]

Shrader, J. W. *Bone marrow differentiation in vitro.* 425 references.[1576]

Published in 1984

Butterfield, J. H., Maddox, D. E., and Gleich, G. J. *The eosinophil leukocyte: maturation and function.* 433 references.[246]

Butterworth, A. E. *Cell-mediated damage to helminths.* 310 references.[249]

Gleich, G. J. and Loegering, D. A. *Immunobiology of eosinophils.* 176 references.[659]

Hayashi, H., Honda, M., Shimokawa. Y., and Hirashima, M. *Chemotactic factors associated with leukocyte emigration in immune tissue injury: their separation, characterization, and functional specificity.* 278 references.[772]

Kay, A. B. *Eosinophils.* 109 references.[928]

Malmsten, C. L. *Leukotrienes: mediators of inflammation and immediate hypersensitivity reactions.* 341 references.[1149]

Schwartz, L. B. *Hypereosinophilic syndrome: a review.* 34 references.[1578]

Weller, P. F. *Eosinophilia.* 31 references.[1905]

Published in 1985

Kay, A. B. *Eosinophils as effector cells in immunity and hypersensitivity disorders.* 89 references.[929]

Olsen, E. G. and Spry, C. J. *Relation between eosinophilia and endomyocardial disease.* 82 references.[1319]

Spry, C. J. *Synthesis and secretion of eosinophil granule substances.* 44 references.[1687]

Published in 1986

Colley, D. G., Stewart, S. J., Duncan, E. K., and Secor, W. E. *The role of the eosinophil in host defense.* 23 references.[344]

Frigas, E. and Gleich, G. J. *The eosinophil and the pathophysiology of asthma.* 81 references.[604]

Gleich, G. J. *The functions of eosinophils.* 34 references.[653]

Gleich, G. J. *The role of the eosinophilic leukocyte in bronchial asthma.* 45 references.[654]

Gleich, G. J. and Adolphson, C. R. *The eosinophilic leukocyte: structure and function.* 450 references.[656]

Rocco, V. K. and Hurd, E. R. *Scleroderma and scleroderma-like disorders.* 430 references.[1507]

Published in 1987

Capron, M. and Capron, A. *The IgE receptor of human eosinophils.* 20 references.[269]

Denburg, J. A., Otsuka, H., Ohnisi, M., Ruhno, J., Bienenstock, J., and Dolovich, J. *Contribution of basophil/mast cell and eosinophil growth and differentiation to the allergic tissue inflammatory response.* 59 references.[431]

Gleich, G. J., Adolphson, C. R., Slifman, N. R., Loegering, D. A., and McKeen, D. J. *Purification, neurotoxic and enzymatic activities of human eosinophil-derived neurotoxin and human eosinophil cationic protein.* 31 references.[657]

Hogan, T. F., Koss, W., Murgo, A. J., Amato, R. S., Fontana, J. A., and VanScoy, F. L. *Acute lymphoblastic leukemia with chromosomal 5;14 translocation and hypereosinophilia: case report and literature review.* 41 references.[806]

Koeffler, H. P. *Syndromes of acute nonlymphocytic leukemia.* 102 references.[987]

Reynolds, H. Y. *Bronchoalveolar lavage.* 226 references.[1488]

Silberstein, D. S. and David, J. R. *The regulation of human eosinophil function by cytokines.* 64 references.[1627]

Spry, C. J. *Eosinophils and endomycardial fibrosis: a review of clinical and experimental studies 1980–86.* 115 references.[1691]

References

1. Abelson, M. B., Madiwale, N., and Weston, J. H. (1983). Conjunctival eosinophils in allergic ocular disease. *Arch. Ophthalmol* **101**, 555–6. [p. 218]
2. Abrishami, M. A. and Thomas, J. (1977). Aspirin intolerance – a review. *Ann. Allergy*. **39**, 28–37. [p. 202]
3. Ackerman, G. A. (1964). Eosinophilic leukemia. A morphologic and histochemical study. *Blood* **24**, 372–88. [p. 280]
4. Ackerman, S. J., Durack, D. T., and Gleich, G. J. (1982). Eosinophil effector mechanisms in health and disease. In *Advances in host defence mechanisms. 1. Phagocytic cells* (ed. J. I. Gallin and A. S. Fauci), Raven Press, New York. pp. 269–93. [p. 324]
5. Ackerman, S. J., Gleich, G. J., Loegering, D. A., Richardson, B. A., and Butterworth, A. E. (1985). Comparative toxicity of purified human eosinophil granule cationic proteins for schistosomula of Schistosoma mansoni. *Am. J. Trop. Med. Hyg.* **34**, 735–45. [p. 47, 52, 55, 115]
6. Ackerman, S. J., Gleich, G. J., Weller, P. F., and Ottesen, E. A. (1981). Eosinophilia and elevated serum levels of eosinophil major basic protein and Charcot–Leyden crystal protein (lysophospholipase) after treatment of patients with Bancroft's filariasis. *J. Immunol.* **127**, 1093–8. [p. 142]
7. Ackerman, S. J., Kephart, G. M., Habermann, T. M., Greipp, P. R., and Gleich, G. J. (1983). Localization of eosinophil granule major basic protein in human basophils. *J. Exp. Med.* **158**, 946–61. [p. 45, 282]
8. Ackerman, S. J., Loegering, D. A., and Gleich, G. J. (1980). The human eosinophil Charcot–Leyden crystal protein: biochemical characteristics and measurement by radioimmunoassay. *J. Immunol.* **125**, 2118–26.[p. 63, 64, 65]
9. Ackerman, S. J., Loegering, D. A., Venge, P., Olsson, I., Harley, J. B., Fauci, A. S., and Gleich,, G. J. (1983). Distinctive cationic proteins of the human eosinophil granule: major basic protein, eosinophil cationic protein, and eosinophil-derived neurotoxin. J. Immunol. **131**, 2977–82. [p. 281]
10. Ackerman, S. J., Wassom, D. L., Loegering, D. A., and Gleich, G. J. (1981). Elevated levels of human eosinophil Charcot–Leyden crystal protein (lysophospholipase) in sera of patients with eosinophilia (abstract). *Fed. Proc.*, 4753. [p. 65]
11. Ackerman, S. J., Weil, G. J., and Gleich, G. J. (1982). Formation of Charcot–Leyden crystals by human basophils. *J. Exp. Med.* **155**, 1597–609. [p. 45]
12. Ackerman, S. J., Weil, G. J., and Gleich, G. J. (1983). The Charcot–Leyden crystal protein (lysophospholipase): biochemical characteristics, measurement by radioimmunoassay and detection in human basophils. In *Immunobiology of the eosinophil* (eds. T. Yoshida and M. Torisu), pp. 121–44. Elsevier Biomedical, New York. [p. 65]
13. Ackerman, S. J. and Weller, P. F. Charcot–Leyden crystal protein: myristyla-

tion in HL–60 cells and eosinophils (abstract). Presented to the 6th International Congress of Immunology, Toronto, Canada, 1986. [p. 26, 63]

14. Acquatella, H., Schiller, N.B., Puigbo, J. J., Gomez Mancebo, J. R., Suarez, C., and Acquatella, G. (1983). Value of two-dimensional echocardiography in endomyocardial disease with and without eosinophilia. A clinical and pathologic study. *Circulation* **67**, 1219–26. [p. 251,256]
15. Adams, H. W., Mainz, D. L. (1977). Eosinophilic ascites. A case report and review of the literature. *Am. J. Dig. Dis.* **22**, 40–2. [p. 186, 245]
16. Adams, W. H. and Liu, Y. K. (1982). Periodic neutropenia and monocytopenia. *Am. J. Hematol.* **13**, 73–82. [p. 11, 261]
17. Adelman, M., Albelda, S. M., Gottlieb, J. and Haponik, E. F. (1984). Diagnostic utility of pleural fluid eosinophilia. *Am J. Med.* **77**, 915–20. [p. 212]
18. Aderele, W. I. and Oduwole, O. (1982). Ascaris and bronchial asthma in children. *Afr. J. Med. Med. Sci.* **11**, 161–6. [p. 201]
19. Adewusi, K. and Goven, A. J. (1986). Enhancement of lysophospholipase activity with Trichinella spiralis antigen: evidence for cell cooperation. *J. Parasitol.* **72**, 716–22. [p. 63]
20. Adewusi, K. and Goven, A. J. (1987). Enhanced lysophospholipase activity in sensitized mice challenged with Trichinella spiralis: a role for cell-cooperation. *Dev. Comp. Immunol.* **11**, 215–25. [p. 66, 111, 116]
21. Adewusi, K. and Goven, A. J. (1987). Effect of anti-thymocyte serum on the eosinophil and lysophospholipase responses in mice infected with Trichinella spiralis. *Parasitology* **94**, 115–22. [p. 66]
22. Adrouny, A., Seraydarian, A., Levine, A. M., Hungerford, G. F. and Carmel, R. (1984). Cyclic eosinophilic leukocytosis in eosinophilic leukemia with observations on transcobalamin I and eosinophils. *Cancer* **54**, 1374–8. [p. 284]
23. Aftandelians, R., Raafat, F., Taffazoli, M. and Beaver, P. C. (1977). Pulmonary capillariasis in a child in Iran. *Am. J. Trop. Med. Hyg.* **26**, 64–71. [p. 144]
24. Agosti, J. M., Altman, L. C., Ayars, G. H., Loegering, D. A., Gleich, G. J. and Klebanoff, S. J. (1987). The injurious effect of eosinophil peroxidase, hydrogen peroxide, and halides on pneumocytes *in vitro*. *J. Allergy. Clin. Immunol.* **79**, 496–504. [p. 47, 118, 193]
25. Agrawal, B. L. and Giesen, P. C. (1981). Eosinophilic myositis. An unusual cause of pseudotumor and eosinophilia. *JAMA* **246**, 70–1. [p. 179]
26. Al Dabbagh, A. I. and Al Irhayim, B. (1983). Eosinophilic transient synovitis. *Ann. Rheum. Dis.* **42**, 462–5. [p. 178]
27. Alfaham, M. A., Ferguson, S. D., Sihra, B. and Davies, J. (1987). The idiopathic hypereosinophilic syndrome. *Arch. Dis. Child.* **62**, 601–13. [p. 268, 290]
28. Ali Khan, Z., Siboo, R., Meerovitch, E., Faubert, G., and Faucher, M. G. (1981). Cysticercus racemosus in an eosinophilic phlegmon in the brain. *Trans. R. Soc. Trop. Med. Hyg.* **75**, 774–9. [p. 138]
29. Alipour, M., Tarbiat, C., and Nazarian, I. (1980). Right ventricular endomyocardial fibrosis simulating Ebstein's anomaly. *Am. Heart. J.* **100**, 859–65. [p. 251]
30. Allansmith, M. R., Baird, R. S., and Greiner, J. V. (1979). Vernal conjunctivitis and contact lens-associated giant papillary conjunctivitis compared and contrasted. *Am. J. Ophthalmol.* **87**, 544–5. [p. 218]
31. Allansmith, M. R., Korb, D.R., and Greiner, J. V. (1978). Giant papillary

conjunctivitis induced by hard or soft contact lens wear: quantitative histology. *Ophthalmology* **85**, 766–78. [p. 218]

32. Allen, B. V., Kane, C. E., Powell, D. G. (1984). Leucocyte counts in the healthy English thoroughbred in training. *Equine Vet. J.* **16**, 207–9. [p. 126]
33. Allen, D. H., Basten, A., and Woolcock, A. J. (1976). Family studies in hypersensitivity pneumonitis. *Chest* **69**, 283–4. [p. 204]
34. Allen, S. C. (1984). Eosinophilic fasciitis in an African – possible benefit of chloroquine treatment. *Postgrad. Med. J.* **60**, 685–6. [p. 181]
35. Alonso Ruiz, A., Zea Mendoza, A. C., Salazar Vallinas, J. M., Rocamora Ripoll, A., and Beltran Gutierrez, J. (1986). Toxic oil syndrome: a syndrome with features overlapping those of various forms of schleroderma. *Semin. Arthritis Rheum.* **15**, 200–12. [p. 182]
36. Andersen, V., Bro Rasmussen, F., and Hougaard, U. (1969). Autoradiographic studies of eosinophil kinetics: effect of cortisol. *Cell Tissue Kinet.* **2**, 139–46. [p. 290]
37. Andersson, L. C. and Gahmberg, C. G. (1978). Surface glycoproteins of human white blood cells: analysis by surface labeling. *Blood* **52**, 57–67. [p. 84]
38. Andy, J. J., Bishara, F. F., and Soyinka, O. O. (1981). Relation of severe eosinophilia and microfilariasis to chronic African endomyocardial fibrosis. *Br. Heart. J.* **45**, 672–80. [p. 257]
39. Andy, J. J., Bishara, F. F., Soyinka, O. O., and Odesanmi, W. O. (1981). Loiasis as a possible trigger of African endomyocardial fibrosis: a case report from Nigeria. *Acta. Trop. (Basel)* **38,** 179–86. [p. 256, 257]
40. Andy, J. J., O'Connell, J. P., Daddario, R. C., and Roberts, W. C. (1977). Trichinosis causing extensive ventricular mural endrocarditis with superimposed thrombosis. Evidence that severe eosinophilia damages endocardium. *Am. J. Med.* **63**, 824–9. [p. 145, 230]
41. Angelillo, V. A., Kanner, R. E., and Renzetti, A. D. Jr. (1977). Chronic eosinophilic pneumonia: a report of four cases and a review of the literature. *Am. J. Med. Sci.* **273**, 279–87. [p. 206, 248]
42. Anteunis, A., Astesano, A., and Robineaux, R. (1977). Ultrastructural characteristics of developing eosinophil leukocytes in human bone marrow during acute leukemia: evidence for extracellular granule release from human eosinophils. *Inflammation* **2**, 17–26. [p. 13]
43. Antia, A. U., Effiong, C. E., and Dawodu, A. H. (1972). The pattern of acquired heart disease in Nigerian children. *Afr. J. Med. Med. Sci.* **3**, 1–12. [p. 249]
44. Antonakopoulos, G. N. and Newman, J. (1984). Eosinophilic cystitis with giant cells. A light microscopic and ultrastructural study. *Arch. Pathol. Lab. Med.* **108**, 728–31. [p. 223]
45. Anwar, A. R. and Kay, A. B. (1977). The ECF-A tetrapeptides and histamine selectively enhance human eosinophil complement receptors. *Nature* **269**, 522–4. [p. 82]
46. Anwar, A. R. and Kay, A. B. (1980). H1-receptor dependence of histamine-induced enhancement of human eosinophil C3b rosettes. *Clin. Exp. Immunol.* **42**, 196–9. [p. 82]
47. Anwar, A. R., McKean J. R., Smithers, S. R., and Kay, A. B. (1980). Human eosinophil- and neutrophil-mediated killing of schistosomula of Schistosoma mansoni in vitro. I. Enhancement of complement-dependent damage by mast-

cell derived mediators and formyl methionyl peptides. *J. Immunol* **124**, 1122–9. [p. 120]
48. Anwar, A. R., Smithers, S. R. and Kay, A. B. (1979). Killing of schistosomula of Schistosoma mansoni coated with antibody and/or complement by human leukocytes in vitro: requirement for complement in preferential killing by eosinophils. *J. Immunol.* **122**, 628–37. [p. 114]
49. Appel, G. B. and Neu, H. C. (1977). The nephrotoxicity of antimicrobial agents. *N. Engl. J. Med.* **296**, 663–70. [p. 220, 309]
50. Appel, J. (1972). Loeffler's endocarditis in the organism hypersensitized by Taenia saginata. *Acta. Morphol. Acad. Sci. Hung.* **20**, 133–7. [p. 236]
51. Archer, C. B., Page, C. P., Morley, J. and MacDonald, D. M. (1985). Accumulation of inflammatory cells in response to intracutaneous platelet activating factor (Paf-acether) in man. *Br. J. Dermatol.* **112**, 285–90. [p. 97]
52. Archer, G. T. (1968). The function of the eosinophil. *Bibl. Hemat.* **29** Part 1, 71–85. [p. 9]
53. Archer, G. T., Air, G., Jackas, M., and Morell, D. B. (1965). Studies on rat eosinophil peroxidase. *Biochim. Biophys. Acta.* **99**, 96–101. [p. 57, 58]
54. Archer, G. T. and Blackwood, A. (1965). Formation of Charcot–Leyden crystals in human eosinophils and basophils and study of the composition of isolated crystals. *J. Exp. Med.* **122**, 173–80. [p. 64]
55. Archer, G. T. and Hirsch J. G. (1963). Isolation of granules from eosinophil leucocytes and study of their enzyme content. *J. Exp. Med.* **118**, 277–84. [p. 6]
56. Archer, G. T., and Hirsch, J. G. (1963). Motion picture studies on degranulation of horse eosinophils during phagocytosis. *J. Exp. Med.* **118**, 287–93. [p. 6, 90]
57. Archer, G. T. and Jackas, M. (1965). Disruption of mast cells by a component of eosinophil granules. *Nature.* **205**, 599–600. [p. 60]
58. Archer, G. T., Nelson, M., and Johnston, J. (1969). Eosinophil granule lysis in vitro induced by antigen-antibody complexes. *Immunology* **17**, 777–87.[p. 80, 90]
59. Archer, R. K. (1965). On the functions of eosinophils in the antigen-antibody reaction. *Br. J. Haematol.* **11**, 123–9. [p. 42]
60. Archer, R. K. (1968). The eosinophil leukocytes. *Ser. Haemat.* **1**, 3–32. [p. 6]
61. Archer, R. K. and Broome, J. (1963). Studies on the peroxidase reaction of living eosinophils and other leucocytes. *Acta. Haematol. (Basel)* **29**, 147–56. [p. 57]
62. Archer, R. K., Engisch, H. J. C., Gaha, T., and Ruxton, J. (1971). The eosinophil leucocytes in the blood and bone marrow of patients with Down's anomaly. *Br. J. Haematol.* **21**, 271–6. [p. 295]
63. Archimbaud, E., Coiffier, B., and Bryon, P. A., Vasselon, C., Brizard, C. P., and Viala, J. J. (1987). Prognostic factors in angioimmunoblastic lymphadenopathy. *Cancer* **59**, 208–12. [p. 163]
64. Arenzana Seisdedos, F., Barbey, S., Virelizier, J. L., Kornprobst, M., and Nezelof, C. (1986). Histiocytosis X. Purified (T6+) cells from bone granuloma produce interleukin 1 and prostaglandin E2 in culture. *J. Clin. Invest.* **77**, 326–9. [p. 164]
65. Arkin, C. F., Sherry, M.A., Gough, A. G., and Copeland, B. E. (1977). An automatic leukocyte analyzer. Validity of its results. *Am. J. Clin. Pathol.* **67**, 159–69. [p. 30]

66. Arnason, B. G. and Waksman, B. H. (1963). The retest reaction in delayed sensitivity. *Lab. Invest.* **12**, 737–47. [p. 100]
67. Arthur, D. C. and Bloomfield, C. D. (1983). Partial deletion of the long arm of chromosome 16 and bone marrow eosinophilia in acute nonlymphocytic leukemia: a new association. *Blood* **61**, 994–8. [p. 156, 158]
68. Arvay, A. and Lengyel M. (1983). Endomyocardial fibrosis with successful surgical treatment in a Hungarian woman. *Cor. Vasa.* **25**, 191–5. [p. 244]
69. Arvay, A., Lengyel, M., Meszaros, R., and Palik, I. (1985). Surgical experience with thrombotic and fibrotic forms of non-tropical eosinophilic endomyocardial disease. *Thorac. Cardiovasc. Surg.* **33**, 314–6. [p. 240, 244, 253, 254]
70. Ascensao, J. L., Oken, M. M., Ewing, S. L., Goldberg, R. J., and Kaplan, M. E. (1987). Leukocytosis and large cell lung cancer: a frequent association. *Cancer* **60**, 903–5. [p. 174]
71, Ascensao, J. L., Vercellotti, G. M., Jacob, H. S. and Zanjani, E. D. (1984). Role of endothelial cells in human hematopoiesis: modulation of mixed colony growth *in vitro. Blood* **63**, 553–58. [p. 18]
72. Ashok, P. P., Sapru, R. P., Radhakrishnan, V. V., and Virmani, V. (1982). Skeletal muscle involvement in tropical endomyocardial fibrosis. *J. Neurol. Sci.* **54**, 1–12. [p. 253]
73. Askin, F. B., McCann, B. G., and Kuhn, C. (1977). Reactive eosinophilic pleuritis: a lesion to be distinguished from pulmonary eosinophilic granuloma. *Arch. Pathol. Lab. Med.* **101**, 187–91. [p. 212]
74. Atkinson, J. B., Robinowitz, M., McAllister, H. A., and Virmani, R. (1985). Association of eosinophils with cardiac rupture. *Hum. Pathol.* **16**, 562–8. [p. 229]
75. Aubertin, C. and Giroux, L. (1912). Action des rayons X sur les eosinophiles. *Presse Med.* **20**, 597–8. [p. 289]
76. Aufdemorte, T. B., Huntington, H. W., Ripley, J. F., and Ramzy, I. (1983). Localized eosinophilic myositis of the masseter muscle associated with actinomycosis. *J. Oral Maxillofac. Surg.* **41**, 196–200. [p. 179]
77. Aumuller, G. and Seitz, J. (1985). Cytochemistry and biochemistry of acid phosphatases. VI: Immunoelectron microscopic studies on human prostatic and leukocytic acid phosphatases. *Prostate* **7**, 161–9. [p. 60]
78. Auriault, C., Capron M. and Capron, A. (1982). Activation of rat and human eosinophils by soluble factor(s) released by Schistosoma mansoni schistosomula. *Cell. Immunol.* **66**, 59–69. [p. 78, 110]
79. Auriault, C., Capron, M., Cesari, I. M. and Capron, A. (1983). Enhancement of eosinophil effector function by soluble factors released by S. mansoni: role of proteases. *J. Immunol.* **131**, 464–70. [p. 110]
80. Austen, K. F. (1978). Homeostasis of effector systems which can also be recruited for immunologic reactions. *J. Immunol.* **121**, 793–805. [p. 9, 83, 99]
81. Austen, K. F. (1987). The role of arachidonic acid metabolites in local and systemic inflammatory processes. *Drugs* **33** Suppl. 1, 10–17. [p. 70]
82. Avgerinos, P. C., Papadimitriou, C. S., Kokkini, G., and Moutsopoulos, H. M. (1982). Asymptomatic diffuse fasciitis with eosinophilia. *Ann. Rheum. Dis.* **41**, 621–2. [p. 181]
83. Ayars, G. H., Altman, L. C., Gleich, G. J., Loegering, D. A., and Baker, C. B. (1985). Eosinophil- and eosinophil granule-mediated pneumocyte injury. *J. Allergy Clin. Immunol.* **76**, 595–604. [p. 47, 119]

84. Aylesworth, R. and Vance, J. C. (1982). Demodex folliculorum and Demodex brevis in cutaneous biopsies. *J. Am. Acad. Dermatol.* **7**, 583–9. [p. 149]
85. Azuma, C., Tanabe, T., Konishi, M., Kinashi, T., Noma, T., Matsuda, F., Yaoita, Y., Takatsu, K., Hammarstrom, L., Smith, C. L., and Honjo, T. (1986). Cloning of cDNA for human T-cell replacing factor (interleukin-5) and comparison with the murine homologue. *Nucleic Acids Res.* **14**, 9149–58. [p. 19]
86. Baandrup, U. (1977). Loffler's endocarditis and endomyocardial fibrosis – a nosologic entity? *Acta Pathol. Microbiol. Scand. (A)* **85**, 869–74. [p. 242]
87. Baandrup, U. and Olsen, E. G. (1981). Critical analysis of endomyocardial biopsies from patients suspected of having cardiomyopathy. 1. Morphological and morphometric aspects. *Br. Heart. J.* **45**, 475–86. [p. 242]
88. Bach, M. K. (1982). Mediators of anaphylaxis and inflammation. *Annu. Rev. Microbiol.* **36**, 371–413. [p. 100]
89. Back, O., Liden, S., and Ahlstedt, S. (1977). Adverse reactions to nitrofurantoin in relation to cellular and humoral immune responses. *Clin. Exp. Immunol.* **28**, 400–6. [p. 313]
90. Backenroth, R., Spinowitz, B. S., Galler, M., Golden, R. A., Rascoff, J. H., and Charytan, C. (1986). Comparison of eosinophilia in patients undergoing peritoneal dialysis and hemodialysis. *Am. J. Kidney Dis.* **8**, 186–91. [p. 222]
91. Badley, J. E., Grieve, R. B., Rockey, J. H., and Glickman, L. T. (1987). Immune-mediated adherence of eosinophils to Toxocara canis infective larvae: the role of excretory-secretory antigens. *Parasite Immunol.* **9**, 133–43. [p. 140]
92. Baehner, R. L. and Johnston, R. B. Jr. (1971). Metabolic and bactericidal activities of human eosinophils. *Br. J. Haematol.* **20**, 277–85. [p. 120]
93. Baggen, M. G., Krenning, E. P., Witte, R., and Hennemann, G. (1982). The hypereosinophilic syndrome. *Neth. J. Med.* **25**, 154–8. [p. 272, 291]
94. Baggiolini, M. (1984). Phagocytes use oxygen to kill bacteria. *Exper.* **40**, 906–9. [p. 69, 119]
95. Baigelman, W., Chodosh, S., Pizzuto, D., and Cupples, L. A. (1983). Sputum and blood eosinophil during corticosteroid treatment of acute exacerbations of asthma. *Am. J. Med.* **75**, 929–36. [p. 198, 199]
96. Bailey, C. C. and Campbell, R. H. (1973). Lymphosarcoma presenting as Löffler's syndrome. *Br. Med. J.* **1**, 460–61. [p. 163]
97. Bain, B., Seed, M., and Godsland, I. (1984). Normal values for peripheral blood white cell counts in women of four different ethnic origins. *J. Clin. Pathol.* **37,** 188–93. [p. 31]
98. Bain, B. J. (1986). An assessment of the three-population differential count on the Coulter Counter Model S Plus IV. *Clin. Lab. Haematol.* **8**, 347–59. [p. 31]
99. Bain, B. J., Neill, P. J., Scott, D., Scott, T. J., and Innis, M. D. (1980). Automated differential leucocyte counters: an evaluation of the Hemalog D and A comparison with the Hematrak. I. Principles of operation; reproducibility and accuracy on normal blood samples. *Pathology* **12**, 83–100. [p. 31]
100. Bainton, D. F. and Farquhar, M. G. (1970). Segregation and packaging of granule enzymes in eosinophilic leukocytes. *J. Cell. Biol.* **45**, 54–73. [p. 57, 59, 61]

101. Baker, J. R., Bassett, E. G., and de Souza, P. (1976). Eosinophils in healing dermal wounds. *J. Anat.* **121**, 401a. [p. 9]

102. Balakrishnan, K. G., Sapru, R. P., Sasidharan, K., and Venkitachalam, C. G. (1982). A comparison of the clinical, haemodynamic and angiographic features in right ventricular endomyocardial fibrosis and Ebstein's anomaly of the tricuspid valve. *Cardiology* **69**, 265–75. [p. 251]

103. Balakrishnan, K. G., Sasidharan, K., Venkitachalam, C. G., and Sapru, R. P. (1983). Coronary angiographic features in endomyocardial fibrosis. *Cardiology* **70**, 121–6. [p. 252]

104. Balakrishnan, K. G., Venkitachalam, C. G., Pillai, V. R., Subramanian, R., and Valiathan, M. S. (1986). Postoperative evaluation of endomyocardial fibrosis. *Cardiology* **73**, 73–84. [p. 234, 255]

105. Baldwin, D. S., Levine, B. B., McCluskey, R. T., and Gallo, G. R. (1968). Renal failure and interstitial nephritis due to penicillin and methicillin. *N. Engl. J. Med.* **279**, 1245–52. [p. 309]

106. Baler, G. R. (1981). Angiolymphoid hyperplasia with eosinophilia. A report of two cases. *J. Dermatol. Surg. Oncol.* **7**, 229–34. [p. 168]

107. Ball, E. D., Graziano, R. F., and Fanger, M. W. (1983). A unique antigen expressed on myeloid cells and acute leukemia blast cells defined by a monoclonal antibody. *J. Immunol.* **130**, 2937–41. [p. 87]

108. Ballin, A., Meytes, D., Lieberman, D., and Ramot, B. (1983). Extreme transient eosinophilia in a healthy infant: eosinophil colonies (CFU-EO) studied in culture. *Br. J. Haematol.* **53**, 168–70. [p. 295]

109. Baraff, L. J., Wilkins, J., and Overturf, G. D. (1977). Oral cefatrizine in pediatric infections. *Curr. Ther. Res.* **21**, 187–91. [p. 310]

110. Barber, F. A. and Roach, J. W. (1986). Torticollis: a presentation of eosinophilic granuloma. A case report. *Orthopedics* **9**, 1237–9. [p. 165]

111. Barnes, L., Koss, W., and Nieland, M. L. (1980). Angiolymphoid hyperplasia with eosinophilia: a disease that may be confused with malignancy. *Head Neck Surg.* **2**, 425–34. [p. 168]

112. Barnes, L., Rodnan, G. P., Medsger, T. A., and Short, D. (1979). Eosinophilic fasciitis. A pathologic study of twenty cases. *Am. J. Pathol.* **96**, 493–517. [p. 181]

113. Barnes, N., Gray, B. J., Heaton, R., and Costello, J. F. (1983). Pulmonary eosinophilia in identical twins. *Thorax* **38**, 318–9. [p. 207]

114. Barr, R. D., Koekebakker, M., Brown, E. A., and Falbo, M. C. (1987). Putative role for lithium in human hematopoiesis. *J. Lab. Clin. Med.* **109**, 159–63. [p. 24]

115. Barr, R. D., Volaric, Z., and Koekebakker, M. (1987). Stimulation of human eosinophilopoiesis by hydrocortisone in vitro. *Acta Haematol. (Basel)* **77**, 20–4. [p. 24]

116. Barresi, G., Inferrera, C., and De Luca, F. (1978). Eosinophilic pancreatitis in the newborn infant of a diabetic mother. *Virchows Arch. (Pathol. Anat.)* **380**, 341–8. [p. 306]

117. Barrett, A. J. and Barrett, A. (1975). Bronchial carcinoma with eosinophilia and cardiomegaly. *Br. J. Dis. Chest* **69**, 287–92. [p. 22, 246, 271]

118. Bartelmez, S. H., Dodge, W. H., and Bass, D. A. (1980). Differential regulation of spleen cell-mediated eosinophil and neutrophil-macrophage production. *Blood* **55**, 489–93. [p. 16, 18]

119. Bartelmez, S. H. Dodge, W. H. Mahmoud, A. A., and Bass, D. A. (1980). Stimulation of eosinophil production in vitro by eosinophilopoietin and spleen-cell-derived eosinophil growth-stimulating factor. *Blood* **56**, 706–11. [p. 17, 18]
120. Barton, J. C., Parmley, R. T., Carroll, A. J., Huang, S. T., Goodnough, L. T., Findley, H. W. Jr., and Ragab, A. H. (1987). Preleukemia in Fanconi's anemia: hematopoietic cell multinuclearity, membrane duplication, and dysgranulogenesis. *J. Submicrosc. Cytol.* **19**, 355–64. [p. 261]
121. Bass, D. A. (1975). Behaviour of eosinophil leukocytes in acute inflammation. I. Lack of dependence on adrenal function. *J. Clin. Invest.* **55**, 1229–36. [p. 28]
122. Bass, D. A. (1975). Behaviour of eosinophil leukocytes in acute inflammation. II. Eosinophil dynamics during acute inflammation. *J. Clin. Invest.* **56**, 870–9. [p. 28]
123. Bass, D. A. (1977). Reproduction of the eosinophilia of acute infection by passive transfer of a material obtained from inflammatory exudate. *Infect. Immun.* **15**, 410–16. [p. 28]
124. Bass, D. A., (1982). Eosinophil behaviour during host defense reactions. In *Advances in host defense mechanisms. 1.* (eds. J. I. Gallin and A. S. Fauci) pp. 211–41. Raven Press, New York. [p. 9, 18, 28, 84, 89, 111, 113, 285, 324.]
125. Bass, D. A., Gonwa, T. A., Szejda, P., Cousart, M. S., DeChatelet, L. R., and McCall, C. E. (1980). Eosinopenia of acute infection: production of eosinopenia by chemotactic factors of acute inflammation. *J. Clin. Invest.* **65**, 1265–71. [p. 28, 75, 220]
126. Bass, D. A., Grover, W. H., Lewis, J. C., DeChatelet, L. R., and McCall, C. E. (1982). Stimulation or activation of eosinophils in vivo during eosinophilia: possible role of arachidonic acid metabolism. *Adv. Exp. Med. Biol.* **141**, 509–18. [p. 67]
127. Bass, D. A., Grover, W. H. Lewis, J. C., Szejda, P., DeChatelet, L. R., and McCall, C. E. (1980). Comparison of human eosinophils from normals and patients with eosinophilia. *J. Clin. Invest.* **66**, 1265–73. [p. 34, 61, 67, 74, 105, 281, 282]
128. Bass, D. A., Lewis, J. C., Szejda, P., Cowley, L., and McCall, C. E. (1981). Activation of lysosomal acid phosphatase of eosinophil leukocytes. *Lab. Invest.* **44**, 403–9. [p. 61]
129. Bass, D. A. and Szejda, P. (1979). Eosinophils versus neutrophils in host defense. Killing of newborn larvae of Trichinella spiralis by human granulocytes in vitro. *J. Clin. Invest.* **64**, 1415–22. [p. 115]
130. Bass, D. A. and Szejda P. (1979). Mechanisms of killing of newborn larvae of Trichinella spiralis by neutrophils and eosinophils. Killing by generators of hydrogen peroxide in vitro. *J. Clin Invest* **64**, 1558–64. [p. 60]
131. Bass, D. A., Szejda, P., Goetzl, E. J., Love, S., O Flaherty, J. T., and McCall, C. E. (1981). Stimulation of hexose uptake by human eosinophils with chemotactic factors. *J. Infect. Dis.* **143**, 719–25. [p. 67]
132. Bass, J. L., Mehta, K. A., Glickman, L. T., Blocker, R., and Eppes, B. M. (1987). Asymptomatic toxocariasis in children. A prospective study and treatment trial. *Clin. Pediatr. (Phila)* **26**, 441–6. [p. 140]
133. Bassett, E. G. (1962). Infiltration of eosinophils into the modified connective tissue of oestrous and pregnant animals. *Nature* **194**, 1259–61. [p. 9]

134. Bassett, E. G., Baker, J. R., Baker, P. A., and Myers, D. B. (1976). Comparison of collagenase activity in eosinophil and neutrophil fractions from rat peritoneal exudates. *Aust. J. Exp. Biol. Med. Sci.* **54**, 459–65. [p. 61]

135. Bassett, E. G., Baker, J. R., and de Souza, P. (1977). A light microscopical study of healing incised dermal wounds in rats, with special reference to eosinophil leucocytes and to the collagenous fibres of the periwound areas. *Br. J. Exp. Pathol.* **58**, 581–605. [p. 9]

136. Basten, A. and Beeson, P. B. (1970). Mechanisms of eosinophilia. II. Role of the lymphocyte. *J. Exp. Med.* **131**, 1288–305. [p. 7, 18, 137, 313]

137. Bauke, J. and Rottger, P. (1966). Hochgradige eosinophil Reaktion bei Hypernephrom. *Med. Welt.* **16**, 865–74. [p. 169, 175]

138. Baum, E. W., Sams, W. M. Jr., and Monheit, G. D. (1982). Angiolymphoid hyperplasia with eosinophilia. The disease and a comparison of treatment modalities. *J. Dermatol. Surg. Oncol.* **8**, 966–70. [p. 167]

139. Baybick, J. H. (1987). Reticuloendotheliosis with eosinophilia (Omenn's syndrome). Findings in fine needle aspirate of a lymph node. *Acta Cytol. (Baltimore)* **31**, 20–4. [p. 166]

140. Bayever, E., Rosove, M. H., and Lenarsky, C. (1984). Nonthrombocytopenic purpura with eosinophilia. *J. Pediatr.* **105**, 277–8. [p. 262]

141. Beauvais, F. and Mencia Huerta, J. M. (1986). Role of eosinophils in the IgG4-dependent human basophil degranulation (abstract). *Fed. Proc.* **45**, 1105. [p. 79]

142. Beaver, P. C. (1962). Observations on the nature of Charcot–Leyden crystals. *Bull. Soc. Pathol. Exot. Filiales* **55**, 471–6. [p. 64]

143. Beaver. P. C., Snyder, C. H., Carrera, G. M., Dent. J. H., and Lafferty, J. W. (1952). Chronic eosinophilia due to visceral larva migrans. Report of three cases. *Pediatrics* **9**, 7–19. [p. 139]

144. Beck, B., Friis, B., Heilmann, C., Pedersen, F. K., and Valerius, N. H. (1980). Severe combined immunodeficiency associated wtih hyperimmunoglobulinaemia E, eosinophilia and impaired neutrophil chemotaxis. *Acta Paediatr. Scand.* **69**, 797–801. [p. 317]

145. Bedford, D. E. and Konstam, G. L. S. (1946). Heart failure of unknown aetiology in Africans. *Br. Heart. J.* **8**, 236–7. [p. 232, 249]

146. Beeken, W. L., Northwood, I., Beliveau, C., Baigent, G., and Gump, D. (1987). Eosinophils of human colonic mucosa: C3b and Fc gamma receptor expression and phagocytic capabilities. *Clin. Immunol. Immunopathol.* **43**, 289–300. [p. 89, 105, 172]

147. Beeson, P. B., and Bass, D. A. (1977). The eosinophil. *Major Probl Intern Med.* **14**. pp. 269. Saunders, Philadelphia. [p. 18, 315, 321, 322]

148. Begley, C. G., Lopez, A. F., Nicola, N. A., Warren, D. J., Vadas, M. A., Sanderson, C. J., and Metcalf, D. (1986). Purified colony-stimulating factors enhance the survival of human neutrophils and eosinophils *in vitro*: a rapid and sensitive microassay for colony-stimulating factors. *Blood* **68**, 162–6. [p. 28, 36]

149. Beintema J. J., Wietzes, P., Weickmann, J. L., and Glitz, D. G. (1984). The amino acid sequence of human pancreatic ribonuclease. *Anal Biochem* **136**, 48–64. [p. 49]

150. Belding, M. E., Klebanoff, S. J., and Ray, C. G. (1970). Peroxidase-mediated viracidal systems. *Science* **167**, 195–6. [p. 120]

151. Bell, D., Mackay, I. G., and Pentland, B. (1985). Hypereosinophilic syndrome presenting as peripheral neuropathy. *Postgrad. Med. J.* **61**, 429–32. [p. 270, 275]

152. Bell, J. A., Jenkins, B. S., and Webb-Peploe, M. M. (1976). Clinical, haemodynamic and angiography findings in Löffler's eosinophilic endocarditis. *Br. Heart J.* **38**, 541–8. [p. 240, 241, 244, 286]

153. Bell, R. J. (1964). Pulmonary infiltration with eosinophils caused by chlorpropamide. *Lancet* **1**, 1249–50. [p. 309]

154. Ben-Bassat, I. and Gale, R. P. (1984). Hybrid acute leukemia (Editorial). *Leuk. Res.* **8**, 929–36. [p. 12]

155. Benfield, G. F. and Asquith, P. (1986). Blood eosinophilia and ulcerative colitis – influence of ethnic origin. *Postgrad. Med. J.* **62**, 1101–5. [p. 190]

156. Bentley, H. P. Jr, Reardon, A. E., Knoedler, J. P., and Krivit, W. (1961). Eosinophilic leukemia. Report of a case, with review and classification. *Am. J. Med.* **30**, 310–22. [p. 151, 153, 236]

157. Benvenisti, D. S. and Ultmann, J. E. (1969). Eosinophilic leukemia. Report of five cases and review of the literature. *Ann. Intern Med.* **71**, 731–45. [p. 263, 285]

158. Berblinger, W. (1948). Zur kenntnis der Endocarditis parietalis fibroplastica. *Schweiz Med. Wochenschr.* **78**, 829–32. [p. 232]

159. Berger, R., Bernheim, A., Daniel, M. T., Valensi, F., Sigaux, F., and Flandrin, G. (1985). Cytogenetic studies on acute myelomonocytic leukaemia (M4) with eosinophilia. *Leuk. Res.* **9**, 279–88. [p. 158]

160. Bergner, R. K. and Bergner, A. (1985). Marked peripheral eosinophilia: a clue to allergic bronchopulmonary aspergillosis in office practice. *New Engl. Reg. Allergy Proc.* **6**, 367–73. [p. 132]

161. Bergstrand, H., Lungquist, B., Petersson, B. A., Petersson, C., and Venge, P. (1985). Eosinophil-derived cationic proteins in human leukocyte histamine release. In *Inflammation: basic mechanisms, tissue injuring principles and clinical models* (Eds. P. Venge and A. Lindblom) Almqvist and Wisbell International, Stockholm. [p. 48, 52, 56]

162. Berretty, P. J. and Cormane, R. H. (1978). The aniline blue fluorescence staining of eosinophilic granulocytes. *Br. J. Dermatol.* **99**, 377–82. [p. 38]

163. Bertrand, E., Chauvet, J., Assamoi, M. O., Charles, D., Ekra, E., Dienot, B. B., Caileau, G., Burdin, J., Longechaud, A., Millet, P., *et al.* (1985). Results, indications and contra-indications of surgery in restricive endomyocardial fibrosis: comparative study on 31 operated and 30 non-operated patients. *East Afr. Med. J.* **62**, 151–60. [p. 234, 254]

164. Bevilacqua, M. P., Pober, J. S., Majeau, G. R., Cotran, R. S., and Gimbrone, M. A. (1984). Interleukin 1 (IL-I) induces biosynthesis and cell surface expression of procoagulant activity in human vascular edothelial cells. *J. Exp. Med.* **160**, 618–23. [p. 271]

165. Bevilacqua, M. P., Pober, J. S., Wheeler, M. E., Mendrick, D. L., Fiers, W., and Gimbrone, M. A. Jr. (1986). Interleukin 1 (IL-1) and tumor necrosis factor (TNF) independently activate vascular endothelial cell functions (abstract). *Fed. Proc.* **45**, 941. [p. 98]

166. Bhat, A. M. and Scanlon, J. W. (1981). The pattern of eosinophilia in

premature infants. A prospective study in premature infants using the absolute eosinophil count. *J. Pediatr.* **98**, 612. [p. 294]

167. Bia, F. J. and Barry, M. (1986). Parasitic infections of the central nervous system. *Neurol. Clin.* **4**, 171–206. [p. 216]
168. Bianco, P., Papa, G., Martelli, M., and Bonucci, E. (1984). Eosinophilic leukemia with prominent visceral involvement: histopathological and histochemical observations. *Appl. Pathol.* **2**, 247–54. [p. 154]
169. Bielek, E. (1981). Developmental stages and localization of peroxidatic activity in the leucocytes of three teleost species (Cyprinus carpio L.; Tinca tinca L.; Salmo gairdneri Richardson). *Cell Tissue Res.* **220**, 163–80. [p. 124]
170. Billingham, M. E. (1985). Pharmacotoxic myocardial disease: an endomycardial study. *Heart Vessels Suppl.* **1**, 278–82. [p. 229]
171. Binder, E., Holopainen, E., Malmberg, H., and Salo, O. P. (1984). Clinical findings in patients with allergic rhinitis. *Rhinology* **22**, 255–60. [p. 213]
172. Bindseil, E. (1987). Eosinophilic leucocyte infiltration in ruptured necrotic thigh muscle of downer cows. *Vet. Rec.* **120**, 183–4. [p. 180]
173. Bisgaard, H., Helqvist, S., Boudet, L., Venge, P., Dahl, R., and Sondergaard, J. (1986). Chemotactic activity of LTB4 in man. *Allergy* **41**, 365–72. [p. 101]
174. Bissonnette, B. and Beaudet, F. (1983). Reactive arthritis with eosinophilic synovial infiltration. *Ann. Rheum. Dis.* **42**, 466–8. [p. 177]
175. Bjornson, B. H., Andre Schwartz, J., and Desforges, J. F. (1982). In vitro culture of circulating CFUEOS from normal donors. *Exp. Hematol.* **10**, 271–6. [p. 15]
176. Bjornson, B. H., Harley, J. B., Andre Schwartz, J., Fauci, A. S., and Desforges, J. F. (1982). Peripheral blood myeloid progenitor cell cultures in patients with hypereosinophilic syndrome (CFU-eos in hypereosinophilic syndrome). *Blood* **60**, 721–6. [p. 286]
177. Bjornson, B. H., Harvey, J. M., and Rose, L. (1985). Differential effect of hydrocortisone on eosinophil and neutrophil proliferation. *J. Clin. Invest.* **76**, 924–9. [p. 16]
178. Blacklock, H. A., Cleland, J. F., Tan, P., and Pilai, V. M. (1979). The hypereosinophilic syndrome and leukapheresis (letter). *Ann. Intern. Med.* **91**, 650–1. [p. 292]
179. Blair, H. T., Chahine, R. A., Raisner, A. E., Gyorkey, F., and Luchi, R. J. (1974). Unusual hemodynamics in Löffler's endomyocarditis. *Am. J. Cardiol.* **34**, 606–9. [p. 241]
180. Blatt, P. M., Rothstein, G., Miller, H. L., and Cathey, W. J. (1974). Löffler's endomyocardial fibrosis with eosinophilia in association with acute lymphoblastic leukemia. *Blood* **44**, 489–93. [p. 161, 237]
181. Blenkinsopp, W. K., Haffenden, G. P., Fry, L., and Leonard, J. N. (1983). Histology of linear IgA disease, dermatitis herpetiformis, and bullous pemphigoid. *Am. J. Dermatopathol.* **5**, 547–54. [p. 303]
182. Bletry, O., Scheuble, C., Cereze, P., Masquet, C., Priollet, P., Balafrej, M., and Godeau, P. (1984). (Cardiac manifestations of the hypereosinophilic syndrome. The value of 2-dimensional echography (12 cases).) *Arch. Mal. Coeur* **77**, 633–41. [p. 239]
183. Bloss, R. S., Miller, T. A., and Duke, J. H. Jr. (1980). Eosinophilic infiltration of the stomach. *South. Med. J.* **73**, 672–4. [p. 187]

184. Bodammer, J. E. (1986). Ultrastructural observations on peritoneal exudate cells from the striped bass. *Vet. Immunol. Immunopathol.* **12**, 127–40. [p. 124]
185. Bolarin, D. M. and Andy, J. J. (1982). Clinical feminization and serum testosterone levels in male patients with chronic African endomyocardial fibrosis. *Trop. Geogr. Med.* **34**, 309–12. [p. 253]
186. Bolarin, D. M. and Andy, J. J. (1983). Enzymes of collagen synthesis and type III procollagen amino- propeptide in serum from Nigerians with chronic endomyocardial fibrosis. *Ann. Clin. Res.* **15**, 123–7. [p. 253]
187. Bollinger, A., Leu, H. J., and Brunner, U. (1986). Juvenile arteritis of extracranial arteries with hypereosinophilia. *Klin. Wochenschr.* **64**, 526–9. [p. 231]
188. Bolscher, B. G., Plat, H., and Wever, R. (1984). Some properties of human eosinophil peroxidase, a comparison with other peroxidases. *Biochim Biophys. Acta* **784**, 177–86. [p. 58]
189. Boongird, P., Phuapradit, P., Siridej, N., Chirachariyavej, T., Chuahirun, S., and Vejjajiva, A. (1977). Neurological manifestations of gnathostomiasis. *J. Neurol. Sci.* **31**, 279–91. [p. 146]
190. Border, W. A., Lehman, D. H., Egan, J. D., Sass, H. J., Glode, J. E., and Wilson, C. B. (1974). Antitubular basement-membrane antibodies in methicillin-associated interstitial nephritis. *N. Engl. J. Med.* **291**, 381–84. [p. 309]
191. Borer, J. S., Henry, W. L., and Epstein, S. E. (1977). Echocardiographic observations in patients with systemic infiltrative disease involving the heart. *Am. J. Cardiol.* **39**, 184–8. [p. 239]
192. Bos, A. J., Wever, R., Hamers, M. N., and Roos, D. (1981). Some enzymatic characteristics of eosinophil peroxidase from patients with eosinophilia and from healthy donors. *Infect. Immun.* **32**, 427–31. [p. 59]
193. Bostrom, S. G., and Hart, W. R. (1981). Carcinomas of the cervix with intense stromal eosinophilia. *Cancer* **47**, 2887–93. [p. 174]
194. Boswell, R. N., Austen, K. F., and Goetzl., E. J. (1976). A chemotactic receptor for val(ala)-gly-ser-glu on human eosinophil polymorphonuclear leukocytes. *Immunol. Comm.* **5**, 469–79. [p. 83]
195. Botma, J. P., Burger, E. G., and de Kock, M. L. (1987). Eosinophilic cystitis associated with Glanzmann's thrombasthenia. A case report. *S. Afr. Med. J.* **71**, 533–4. [p. 223]
196. Bottone, E., Macchia, P., and Consolini, R. (1982). Acute lymphoblastic leukemia first appearing as hypereosinophilia. *Eur. J. Pediatr.* **138**, 85–8. [p. 161]
197. Bouree, P., Bouvier, J. B., Passeron, J., Galanaud, P., and Dormont, J. (1979). Outbreak of trichinosis near Paris. *Br. Med. J.* **I**, 1047–9. [p. 145]
198. Bousser, J. (1957). Eosinophilie et leucemie. *Sang.* **28**, 553–80. [p. 151, 264]
199. Bowers, T. K., Craddock, R. R., and Jacob, H. S. (1977). Acquired granulocyte abnormality during drug allergic reactions. Possible role of complement activation. *Blood* **49**, 3–8. [p. 312]
200. Bozdech, M. J., Bainton, D. F., and Mustacchi, P. (1980). Partial peroxidase deficiency in neutrophils and eosinophils associated with neurologic disease. Histochemical, cytochemical and biochemical studies. *Am. J. Clin. Pathol.* **73**, 409–16. [p. 260]
201. Brehmer Andersson, E., Kaaman, T., Skog, E., and Frithz, A. (1986). The

histopathogenesis of the flame figure in Wells' syndrome based on five cases. *Acta Derm. Venereol. (Stockh)* **66**, 213–9. [p. 168]

202. Brenner, B. E. and Thorgeirsson, G. (1979). An association between chronic eosinophilic pneumonia and histiocytic lymphoma. *Am. J. Med. Sci.* **278**, 83–8. [p. 162, 174]
203. Breslin, A. B. and Jenkins, C. R. (1984). Experience with allergic bronchopulmonary aspergillosis: some unusual features. *Clin. Allergy* **14**, 21–8. [p. 133]
204. Breton Gorius, J. and Reyes F. (1976). Ultrastructure of human bone marrow cell maturation. *Int. Rev. Cytol.* **46**, 251–321. [p. 12]
205. Brettle, R. P., Curtis, L., Pinching, A. J., and Spry, C. J. (1979). Tartrazine sensitivity in renal failure (letter). *Lancet* **1**, 167. [p. 311]
206. Brewer, J. M. and Bignold, L. P. (1980). Multiple coronary artery aneurysms with aortic sinus aneurysms. A case report. *Arch. Pathol. Lab. Med.* **104**, 592–4. [p. 231]
207. Brink, A. J. and Weber, H. W. (1963). Fibroplastic parietal endocarditis with eosinophilia. Loeffler's endocarditis. *Am. J. Med.* **34**, 52–70.[p. 234]
208. Brockington, I. F., Luzzatto, L., and Osunkoya, B. O. (1970). The heart in eosinophilic leukaemia. *Afr. J. Med. Med. Sci.* **1**, 343–52. [p. 3, 154, 245]
209. Brockington, I. F. and Olsen, E. G. (1973). Löffler's endocarditis and Davies' endomyocardial fibrosis. *Am. Heart. J.* **85**, 308–22. [p. 233]
210. Brockington, I. F., Olsen, E. G., and Goodwin, J. F. (1967). Endomyocardial fibrosis in European resident in tropical Africa. *Lancet* **1**, 583–8.[p. 249, 255]
211. Brogadir, S. P., Goldwein, M. I., and Schumacher, H. R. (1980). A hypereosinophilic syndrome mimicking rheumatoid arthritis. *Am. J. Med.* **69**, 799–802. [p. 177]
212. Brostoff, J., Craig, O., and Everest, M. (1970). Eosinophilic gastro-enteritis. *Br. J. Surg.* **57**, 653–7. [p. 184]
213. Broudy, V. C., Kaushansky, K., Harlan, J. M., and Adamson, J. W. (1987). Interleukin 1 stimulates human endothelial cells to produce granulocyte-macrophage colony-stimulating factor and granulocyte colony-stimulating factor. *J. Immunol.* **139**. 464–08. [p. 109, 164]
214. Broustet, A., Bernard, P., Dachary, D., David, B., Marit, G., Lacombe, F., Issanchou, A. M., and Reiffers, J. (1986). Acute eosinophilic leukemia with a translocation (10p+; 11q−). *Cancer Genet. Cytogenet.* **21**, 327–33. [p. 156]
215. Brown, J. P., Rola Pleszczynski, M., and Menard, H. A. (1986). Eosinophilic synovitis: clinical observations on a newly recognized subset of patients with dermatographism. *Arthritis Rheum.* **29**, 1147–51. [p. 178]
216. Brown, L. F., Goldman, H., and Antonioli, D. A. (1984). Intraepithelial eosinophils in endoscopic biopsies of adults with reflux esophagitis. *Am. J. Surg. Pathol.* **8**, 899–905. [p. 184]
217. Brown, R. D., Yuen, E., Rickard, K. A., and Kronenberg, H. (1987). Persisting colonies in agar cultures containing serum from patients with CML in blastic transformation. *Leuk. Res.* **11**, 545–7. [p. 23]
218. Brown, S. J., Galli, S. J., Gleich, G. J., and Askenase, P. W. (1982). Ablation of immunity to Amblyomma americanum by anti-basophil serum: cooperation between basophils and eosinophils in expression of immunity to ectoparasites (ticks) in guinea pigs. *J. Immunol.* **129**, 790–6. [p. 84]
219. Brown, T. R. (1898). Studies on trichinosis with especial reference to the

increase of the eosinophilic cells in the blood and muscle, the origin of these cells and their diagnostic importance. *J. Exp. Med.* **3**, 315–47. [p. 4, 5]

220. Bruijnzeel, P. L., de Monchy, J. G., Verhagen, J., and Kauffman, H. F. (1986). The eosinophilic granulocyte an active participant in the late phase asthmatic reaction? *Bull. Eur. Physiopathol. Respir.* **22** Suppl 7, 54–61. [p. 69, 70, 71, 200]
221. Bruijnzeel, P. L., Hamelink, M. L., Prins, K., Remmert, G., and Meyling, F. H. (1987). Blood lumphocyte subpopulations in extrinsic and intrinsic asthmatics. *Ann. Allergy* **58**, 179–82. [p. 197]
222. Bruynzeel Koomen, C., van Wichen, D. F., Spry, C. J., Venge, P., and Bruynzeel, P. (1988). Active participation of eosinophils in patch test reactions to inhalant allergens in patients with atopic dermatitis. *Br. J. Dermatol.*, **118**, 229–38. [p. 299]
223. Bruynzeel, P. L., Koenderman, L., Kok, P. T., Hameling, M. L., and Verhagen, J. (1986). Platelet-activating factor (PAF-acether) induced leukotriene C4 formation and luminol dependent chemiluminescence by human eosinophils. *Pharmacol Res Commun* **18** Suppl, 61–9. [p. 71]
224. Bruynzeel, P. L., Kok, P. T., Vietor, R. J., and Verhagen, J. (1985). On the optimal conditions of LTC4 formation by human eosinophils in vitro. *Prostaglandins Leukotrienes Med.* **20**, 11–22. [p. 70]
225. Bryant. D. H., and Kay, A. B. (1977). Cutaneous eosinophil accumulation in atopic and non-atopic individuals: the effect of an ECF-A tetrapeptide and histamine. *Clin. Allergy* **7**, 211–7. [p. 99]
226. Bryceson, A. D. M. Ed. (1980). The eosinophil in tropical disease. *Trans. R. Soc. Trop. Med. Hyg.* **74** Suppl., 1–63. [p. 322]
227. Buckley, R. H., Wray, B. B., and Belmaker, E. B. (1972). Extreme hyperimmunoglobulinemia E and undue susceptibility to infection. *Pediatrics* **49**, 59–70. [p. 316]
228. Buddecke, E., Essellier, A. F., and Marti, H. R. (1956). Uber die chemische Natur der Charcot–Leydenschen Kristalle. *Z. Physiol. Chem. (Hoppe Seyler)* **305**, 203–6. [p. 64]
229. Bujak, J. S. and Root, R. K. (1974). The role of peroxidase in the bactericidal activity of human blood eosinophils. *Blood* **43**, 727–36. [p. 89]
230. Bullock, W. E., Artz, R. P., Bhathena, D., and Tung, K. S. (1979). Histoplasmosis. Association with circulating immune complexes, eosinophilia, and mesangiopathic glomerulonephritis. *Arch. Intern. Med.* **139**, 700–2. [p. 133]
231. Bunnag, C., Pacharee, P., Vipulakom, P., and Siriyananda, C. (1983). A study of allergic factor in nasal polyp patients. *Ann. Allergy* **50**, 126–32. [p. 214]
232. Burgess, A. W., Begley, C. G., Johnson, G. R., Lopez, A. F., Williamson, D. J., Mermod, J. J., Simpson, R. J., Schmitz, A., and DeLamarter, J. F. (1987). Purification and properties of bacterially synthesized human granulocyte-macrophage colony stimulating factor. *Blood* **69**, 43–51. [p. 21]
233. Burgess, A. W., Cruise, K. M., Mitchell, G. F., and Watt, S. M. (1980). Preparation and surface labeling of murine eosinophils. *Exp. Hematol.* **8**, 108–9. [p. 75]
234. Burkle, W. S. (1979). Allopurinol hypersensitivity. *Drug Intell. Clin. Pharm.* **130**, 218–23. [p. 308]

235. Burns, C. P. and Hoak, J. C. (1975). Freeze-etch studies of the granules of human mast-cells and eosinophils. *J. Ultrastruct. Res.* **50**, 143–9. [p. 75]

236. Bush, M., Custer, R. S., Whitla, J. C., and Smith, E. E. (1982). Hematologic values of captive golden lion tamarins (Leontopithecus rosalia): variations with sex, age, and health status. *Lab. Anim. Sci.* **32**, 294–7. [p. 126]

237. Bush, R. K., Geller, M., Busse, W. W., Flaherty, D. K., and Dickie, H. A. (1978). Response to corticosteroids in the hypereosinophilic syndrome. Association with increased serum IgE levels. *Arch. Intern. Med.* **138**, 1244–6. [p. 177, 290]

238. Bushkell, L. L. and Jordon, R. E. (1983). Bullous pemphigoid: a cause of peripheral blood eosinophilia. *J. Am. Acad. Dermatol.* **8**, 648–51. [p. 303]

239. Businco, L., Di Fazio, A., Ziruolo, M. G., Boner, A. L., Valletta, E. A., Ruco, L. P., Vitolo, D., Ensoli, B., and Paganelli, R. (1987). Clinical and immunological findings in four infants with Omenn's syndrome: a form of severe combined immunodeficiency with phenotypically normal T cells, elevated IgE, and eosinophilia. *Clin. Immunol. Immunopathol.* **44**, 123–33. [p. 166]

240. Butland, R. J. and Coulson, I. H. (1985). Pulmonary eosinophilia associated with cutaneous larva migrans. *Thorax* **40**, 76–7. [p. 144]

241. Butler, T. W., Feintuch, T. A., and Caine, W. P. Jr. (1985). Eosinophilic cholangitis, lymphadenopathy, and peripheral eosinophilia: a case report. *Am. J. Gastroenterol.* **80**, 572–4. [p. 191]

242. Butterfield, J. H., Ackerman, S. J., Scott, R. E., Pierre, R. V., and Gleich, G. J. (1984). Evidence for secretion of human eosinophil granule major basic protein and Charcot–Leyden crystal protein during eosinophil maturation. *Exp. Hematol.* **12**, 163–70. [p. 13]

243. Butterfield, J. H., Ackerman, S. J., Weiler, D., Eisenbrey, A. B., and Gleich, G. J. (1986). Effects of glucocorticoids on eosinophil colony growth. *J. Allergy Clin. Immunol.* **78** (3 Pt 1), 450–7. [p. 28]

244. Butterfield, J. H., Eisenbrey, A. B., and Gleich, G. J. (1982). Membrane marker characterization of the eosinophil colony-forming cell. *Br. J. Haematol.* **51**, 209–16. [p. 16]

245. Butterfield, J. H., Kephart, G. M., Banks, P. M., and Gleich, G. J. (1986). Extracellular deposition of eosinophil granule major basic protein in lymph nodes of patients with Hodgkin's disease. *Blood* **68**, 1250–6. [p. 163]

246. Butterfield, J. H., Maddox, D. E., and Gleich, G. J. (1983–84). The eosinophil leukocyte: maturation and function. *Clin. Immunol. Rev.* **2**, 187–306. [p. 115, 325]

247. Butterfield, J. H. and Weiler, D. (1986). Giant eosinophil colonies from cultures of bone marrow cells. *In Vitro Cell Dev. Biol.* **22**, 157–63. [p. 17]

248. Butterworth, A. E. (1977). The eosinophil and its role in immunity to helminth infection. *Curr. Top. Microbiol. Immunol.* **77**, 127–68. [p. 323]

249. Butterworth, A. E. (1984). Cell-mediated damage to helminths. *Adv. Parasitol.* **23**, 143–235. [p. 112, 325]

250. Butterworth, A. E., Bensted Smith, R., Capron, A., Capron, M., Dalton, P. R., Dunne, D. W., Grzych, J. M., Kariuki, H. C., Khalife, J., Koech, D., et al. (1987). Immunity in human schistosomiasis mansoni: prevention by blocking antibodies of the expression of immunity in young children. *Parasitology* **94**, 281–300. [p. 148]

251. Butterworth, A. E., Capron, M., Cordingley, J. S., Dalton, P. R., Dunne, D. W., Kariuki, H. C., Kimani, G., Koech, D., Mugambi, M., Ouma, J. H., Prentice, M. A., Richardson, B. A., Arap Siongkok, T. K., Sturrock, R. F., and Taylor, D. W. (1985). Immunity after treatment of human schistosomiasis mansoni. II. Identification of resistant individuals, and analysis of their immune responses. *Trans. R. Soc. Trop. Med. Hyg.* **79**, 393–408. [p. 148]

252. Butterworth, A. E. and David, J. R. (1981). Eosinophil function. *N. Engl. J. Med.* **304**, 154–6. [p. 324]

253. Butterworth, A. E. and Richardson, B. A. (1985). Factors affecting the levels of antibody- and complement-dependent eosinophil-mediated damage to schistosomula of Schistosoma mansoni in vitro. *Parasite Immunol.* **7**, 119–31. [p. 114]

254. Butterworth, A. E., Sturrock, R. F., and Houba, V. (1974). Antibody-dependent cell-mediated damage to schistosomula in vitro. *Nature* **252**, 503–5. [p. 114]

255. Butterworth, A. E., Sturrock, R. F., Houba, V., Mahmoud, A. A., Sher, A., and Rees, P. H. (1975). Eosinophils as mediators of antibody-dependent damage to schistosomula. *Nature* **256**, 727–9. [p. 8, 111]

256. Butterworth, A. E., Vadas, M. A., Wassom, D. L., Dessein, A., Hogan, M., Sherry, B., Gleich, G. J., and David, J. R. (1979). Interactions between human eosinophils and schistosomula of Schistosoma mansoni. II. The mechanism of irreversible eosinophil adherence. *J. Exp. Med.* **150**, 1456–71. [p. 112]

257. Butterworth, A. E., Wassom, D. L., Gleich, G. J., Loegering, D. A., and David, J. R. (1979). Damage to schistosomula of Schistosoma mansoni induced directly by eosinophil major basic protein. *J. Immunol.* **122**, 221–9. [p. 47, 113, 115]

258. Buurman, W. A., Vegt, P. A., Groenewegen, G., van der Linden, C. J., and Jeunhomme, G. M. (1982). Analysis of buoyant density of canine peripheral blood leukocytes with PVP-Silica (Percoll) density gradients. *Vet. Immunol. Immunopathol.* **3**, 547–56. [p. 125]

259. Buys, J., Wever, R., and Ruitenberg, E. J. (1984). Myeloperoxidase is more efficient than eosinophil peroxidase in the *in vitro* killing of newborn larvae of Trichinella spiralis. *Immunology* **51**, 601–7. [p. 47, 60]

260. Calame, J. J., van t Wout, J. W., van Dijk, J. G., and Bots, G. T. (1986). A case of eosinophilic meningo-encephalitis accompanied by eosinophilic inflammation of the myenteric plexus in Hodgkin's disease. *Histopathology* **10**, 535–9. [p. 216]

261. Calvo, F., Dresch, C., Zittoun, J., Boiron, M., and Bernard, J. (1987). Cyclical eosinophilia: a case report of a non-malignant disorder with abnormal regulation of eosinophil production and maturation. Submitted. [p. 301]

262. Cameron, J., Radford, D. J., Howell, J., and O Brien, M. F. (1985). Hypereosinophilic heart disease. *Med. J. Aust.* **143**, 408–10. [p. 235]

263. Campbell, E. W. and Beals, C. (1977). Striking eosinophil in sparganosis. *Postgrad Med* **62**, 138–40. [p.137]

264. Campbell, H. D., Tucker, W. Q., Hort, Y., Martinson, M. E., Mayo, G., Clutterbuck, E. J., Sanderson, C. J., and Young, I. G. (1987). Molecular cloning, nucleotide sequence, and expression of the gene encoding human

eosinophil differentiation factor (interleukin 5). *Proc. Natl. Acad. Sci. USA.* **84**, 6629–33. [p. 19]

265 Candell Riera, J., Permanyer Miralda, G., and Soler Soler, J. (1982). Echocardiographic findings in endomyocardial fibrosis. *Chest* **82**, 88–90. [p. 251]

266. Canon, P. (1892). Über eosinophile Zellen und Mastzellen im Blute Gesunder und Kranker. *Dtsch. Med. Wochenschr.* **10**, 206. [p. 5]

267. Capron, A., Dessaint, J. P., Capron, M., Joseph, M., Amiesen, J. C., and Tonnel, A. B. (1986). From parasites to allergy: the second receptor for IgE (FcεR2). *Immunol. Today* **7**, 15–18. [p. 79]

268. Capron, M., Bazin, H., Joseph, M., and Capron, A. (1981). Evidence for IgE-dependent cytotoxicity by rat eosinophils. *J. Immunol.* **126.**, 1764–8. [p. 80]

269. Capron, M. and Capron, A. (1987). The IgE receptor of human eosinophils. In *Allergy and inflammation* (Ed. A. B. Kay) pp. 151–9. Academic Press, London. [p. 79, 80, 81, 326]

270. Capron, M., Capron, A., Dessaint, J. P., Torpier, G., Johansson, S. G., and Prin, L. (1981). Fc receptors for IgE on human and rat eosinophils. *J. Immunol.* **126**, 2087–92. [p. 79]

271. Capron, M., Capron, A., Goetzl, E. J., and Austen, K. F. (1981). Tetrapeptides of the eosinophil chemotactic factor of anaphylaxis (ECF-A) enhance eosinophil Fc receptor. *Nature* **289**, 71–3 [p. 78, 120]

272. Capron, M. and Jouault, T. (1986). IgE receptors on human eosinophils and eosinophil heterogeneity. *Ann. Inst. Pasteur Immunol.* **137C**, 371–4. [p. 80]

273. Capron, M., Jouault, T., Prin, L., Joseph, M., Ameisen, J. C., Butterworth, A. E., Papin, J. P., Kusnierz, J. P., and Capron, A. (1986). Functional study of a monoclonal antibody to IgE Fc receptor (FcεR2) of eosinophils, platelets, and macrophages. *J. Exp. Med.* **164**, 72–89. [p. 79]

274. Capron, M., Kazatchkine, M. D., Fischer, E., Joseph, M., Butterworth, A. E., Kusnierz, J. P., Prin, L., Papin, J. P., and Capron, A. (1987). Functional role of the alpha-chain of complement receptor type 3 in human eosinophil-dependent antibody-mediated cytotoxicity against schistosomes. *J. Immunol.* **139**, 2059–65. [p. 79]

275. Capron, M., Kusnierz, J. P., Prin, L., Spiegelberg, H. L., Khalife, J., Tonnel, A. B., and Capron, A. (1985). Cytophilic IgE on human blood and tissue eosinophils. *Int. Arch. Allergy. Appl. Immunol.* **77** (1–2), 246–8. [p. 79]

276. Capron, M., Kusnierz, J. P., Prin, L., Spiegelberg, H. L., Ovlaque, G., Gosset, P., Tonnel, A. B., and Capron, A. (1985). Cytophilic IgE on human blood and tissue eosinophils: detection by flow microfluorometry. *J. Immunol.* **134,** 3013–8. [p. 79, 80]

277. Capron, M., Spiegelberg, H. L., Prin, L., Bennich, H., Butterworth, A. E., Pierce, R. J., Ouaissi, M. A., and Capron, A. (1984). Role of IgE receptors in effector function of human eosinophils. *J. Immunol.* **132**, 462–8. [p. 80, 81]

278. Carey, J. P. and Burke, A. C. (1982). Transient hypereosinophilia in the infant of a mother with hypereosinophilic syndrome (letter). *Arch. Intern. Med.* **142**, 1754–5. [p. 266]

279. Carlisle, R., Ogunba, E. O., McFarlane, H., Onayemi, O. A., and Oyeleye,

V. O. (1972). Immunoglobulins and antibody to Loa loa in Nigerians with endomyocardial fibrosis and other heart diseases. *Br. Heart J.* **34**, 678–80. [p. 255]

280. Carlson, M. G., Peterson, C. G., and Venge, P. (1985). Human eosinophil peroxidase: purification and characterization. *J. Immunol.* **134**, 1875–9. [p. 58, 59]
281. Carrington, C., Addington, W., Goff, A., Madoff, L., Marks, A., Schwaber, J., and Gaensler, E. (1969). Chronic eosinophilic pneumonia. *N. Engl. J. Med.* **280**, 787–98. [p. 206, 207]
282. Carroll, S. M. and Grove, D. I. (1986). Response of dogs to challenge with Ancylostoma ceylanicum during the tenure of a primary hookworm infection. *Trans. R. Soc. Trop. Med. Hyg.* **80**, 406–11. [p. 144]
283. Carroll, S. M. and Grove, D. I. (1986). Experimental infection of humans with Ancylostoma ceylanicum: clinical, parasitological, haematological and immunological findings. *Trop. Geogr. Med.* **38**, 38–45. [p. 144]
284. Carvalho, F. R, Matos, S., Victor, E. G., Saraiva, L., Brindeiro Filho, D., Maranhao, E., and Moraes, C. R. (1984). Phonomechanocardiographic findings in endomyocardial fibrosis. *Angiology* **35**, 63–70. [p. 234]
285. Casley Smith, J. R. (1968). Transformation of the granules of intestinal eosinophilic polymorphonuclear leukocytes by helminthic infestation. *J. Path. Bact.* **95**, 299–301. [p. 111]
286. Casslen, B., Kobayashi, T. K., and Stormby, N. (1982). Cyclic variation of the cellular components in human uterine fluid. *J. Reprod. Fertil.* **66**, 213–18. [p. 226]
287. Castells, M. C., Irani, A. M., and Schwartz, L. B. (1987). Evaluation of human peripheral blood leukocytes for mast cell tryptase. *J. Immunol.* **138**, 2184–9. [p. 45]
288. Castro Garcia, M., Posada, M., Diaz de Rojas, F., Abaitua Borda, I., and Tabuenca Oliver, J. M. (1986). Hypercoagulable states and the toxic oil syndrome (letter). *Ann. Intern. Med.* **104**, 730. [p. 182]
289. Catovsky, D., Bernasconi, C., Verdonck, P. J., Postma, A., Hows, J., van der Does van den Berg, A., Rees, J. K., Castelli, G., Morra, E., and Galton, D. A. (1980). The association of eosinophilia with lymphoblastic leukaemia or lymphoma: a study of seven patients. *Br. J. Haematol.* **45**, 523–34. [p. 161]
290. Caulfield, J. P., Korman, G., Butterworth, A. E., Hogan, M., and David, J. R. (1980). The adherence of human neutrophils and eosinophils to schistosomula: evidence for membrane fusion between cells and parasites. *J. Cell. Biol.* **86**, 46–63. [p. 115]
291. Caulfield, J. P., Korman, G., Butterworth, A. E., Hogan, M., and David, J. R. (1980). Partial and complete detachment of neutrophils and eosinophils from schistosomula: evidence for the establishment of continuity between a fused and normal parasite membrane. *J. Cell Biol.* **86**, 64–76. [p. 115]
292. Caulfield, J. P., Lenzi, H. L., Elsas, P., and Dessein, A. J. (1985). Ultrastructure of the attack of eosinophils stimulated by blood mononuclear cell products on schistosomula of Schistosoma mansoni. *Am. J. Pathol.* **120**, 380–90. [p. 107]
293. Cazzadori, A., Braggio, P., and Bontempini, L. (1985). Salazopyrin-induced eosinophilic pneumonia. *Respiration* **47**, 158–60. [p. 309]

294. Cello, J. P. (1979). Eosinophilic gastroenteritis – a complex disease entity. *Am. J. Med.* **67**, 1097–104. [p. 183, 184]

295. Cervantes, F., Montserrat, E., and Rozman, C. (1979). Eosinophilic meningitis in Hodgkin's disease (letter). *Ann. Intern. Med.* **91**, 930. [p. 216]

296. Chaine, G., Davies, J., Kohner, E. M., Hawarth, S., and Spry, C. J., (1982). Ophthalmologic abnormalities in the hypereosinophilic syndrome. *Ophthalmology* **89**, 1348–56. [p. 271, 275]

297. Challacombe, D. N., Wheeler, E. E., and Campbell, P. E. (1986). Morphometric studies and eosinophil cell counts in the duodenal mucosa of children with chronic nonspecific diarrhoea and cow's milk allergy. *J. Pediatr. Gastroenterol. Nutr.* **5**, 887–91. [p. 188]

298. Chambers, W. H., Washburn, S. M., Campos, M., and Klesius, P. H. (1985). Isolation of bovine eosinophils by density gradient centrifugation. *Am. J. Vet. Res.* **46**, 154–6. [p. 125]

299. Chamone, D. F., Fujimura, A. Y., and Jamra, M. (1986). Increased levels of eosinophil-derived PAF-acether activity in a patient with idiopathic hypereosinophilic syndrome. *Braz. J. Med. Biol. Res.* **19**, 135–6. [p. 282]

300. Chan, H. L., Ku, G., and Khoo, O. T. (1977). Allopurinol associated hypersensitivity reactions: cutaneous and renal manifestations. *Aust. N.Z. J. Med.* **7**, 518–22. [p. 311]

301. Chan, P. C., Hayes, L., and Bain, B. J. (1985). A comparison of the white cell counts of cord blood from babies of different ethnic origins. *Ann. Trop. Paediatr.* **5**, 153–5. [p. 294]

302. Chanalet, G. and Chastel, F. (1964). Un cas de meningite a pneumocoques avec eosinophilie rachidienne. *Medicine Tropicale* **24**, 203–5. [p. 216]

303. Chandler, M. J., Grammer, L. C., and Patterson, R. (1986). Eosinophilic vasculitis with atypical features (clinical conference). *J. Allergy Clin. Immunol.* **77**, 741–5. [p. 231]

304. Chandran, P. K., Humayun, H. M., Daugirdas, J. T., Nawab, Z. M., Gandhi, V. C., and Ing, T. S. (1985). Blood eosinophilia in patients undergoing maintenance peritoneal dialysis. *Arch. Intern. Med.* **145**, 114–16. [p. 221]

305. Chapman, J. S. and Clark, J. (1968). Components of fungi in relation to eosinophilia. *Am. Rev. Respir. Dis.* **97**, 399–405. [p. 132]

306. Charcot, J. M. and Robin, C. (1853). Observation de Leucocythemie. *C. R. Mem. Soc. Biol.* **5**, 44–50. [p. 64]

307. Charnoff, S. K. (1985). Radiology notes. Case 1. Eosinophilic granuloma of the spine. *Mt. Sinai J. Med. (NY)* **52**, 133–5. [p. 165]

308. Chen, H. P. and Smith, H. S. (1960). Eosinophilic leukemia. *Ann. Intern. Med.* **52**, 1343–52. [p. 151, 277, 279]

309. Chen, K. T. and Marsh, H. H. (1984). Philadelphia chromosome-negative chronic myelogenous leukemia with prominent eosinophilic component. *Am. J. Clin. Pathol.* **81**, 789–91. [p. 159]

310. Cherian, G., Vijayaraghavan, G., Krishnaswami, S., Sukumar, I. P., John, S., Jairaj, P. S., and Bhaktaviziam A. (1983). Endomyocardial fibrosis: report on the hemodynamic data in 29 patients and review of the results of surgery. *Am. Heart. J.* **105**, 659–66. [p. 234, 252]

311. Cherian, K. M., John, T. A., and Abraham, K. A. (1983). Endomyocardial fibrosis: clinical profile and role of surgery in management. *Am. Heart J.* **105**, 706–9. [p. 254]

312. Chervenick, P. A. and Boggs, D. R. (1971). In vitro growth of granulocytic and mononuclear cell colonies from blood of normal individuals. *Blood* **37**, 131–5. [p. 8, 15]
313. Chesney, J. C., Hoganson, G. E., and Wilson, M. H. (1980). CSF eosinophilia during an acute coxsackie B4 viral meningitis. *Am. J. Dis. Child.* **134**, 703. [p. 135, 216]
314. Chester, A. C., Diamond, L. H., and Schreiner, G. E. (1978). Hypersensitivity to salicylazosulfapyridine: renal and hepatic toxic reactions. *Arch. Intern. Med.* **138**, 1138–9. [p. 309]
315. Chi, E. Y. and Henderson, W. R. (1984). Ultrastructure of mast cell degranulation induced by eosinophil peroxidase: use of diaminobenzidine cytochemistry by scanning electron microscopy. *J. Histochem. Cytochem.* **32**, 337–41. [p. 60]
316. Chihara, J., Kino, T., Yashuba, H., Furue, M., Fukuda K., Izumi, T., and Oshima, S. Increases of pulmonary hypodense eosinophils and eosinophils with hypersegmented nuclei in patients with PIE syndrome (abstract). Presented to the 6th International Congress of Immunology, Toronto, Canada, 1986. [p. 35, 40]
317. Christensen, R. D. and Hill, H. R. (1987). Exercise-induced changes in the blood concentration of leukocyte populations in teenage athletes. *Am. J. Pediatr. Hematol. Oncol.* **9**, 140–2. [p. 31]
318. Christensen, W. N. and Hutchins, G. M. (1985). Hypereosinophilic mucoid impaction of bronchi in two children under two years of age. *Pediatr. Pulmonol.* **1**, 278–80. [p. 133]
319. Chudwin, D. S., Ammann, A. J., Wara, D. W., Cowan, M. J., and Phibbs, R. H. (1982). Posttransfusion syndrome: rash, eosinophilia, and thrombocytopenia following intrauterine and exchange transfusions. *Am. J. Dis. Child.* **136**, 612–4. [p. 295]
320. Chumbley, L. C., Harrison, E. G. Jr., and DeRemee, R. A. (1977). Allergic granulomatosis and angiitis (Churg-Strauss syndrome): report and analysis of 30 cases. *Mayo Clin. Proc.* **52**, 477–84. [p. 203]
321. Church, J. A., Wang, D. W., Swanson, V., Thomas, D., and Sinatra, F. (1978). Cow's milk allergy in a premature infant with hypereosinophilia and hyperimmunoglobulinemia E. *Ann. Allergy* **41**, 307–10. [p. 189, 224]
322. Churg, A. (1983). Pulmonary angiitis and granulomatosis revisited. *Hum. Pathol.* **14**, 868–83. [p. 209]
323. Churg, J. and Strauss, L. (1951). Allergic granulomatosis, allergic angiitis, and periarteritis nodosa. *Am. J. Pathol.* **27**, 277–301. [p. 202]
324. Chusid, M. J. and Dale, D. C. (1975). Eosinophilic leukemia: remission with vincristine and hydroxyurea. *Am. J. Med.* **59**, 297–9. [p. 157]
325. Chusid, M. J., Dale, D. C., West, B. C., and Wolff, S. M. (1975). The hypereosinophilic syndrome: analysis of fourteen cases with review of the literature. *Medicine (Baltimore)* **54**, 1–27. [p. 7, 263, 265, 266, 268, 270, 273, 276, 300, 323]
326. Citino, S. B., Bush, M., Phillips, L. G., Montali, R. J., Wang, K. P., and Ravich, W. J. (1985). Eosinophilic enterocolitis in a juvenile orangutan. *J. Am. Vet. Med. Assoc.* **187**, 1279–80. [p. 190]
327. Clark, G. M., Valentine, E., and Blount, S. G. (1956). Endocardial fibrosis

simulating constrictive pericarditis: report of a case with determinations of pressure in the right side of the heart and eosinophilia. *N. Engl. J. Med.* **254**, 349–55. [p. 240]

328. Clark, R. A., Gallin, J. I., and Kaplan, A. P. (1975). The selective eosinophil chemotactic activity of histamine. *J. Exp. Med.* **142**, 1462–76. [p. 283]
329. Clark, R. A., Sandler, J. A., Gallin, J. I., and Kaplan, A. P. (1977). Histamine modulation of eosinophil migration. *J. Immunol.* **118**, 137–45. [p. 100]
330. Claudatus, J. C. Jr, d Ovidio, R., Lospalluti, M., and Meneghini, C. L. (1986). Skin tumors and reactive cellular infiltrate: further studies. *Acta Derm. Venereol (Stockh)* **66**, 29–34. [p. 173]
331. Clement, L. T., Lehmeyer, J. E., and Gartland, G. L. (1983). Identification of neutrophil subpopulations with monoclonal antibodies. *Blood* **61**, 26–32. [p. 85]
332. Cline, M. J. and Golde, D. W. (1979). Cellular interactions in haematopoiesis. *Nature* **277**, 177–81. [p. 12]
333. Cluzel, M., Damon, M., Chanez, P., Bousquet, J., Crastes de Paulet, A., Michel, F. B., and Godard, P. (1987). Enhanced alveolar cell luminol-dependent chemiluminescence in asthma. *J. Allergy Clin. Immunol.* **80**, 195–201. [p. 199]
334. Cofrancesco, E., Cortellaro, M., Pogliani, E., Boschetti, C., Salvatore, M., and Polli, E. E. (1984). Response to vincristine treatment in a case of idiopathic hypereosinophilic syndrome with multiple clinical manifestations. *Acta Haematol. (Basel)* **72**, 21–5. [p. 270, 291]
335. Cohen, G. A., MacPherson, G. A., Golembesky, H. E., Jalowayski, A. A., and O'Connor, R. D. (1985). Normal nasal cytology in infancy. *Ann. Allergy* **54**, 112–14. [p. 213]
336. Cohen, J., Davies, J., Goodwin, J. F., and Spry, C. J. (1980). Arrhythmias in patients with hypereosinophilia: a comparison of patients with and without Löffler's endomyocardial disease. *Postgrad. Med. J.* **56**, 828–32. [p. 238]
337. Cohen, J. and Spry, C. J. (1979). Strongyloides stercoralis infection and small intestinal lymphoma. *Parasite Immunol.* **1**, 167–78, [p. 171]
338. Cohen, M. S., Jaques, P. F., Wall, S. D., and Walker, D. H. (1983). A fatal eosinophilic process in a Laotian refugee. *Am. J. Clin. Pathol.* **80**, 738–43. [p. 187]
339. Cohen, S. G. and Ottesen, E. A. (1983). The eosinophil, eosinophilia, and eosinophil-related disorders. In *Allergy. Principles and Practice.* 2nd Edition (eds. E. Middleton Jr, C. E. Reed and E. F. Ellis), pp. 701–69. C. V. Mosby Co., New York. [p. 324]
340. Coimbra, A. and Lopes Vaz, A. (1971). The presence of lipid droplets and the absence of stable sudanophilia in osmium-fixed human leukocytes. *J. Histochem. Cytochem.* **19**, 551–9. [p. 40]
341. Colby, T. V. and Lombard, C. (1983). Histiocytosis X in the lung. *Hum. Pathol.* **14**, 847–56. [p. 211]
342. Colley, D. G. (1973). Eosinophils and immune mechanisms: I. Eosinophil stimulation promoter (ESP); a lymphokine induced by specific antigen or phytohaemagglutinin. *J. Immunol.* **110**, 1419–23. [p. 18, 100]
343. Colley, D. G. (1976). Eosinophils and immune mechanisms: IV. Culture conditions, antigen requirements, production kinetics and immunologic spec-

ificity of the lymphokine eosinophil stimulation promoter. *Cell Immunol.* **24**, 328–35. [p. 100]

344. Colley, D. G., Stewart, S. J., Duncan, E. K., and Secor, W. E. (1986). The role of the eosinophil in host defense. In *Leukocytes and host defense* (eds. Oppenheim and Jacobs), pp. 357–64. Arnold Liss, New York. [p. 325]
345. Colon, A. R., Sorkin, L. F., Stern, W. R., Lessinger, V. S., Hefter, L. G. and Hodin, E. (1983). Eosinophilic gastroenteritis. *J. Pediatr Gastroenterol. Nutr.* **2**, 187–9. [p. 184]
346. Colton, A. S., Schachner, L., and Kowalczyk, A. P. (1986). Eosinophilic pustular folliculitis. *J. Am. Acad. Dermatol.* **14**, 469–74. [p. 304]
347. Connell, J. T. (1969). Abnormal eosinophils, eosinophilia and basophilia in methimazole neutropenia. *Ann. Allergy* **27**, 595–602. [p. 314]
348. Connor, D. H., George, G. H., and Gibson, D. W. (1985). Pathologic changes of human onchocerciasis: implications for future research. *Rev. Infect. Dis.* **7**, 809–19. [p. 143]
349. Connor, D. H., Palmieri, J. R., and Gibson, D. W. (1986). Pathogenesis of lymphatic filariasis in man. *Z. Parasitenkd.* **72**, 13–28. [p. 141]
350. Connor, D. H., Somers, K., Hutt, M. S., Manion, W. C., and d'Arbela, P. C. (1967). Endomyocardial fibrosis in Uganda (Davies' disease): an epidemiologic, clinical and pathologic study. Part I. *Am. Heart. J.* **74**, 687–709. [p. 256]
351. Connor, D. H., Somers, K., Hutt, M. S., Manion, W. C., and d'Arbela, P. C. (1968). Endomyocardial fibrosis in Uganda (Davies' disease): an epidemiologic, clinical and pathologic study. Part II. *Am. Heart J.* **75**, 107–24. [p. 256]
352. Conrad, K. A., Gross, J. L., and Trojanowski, J. Q. (1986). Leptomeningeal carcinomatosis presenting as eosinophilic meningitis. *Acta Cytol. (Baltimore)* **30**, 29–31. [p. 217]
353. Contamin, F., Bantman, C., Lancastre, L., Koubi, G., and Strul, J. (1972). Hypereosinophilie sanguine et eosinophilie du L.C.R. accompagnant l'evolution d'un glioblastome cerebral. *Ann. Med. Interne* **123**, 895–9. [p. 172]
354. Cook, R. M., Ashworth, R. F., and Musgrove, N. R. (1987). Eosinophil- and neutrophil-mediated injury of human lung fibroblast cells. *Int. Arch. Allergy Appl. Immunol.* **83**, 428–31. [p. 118]
355. Cook, R. M., Musgrove, N. R., and Ashworth, R. F. (1987). Activity of rat peritoneal eosinophils following induction by different methods. *Int. Arch. Allergy Appl. Immunol.* **83**, 423–7. [p. 105, 127]
356. Cook, R. M. and Smith, H. Ability of drugs to affect the activity of rat peritoneal eosinophils and neutrophils *in vitro* (abstract). Presented to the 6th International Congress of Immunology, Toronto, Canada, 1986. [p. 95]
357. Cooney, T. P. (1981). Interrelationship of chronic eosinophilic pneumonia, bronchiolitis obliterans, and rheumatoid disease: a hypothesis. *J. Clin. Pathol.* **34**, 129–37. [p. 177]
358. Cooper, D. K., Cleland, W. P., and Bentall, H. H. (1978). Collagen diseases as a cause of constrictive pericarditis. *Thorax* **33**, 368–71. [p. 228]
359. Corwin, H. L., and Haber, M. H. (1987). The clinical significance of eosinophiluria. *Am. J. Clin. Pathol.* **33**, [p. 224]
360. Corwin, H. L., Korbet, S. M., and Schwartz, M. M. (1985). Clinical correlates of eosinophiluria. *Arch. Intern. Med.* **145**, 1097–9. [p. 224]
361. Cotran, R. S., Gimbrone, M. A. Jr, Bevilacqua, M. P., Mendrick, D. L.,

and Pober, J. S. (1986). *In situ* induction and detection of a human endothelial cell activation antigen in immunologic inflammation (abstract). *Fed. Proc.* **45**, 379. [p. 98]

362. Cotran, R. S. and Litt, M. (1969). The entry of granule-associated peroxidase into the phagocytic vacuoles of eosinophils. *J. Exp. Med.* **129**, 1291–9. [p. 90]
363. Couto, C. G. (1984). Tumor-associated eosinophilia in a dog. *J. Am. Vet. Med. Assoc.* **184**, 837. [p. 175]
364. Crabtree, J. E. and Wilson, R. A. (1984). Schistosoma mansoni: cellular reactions to challenge infections in the cheek pouch skin of chronically infected Chinese hamsters. *Parasitology* **89**, 59–69. [p. 126]
365. Cramer, R., Soranzo, M. R., Dri, P., Menegazzi, R., Pitotti, A., Zabucchi, G., and Patriarca, P., (1984). A simple reliable assay for myeloperoxidase activity in mixed neutrophil-eosinophil cell suspensions: application to detection of myeloperoxidase deficiency. *J. Immunol. Methods* **70**, 119–25. [p. 59]
366. Cranendonk, E., van Gennip, A. H., Abeling, N. G., Behrendt, H., and Hart, A. A. (1985). Reference values for automated cytochemical differential count of leukocytes in children 0–16 years old: comparison with manually obtained counts from Wright-stained smears. *J. Clin. Chem. Clin. Biochem.* **23**, 663–7. [p. 30]
367. Crennan, J. M. and Van Scoy, R. E. (1986). Eosinophilic meningitis caused by Rocky Mountain spotted fever. *Am. J. Med.* **80**, 288–9. [p. 216]
368. Crisp, A. J., Armstrong, R. D., Grahame, R., and Dussek, J. E. (1982). Rheumatoid lung disease, pneumothorax, and eosinophilia. *Ann. Rheum. Dis.* **41**, 137–40. [p. 177]
369. Crofton, J. W., Livingstone, J. L., Oswald, N. C., and Roberts, A. T. M. (1952). Pulmonary eosinophilia. *Thorax* **7**, 1–35. [p. 194, 205]
370. Croker, B. P., Lee, T., and Gunnells, J. C. (1987). Clinical and pathologic features of polyarteritis nodosa and its renal-limited variant: primary crescentic and necrotizing glomerulonephritis. *Hum. Pathol.* **18**, 38–44. [p. 231]
371. Cromwell, O., Fitzharris, P., Harvey, C., Moqbel, R., Shaw, R. J., and Kay, A. B. Antigen specific IgG-dependent release of LTC4 from human eosinophils (abstract). Presented to the 6th International Congress of Immunology, Toronto, Canada, 1986. [p. 71]
372. Crosby, W. H. (1985). The hematology of hookworm disease: contribution of Bailey K. Ashford. *P. R. Health Sci. J.* **4**, 113–9. [p. 5, 143]
373. Crowley, J. P. and Myers, T. J. (1983). Humoral and cellular studies of eosinophils in reactive and myeloproliferative syndromes with marked eosinophilia. *Am. J. Clin. Pathol.* **79**, 301–5. [p. 68]
374. Cunningham, A. S. (1975). Eosinophil counts: age and sex differences. *J. Pediatr.* **87**, 426–7. [p. 31]
375. Cutts, J. H. and Krause, W. J. (1980). Leukocytes in the peripheral blood of the developing opossum. *J. Anat.* **130**, 113–20. [p. 126]
376. Czarnetzki, B. M., Meentken, J., Kolde, G., and Brocker, E. B. (1985). Morphology of the cellular infiltrate in delayed pressure urticaria. *J. Am. Acad. Dermatol.* **12**, 253–9. [p. 97, 299]
377. d'Ablaing, G. 3d. and Beck, M. (1977). Congenital neonatal eosinophilic cervicitis. *Am. J. Obstet. Gynecol.* **129**, 345–6. [p. 226]
378. Dachary, D., Bernard, P., Lacombe, F., Reiffers, J., David, B., Marit, G., Boisseau, M. R., and Broustet, A. (1986). Acute myeloid leukemia with

marrow hypereosinophilia and chromosome 16 abnormality. *Cancer Genet. Cytogenet.* **20** (3–4), 241–6. [p. 158]

379. Dahl, M. V., Greene, W. H. Jr., and Quie, P. G. (1976). Infection, dermatitis, increased IgE, and impaired neutrophil chemotaxis: a possible relationship. *Arch. Dermatol.* **112**, 1387–90. [p. 317]
380. Dahl, R., Fredens, K., and Venge, P. (1988). In vitro studies of the interaction between heparin and the eosinophil cationic protein. Submitted. [p. 53]
381. Dahl, R. and Venge, P. (1979). Enhancement of urokinase-induced plasminogen activation by the cationic protein of human eosinophil granulocytes. *Thromb. Res.* **14**, 599–608. [p. 53, 247]
382. Dahl, R., Venge, P., and Olsson, I. (1978). The content of eosinophil cationic protein in eosinophil leucocytes. Study on normal controls and patients with bronchial asthma. *Allergy* **33**, 152–4. [p. 198]
383. Dahl, R., Venge, P., and Olsson, I. (1978). Variations of blood eosinophils and eosinophil cationic protein in serum in patients with bronchial asthma: studies during inhalation challenge test. *Allergy* **33**, 211–5. [p. 198, 200]
384. Dahl, R., Venge, P., and Olsson, I. (1978). Blood eosinophil leucocytes and eosinophil cationic protein. Diurnal variation in normal subjects and patients with bronchial asthma. *Scand. J. Respir, Dis.* **59**, 323–5. [p. 198]
385. Dale, D. C., Hubert, R. T., Fauci, A. S. (1976). Eosinophil kinetics in the hypereosinophilic syndrome. *J. Lab. Clin. Med.* **87**, 487–95. [p. 284]
386. Dallocchio, M., Clementy, J., Mullen, P., Jacquinet, J. P., Bricaud, D. H., and Broustet P. (1975). Fibrose endomyocardique autochtone observee aucours d'une distomatose. *Arch. Mal. Coeur* **68**, 329–32. [p. 236]
387. Dalvi, A. N., Shenoy, S. G., Satoskar, R. R., Vora, I. M., and Candes, F. P. (1986). Eosinophilic granulomatous polyp and intussusception (a case report). *J. Postgrad. Med.* **32**, 171–2, 170B. [p. 187]
388. Danielson, B. G., Hallgren, R., and Venge, P. (1984). Neutrophil and eosinophil degranulation by hemodialysis membranes. *Contrib. Nephrol.* **37**, 83–8. [p. 222]
389. Darbyshire, P. G., and Chandler, G. N. (1984). Pleural fluid eosinophilia in association with trauma. *Br. J. Clin. Pract.* **38**, 326. [p. 212]
390. Darbyshire, P. J., Shortland, D., Swansbury, G. J., Sadler, J., Lawler, S. D., and Chessells, J. M. (1987). A myeloproliferative disease in two infants associated with eosinophilia and chromosome t(1;5) translocation. *Br. J. Haematol.* **66**, 483–6. [p. 25, 152, 156]
391. Darrow, D. and Linzer, M. (1987). Eosinophilic granuloma: I need this like a hole in the head. *N.C. Med. J.* **48**, 15–7. [p. 165]
392. Dart, J. K., Buckley, R. J., Monnickendan, M., and Prasad, J. (1986). Perennial allergic conjunctivitis: definition, clinical characteristics and prevalence: a comparison with seasonal allergic conjunctivitis. *Trans. Ophthalmol. Soc. UK.* **105**, 513–20. [p. 219]
393. Date, A., Parameswaran, A., and Bhaktaviziam, A. (1983). Renal lesions in the obliterative cardiomyopathies: endomyocardial fibrosis and Löffler's endocarditis. *J. Pathol.* **140**, 113–22. [p. 253]
394. Daugirdas, J. T., Leehey, D. J., Popli, S., Gandhi, V. C., Zayas, I., Hoffman, W., and Ing, T. S. (1985). Induction of peritoneal-fluid eosinophilia

by intraperitoneal air in patients on continuous ambulatory peritoneal dialysis (letter). *N. Engl. J. Med.* **313**, 1481. [p. 222]

395. Daugirdas, J. T., Leehey, D. J., Popli, S., Hoffman, W., Zayas, I., Gandhi, V. C., and Ing, T. S. (1987). Induction of peritoneal-fluid eosinophilia and/or monocytosis by intraperitoneal air injection. *Am. J. Nephrol.* **7**, 116–20. [p. 222]
396. David, J. R., Vadas, M. A., Butterworth, A. E., de Brito, P. A., Carvalho, E. M., David, R. A., Bina, J. C., and Andrade, Z. A. (1980). Enhanced helminthotoxic capacity of eosinophils from patients with eosinophilia. *N. Engl. J. Med.* **303**, 1147–52. [p. 105]
397. Davies, J., Gibson, D. G., Foale, R., Heer, K., Spry, C. J., Oakley, C. M., and Goodwin, J. F. (1982). Echocardiographic features of eosinophilic endomyocardial disease. *Br. Heart J.* **48**, 434–40. [p. 240]
398. Davies, J., Powell, D., McCall, E., Hegde, G., Spry, C. J. (1988). Thrombogenic mechanisms in the hypereosinophilic syndrome. Submitted. [p. 230, 248, 287]
399. Davies, J., Sapsford, R., Brooksby, I., Olsen, E. G., Spry, C. J., Oakley, C. M., and Goodwin, J. F. (1981). Successful surgical treatment of two patients with eosinophilic endomyocardial disease. *Br. Heart J.* **46**, 438–45. [p. 244]
400. Davies, J. and Spry, C. J. (1982). Plasma exchange or leukapheresis in the hypereosinophilic syndrome (letter). *Ann. Intern. Med.* **96,** 791. [p. 292]
401. Davies, J., Spry, C. J., Sapsford, R., Olsen, E. G., de Perez, G., Oakley, C. M., and Goodwin, J. F. (1983). Cardiovascular features of 11 patients with eosinophilic endomyocardial disease. *Q. J. Med.* **52**, 23–39. [p. 240]
402. Davies, J., Spry, C. J., Vijayaraghavan, G., and De Souza, J. A. (1983). A comparison of the clinical and cardiological features of endomyocardial disease in temperate and tropical regions. *Postgrad. Med. J.* **59**, 179–85. [p. 234, 258]
403. Davies, J. N. (1948). Endocardial fibrosis in Africans. *East Afr. Med. J.* **25**, 10–14. [p. 256]
404. Davies, J. N. (1960). Some considerations regarding obscure diseases affecting the mural endocardium. *Am. Heart. J.* **59**, 600–31. [p. 234]
405. Davies, J. N. (1972). African endomyocardial fibrosis. *Cardiovasc. Clin.* **4**, 345–59. [p. 250]
406. Davies, J. N. and Ball, J. D. (1955). The pathology of endomyocardial fibrosis in Uganda. *Br. Heart. J.* **17**, 337–59. [p. 232]
407. Davies, J. R., Geary, C. G., Testa, N. G., and Pumphrey, R. S., (1985). Cyclical eosinophilia: a manifestation of periodic haemopoiesis? *Br. J. Haematol.* **61**, 65–70. [p. 301]
408. Davis, P. and Hughes, G. R. (1974). Significance of eosinophilia during gold therapy. *Arthritis Rheum.* **17**, 964–8. [p. 312]
409. Davis, W. B., Fells, G. A., Sun, X. H., Gadek, J. E., Venet, A., and Crystal, R. G. (1984). Eosinophil-mediated injury to lung parenchymal cells and interstitial matrix: a possible role for eosinophils in chronic inflammatory disorders of the lower respiratory tract. *J. Clin. Invest.* **74**, 269–78. [p. 61, 118, 194]
410. Davison, A. G., Thompson, P. J., Davies, J., Corrin, B., and Turner Warwick, M. (1983). Prominent pericardial and myocardial lesions in the

Churg-Strauss syndrome (allergic granulamatosis and angiitis). *Thorax* **38**, 793–5. [p. 203]

411. Dawes, P. T., Smith, D. H., and Scott, D. L. (1986). Massive eosinophilia in rheumatoid arthritis: report of four cases. *Clin. Rheumatol.* **5**, 62–5. [p. 177]
412. de Bruijn, W. C., van der Meulen, J., Brederoo, P., and Daems, W. T. (1986). Pt-staining of peroxidatic reaction products at the ultrastructural level. *Histochemistry* **84**, 492–500. [p. 59]
413. de Korte, D., Haverkort, W. A., Behrendt, H., Roos, D., and van Gennip, A. H. (1986). Abnormal nucleotide pattern in the eosinophils of a patient with acute lymphoblastic leukemia associated with eosinophilia. *Leuk. Res.* **10**, 1419–24. [p. 160]
414. de Korte, D., Haverkort, W. A., van Gennip, A. H., and Roos, D. (1985). Nucleotide profiles of normal human blood cells determined by high-performance liquid chromatography. *Anal. Biochem.* **147**, 197–209. [p. 66]
415. de Messias, I. T., Telles, F. Q., Boaretti, A. C., Sliva, S., Guimarres, L. M., and Genta R. M. (1987). Clinical, immunological and epidemiological aspects of strongyloidiasis in an endemic area of Brazil. *Allergol. Immunopathol. (Madr)* **15**, 37–41. [p. 145]
416. De Monchy, J. G., Kauffman, H. F., Venge, P., Koeter, G. H., Jansen, H. M., Sluiter, H. J., and De Vries, K. (1985). Bronchoalveolar eosinophilia during allergen-induced late asthmatic reactions. *Am. Rev. Respir. Dis.* **131**, 373–6. [p. 200, 201]
417. De Simone, C., Donelli, G., Mango, G., Salvi, M. C., Rosati, F., and Sorice, F. Demonstration and ultrastructural morphology of a subpopulation of human eosinophils expressing surface antigens of activated T-lymphocytes (abstract). Presented to the 6th International Congress of Immunology, Toronto, Canada, 1986. [p. 87]
418. De Simone, C., Donelli, G., Meli, D., Molinari, A., Rosati, F., and Sorice, F. (1982). Human peripheral eosinophils with receptors for IgM: demonstration and ultrastructural morphology. *Immunobiology* **162**, 116–27. [p. 76]
419. De Simone, C., Donelli, G., Meli, D., Rosati, F., and Sorice, F. (1980). Human eosinophils and parasitic diseases: light and electron microscopy evidence of interaction with sheep erythrocyte. *Clin. Exp. Immunol.* **39**, 247–53. [p. 76]
420. De Simone, C., Doneli, G., Meli, D., Rosati, F., and Sorice, F. (1982). Human eosinophils and parasitic diseases: II. Characterization of two cell fractions isolated at different densities. *Clin. Exp. Immunol.* **48**, 249–55. [p. 33, 34]
421. De Simone, C., Ferrari, M., Ferrarelli, G., Rumi, C., Pugnaloni, L., and Sorice, F. (1987). The effects of substance P on human eosinophil receptors and functions. *Ann. NY. Acad. Sci.* **496**, 226–32. [p. 109]
422. De Simone, C., Ferrari, M., Pugnaloni, L., Ferrarelli, G., Rumi, C., and Sorice, F. (1986). Eosinophil-mediated cellular cytotoxicity induced by zymosan-activated serum. *Immunol. Lett.* **12**, 37–41. [p. 82]
423. De Simone, C., Salvi, M. C., Ferrarelli, G., De Santis, G., Mango, G., and Sorice, F. (1986). Human eosinophils and parasitic diseases – III. Beta-interferon increases eosinophil IgG-Fc receptor expression and capacity. *Int. J. Immunopharmacol.* **8**, 479–85. [p. 78, 109, 121]
424. de Vaan, G. A., van Haelst, U. J. (1979). Hypereosinophilia syndrome or

eosinophilic leukaemia. A case report of a one-year-old infant. *Helv. Paediatr. Acta* **34**, 271–9. [p. 153, 295]

425. DeChatelet, L. R., Migler, R. A., Shirley, P. S., Bass, D. A., and McCall, C. E. (1978). Enzymes of oxidative metabolism in the human eosinophil. *Proc. Soc. Exp. Biol. Med.* **158**, 537–41. [p. 69]
426. DeChatelet, L. R., Migler, R. A., Shirley, P. S., Muss, H. B., Szejda, P., and Bass, D. A. (1978). Comparison of intracellular bactericidal activities of human neutrophils and eosinophils. *Blood* **52**, 609–17. [p. 89]
427. DeChatelet, L. R., Shirley, P. S., McPhail, L. C., Huntley, C. C., Muss, H. B., and Bass, D. A. (1977). Oxidative metabolism of the human eosinophil. *Blood* **50**, 525–35. [p. 67]
428. Defendini, R., Hunter, S. B., Schlesinger, E. B., Leifer, E., and Rowland, L. P. (1981). Eosinophilic meningitis in a case of disseminated glioblastoma. *Arch. Neurol.* **38**, 52–3. [p. 172]
429. Dejaegher, P. and Demedts, M. (1984). Bronchoalveolar lavage in eosinophilic pneumonia before and during corticosteroid therapy. *Am. Rev. Respir. Dis.* **129**, 631–2. [p. 194, 207]
430. Delafuente, J. C., Panush, R. S., and Caldwell, J. R. (1979). Pencillin and cephalosporin immunogenicity in man. *Ann. Allergy* **43**, 337–40. [p. 310]
431. Denburg, J. A., Otsuka, H., Ohnisi, M., Ruhno, J., Bienenstock, J., and Dolovich, J. (1987). Contribution of basophil/mast cell and eosinophil growth and differentiation to the allergic tissue inflammatory response. *Int. Arch. Allergy. Appl. Immunol.* **82** (3–4), 321–6. [p. 22, 326]
432. Denburg, J. A., Richardson, M., Telizyn, S., and Bienenstock, J. (1983). Basophil/mast cell precursors in human peripheral blood. *Blood* **61**, 775–80. [p. 12]
433. Denburg, J. A., Telizyn, S., Messner, H., Lim, B., Jamal, N., Ackerman, S. J., Gleich, G. J., and Bienenstock, J. (1985). Heterogeneity of human peripheral blood eosinophil-type colonies: evidence for a common basophil-eosinophil pregenitor. *Blood* **66**, 312–8. [p. 11, 12]
434. DePace, N. L., Nestico, P. F., Morganroth, J., Ross, J., Fox, R., Kotler, M. N., Mintz, G. S., and Vassallo, R. (1983). Dilated cardiomyopathy in the idiopathic hypereosinophilic syndrome. *Am. J. Cardiol.* **52**, 1359–60. [p. 239]
435. Der Goukassian, P. (1983). Hematology of the lesser mouse lemur (Microcebus murinus): a preliminary study. *Folia Primatol. (Basel)* **41**, 129–36. [p. 126]
436. Desakorn, V., Suntharasamai, P., Pukrittayakamee, S., Migasena, S., and Bunnag, D. (1987). Adherence of human eosinophils to infective filariform larvae of Necator americanus in vitro. *Southeast Asian J. Trop. Med. Public Health* **18**, 66–72. [p. 144]
437. DeSchryver Kecskemeti, K. and Clouse, R. E. (1984). A previously unrecognized subgroup of 'eosinophilic gastroenteritis': association with connective tissue diseases. *Am. J. Surg. Pathol.* **8**, 171–80. [p. 183]
438. DeSimone, P. A. (1980). Grand rounds; hypereosinophilic syndrome: a review of clinical manifestations and therapy. *J. Ky. Med. Assoc.* **78**, 87–8. [p. 264]
439. Dessein, A., Samuelson, J. C., Butterworth, A. E., Hogan, M., Sherry, B. A., Vadas, M. A., and David, J. R. (1981). Immune evasion by Schistosoma mansoni: loss of susceptibility to antibody or complement-dependent eosino-

phil attack by schistosomula cultured in medium free of macromolecules. *Parasitology* **82**, 357–74. [p. 114]

440. Dessein, A. J. and David, J. R., (1982). The eosinophil in parasitic diseases. In *Advances in Host Defense Mechanisms, Phagocytic Cells. 1.* (eds. J. I. Gallin and A. S. Fauci) pp. 243–67. Raven Press. New York. [p. 324]
441. Dessein, A. J., Lee, T. H., Elsas, P., Ravalese, J. 3d, Silberstein, D., David, J. R., Austen, K. F., and Lewis, R. A. (1986). Enhancement by monokines of leukotriene generation by human eosinophils and neutrophils stimulated with calcium ionophore A23187. *J. Immunol.* **136**, 3829–38. [p. 71]
442. Dessein, A. J., Lenzi, H. L., Bina, J. C., Carvalho, E. M., Weiser W. Y., Andrade, Z. A., and David, J. R. (1984). Modulation of eosinophil cytotoxicity by blood mononuclear cells from healthy subjects and patients with chronic schistosomiasis mansoni. *Cell Immunol.* **85**, 100–13. [p. 107]
443. Dessein, A. J., Lenzi, H. L., Vadas, M. A., and David, J. R. (1983). A new class of eosinophil activators that enhance eosinophil helminthotoxicity. In *Immunobiology of the eosinophil* (eds. T. Yoshida and M. Torisu), pp. 369–83. Elsevier Biomedical, New York. [p. 107]
444. Dessein, A. J., Vadas, M. A., Nicola, N. A., Metcalf, D., and David, J. R. (1982). Enhancement of human blood eosinophil cytotoxicity by semi-purified eosinophil colony-stimulating factor(s). *J. Exp. Med.* **156**, 90–103. [p. 108]
445. Desser, R. K., Himmelhoch, Sr., Evans, W. H., Januska, M., Mage, M., and Shelton, E. (1972). Guinea pig heterophil and eosinophil peroxidase. *Arch. Biochem. Biophys.* **148**, 452–65. [p. 58]
446. Desser, S. S. and Weller, I. (1979). Ultrastructural observations on the granular leucocytes of the tuatara Sphenodon punctatus (Gray). *Tissue Cell* **11**, 703–15. [p. 127]
447. Detlefs, R. L., Frieden, I. J., Berger, T. G., and Westrom, D. (1987). Eosinophil fluorescence: a cause of false positive slide tests for herpes simplex virus. *Pediatr. Dermatol.* **4**, 129–33. [p. 36]
448. Diaz, P., Galleguillos, F. R., Gonzalez, M.C., Pantin, C. F., and Kay, A. B. (1984). Bronchoalveolar lavage in asthma: the effect of disodium cromoglycate (cromolyn) on leukocyte counts, immunoglobulins, and complement. *J. Allergy Clin. Immunol.* **74**, 41–8. [p. 199]
449. Diaz, P., Gonzalez, C., Galleguillos, F., Ancic, P., and Kay, A. B. Eosinophils and macrophages in bronchial mucus and bronchoalveolar lavage during allergen-induced late-phase asthmatic reactions (abstract). Presented to the 6th International Congress of Immunology, Toronto, Canada, 1986. [p. 201]
450. Dierksmeier, U., Frosch, P. J., and Czarnetszki, B. M. (1980). Eosinophil chemotactic factor (ECF) in blister fluid of dermatological diseases. *Br. J. Dermatol.* **102**, 43–8. [p. 102]
451. Dikeakou, T., Garelly, E., and Gervais, P. (1970). The vacuolisation of eosinophils and its significance in the skin window test. *Acta Allergol. (Kbh)* **25**, 341–6. [p. 314]
452. Dincsoy, H. P., Burton, T. J., and van der Bel Kahn, J. M. (1981). Circulating Charcot–Leyden crystals in the hypereosinophilic syndrome. *Am. J. Clin. Pathol.* **75**, 236–43. [p. 64]
453. Dinehart, S. M., Noppakun, N., Solomon, A. R., and Smith, E. B. (1986). Eosinophilic pustular folliculitis. *J. Am. Acad. Dermatol.* **14**, 475–9. [p. 304]
454. Discombe, G. (1946). Criteria of eosinophilia. *Lancet* **1**, 195–6. [p. 30]

455. Djaldetti, M., Fishman, D., and Pinkhas, J. (1975). Ultrastructural alterations of the eosinophils in hypereosinophilic syndrome. *Harefuah* **88**, 267–70. [p. 281]

456. Don, I. J., Khettry, U., and Canoso, J. J. (1978). Progressive systemic sclerosis with eosinophilia and a fulminating course. *Am. J. Med.* **65**, 346–8. [p. 212]

457. Donabedian, H. and Gallin, J. I. (1983). The hyperimmunoglobulin E recurrent-infection (Job's) syndrome: a review of the NIH experience and the literature. *Medicine (Baltimore)* **62**, 195–208. [p. 317]

458. Donohue, W. L., Snelling, C. E., Jackson, S. H., Keith, J. D., Chute, A. L., Laski, B., and Silverthorne, N. (1950). Pituitary adrenocorticotropic hormone (ACTH) therapy in eosinophilic leukemia. JAMA **143**, 154–7. [p. 268]

459. Donohugh, D. L. (1963). Tropical eosinophilia: an etiologic inquiry. *N. Engl. J. Med.* **269**, 1357–64. [p. 141]

460. Dor, P. J., Ackerman, S. J., and Gleich, G. J. (1984). Charcot–Leyden crystal protein and eosinophil granule major basic protein in sputum of patients with respiratory diseases. *Am. Rev. Respir. Dis.* **130**, 1072–7. [p. 199]

461. Dorfman, L. J. and Forno, L. S. (1986). Multiple mononeuropathy and hypereosinophilia (letter). *Muscle Nerve* **9**, 757–8. [p. 217]

462. Dorfman, L. J., Ransom, B. R., Forno, L. S., and Kelts, A. (1983). Neuropathy in the hypereosinophilic syndrome. *Muscle Nerve* **6**, 291–8. [p. 275, 276]

463. Douglas, S. D. and Ooka, M. P. (1977). Freeze-fracture of circulating human eosinophils. *Acta Haematol. (Basel)* **57**, 129–34. [p. 75]

464. Dowse, G. K., Turner, K. J., Stewart, G. A., Alpers, M. P., and Woolcock, A. J. (1985). The association between Dermatophagoides mites and the increasing prevalence of asthma in village communities within the Papua New Guinea highlands. *J. Allergy. Clin. Immunol.* **75**, 75–83. [p. 201]

465. Doyle, J. A. (1984). Eosinophilic fasciitis: extracutaneous manifestations and associations. *Cutis* **34**, 259–61. [p. 181]

466. Doyle, J. A., Connolly, S. M., and Hoagland, H. C. (1985). Hematologic disease in scleroderma syndromes. *Acta Derm-Venereol (Stockh)* **65**, 521–5. [p. 181]

467. Drutz, D. J. and Catanzaro, A. (1978). Coccidioidomycosis: Part II. *Am. Rev. Respir. Dis.* **117**, 727–71. [p. 133]

468. Dubertret, L., Bertaux, B., Fosse, M., and Touraine, R. (1980). Cellular events leading to blister formation in bullous pemphigoid. *Br. J. Dermatol.* **103**, 615–24. [p. 303]

469. Dubost, C., Maurice, P., Gerbaux, A., Bertrand, E., Rulliere, F., Vial, F., Barrillon, A., Prident, C., Carpentier, A., and Soyer, R. (1976). The surgical treatment of constrictive fibrose endocarditis. *Ann. Surg.* **184**, 303–7. [p. 254]

470. Dubost, C., Maurice, P., Gerbaux, A., Rulliere, R., Bertrand, E., Barrilion, A., Vial, F., Prigent, C. P., Carpentier, A., and Soyer, R. (1977). L'endocardite fibreuse constrictive: traitement chirurgical. *Arch. Mal. Coeur.* **70**, 155–62. [p. 254]

471. Dubost, C., Prigent, C., Gerbaux, A., Maurice, P., Passelecq, J., Rulliere, R., Carpentier, A., and DeLoche, A. (1983). Surgical approaches in endomyocardial disease (abstract). *Postgrad. Med. J.* **59**, 160–1. [p. 234]

472. Dufer, J. (1985). An improved cytochemical method for the evaluation of eosinophil colonies in soft-agar cultures from human blood or bone marrow. *Acta Histochem. (Jena)* **76**, 219–23. [p. 15]

473. Duffus, W. P., Thorne, K., and Oliver, R. (1980). Killing of juvenile Fasciola hepatica by purified bovine eosinophil proteins. *Clin. Exp. Immunol.* **40**, 336–40. [p. 47, 125]

474. Dufresne, R. G. Jr., Malcomb, A. W., Salhany, K. E., and King, L. E. Jr. (1987). Histiocytosis X mimicking the follicular occlusion syndrome: response to local therapy (letter). *J. Am. Acad. Dermatol.* **16** (2 Pt 1), 385–6. [p. 165]

475. Dunger, R. (1910). Eine einfache Methode der Sahlung der eosinophilen Leukozyten und der praktische Wert dieser Untersuchung. *Munch. Med. Wschr.* **57**, 1942–4. [p. 5, 30]

476. Dunne, D. W., Bickle, Q. D., Butterworth, A. E., and Richardson, B. A. (1987). The blocking of human antibody-dependent, eosinophil-mediated killing of Schistosoma mansoni schistosomula by monoclonal antibodies which cross-react with a polysaccharide-containing egg antigen. *Parasitology* **94**, 269–80. [p. 148]

477. Dupre, A. and Viraben, R. (1987). Coexistence of angiolymphoid hyperplasia with eosinophilia and pulmonary neoplasia (letter). *J. Am. Acad. Dermatol.* **16**, 142–4. [p. 169]

478. Durack, D. T., Ackerman, S. J., Loegering, D. A., and Gleich, G. J. (1981). Purification of human eosinophil-derived neurotoxin. *Proc. Natl. Acad. Sci. USA* **78**, 5165–9. [p. 54, 55]

479. Durack, D. T., Sumi, S. M., and Klebanoff, S. J. (1979). Neurotoxicity of human eosinophils. *Proc. Natl. Acad. Sci. USA* **76**, 1443–7. [p. 53, 54, 55]

480. Durand, D. V., Dellinger, A., Guerin, C., Guerin, J. C., and Levrat, R. (1984). Pleural sarcoidosis: one case presenting with an eosinophilic effusion. *Thorax* **39**, 468–9. [p. 212]

481. Durham, S. R. and Kay, A. B. (1985). Eosinophils, bronchial hyperreactivity and late-phase asthmatic reactions. *Clin. Allergy* **15**, 411–8. [p. 200]

482. Duschet, P., Schwarz, T., and Gschnait, F. (1986). Erythromelanoderma with eosinophilic spongiosis and epidermal intercellular antibodies: differentiation from pemphigus. *J. Cutan. Pathol.* **13**, 40–5. [p. 302]

483. Dvilansky, A., Alkan, M. L., Ho, W., Kaplan, H., Tiberin, P., and Rachmilewitz, B. (1975). Chronic eosinophilic leukemia complicated by epidural myeloblastoma. *Acta Haematol. (Basel)* **53**, 356–61. [p. 152, 155]

484. Dvorak, A. M. (1980). Ultrastructural evidence for release of major basic protein- containing crystalline cores of eosinophil granules in vivo: cytotoxic potential in Crohn's disease. *J. Immunol.* **125**, 460–2. [p. 189]

485. Dvorak, A. M., Ishizaka, T., and Galli, S. J. (1985). Ultrastructure of human basophils developing in vitro: evidence for the acquisition of peroxidase by basophils and for different effects of human and murine growth factors on human basophil and eosinophil maturation. *Lab. Invest.* **53**, 57–71. [p. 45]

486. Dvorak, A. M., Klebanoff, S. J., Henderson, W. R., Monahan, R. A., Pyne, K., and Galli, S. J. (1985). Vesicular uptake of eosinophil peroxidase by guinea pig basophils and by cloned mouse mast cells and granule-containing lymphoid cells. *Am. J. Pathol.* **118**, 425–38. [p. 45]

487. Dvorak, A. M., Mihm, M. C. Jr., Osage, J. E., Kwan, T. H., Austen, K. F., and Wintroub, B. U. (1982). Bullous pemphigoid, an ultrastructural study of

the inflammatory response: eosinophil, basophil and mast cell granule changes in multiple biopsies from one patient. *J. Invest. Dermatol.* **78**, 91–101. [p. 303]

488. Dvorak, A. M., Monahan, R. A., Osage, J. E., and Dickersin, G. R. (1980). Crohn's disease; transmission electron microscopic studies: II. Immunologic inflammatory response; alterations of mast cells, basophils, eosinophils, and the microvasculature. *Hum. Pathol.* **11**, 606–19. [p. 189]
489. Eakin, D. L., Gill, D. P., and Weiss, G. B. (1982). Response of hypereosinophilic syndrome to 6-thioguanine and cytarabine. *Cancer Treat. Rep.* **66**, 545–7. [p. 291]
490. Echols, R. M., Palmer, D. L., and Long, G. W. (1982). Tissue eosinophilia in human coccidioidomycosis. *Rev. Infect. Dis.* **4**, 656–64. [p. 133]
491. Edelman, J., David, P., and Owen, E. T. (1983). Prevalence of eosinophilia during gold therapy for rheumatoid arthritis. *J. Rheumatol.* **10**, 121–3. [p. 307]
492. Edge, J. R. (1946). Myocardial fibrosis following arsenical therapy. *Lancet* **2**, 675–7. [p. 237]
493. Edwards, D., Wald, J. A., Dobozin, B. S., and Kirkpatrick, C. H. (1987). Troleandomycin and methylprednisolone for treatment of the hypereosinophilic syndrome (letter). *N. Engl. J. Med.* **317**, 573–4. [p. 272, 291]
494. Efstratopoulos, A. D., Spantideas, A. N., and Komninos, Z. D. (1980). Extreme eosinophilia due to common streptococcal infection in an adult. *Br. Med. J.* **281**, 588. [p. 132]
495. Egesten, A., Alumets, J., von Mecklenburg, C., Palmegren, M., and Olsson, I. (1986). Localization of eosinophil cationic protein, major basic protein, and eosinophil peroxidase in human eosinophils by immuneolectron microscopic technique. *J. Histochem. Cytochem.* **34**, 1399–403. [p. 46, 50]
496. Eggert, F. M. and Germain, J. P. (1980). Stable acid phosphatase: I. Demonstration and distribution. *Histochemistry* **66**, 307–17. [p. 126]
497. Ehrlich, P. (1879). Beitrage zur Kenntniss der granulirten bindergewebszellen und der eosinophilen leukocyten. *Arch. Anat. Physiol. Lpz. 3 Physiol. Abt.*, 166–9. [p. 5]
498. Ehrlich, P. (1879). Ueber die specifischen granulationen des Blutes. *Arch. Anat. Physiol. Lpz. 3 Physiol. Abt.*, 571–9. [p. 4]
499. Ehrlich, P. and Lazarus, A. (1900). *Histology of the blood: normal and pathological.* (ed: W. Myers). Cambridge University Press, Cambridge. pp. 216. [p. 5, 36]
500. Eidinger, D., Wilkinson, R., and Rose, B. (1964). A study of cellular responses in immune reactions utilizing the skin window technique. I. Immediate hypersensitivity reactions. *J. Allergy.* **35**, 77–85. [p. 97]
501. el Garf, A. (1985). Parasitic rheumatism: rheumatic manifestations associated with calcified guinea worm. *J. Rheumatol.* **12**, 976–9. [p. 177]
502. El Hashimi, W. (1971). Charcot–Leyden crystals: formation from primate and lack of formation from non-primate eosinophils. *Am. J. Pathol.* **65**, 311–24. [p. 64]
503. Eling, W. M., Jerusalem, C. R., and Heinen Borries, U. (1984). Role of macrophages in the pathogenesis of endomyocardial fibrosis in murine malaria. *Trans. R. Soc. Trop. Med. Hyg.* **78**, 43–8. [p. 257]
504. Ellis, W. M., Georgiou, G. M., Roberton, D. M., and Johnson, G. R. (1984). The use of discontinuous Percoll gradients to separate populations of

cells from human bone marrow and peripheral blood. *J. Immunol. Methods.* **66**, 9–16. [p. 33]

505. Ellman, L., Hammond, D., and Atkins, L. (1979). Eosinophilia, chloromas and a chromosome abnormality in a patient with a myeloproliferative syndrome. *Cancer* **43**, 2410–3. [p. 152]
506. Ellman, L., Miller, L., and Rappeport, J. (1974). Leukopheresis therapy of a hypereosinophilic disorder. JAMA **230**, 1004–5. [p. 292]
507. Ellul Micallef, R., Mohammed, D. E., and Fenech, F. F. (1980). The hypereosinophilic syndrome – a diagnostic enigma. *Postgrad. Med. J.* **56**, 506–8. [p. 276]
508. Elmalek, M. and Hammel, I. (1987). Morphometric evidence that the maturation of the eosinophil granules is independent of volume change. *J. Submicrosc. Cytol.* **19**, 265–8. [p. 13]
509. Elouaer Blanc, L., Zafrani, E. S., Farcet, J. P., Saint Marc Girardin, M. F., Mathieu, D., and Dhumeaux, D. (1985). Hepatic vein obstruction in idiopathic hypereosinophilic syndrome. *Arch. Intern. Med.* **145**, 751–3. [p. 270, 273]
510. Elsas, P., Lee, T. H., Lenzi, H. L., and Dessein, A. J. (1987). Monocytes activate eosinophils for enhanced helminthotoxicity and increased generation of leukotriene C4. *Ann. Inst. Pasteur Immunol.* **138**, 97–116. [p. 107]
511. Elzay, R. P. (1983). Traumatic ulcerative granuloma with stromal eosinophilia (Riga-Fede's disease and traumatic eosinophilic granuloma). *Oral Surg. Oral Med. Oral Pathol.* **55**, 497–506. [p. 192]
512. Engbaek, H. C., Heerup, L., and Thomsen, S. (1942). Eosinophilic leukaemia or eosinophilic leukaemoid reaction. *Nord Medicin.* **14**, 1535–51. [p. 268]
513. Engelhard, D., Landreth, K. S., Kapoor, N., Kincade, P. W., De Bault, L. E., Theodore, A., and Good, R. A. (1983). Cycling of peripheral blood and marrow lymphocytes in cyclic neutropenia. *Proc. Natl. Acad. Sci. USA* **80**, 5734–8. [p. 261]
514. Engfeldt, B. and Zetterstrom, R. (1956). Disseminated eosinophilic 'collagen disease': a clinical and pathological study of a clinical entity related to Löffler's syndrome. *Acta Med. Scand.* **153**, 337–53. [p. 269]
515. Engle, W. A., Schreiner, R. L., and Baehner, R. L. (1983). Neonatal white blood cell disorders. *Semin. Perinatol.* **7**, 184–200. [p. 294, 324]
516. English, A. W. and Lepherd, E. E. (1981). The haematology and serum biochemistry of wild fallow deer (Dama dama) in New South Wales. *J. Wildl. Dis.* **17**, 289–95. [p. 125]
517. Enokihara, H., Furusawa, S., and Kajitani, H., Hamaguchi, H., Saito, K., Fukuda, T., and Shishido, H. (1988). Interleukin 2 stimulates the T-cells from patients with an eosinophilia to produce Eo-CSF. Submitted. [p. 20]
518. Enokihara, H., Hamaguchi, H., Sakamaki, H., Hazama, S., Saito, K., Furusawa, S., and Shishido, H. (1985). Specific production of eosinophil colony stimulating factor from sensitized T-cells from a patient with allergic eosinophilia. *Br. J. Haematol.* **59**, 85–91. [p. 19]
519. Enokihara, H., Kajitani, H., Hamaguchi, H., Saito, K., Furusawa, S., and Shishido, H. Antigenic stimulation of T-lymphocytes for production of eosinophilopoiesis-stimulating factors in patients with eosinophilia (abstract). Presented to the 6th International Congress of Immunology, Toronto, Canada, 1986. [p. 19]

520. Enomoto, T. and Kitani, T. (1966). Electron microscopic studies on peroxidase and acid phosphatase reaction in human leukocytes in normal and leukemic cells and on phagocytosis. *Acta Haematol. Jap.* **29**, 554–70. [p. 44, 59, 60]

521. Epstein, D. M., Taormina, V., Gefter, W. B., and Miller, W. T. (1981). The hypereosinophilic syndrome. *Radiology* **140**, 59–62. [p. 272]

522. Epstein, J. I. and Hutchins, G. M. (1984). Granulomatous prostatitis: distinction among allergic, nonspecific, and post-transurethral resection lesions. *Hum. Pathol.* **15**, 818–25. [p. 224]

523. Eriksen, L. and Nielsen, K. (1977). A study of blood eosinophil counting in calves. *Nord. vet. Med.* **29**, 144–50. [p. 125]

524. Ernstoff, M. S. and Kirkwood, J. M. (1984). Changes in the bone marrow of cancer patients treated with recombinant interferon alpha-2. *Am. J. Med.* **76**, 593–6. [p. 109]

525. Eschenbacher, W. L. and Gravelyn, T. R. (1987). A technique for isolated airway segment lavage. *Chest* **92**, 105–9. [p. 194, 199]

526. Eugene, C., Gury, B., Bergue, A., and Quevauvilliers, J. (1984). (Icterus disclosing pancreatic involvement in idiopathic hypereosinophilic syndrome). *Gastroenterol. Clin. Biol.* **8**, 966–9. [p. 270, 272]

527. Fabbri, L. M., Boschetto, P., Zocca, E., Milani, G., Pivirotto, F., Plebani, M., Burlina, A., Licata, B., and Mapp, C. E. (1987). Bronchoalveolar neutrophilia during late asthmatic reactions induced by toluene disocyanate. *Am. Rev. Respir. Dis.* **136**, 36–42. [p. 201]

528. Fabian, I. and Aronson, M. (1975). Deamination of histamine by peroxidase of neutrophils and eosinophils. *J. Reticuloendothel. Soc.* **17**, 141–5. [p. 57]

529. Fadel, R., Herpin Richard, M., Rihoux, J. P., and Henocq, E. (1987). Inhibitory effect of cetirizine 2HC1 on eosinophil migration in vivo. *Clin. Allergy.* **17**, 373–9. [p. 100]

530. Fadell, E. J., Crone, R. I., Leonard, M. E. and Altimirano, M. D. (1957). Eosinophilic leukemia. *Arch. Intern. Med.* **99**, 819–23. [p. 270]

531. Fagerland, J. A., Hagemoser, W. A., and Ireland, W. P. (1987). Ultrastructure and stereology of leukocytes and platelets of normal foxes and a fox with a Chediak-Higashi-like syndrome. *Vet. Pathol.* **24**, 164–9. [p. 261]

532. Falanga, V., Medsger, T. A. Jr., Reichlin, M., and Rodnan, G. P. (1986). Linear schleroderma: clinical spectrum, prognosis, and laboratory abnormalities. *Ann. Intern. Med.* **104**, 849–57. [p. 181]

533. Falase, A. O. (1983). Endomyocardial fibrosis in Africa. *Postgrad. Med. J.* **59**, 170–8. [p. 255]

534. Falase, A. O. (1985). Are eosinophils the cause of endomyocardial fibrosis in the tropics? *Afr. J. Med. Med. Sci.* **14**, 1–2. [p. 256]

535. Falase, A. O., Kalawole, T. M., and Lagundoye, S. B. (1976). Endomyocardial fibrosis: problems in differential diagnosis. *Br. Heart. J.* **38**, 369–74. [p. 250]

536. Falk, E. S., and Eide, T. J. (1981). Histologic and clinical findings in human scabies. *Int. J. Dermatol.* **20**, 600–5. [p. 149]

537. Faller, A. (1966). Zur Frage von Struktur und Aufbau der Eosinophilen Granula. *Z. Zellforsch. Mikrosk. Anat.* **69**, 551–65. [p. 39]

538. Farag, H. M., Naguib, M., Gyasi, H., and Ibrahim, A. W. (1986). Anesthesia for a patient with eosinophilic myositis. *Anesth. Analg.* **65**, 903–4. [p. 180]

539. Faravelli, A., Gromo, G., and Besana, C. (1984). Fibroplastic endomyocar-

ditis with eosinophilia: presentation of a fatal case and diagnostic considerations on eosinophilic leukemia. *Haematologica (Pavia)* **69**, 218–26. [p. 153]

540. Farcet, J. P., Binaghi, M., Kuentz, M., Merlier, J. F., Mayaud, C., Nebout, T., Nass, P., and Ferret, J. (1982). A hypereosinophilic syndrome with retinal arteritis and tuberculosis. *Arch. Intern. Med.* **142**, 625–7. [p. 275, 290]
541. Farnam, J., Jorizzo, J. L., Grant, J. A., Lavastida, M. T., Ichikawa, Y., and Daniels, J. C. (1984). Sjögren's syndrome presenting with hypereosinophilia, lymphopenia and circulating immune complexes. *Clin. Exp. Rheumatol.* **2**, 41–6. [p. 182]
542. Fattah, D. I. Maizels, R. M., McLaren, D. J., and Spry, C. J. (1986). Toxocara canis: interaction of human blood eosinophils with the infective larvae. *Exp. Parasitol.* **61**, 421–31. [p. 113, 140]
543. Fauci, A. S. (1983). Vasculitis. *J. Allergy Clin. Immunol.* **72**, 211–23. [p. 231]
544. Fauci, A. S., Harley, J. B., Roberts, W. C., Ferrans, V. J., Gralnick, H. R., and Bjornson, B. H. (1982). NIH conference: the idiopathic hypereosinophilic syndrome: clinical, pathophysiologic, and therapeutic considerations. *Ann. Intern. Med.* **97**, 78–92. [p. 241, 265, 270, 276]
545. Fauci, A. S., Haynes, B. F., and Katz, P. (1978). The spectrum of vasculitis. Clinical, pathologic, immunologic, and theraputic considerations. *Ann. Intern. Med.* **89**, 660–76. [p. 209, 231]
546. Fauci, A. S., and Wolff, S. M. (1973). Wegener's granulomatosis: studies in eighteen patients and a review of the literature. *Medicine (Baltimore)* **52**, 535–61. [p. 210]
547. Favara, B. E., McCarthy, R. C., and Mierau, G. W. (1983). Histiocytosis X. *Hum. Pathol.* **14**, 663–76. [p. 324]
548. Fawaz Estrup, F. and Kaplan, S. R. (1987). Synovial fluid eosinophilia (letter). *Clin. Exp. Rheumatol.* **5**, 90–2. [p. 178]
549. Fawzy, M. E., Ziady, G., Halim, M., Guindy, R., Mercer, E. N., and Feteih, N. (1985). Endomyocardial fibrosis: report of eight cases. *J. Am. Coll. Cardiol.* **5**, 893–8. [p. 234]
550. Fearon, D. T. (1985). Human complement receptors for C3b (CR1) and C3d (CR2). *J. Invest. Dermatol.* **85** (1 Suppl.), 53s–57s. [p. 81]
551. Feczko, P. J., Halpert, R. D., and Zonca, M. (1985). Radiographic abnormalities in eosinophilic esophagitis. *Gastrointest. Radiol.* **10**, 321–4. [p. 183, 185]
552. Fedorko, M. E. (1968). Formation of cytoplasmic granules in human eosinophilic myelocytes: an electron microscope autoradiographic study. *Blood* **31**, 188–94. [p. 42]
553. Feldman, R. B., Moore, D. M., Hood, C. I., Hiles, D. A., and Romano, P. E. (1985). Solitary eosinophilic granuloma of the lateral orbital wall. *Am. J. Ophthalmol.* **100**, 318–23. [p. 219]
554. Feltelius, N., Hallgren, R., and Venge, P. (1987). Raised circulating levels of the eosinophil cationic protein in ankylosing spondylitis: relation with the inflammatory activity and the influence of sulphasalazine treatment. *Ann. Rheum. Dis.* **46**, 403–7. [p. 179]
555. Fenoglio, J. J. Jr, McAllister, J. A. Jr, and Mullick, F. G. (1981). Drug related myocarditis. I. Hypersensitivity myocarditis. *Hum. Pathol.* **12**, 900–7. [p. 309]
556. Ferguson, G. T. and Starkebaum, G. (1985). Thromboangiitis obliterans

associated with idiopathic hypereosinophilia. *Arch. Intern. Med.* **145**, 1726–8. [p. 272]

557. Fernandez, L. A., Olsen, T. G., Barwick, K. W., Sanders, M., Kaliszewski, C., and Inagami, T. (1986). Renin in angiolymphoid hyperplasia with eosinophilia: its possible effect on vascular proliferation. *Arch. Pathol. Lab. Med.* **110**, 1131–5. [p. 168]
558. Fernandez, N., Torres, A., and Ackerman, A. B. (1977). Pathologic findings in human scabies. *Arch. Dermatol.* **113**, 320–4. [p. 149]
559. Ferrer, J. M., Gonzalez Garrigues, M., and Stockert, J. C. (1983). Meruro-chrome: a fluorescent and electron opaque dye. *Microsc. Acta* **87**, 293–300. [p. 38]
560. Ferrer, J. M., Tato, A., and Stockert, J. C. (1986). Electronmicroscopical contrast by palladium chloride. Z. Naturforsch (C) **41**, 483–4. [p. 38]
561. Fialkow, P. J., Jacobson, R. J., Singer, J. W., Sacher, R. A., McGuffin, R. W., and Neefe, J. R. (1980). Philadelphia chromosome (Phl)-negative chronic myelogenous leukemia (CML): a clonal disease with origin in a multipotent stem cell. *Blood* **56**, 70–3. [p. 159]
562. Filley, W. V., Ackerman, S. J., and Gleich, G. J. (1981). An immunofluores-cent method for specific staining of eosinophil granule major basic protein. *J. Immunol. Methods* **47**, 228–38. [p. 46]
563. Filley, W. V., Holley, K. E., Kephart, G. M., and Gleich, G. J. (1982). Identification by immunofluorescence of eosinophil granule major basic protein in lung tissues of patients with bronchial asthma. *Lancet* **2**, 11–16. [p. 197]
564. Fine, S. R. (1986). Evaluation of the eosinophil. *Bull. NY Acad. Med.* **62**, 766–7. [p. 30]
565. Finlay, D. (1985). Eosinophilic leukaemia in the cat: a case report. *Vet. Rec.* **116**, 567. [p. 157]
566. Fischer, E., Capron, M., Prin, L., Kusnierz, J. P., and Kazatchkine, M. D. (1986). Human eosinophils express CR1 and CR3 complement receptors for cleavage fragments of C3. *Cell Imunol.* **97**, 297–306. [p. 81]
567. Fischkoff, S. A., Brown, G. E., and Pollak, A. (1986). Synthesis of eosinophil-associated enzymes in HL–60 promyelocytic leukemia cells. *Blood* **68**, 185–92. [p. 26, 27]
568. Fischkoff, S. A. and Condon, M. E. (1985). Switch in the differentiative response to maturation inducers of human promyelocytic leukemia cells by prior exposure to alkaline conditions. *Cancer Res.* **45**, 2065–9. [p. 26]
569. Fischkoff, S. A., Pollak, A., Gleich, G. J., Testa, J. R., Misawa, S., and Reber, T. J. (1984). Eosinophilic differentiation of the human promyelocytic leukemia cell line, HL–60. *J. Exp. Med.* **160**, 179–96. [p. 15, 26]
570. Fitzharris, P., Moqbel, R., Thorne, K. J., Richardson, B. A., Butterworth, A. E., Hartnell, A., Cromwell, O., and Kay, A. B. Monocyte-derived eosinophil activating factor (EAF) enhances LTC4 production by human eosinophils (abstract). Presented to the 6th International Congress of Immunology, Toronto, Canada, 1986. [p. 71]
571. Fitzharris, P., Moqbel, R., Thorne, K. J., Richardson, B. A., Hartnell, A., Cromwell, O., Butterworth, A. E., and Kay, A. B. (1986). The effects of eosinophil activating factor on IgG-dependent sulphidopeptide leukotriene generation by human eosinophils. *Clin. Exp. Immunol.* **66**, 673–80. [p. 71]
572. Flannery, E. P., Dillon, D. E., Freeman, M. V., Levy, J. D., Ambrosio, V.,

and Bedynek, J. L. (1972). Eosinophilic leukemia with fibrosing endocarditis and short Y chromosome. *Ann. Intern. Med.* **77**, 223–8. [p. 152, 155, 156, 285]

573. Flaum, M. A., Schooley, R. T., Fauci, A. S., and Gralnick, H. R. (1981). A clinicopathologic correlation of the idiopathic hypereosinophilic syndrome. I. Hematologic manifestations. *Blood* **58**, 1012–20. [p. 284, 285, 290]
574. Flavahan, N. A., Aarhus, L. L., Rimele, T. J., and VanHoutte, P. M. (1985). Respiratory epithelium inhibits bronchial smooth muscle tone. *J. Appl. Physiol.* **58**. 834–8. [p. 196]
575. Fledelius, H. (1970). Extreme persistent eosinophilia with high serum B12 values. A report of two cases. *Acta Med. Scand.* **187**, 235–40. [p. 284]
576. Fleischmajer, R., Jacotot, A. B,. Shore, S., and Binnick, S. A. (1978). Scleroderma, eosinophilia, and diffuse fasciitis. *Arch. Dermatol.* **114**, 1320–5. [p. 181]
577. Fleit, H. B., Wright, S. D., Durie, C. J., Valinsky, J. E., and Unkeless, J. C. (1984). Ontogeny of Fc receptors and complement receptor (CR3) during human myeloid differentiation. *J. Clin. Invest.* **73**, 516–25. [p. 77]
578. Flint, K. C. and Johnson, N. M. (1987). Pulmonary eosinophilia associated with naproxen therapy. *J. R. Soc. Med.* **80**, 120–1. [p. 309]
579. Flint, K. C., Leung, K. B., Hudspith, B. N., Brostoff, J., Pearce, F. L., and Johnson, N. M. (1985). Bronchoalveolar mast cells in extrinsic asthma: a mechanism for the initiation of antigen specific bronchoconstriction. *Br. Med. J. (Clin. Res.)* **291**, 923–6. [p. 199]
580. Flores, M., Merino Angulo, J., Tanago, J. G., and Aquirre, C. (1983). Late generalized tuberculosis and eosinophilia (letter). *Arch. Intern. Med.* **143**, 182. [p. 131]
581. Floyd, K., Suter, P. F., and Lutz, H. (1983). Granules of blood eosinophils are stained directly by anti-immunoglobulin fluorescein isothiocyanate conjugates. *Am. J. Vet. Res.* **44**, 2060–3. [p. 36]
582. Foasso, M. F., Hermierm, M., Age, C., Mermillon, M., and Franccois, R. (1984). (Hypereosinophilic syndrome with endomyocardial involvement in children. Critical analysis of the literature apropos of a case). *Pediatrie* **39**, 147–155. [p. 269]
583. Feogh, M. L., Maddox, Y. T., and Ramwell, P. W. (1986). Human peritoneal eosinophils and formation of arachidonate cyclooxygenase products. *Scand. J. Immunol.* **23**, 599–603. [p. 71, 221]
584. Foon, K. A., Buescher, S., Kimball, E. S., Huang, L. C., Stevenson, H. C., Clarke, G., Gregorio, T., and Harley, J. B. (1983). Monoclonal antibody to human eosinophils recognizing 95 kD surface membrane antigen. *Hybridoma* **2**, 393–402. [p. 87]
585. Forget, P., Eggermont, E., Marchal, G., Geboes, K., Jaeken, J., and Melchior, S. (1978). Eosinophilic infiltration of the oesophagus in an infant. *Acta Paediatr. Belg.* **31**, 91–3. [p. 183, 185]
586. Forni, G., Giovarelli, M., Santoni, A., Modesti, A., and Forni, M. (1986). Tumour inhibition by interleukin-2 at the tumour/host interface. *Biochim. Biophys. Acta* **865**, 307–27. [p. 20]
587. Forssman, O. and Korsgren, M. (1962). An eosinophilia in a patient with bronchial asthma. *Acta Med. Scand.* **172**, 1–4. [p. 315]

588. Fossaluzza, V. and Tosato, F. (1980). Acquired Pelger-Hüet anomaly limited to eosinophils. *Acta Haematol. (Basel)* **63**, 295. [p. 261]

589. Fournial, G., Schlanger, R., Berthoumieu, F., Pris, J., Marco, J., and Eschapasse, H. (1982). Surgery for cardiac complications caused by endocardial mural fibrin deposits in a hypereosinophilic syndrome. *Circulation* **65**, 1010–4. [p. 243]

590. Fox, A. S., Kazacos, K. R., Gould, N. S., Heydemann, P. T., Thomas, C., and Boyer, K. M. (1985). Fatal eosinophilic meningoencephalitis and visceral larva migrans caused by the raccoon ascarid Baylisascaris procyonis. *N. Engl. J. Med.* **312**, 1619–23. [p. 139]

591. Fox, B. and Seed, W. A. (1980). Chronic eosinophilic pneumonia. *Thorax* **35**, 570–80. [p. 207, 208]

592. Fox, H. and Mainwaring, A. R. (1972). Eosinophilic infiltration of the gallbladder. *Gastroenterology* **63**, 1049–52. [p. 190]

593. Fox, J. L. and Berman, B. (1983). T6-antigen-bearing cells in eosinophilic granuloma of bone. JAMA **249**, 3071–2. [p. 164]

594. Franchi, F., De Rosa, F., Seminara, P., Calvieri, S., Carfagna, G. F., and Bosman, C. (1984). Hypereosinophilic syndrome and plasmocytoma: report of a case and review of the literature. *Acta Haematol. (Basel)* **72**, 14–20. [p. 162]

595. Frandsen, B. and Lose, G. (1986). Determination of eosinophil cationic protein in urine by an enzyme immunoassay. *Scand. J. Clin. Lab. Invest.* **46**, 629–34. [p. 50, 223]

596. Franklin, W. and Goetzl, E. J. (1981). Total absence of eosinophils in a patient with an allergic disorder. *Ann. Intern. Med.* **94**, 352–3. [p. 316]

597. Fredens, K., Dahl, R., and Venge, P. (1982). The Gordon phenomenon induced by the eosinophil cationic protein and eosinophil protein X. *J. Allergy Clin. Immunol.* **70**, 361–6. [p. 52]

598. Fredens, K., Dahl, R., and Venge, P. (1985). Neurotoxic effect of the eosinophil cationic protein (ECP). In *Inflammation: basic mechanisms, tissue injuring principles and clinical models* (eds. P. Venge and A. Lindblom), pp 347–9. Almqvist and Websell International, Stockholm, Sweden. [p. 52]

599. Fredens, K., Dahl, R., and Venge, P. (1986). An immunofluorescent method for a specific demonstration of granulocytes and some of their proteins (ECP and CCP). *Histochemistry* **84**, 247–50. [p. 37]

600. Frenkiel, S., Small, P., Rochon, L., Cohen, C., Darragh, D., and Black, M. (1982). Nasal polyposis – a multidisciplinary study. *J. Otolaryngol.* **11**, 275–8. [p. 214]

601. Friedberg, M., Joffe, P., Nielson, B., and Nielsen, L. P. (1987). Eosinophilia in hemodialysis patients. *Artif. Organs* **11**, 90–2. [p. 220]

602. Friedlaender, M. H., Okumoto, M., and Kelley, J. (1984). Diagnosis of allergic conjunctivitis. *Arch Ophthalmol* **102**, 1198–9. [p. 218]

603. Friedmann, I. and Ferlito, A. (1981). Primary eosinophilic granuloma of the larynx. *J. Laryngol. Otol.* **95**, 1249–54. [p. 215]

604. Frigas, E., and Gleich, G. J. (1986). The eosinophil and the pathophysiology of asthma. *J. Allergy Clin. Immunol.* **77**, 527–37. [p. 195, 325]

605. Frigas, E., Loegering, D. A., and Gleich, G. J. (1980). Cytotoxic effects of the guinea pig eosinophil major basic protein on tracheal epithelium. *Lab. Invest.* **42**, 35–43. [p. 47]

606. Frigas, E., Loegering, D. A., Solley, G. O., Farrow, G. M., and Gleich, G. J. (1981). Elevated levels of the eosinophil granule major basic protein in the sputum of patients with bronchial asthma. *Mayo Clin. Proc.* **56**, 345–53. [p. 199]

607. Fuerst, D. E. and Jannach, J. R. (1965). Autofluorescence of eosinophils: a bone marrow study. *Nature* **205**, 1333–4. [p. 37]

608. Fuggle, W. J., Crocker, J., and Smith, P. J. (1984). A quantitative study of eosinophil polymorphs in Hodgkin's disease. *J. Clin. Pathol.* **37**, 267–71. [p. 162]

609. Fujita, Y., Rubinstein, E., Greco, D. B., Reisman, R. E., and Arbesman, C. E. (1975). Antigen-antibody complexes in or on eosinophils in nasal secretions. *Int. Arch. Allergy Appl. Immunol.* **48**, 577–83. [p. 79]

610. Fukuda, T., Ackerman, S. J., Reed, C. E., Peters, M. S., Dunnette, S. L., and Gleich, G. J. (1985). Calcium ionophore A231287 calcium-dependent cytolytic degranulation in human eosinophils. *J. Immunol.* **135**, 1349–56. [p. 94]

611. Fukuda, T., Dunnette, S. L., Reed, C. E., Ackerman, S. J., Peters, M. S., and Gleich, G. J. (1985). Increased numbers of hypodense eosinophils in the blood of patients with bronchial asthma. *Am. Rev. Respir. Dis.* **132**, 981–5. [p. 34, 198, 200]

612. Gabbas, A. G. and Li, C. Y. (1986). Acute nonlymphocytic leukemia with eosinophilic differentiation. *Am. J. Hematol.* **21**, 29–38. [p. 155]

613. Gabriel, L. C., Escribano, L. M., Villa, E., Leiva, C., and Valdes, M. D. (1986). Ultrastructural study of blood cells in toxic oil syndrome. *Acta Haematol. (Basel)* **75**, 165–70. [p. 41, 182]

614. Gabrilove, J. L., Welte, K., Harris, P., Platzer, E., Lu, L., Levi, E., Mertelsmann, R., and Moore, M. A. (1986). Pluripoietin alpha: a second human hematopoietic colony-stimulating factor produced by the human bladder carcinoma cell line 5637. *Proc. Natl. Acad. Sci. USA.* **83**, 2478–82. [p. 23]

615. Gaensler, E. A. and Carrington, C. B. (1977). Peripheral opacities in chronic eosinophilic pneumonia: the photographic negative of pulmonary edema. *Am. J. Roentgenol.* **128**, 1–13. [p. 207]

616. Galbut, D. L., Benson, J., Blankstein, R. L., Vignola, P. A., and Gentsch, T. O. (1983). Endomyocardial fibrosis: preoperative diagnosis and surgical therapy. *Chest* **84**, 779–82. [p. 241]

617. Gallagher, R., Collins, S., Trujillo, J., McCredie, K., Ahern, M., Tsai, S., Metzgar, R., Aulakh, G., Ting, R., Ruscetti, F., and Gallo, R. (1979). Characterization of the continuous, differentiating myeloid cell line (HL–60) from a patient with acute promyelocytic leukemia. *Blood* **54**, 713–33. [p. 26]

618. Galloway, S. J., Rossiter, G. J., and Pidcock, M. E. (1985). An evaluation of the Coulter Diff3 50, an automated differential leukocyte counter. *Pathology* **17**, 563–7. [p. 31]

619. Gangemi, M., Mayer, M., Sainte Rose, C., and Maiuri, F. (1985). Spinal cord compression by an eosinophilic granuloma: case report and review of the literature. J. Neurosurg. Sci. **29**, 117–21. [p. 164]

620. Gansmuller, A., Anteunis, A., Venturiello, S. M., Bruschi, F., and Binaghi, R. A. (1987). Antibody-dependent in vitro cytotoxicity of newborn Trichi-

nella spiralis larvae: nature of the cells involved. *Parasite Immunol.* **9**, 281–92. [p. 115]

621. Ganz, T. (1987). Extracellular release of antimicrobial defensins by human polymorphonuclear leukocytes. *Infect. Immun.* **55**, 568–71. [p. 119]
622. Garber, S. L., O'Morchoe, P. J., O'Morchoe, C. C. (1980). A simultaneous comparison of the cells of blood, renal hilar and thoracic duct lymph in the dog. *Anat. Rec.* **198**, 255–61. [p. 125]
623. Gardais, J., Fanello, S., Joubaud, F., and Simard, C. (1984). (Leukemoid eosinophilic reaction in angioimmunoblastic adenopathy). *Rev. Med. Interne* **5**, 309–14. [p. 163]
624. Gardiol, D. and Picht, E. (1959). (Encephalopathy and myocarditis with an eosinophilia: a case of urogenital tuberculosis treated with tuberculostatic drugs). *Schweiz. Zeit. Tuberk. Pneumon.* **14**, 212–26. [p. 237]
625. Gardner, J. H., Amonette, R. A., and Chesney, T. M. (1981). Angiolymphoid hyperplasia with eosinophilia. *J. Dermatol. Surg. Oncol.* **7**, 414–8. [p. 167]
626. Gardner, R. V., Tebbi, C. K., Chervinsky, D., and McGarry, M. (1986). The role of eosinophils in regulation of granulopoiesis. *Hematol. Oncol.* **4**, 267–74. [p. 25]
627. Gardner-Thorpe, G., Harriman, D. G., Parsons, M., and Rudge, P. (1971). Löffler's eosinophilic endocarditis with Balint's syndrome (optic ataxia and paralysis of visual fixation). *Q. J. Med.* **40**, 249–60. [p. 274]
628. Gartner, I. (1980). Separation of human eosinophils in density gradients of polyvinylpyrrolidone-coated silica gel (Percoll). Immunology **40**, 133–6. [p. 33]
629. Gaynon, P. S. and Gonzalez Crussi, F. (1984). Exaggerated eosinophilia and acute lymphoid leukemia. *Am. J. Pediatr. Hematol. Oncol.* **6**, 334–7. [p. 160, 237]
630. Geha, R. S. and Akl, K. F. (1976). Skin lesions, angioedema, eosinophilia, and hypocomplementemia. *J. Pediatr.* **89**, 724–7. [p. 301]
631. Gelfand, E. W., McCurdy, D., Rao, C. P., and Cohen, A. (1984). Absence of lymphocyte ecto-5'-nucleotidase in infants with reticuloendotheliosis and eosinophilia (Omenn's syndrome). *Blood* **63**, 1475–80. [p. 166]
632. Geltner, D., Friedman, G., Naparstek, E., Granot, H., and Polliack, A. (1978). Acute lymphoblastic leukemia: its occurrence with hypereosinophilic syndrome and bilateral spontaneous pneumothorax. *Arch. Intern. Med.* **138**, 292–3. [p. 161]
633. Genta, R. M., Douce, R. W., and Walzer, P. D. (1986). Diagnostic implications of parasite-specific immune responses in immunocompromised patients with strongyloidiasis. *J. Clin. Microbiol.* **23**, 1099–103. [p. 146]
634. Genta, R. M., Weesner, R., Douce, R. W., Hvitger O'Connor, T., and Walzer, P. D. (1987). Strongyloidiasis in US veterans of the Vietnam and other wars. *JAMA* **258**, 49–52. [p. 145]
635. George, B. O., Gaba, F. E., and Talabi, A. I, (1982). M-mode echocardiographic features of endomyocardial fibrosis. *Br. Heart J.* **48**, 222–8. [p. 251]
636. Gerbaux, A., de Brux, J., Bennaceur, M., and Lenegre, J. (1956). L'endocardite parietale fibroplastique avec eosinophilie sanguine (endocardite de Löffler). *Bull. Mem. Soc. Med. Hop. Paris* **72**, 456–65. [p. 245]
637. Gerbaux, A., Dubost, C., Maurice, P., Prigent, C., Forman, J., Baculard,

P., and Valty, J. (1973). Endo-myocardite fibreuse observee au cours de la filariose: a propos d'un cas traite chirurgicalement. *Ann. Med. Interne.* **124**, 471–82. [p. 254]

638. Gershwin, M. G., Fatardo, C. F., Gurwith, M., and Kosek, J. C. (1972). Eosinophilia terminating in myeloblastoma. *Am. J. Med.* **53**, 343–53. [p. 152, 154, 285]
639. Ghidoni, J. J. and Goldberg, A. F. (1967). Light and electron microscopic localization of acid phosphatase activity in human eosinophils. *Am J. Clin. Pathol.* **45**, 402–5. [p. 60]
640. Ghosh, K., Shome, D. K., Marwaha, N., Mohanty, D., and Das, K. C. (1985). Normal plasma levels of B12 binding proteins in hypereosinophilic syndrome and secondary hypereosinophilia (letter). *Blood* **65**, 510–11. [p. 62]
641. Gibson, E. L., Vaucher, Y., and Corrigan, J. J. Jr. (1979). Eosinophilia in premature infants: relationship to weight gain. *J. Pediatr.* **95**, 99–101. [p. 294]
642. Giffin, H. Z., (1919). Persistent eosinophilia with hyperleukocytosis and splenomegaly. *Am. J. Med. Sci.* **158**, 618–29. [p. 289]
643. Gilbert, G. J. (1987). Churg-Strauss syndrome: determining adequacy of corticosteroid dosage by the eosinophil count. *South Med. J.* **80**, 266–8. [p. 203]
644. Giraldo, B., Blumenthal, M. N., and Spink, W. W. (1969). Aspirin intolerance and asthma: a clinical and immunological study. *Ann. Intern. Med.* **71**, 479–496. [p. 311]
645. Gitlin, N. and Grant, J. (1977). Raised serum transaminase levels in patients with rheumatic fever treated with salicylates. *S. Afr. Med. J.* **51**, 697–8. [p. 310]
646. Gittman, J. E., Schneider, G., Carnes, R. E., and Arkel, Y. S. (1978). Hypercalcemic crisis associated with the hypereosinophilic syndrome. *Am. J. Med.* **64**, 901–5. [p. 271, 276]
647. Gitzelmann, R., Spycher, M. A., Adank, S., Baerlocher, K., and Steinmann, B. (1985). Anomalous eosinophil granulocytes in blood and bone marrow: a diagnostic marker for infantile GM1-gangliosidosis? *Eur. J. Pediatr.* **144**, 82–4. [p. 259]
648. Glancy, J. J., Elder, J. L., and McAleer, R. (1981). Allergic bronchopulmonary fungal disease without clinical asthma. *Thorax* **36**, 345–9. [p. 133]
649. Glauert, A. M., Butterworth, A. E., Sturrock, R. F., and Houba, V. (1978). The mechanism of antibody-dependent, eosinophil-mediated damage to schistosomula of Schistosoma mansoni in vitro: a study by phase-contrast and electron microscopy. *J. Cell. Sci.* **34**, 173–92. [p. 115]
650. Glauert, A. M., Oliver, R. C., and Thorne, K. J. (1980). The interaction of human eosinophils and neutrophils with non-phagocytosable surfaces: a model for studying cell-mediated immunity in schistosomiasis. *Parasitology* **80**, 525–37. [p. 92]
651. Gleich, G. J. (1977). The eosinophil: structure and biochemical composition. *Am. J. Trop. Med. Hyg.* **26**, 126–33. [p. 323]
652. Gleich, G. J. (1977). The eosinophil: new aspects of structure and function. *J. Allergy Clin. Immunol.* **60**, 73–82. [p. 325]
653. Gleich, G. J. (1986). The functions of eosinophils. *Ann. Inst. Pasteur Immunol.* **137D**, 136–41. [p. 325]

654. Gleich, G. J. (1986). The role of the eosinophilic leukocyte in bronchial asthma. *Bull. Eur. Physiopathol. Respir.* **22** Suppl 7, 62–9. [p. 325]

655. Gleich, G. J., Ackerman, S. J., and Loegering, D. A. (1983). Procurement and purification of eosinophils. In *Cell separation, methods and selected applications. 2.* (eds. T. G. Pretlas and T. P. Pretlow) pp. 15–32. Academic Press, New York. [p. 32, 324]

656. Gleich, G. J. and Adolphson, C. R. (1986). The eosinophilic leukocyte: structure and function. *Adv. Immunol,* **39**, 177–253. [p. 46, 47, 84, 117, 226, 325]

657. Gleich, G. J., Adolphson, C. R., Slifman, N. R., Loegering, D. A., and McKean, D. J. (1987). Purification, neurotoxic and enzymatic activities of human eosinophil-derived neurotoxin and eosinophil cationic protein. In *Allergy and inflammation* (ed. A. B. Kay), pp. 165–78. Academic Press, London. [p. 51, 54, 55, 326]

658. Gleich, G. J., Frigas, E., Loegering, D. A., Wassom, D. L., and Steinmuller, D. (1979). Cytotoxic properties of the eosinophil major basic protein. *J. Immunol.* **123**, 2925–7. [p. 47, 48, 117, 118]

659. Gleich, G. J. and Loegering, D. A. (1984). Immunobiology of eosinophils. *Annu. Rev. Immunol.* **2**, 429–59. [p. 325]

660. Gleich, G. J., Loegering, D. A., and Adolphson, C. R. (1985). Eosinophils and bronchial inflammation. *Chest* **87**, 10S–13S. [p. 195]

661. Gleich, G. J., Loegering, D. A., Bell, M. P., Checkel, J. L., Ackerman, S. J., and McKean, D. J. (1986). Biochemical and functional similarities between human eosinophil-derived neurotoxin and eosinophil cationic protein: homology with ribonuclease. *Proc. Natl. Acad. Sci. USA* **83**, 3146–50. [p. 32, 49, 50, 52, 54, 55, 56, 249]

662. Gleich, G. J., Loegering, D. A., Frigas, E., and Filley, W. V. (1983). The eosinophil granule major basic protein: biological activities and relationship to bronchial asthma. *Monogr. Allergy* **18**, 277–83. [p. 47, 325]

663. Gleich, G. J., Loegering, D. A., Kueppers, F., Bajaj, S. P., and Mann, K. G. (1974). Physicochemical and biological properties of the major basic protein from guinea pig eosinophil granules. *J. Exp. Med.* **140**, 313–31. [p. 46, 48]

664. Gleich, G. J., Loegering, D. A., and Maldonado, J. E. (1973). Identification of a major basic protein in guinea pig eosinophil granules. *J. Exp. Med.* **137**, 1459–71. [p. 7, 46]

665. Gleich, G. J., Loegering, D. A., Mann, K. G., and Maldonado, J. E. (1976). Comparative properties of the Charcot–Leyden crystal protein and the major basic protein from human eosinophils. *J. Clin. Invest.* **57**, 633–40. [p. 7, 46, 47, 63, 65]

666. Gleich, G. J., Loegering, D. A., and Olson, G. M. (1975). Reactivity of rabbit antiserum to guinea pig eosinophils. *J. Immunol.* **115**, 950–4. [p. 84]

667. Gleich, G. J., Motojima, S., Frigas, E., Kephart, G. M., Fujisawa, T., and Kravis, L. P. (1987). The eosinophilic leukocyte and the pathology of fatal bronchial asthma: evidence for pathologic heterogeneity. *J. Allergy Clin. Immunol.* **80** (3 Pt 2), 412–5. [p. 195]

668. Gleich, G. J., Olson, G. M., and Herlich, H. (1979). The effect of antiserum to eosinophils and susceptibility and acquired immunity of the guinea-pig to Trichostronglyus colubriformis. *Immunology* **37**, 873–80. [p. 84]

669. Gleich, G. J., Olson, G. M., and Loegering, D. A. (1979). Eosinophils and hypersensitivity reactions. *Chest* **75** (2 Suppl), 215–8. [p. 314]

670. Gleich, G. J., Olson, G. M., and Loegering, D. A. (1979). The effect of ablation of eosinophils on immediate-type hypersensitivity reactions. *Immunology* **38**, 343–53. [p. 84]

671. Gleich, G. J., Pineda, A. A., Solley, G. O., and Taswell, H. F. (1982). Cytopheresis for procurement of eosinophils for the treatment of diseases associated with eosinophilia. Proceedings of the workshop on therapeutic plasmapheresis and cytopheresis. U.S. Department of Health and Human Services. NIH Publication No. 82. pp. 1165–73. [p. 32]

672. Gleich, G. J., Schroeter, A. L., Marcoux, J. P., Sachs, M. I., O'Connell, E. J., and Kohler, P. F. (1984). Episodic angioedema associated with eosinophilia. *N. Engl. J. Med.* **310**, 1621–6. [p. 47, 122, 300]

673. Gleich, G. J., Schroeter, A. L., Marcoux, J. P., Sachs, M. I., O'Connell, E. J., and Kohler, P. F. (1984). Episodic angioedema associated witih eosinophilia. *Trans. Assoc. Am. Physicians* **97**, 25–32. [p. 300]

674. Glovsky, M. M., Hugli, T. E., Ishizaka, T., Lichtenstein, L. M., and Erickson, B. W. (1979). Anaphylatoxin-induced histamine release with human leukocytes: studies of C3a leukocyte binding and histamine release. *J. Clin. Invest.* **64**, 804–11. [p. 82]

675. Godard, P., Bousquet, J., Lebel, B., and Michel, F. B. (1987). Bronchoalveolar lavage in the asthmatic. *Bull. Eur. Physiopathol. Respir.* **23**, 73–83. [p. 199]

676. Godard, P., Chaintreuil, J., Damon, M., Coupe, M., Flandre, O., Crastes de Paulet, A., and Michel, F. B. (1982). Functional assessment of alveolar macrophages: comparison of cells from asthmatics and normal subjects. *J. Allergy Clin. Immunol.* **70**, 88–93. [p. 195, 199]

677. Godfrey, R. M. and Sloan, P. (1985). Traumatic (eosinophilic) granuloma of oral soft tissues: a report of two cases with pseudo-lymphomatous features. *Br. J. Oral Maxillofac. Surg.* **23**, 351–4. [p. 172]

678. Goers, J. W., Glovsky, M. M. Hunkapiller, M. W., Farnsworth, V., and Richards, J. H. (1984). Studies on C3ahu binding to human eosinophils: characterization of binding. *Int. Arch. Allergy. Appl. Immunol.* **74**, 147–51. [p. 82]

679. Goetzl, E. J. (1982). The conversion of leukotriene C4 to isomers of leukotriene B4 by human eosinophil peroxidase. *Biochem. Biophys. Res. Commun.* **106**, 270–5. [p. 60]

680. Goetzl, E. J. and Austen, K. F. (1975). Purification and synthesis of eosinophilotactic tetrapeptides of human lung tissues: identification as eosinophil chemotactic factor of anaphylaxis. *Proc. Natl. Acad. Sci. USA* **72**, 4123–27. [p. 99]

681. Goetzl, E. J. and Austen, K. F. (1977). Eosinophil chemotactic factor of anaphylaxis (ECF-A): cellular origin, structure and function. *Monogr. Allergy* **12**, 189–97. [p. 99]

682. Goetzl, E. J., Rothenberg, J., Weber, E. L., Sinn, C. M., and Austen, K. F. (1980). A novel eosinophil chemotactic factor derived from a histiocytic lymphoma of the central nervous system. *Clin. Exp. Immunol.* **40**, 249–55. [p. 101]

683. Goetzl, E. J., Tashjian, A. H. Jr, Rubin, R. H., and Austen, K. F. (1978).

Production of a low molecular weight eosinophil polymorphonuclear leukocyte chemotactic factor by anaplastic squamous cell carcinomas of human lung. *J. Clin. Invest.* **61**, 770–80. [p. 101, 174]

684. Goetzl, E. J., Wasserman, S. I., and Austen, K. F. (1975). Eosinophil polymorphonuclear leukocyte function in immediate hypersensitivity. *Arch. Pathol. Lab. Med.* **99**, 1–4. [p. 6]

685. Goffman, T. E., Mulvihill, J. J., Carney, D. N., Triche, T. J., and Whang Peng, J. (1983). Fatal hypereosinophilia with chromosome 15q- in a patient with multiple primary and familial neoplasms. *Cancer Genet. Cytogenet.* **8**, 197–202. [p. 155]

686. Goh, K., Swisher, S. N., and Rosenberg, C. A. (1965). Cytogenetic studies of eosinophilic leukemia and chronic myelocytic leukemia. *Ann. Intern. Med.* **62**, 80–6. [p. 155, 157]

687. Goh, K. O., Ho, F. S., Tso, S. C., and Ma, J. (1985). Is hypereosinophilic syndrome a malignant disease? *Cancer* **55**, 2395–9. [p. 152]

688. Gokal, R., Ramos, J. M., Ward, M. K., and Kerr, D. N. (1981). 'Eosinophilic' peritonitis in continuous ambulatory peritoneal dialysis (CAPD). *Clin. Nephrol.* **15**, 328–30. [p. 221]

689. Goldman, H. and Proujansky, R. (1986). Allergic proctitis and gastroenteritis in children: clinical and mucosal biopsy features in 53 cases. *Am. J. Surg. Pathol.* **10**, 75–86. [p. 188, 189, 190]

690. Goldman, J. M., Najfeld, V., and Th'ng, K. H. (1975). Agar culture and chromosome analysis of eosinophilic leukaemia. *J. Clin. Pathol.* **28**, 956–61. [p. 157]

691. Goldsmith, M. M., Cresson, D. H., and Askin, F. B. (1987). The prognostic significance of stromal eosinophilia in head and neck cancer. *Otolaryngol. Head Neck Surg.* **96**, 319–24. [p. 173]

692. Goldstein, M. F., Freeman, M., and Zweiman, B. (1987). Eosinophilic fasciitis with atypical features. *Cutis* **39**, 214–6. [p. 181]

693. Gollasch. (1889). Zur kenntniss der asthmatischen sputums. *Fortschritte der Medizin (Berlin)* **7**, 361–5. [p. 5, 195]

694. Gomez Perretta, C., Armas Portela, R., Stockert, J. C., Tato, A., and Ferrer, J. M. (1986). Increased acidophilia of eosinophil granules after EDTA treatment. *Histochem. J.* **18**, 1–4. [p. 36]

695. Gonzalez, E. B., Swedo, J. L., Rajaraman, S., Daniels, J. C., and Grant, J. A. (1987). Ultrastructural and immunhistochemical evidence for release of eosinophilic granules *in vivo*: cytotoxic potential in chronic eosinophilic pneumonia. *J. Allergy Clin. Immunol.* **79**, 755–62. [p. 208]

696. Good, R. A. and Varco, R. L. (1955). A clinical and experimental study of agammaglobulinemia. *Lancet* **75**, 245–71. [p. 315]

697. Goodwin, J. F. (1983). Endomyocardial disease – clinical features. *Postgrad. Med. J.* **59**, 154–6. [p. 250]

698. Gopinathan, V. P. (1983). Tropical pulmonary eosinophilia. A clinical study. *Med. J. Aust.* **1**, 69–72. [p. 142]

699. Gordon, M. H. (1933). Remarks on Hodgkin's disease: a pathogenic agent in the glands, and its application in diagnosis. *Br. Med. J.* **i**, 641–4. [p. 53]

700. Gosset, P., Prin, L., Capron, M., Auriault, C., Tonnel, A. B., and Capron, A. (1986). Presence of factors chemotactic for granulocytes in hypereosino-

philic syndrome sera: relation with alterations in eosinophil migration. *Clin. Exp. Immunol.* **65**, 654–63. [p. 283]

701. Gosset, P., Tonnel, A. B., Joseph, M., Prin, L., Mallart, A., Charon, J., and Capron, A. (1984). Secretion of a chemotactic factor for neutrophils and eosinophils by alveolar macrophages from asthmatic patients. *J. Allergy Clin. Immunol.* **74**, 827–34. [p. 101]
702. Goto, N., Kawamura, M., Inoue, M., and Sato, A. (1983). Pathology of two cases of canine disseminated hypereosinophilic disease. *Nippon Juigaku Zasshi* **45**, 305–12. [p. 268]
703. Gottdiener, J. S., Maron, B. J., Schooley, R. T., Harley, J. B., Roberts, W. C., and Fauci, A. S. (1983). Two-dimensional echocardiographic assessment of the idiopathic hypereosinophilic syndrome: anatomic basis of mitral regurgitation and peripheral embolization. *Circulation* **67**, 572–8. [p. 239, 248]
704. Gough, N. M., Gough, J., Metcalf, D., Kelso, A., Grail, D., Nicola, N. A., Burgess, A. W., and Dunn, A. R. (1984). Molecular cloning of cDNA encoding a murine haemopoietic growth regulator, granulocyte-macrophage colony stimulating factor. *Nature* **309**, 763–67. [p. 20]
705. Gould, L., Reddy, C. V., Chua, W., Swamy, C. R., and Dorismond, J. C. (1977). Fibroplastic parietal endocarditis with eosinophilia. *Angiology* **28**, 779–87. [p. 239]
706. Graham, J. M., Lawrie, G. M., Feteih, N. M., and Debakey, M. E. (1981). Management of endomyocardial fibrosis: successful surgical treatment of biventricular involvement and consideration of the superiority of operative intervention. *Am. Heart J.* **102**, 771–82. [p. 245]
707. Grammer, L. C., Greenberger, P. A., and Patterson, R. (1986). Allergic bronchopulmonary aspergillosis in asthmatic patients presenting with allergic rhinitis. *Int. Arch. Allergy Appl. Immunol.* **79**, 246–8. [p. 213]
708. Grammer, L. C., and Patterson, R. (1987). IgE against ethylene oxide-altered human serum albumin (ETO-HSA) as an etiologic agent in allergic reactions of hemodialysis patients. *Artif. Organs* **11**, 97–9. [p. 221]
709. Grandjean, P. and Tarkowski, S., Eds. (1984). *Toxic oil syndrome: mass food poisoning in Spain.* WHO Regional Office for Europe. WHO, Copenhagen. pp. 92. [p. 182]
710. Grant, M. D., Horowitz, H. I., Lazarevic, B. M., and Spielvogel, A. R. (1974). Eosinophilic leukemia and myelofibrosis with acute blastic termination: report of a case with review of literature. *Conn. Med.* **38**, 226–9. [p. 285]
711. Grant, S. C. and Klein, C. (1987). Toxoplasma gondii encephalitis in an immunocompetent adult. a case report. *S. Afr. Med. J.* **71**, 585–7. [p. 149]
712. Grantham, J. G., Meadows, J. A., and Gleich, G. J. (1986). Chronic eosinophilic pneumonia: evidence for eosinophil degranulation and release of major basic protein. *Am. J. Med.* **80**, 89–94. [p. 208]
713. Greenberger, P. A., Patterson, R., Ghory, A., Arkins, J. A., Walsh, T., Graves, T., and Saker, J. (1980). Late sequelae of allergic bronchopulmonary aspergillosis. *J. Allergy Clin. Immunol.* **66**, 327–35. [p. 133]
714. Greene, B. M., Taylor, H. R., and Aikawa, M. (1981). Cellular killing of microfilariae of Onchocerca volvulus: eosinophil and neutrophil-mediated immune serum-dependent destruction. *J. Immunol.* **127**, 1611–8. [p. 116]

715. Greif, J., Struhar, D., Kivity, S., and Topilsky, M. (1986). Bronchoalveolar lavage: a useful tool in the diagnosis of eosinophilic pneumonia. *Isr. J. Med. Sci.* **22**, 479–80. [p. 194, 207]

716. Grimaldi, M. C., D Ippolito, S., Pica A., and Della Corte F. (1983). Cytochemical identification of the leukocytes of torpedoes (Torpedo marmorata Risso and Torpedo ocellata Rafinisque). *Basic Appl. Histochem.* **27**, 311–7. [p. 124]

717. Grisold, W. and Jellinger, K. (1985). Multifocal neoropathy with vasculitis in hypereosinophilic syndrome: an entity or drug-induced effect? *J. Neurol.* **231**, 301–6. [p. 275, 276]

718. Groopman, J. E., Mitsuyasu, R. T., DeLeo, M. J., Oette, D. H., and Golde, D. W. (1987). Effect of recombinant human granulocyte-macrophage colony-stimulating factor on myelopoiesis in the acquired immunodeficiency syndrome. *N. Engl. J. Med.* **317**, 593–8. [p. 22]

719. Grosgogeat, Y. and Nicolas, G. (1977). (Endomyocardial biopsy: its value in tropical pathology. Apropos of 3 new cases). *Arch. Mal Coeur* **70**, 179–83. [p. 253, 255]

720. Grouls, V. and Helpap, B. (1981). Selective staining of eosinophils and their immature precursors in tissue sections and autoradiographs with Congo red. *Stain Technol.* **56**, 323–5. [p. 38]

721. Grove, D. I. (1982). What is the relationship between asthma and worms? *Allergy* **37**, 139–48. [p. 201]

722. Grove, D. I., Mahmoud, A. A., and Warren, K. S. (1977). Eosinophils and resistance to Trichinella spiralis. *J. Exp. Med.* **145**, 755–759. [p. 84]

723. Grover, W. H., Winkler, H. H., and Normansell, D. E. (1978). Phagocytic properties of isolated human eosinophils. *J. Immunol.* **121**, 718–25. [p. 90]

724. Groza, P., Bordeianu, A., and Boca, A. (1983). Modifications of the digestive tract in rats submitted to an orbital flight aboard the Soviet satellite Cosmos 1129. *Physiologie* **20**, 35–44. [p. 183]

725. Gruenwald, H., Kiossoglu, K. A., Mitus, W., and Damashek, W. (1965). Philadelphic chromosome in eosinophilic leukemia. *Am. J. Med.* **39**, 1003–10. [p. 157]

726. Grzych, J. M., Dissous, C., Capron, M., Torres, S., Lambert, P. H., and Capron, A. (1987). Schistosoma mansoni shares a protective carbohydrate epitope with keyhole limpet hemocyanin. *J. Exp. Med.* **165**, 865–78. [p. 114]

727. Guerra-Caceres, J. G., Bryceson, A. D., Quakyi, K., and Spry, C. J. (1980). Studies on the mechanisms of adverse reactions produced by diethylcarbamazine in patients with onchocerciasis: the Mazzotti reaction. *Parasite Immunol.* **2**, 121–31. [p. 143]

728. Guillevin, L., Guittard, T., Bletry, O., Godeau, P., and Rosenthal, P. (1987). Systemic necrotizing angiitis with asthma: causes and precipitating factors in 43 cases. *Lung* **165**, 165–72. [p. 203]

729. Gullberg, U., Widegren, B., Arnason, U., Egesten, A., and Olsson, I. (1986). The cytotoxic eosinophil cationic protein (ECP) has ribonuclease activity. *Biochem. Biophys. Res. Commun.* **139**, 1239–42. [p. 51, 55]

730. Gupta, D. S., Gupta, M. K., and Borle, R. M. (1985). Pan-mandibular keratocyst with eosinophilia. *Int. J. Oral Surg.* **14**, 311–13. [p. 172]

731. Hagan, P., Wilkins, H. A., Blumenthal, U. J., Hayes, R. J., and Greenwood,

B. M. (1985). Eosinophilia and resistance to Schistosoma haematobium in man. *Parasite Immunol.* **7**, 625–32. [p. 148]

732. Hajdu, I., Zhang, W., and Gordon, G. B. (1986). Peanut agglutinin binding as a histochemical tool for diagnosis of eosinophilic granuloma. *Arch. Pathol. Lab. Med.* **110**, 719–21. [p. 165]

733. Hall, J. W., Kozak, M., and Spink, W. W. (1964). Pulmonary infiltrates, pericarditis and eosinophilia: a unique case of the pulmonary infiltration and eosinophil syndrome. *Am. J. Med.* **36**, 135–43. [p. 228]

734. Hall, S. W. Jr, Theologides, A., From, A. H., Gobel, F. L., Fortuny, I. E., Lawrence, C. J., and Edwards, J. E. (1977). Hypereosinophilic syndrome with biventricular involvement. *Circulation* **55**, 217–22. [p. 241]

735. Hallgren, R., Bjelle, A., and Venge, P. (1984). Eosinophil cationic protein in inflammatory synovial effusions as evidence of eosinophil involvement. *Ann. Rheum. Dis.* **43**, 556–62. [p. 178]

736. Hallgren, R., Borg, T., Venge, P., and Modig, J. (1984). Signs of neutrophil and eosinophil activation in adult respiratory distress syndrome. *Crit. Care Med.* **12**, 14–18. [p. 211]

737. Hallgren, R., Feltelius, N., Svenson, K., and Venge, P. (1985). Eosinophil involvement in rheumatoid arthritis as reflected by elevated serum levels of eosinophil cationic protein. *Clin. Exp. Immunol.* **59**, 539–46. [p. 51, 177]

738. Hallgren, R., Grefberg, N., and Venge, P. (1984). Elevated circulating levels of eosinophil cationic protein in uremia as signs of abnormal eosinophil homeostasis. *Nephron.* **36**, 10–4. [p. 220]

739. Hallgren, R., Samuelsson, T., Venge, P., and Modig, J. (1987). Eosinophil activation in the lung is related to lung damage in adult respiratory distress syndrome. *Am. Rev. Respir, Dis.* **135**, 639–42. [p. 212]

740. Hallgren, R., Terent, A., and Venge, P. (1983). Eosinophil cationic protein (ECP) in the cerebrospinal fluid. *J. Neurol. Sci.* **58**, 57–71. [p. 56, 217]

741. Hallgren, R., Venge, P., Cullhed, I., and Olsson, I. (1979). Blood eosinophils and eosinophil cationic protein after acute myocardial infarction or corticosteroid administration. *Br. J. Haematol.* **42**, 147–54. [p. 229]

742. Hallgren, R., Venge, P., and Danielson, B. G. (1982). Neutrophil and eosinophil degranulation during hemodialysis are mediated by the dialysis membrane. *Nephron.* **32**, 329–34. [p. 222]

743. Hallgren, R., Venge, P., and Wistedt, B. (1982). Elevated serum levels of lactoferrin and eosinophil cationic protein in schizophrenic patients. *Br. J. Psychiatry.* **140**, 55–60. [p. 217]

744. Halwig, J. M., Brueske, D. A., Greenberger, P. A., Dreisin, R. B., and Sommers, H. M. (1985). Allergic bronchopulmonary curvulariosis. *Am. Rev. Respir. Dis.* **132**, 186–8. [p. 133]

745. Hamada, A. and Greene, B. M. (1987). Clq enhancement of IgG-dependent eosinophil-mediated killing of schistosomula *in vitro*. *J. Immunol.* **138**, 1240–5. [p. 82]

746. Hamamoto, Y., Kinoshita, K., Hashimoto, K., Matsushita, T., Kogishi, K., and Yasuhira, K. (1983). Experimental production of pulmonary granulomas. IV. Eosinophilic granuloma. *Br. J. Exp. Pathol.* **64**, 177–84. [p. 211]

747. Hamann, K. H., Barker, R. L., Loegering, D. A., and Gleich, G. J. (1987). Comparative toxicity of purified human eosinophil granule proteins for

newborn larvae of Trichinella spiralis. *J. Parasitol.* **73**, 523–9 [p. 47, 51, 52, 55, 116]

748. Handa, S. P. (1986). Drug-induced acute interstitial nephritis: report of 10 cases. *Can. Med. Assoc. J.* **135**, 1278–81. [p. 309]
749. Hanker, J. S., Chandross, R. J., Solic, J. J., Weatherly, N. F., Laszlo, J., Moore, J. O., and Ottolenghi, A. (1981). Medusa cells: cytostructure and cytochemistry of amoeboid eosinophils with pseudopod-like processes. *Histochem. J.* **13**, 905–19. [p. 38]
750. Hanker, J. S., Chandross, R. J., Weatherly, N. F., Laszlo, J., Moore, J. O., Buckley, R. H., and Ottolenghi, A. (1980). Medusa cells: the morphology and cytochemistry of common, amoeboid variants of eosinophils. *Histochem. J.* **12**, 701–15. [p. 59]
751. Hanowell, S. T., Kim, Y. D., Rattan, V., and MacNamara, T. E. (1981). Increased heparin requirement with hypereosinophilic syndrome. *Anesthesiology* **55**, 450–2. [p. 242]
752. Hanson, G., Flor, N., Wells, I., Novey, H., and Galant, S. (1977). Bronchocentric granulomatosis: a complication of allergic bronchopulmonary aspergillosis. *J. Allergy. Clin. Immunol.* **59**, 83–90. [p. 131]
753. Hardy, W. R. and Anderson, R. E. (1968). The hypereosinophilic syndromes. *Ann. Intern. Med.* **68**, 1220–9. [p. 263]
754. Harkavy, J. (1941). Vascular allergy: pathogenesis of bronchial asthma with recurrent pulmonary infiltration and eosinophilic polyserositis. *Arch. Intern. Med.* **67**, 709–34. [p. 202]
755. Harley, J. B., Fauci, A. S., and Gralnick, H. R. (1983). Noncardiovascular findings associated with heart disease in the idiopathic hypereosinophilic syndrome. *Am. J. Cardiol.* **52**, 321–4. [p. 235]
756. Harley, J. B., McIntosh, C. L., Kirklin, J. J., Maron, B. J., Gottdiener, J., Roberts, W. C., and Fauci, A. S. (1982). Atrioventricular valve replacement in the idiopathic hypereosinophilic syndrome. *Am. J. Med.* **73**, 77–81. [p. 243]
757. Harmon, W. A. and Helman, C. A. (1981). Eosinophilic gastroenteritis and ascites. *J. Clin. Gastroenterol.* **3**, 371–3. [p. 186]
758. Harries, A. D., Fryatt, R., Walker, J., Chiodini, P. L., and Bryceson, A. D. (1986). Schistosomiasis in expatriates returning to Britain from the tropics: a controlled study. *Lancet* **1**, 86–8. [p. 147]
759. Harries, A. D., Myers, B., and Bhattacharrya, D. (1986). Eosinophilia in Caucasians returning from the tropics. *Trans. R. Soc. Trop. Med. Hyg.* **80**, 327–8. [p. 136, 137, 143, 145, 146]
760. Harris, A., Twarog, F. J., and Geha, R. S. (1983). Chronic urticaria in childhood: natural course and etiology. *Ann. Allergy* **51**, 161–5. [p. 299]
761. Harris, A. I. and Neugarten, J. (1978). Chronic active hepatitis and ulcerative colitis associated with eosinophilia, nonthrombocytopenic hypergammaglobulinemic purpura and serologic abnormalities. *Am. J. Gastroenterol.* **69**, 191–5. [p. 190]
762. Harth, H., Pees., H., and Zankl, H. (1986). Acute myelomonocytic leukemia (M4) with eosinophilia: problems concerning chromosome 16 abnormality. *Cancer Genet. Cytogenet.* **23**, 127–33. [p. 159]
763. Haruda, F. (1979). Phenytoin hypersensitivity: 38 cases. *Neurology* **29**, 1480–5. [p. 310]

764. Harvey, J. W. (1981). Myeloproliferative disorders in dogs and cats. *Vet. Clin. North Am. (Small Anim Pract)* **11**, 349–81. [p. 157]

765. Hashimoto, K., Takahashi, S., Fligiel, A., and Savoy, L. B. (1985). Eosinophilic granuloma: presence of OKT6-positive cells and good response to intralesional steroid. *Arch. Dermatol.* **121**, 770–4. [p. 164]

766. Hasselbacher, P. and Schumacher, H. R. (1977). Bilateral protusio acetabuli following pelvic irradiation. *J. Rheumatol.* **4**, 189–96. [p. 177]

767. Hasselbacher, P. and Schumacher, H. R. (1978). Synovial fluid eosinophilia following arthrography. *J. Rheumatol.* **5**, 173–6. [p. 177]

768. Hastie, A. T., Loegering, D. A., Gleich, G. J., and Kueppers, F. (1987). The effect of purified human eosinophil major basic protein on mammalian ciliary activity. *Am. Rev. Respir. Dis.* **135**, 848–53. [p. 48]

769. Hathirat, P., Bintadish, P., Isarangkura, P., Sasanakul, W., Chiewsilp, P., and Ratanasirivanich, P. (1982). Platelet transfusion in acquired platelet dysfunctioin with eosinophilia. *Southeast Asian J. Trop. Med. Public Health.* **13**, 220–4. [p. 262]

770. Hauwaert, L. G. van der, Corbeel, L., Maldague, P. (1965). Fibroma of the right ventricle producing severe tricuspid stenosis. *Circulation* **32**, 451–6. [p. 170]

771. Hawkey, C. M., Ashton, D. G., Hart, M. G., Cindery, R. N., and Jones, D. M. (1983). Normal and clinical haematology in the yak (Bos grunniens). *Res. Vet. Sci.* **34**, 31–6. [p. 125]

772. Hayashi, H., Honda, M., Shimokawa, Y., and Hirashima, M. (1984). Chemotactic factors associated with leukocyte emigration in immune tissue injury: their separation, characterization, and functional specificity. *Int. Rev. Cytol.* **89**, 179–250. [p. 325]

773. Heatley, R. V. and James, P. D. (1979). Eosinophils in the rectal mucosa. A simple method of predicting the outcome of ulcerative proctocolitis? *Gut* **20**, 787–91. [p. 190]

774. Hellmann, A., Goldman, J. M., and Spry, C. J. (1981). Increased eosinophil colony formation in agar by haemopoietic cells from patients with the hypereosinophilic syndrome. *Clin. Lab. Haematol.* **3**, 205–13. [p. 285]

775. Hellstrom, H. R., Davis, B. K., Shonnard, J. W., and MacPherson, T. A. (1979). Eosinophilic pyeloureteritis: report of a case *J. Urol.* **122**, 833–4.[p. 223]

776. Henderson, W. R. and Chi, E. Y. (1985). Ultrastructural characterization and morphometric analysis of human eosinophil degranulation. *J. Cell. Sci.* **73**, 33–48. [p. 94]

777. Henderson, W. R., Chi, E. Y., Jorg, A., and Klebanoff, S. J. (1983). Horse eosinophil degranulation induced by the ionophore A23187. Ultrastructure and role of phospholipase A2. *Am. J. Pathol.* **111**, 341–9. [p. 94]

778. Henderson, W. R., Chi, E. Y., and Klebanoff, S. J. (1980). Eosinophil peroxidase-induced mast cell secretion. *J. Exp. Med.* **152**, 265–79. [p. 60, 120]

779. Henderson, W. R., Harley, J. B., and Fauci, A. S. (1984). Arachidonic acid metabolism in normal and hypereosinophilic syndrome human eosinophils: generation of leukotrienes B4, C4, D4 and 15-lipoxygenase products. *Immunolgy* **51**, 679–86. [p. 70]

780. Henderson, W. R., Harley, J. B., Fauci, A. S., and Chi, E. Y. (1988).

Hypereosinophilic syndrome human eosinophil degranulation induced by soluble and particulate stimuli. *Br. J. Haematol.* **69**, 13–21. [p. 32, 75, 280, 281, 283]

781. Henderson, W. R., Jong, E. C., and Klebanoff, S. J. (1980). Binding of eosinophil peroxidase to mast cell granules with retention of peroxidatic activity. *J. Immunol.* **124**, 1383–8. [p. 60]
782. Henderson, W. R., Jorg, A., and Klebanoff, S. J. (1982). Eosinophil peroxidase-mediated inactivation of leukotrienes B4, C4, and D4. *J. Immunol.* **128**, 2609–13. [p. 60]
783. Hendrick, M. (1981). A spectrum of hypereosinophilic syndromes exemplified by six cats with eosinophilic enteritis. *Vet. Pathol.* **18**, 188–200. [p. 268]
784. Henocq, E. and Vargaftig, B. B. (1988). Skin eosinophilia in atopic patients. *J. Allergy. Clin. Immunol.* **81**, 691–5. [p. 97]
785. Henriksen, J. M. (1986). Exercise-induced bronchoconstriction. Seasonal variation in children with asthma and in those with rhinitis. *Allergy* **41**, 499–506. [p. 204]
786. Henry, P. G. and Burnett, J. W. (1978). Angiolymphoid hyperplasia with eosinophilia. *Arch. Dermatol.* **114**, 1168–72. [p. 167]
787. Henson, P. M. (1969). The adherence of leucocytes and platelets induced by fixed IgG or complement. *Immunology* **16**, 107–21. [p. 77, 81]
788. Herborn, H. A., Valdimarsson, H., and Wickramasinghe, S. N. (1979). Development of human granulocyte and monocyte Fc receptors. *Scand. J. Haematol.* **22**, 364–8. [p. 77]
789. Herman, J. J. (1982). Eosinophil diamine oxidase activity in acute inflammation in humans. *Agents Actions* **12**, 46–8. [p. 62]
790. Herman, J. J., Rosner, I. K., Davis, A. E., Zeiger, R. S., Arnaout, M. A., and Colten, H. R. (1979). Complement-dependent histaminase release from human granulocytes. *J. Clin. Invest.* **63**, 1195–202. [p. 62]
791. Herrera Goepfert, R. and Larraza Hernandez, O. (1985). (Hypereosinophilic syndrome). *Bol. Med. Hosp. Infant. Mex.* **42**, 201–6. [p. 269]
792. Herskowitz, A., Soule, L. M., Mellits, E. D., Traill, T. A., Achuff, S. C., Reitz, B. A., Borkon, A. M., Baumgartner, W. A., and Baughman, K. L. (1987). Histologic predictors of actute cardiac rejection in human endomyocardial biopsies: a multivariate analysis. *J. Am. Coll. Cardiol.* **9**, 802–10. [p. 229]
793. Herzog, C. A., Snover, D. C., and Staley, N. A. (1984). Acute necrotising eosinophilic myocarditis. *Br. Heart J.* **52**, 343–8. [p. 229]
794. Hibbs, M. S., Mainardi, C. L., and Kang, A. H. (1982). Type-specific collagen degradation by eosinophils. *Biochem. J.* **207**, 621–4. [p. 61]
795. Hickling, P., Buksh, K., and Beck, P. (1980). A case of leiomyoma of the oesophagus complicated by superior vena cava obstruction and associated eosinophilia. *Postgrad. Med. J.* **56**, 431–4. [p. 171]
796. Hill, D. J., Ekert, H., and Bryant, D. H. (1986). Episodic angioedema and hypereosinophilia in childhood (letter). *J. Allergy Clin. Immunol.* **78**, 122–3. [p. 301]
797. Hill, R., Wang, N. S., and Berry, G. (1984). Hypereosinophilic syndrome with pulmonary vascular involvement. *Angiology* **35**, 238–44. [p. 272]
798. Hillerdal, G., Marjanovic, B., and Aberg, H. (1979). Rheumatoid arthritis,

immune complex disease, and hypereosinophilic syndrome: report on a case. *Acta Med. Scand.* **206**, 429–32. [p. 177]

799. Hirashima, M., Tashiro, K., Sakata, K., Muramoto, K., and Iyama, K. (1986). Eosinophil chemotactic factors from granuloma of Kimura's disease, with special reference to T lymphocyte-derived factors. *J. Leukocyte. Biol.* **40**, 393–405. [p. 168]
800. Hirose, Y., Konda, S., Sugai, S., Takiguchi, T., Shimizu, S., Matsushima, K., and Annen, Y. (1981). A case of eosinophilic leukemia associated with Löffler's endocarditis: clinical course and autopsy findings. *Nippon Ketsueki Gakkai Zasshi* **44**, 902–9. [p. 154]
801. Hirsch, J. G., and Hirsch, B. I. (1980). Paul Ehrlich and the discovery of the eosinophil. In *The Eosinophil in Health and Disease* (eds. A. A. Mahmoud, K. F. Austen, and A. S. Simon), pp. 3–23. Grune and Stratton, New York. [p. 4, 90, 123, 155]
802. Hocking, W. G. and Swanson, M. (1986). Multifocal eosinophilic granuloma: response of a patient to etoposide. *Cancer* **58**, 840–2. [p. 166]
803. Hoefer, R. A., Ziegler, M. M., Koop, C. E., and Schnaufer, L. (1977). Surgical manifestations of eosinophilic gastroenteritis in the pediatric patient. *J. Pediatr. Surg.* **12**, 955–62. [p. 184]
804. Hoffman, F. G., Rosenbaum, D., and Genovese, P. D. (1955). Fibroplastic endocarditis with eosinophilia (Löffler's endocarditis parietalis fibroplastica): case report and review of literature. *Ann. Intern. Med.* **42**, 668–80. [p. 234]
805. Hoffmann, J. J. and Tielens, A. G. (1987). Partial deficiency of eosinophil peroxidase. *Blut* **54**, 165–9. [p. 260]
806. Hogan, T. F., Koss, W., Murgo, A. J., Amato, R. S., Fontana, J. A., and VanScoy, F. L. (1987). Acute lymphoblastic leukemia with chromosomal 5;14 translocation and hypereosinophilia: case report and literature review. *J. Clin. Oncol.* **5**, 382–90. [p. 23, 160, 326]
807. Hogg, N., MacDonald, S., Slusarenko, M., and Beverley, P. C. (1984). Monoclonal antibodies specific for human monocytes, granulocytes and endothelium. *Immunology* **53**, 753–67. [p. 87]
808. Hogge, D. E., Misawa, S., Parsa, N. Z., Pollak, A., and Testa, J. R. (1984). Abnormalities of chromosome 16 in association with acute myelomonocytic leukemia and dysplastic bone marrow eosinophils. *J. Clin. Oncol.* **2**, 550–7. [p. 158]
809. Hollister, D. Jr., Clements, M., Coleman, M., and Petito, F. (1983). Eosinophilic meningitis in Hodgkin's disease: report of a case and review of the literature. *Arch. Intern. Med.* **143**, 590–2. [p. 216]
810. Holmes, R., Keating, M. J., Cork, A., Broach, Y., Trujillo, J., Dalton, W. T. Jr, McCredie, K. B., and Freireich, E. J. (1985). A unique pattern of central nervous system leukemia in acute myelomonocytic leukemia associated with inv(16)(pl3q22). *Blood* **65**, 1071–8. [p. 158]
811. Holopainen, E., Makinen, J., Paavolainen, M., Palva, T., and Salo, O. P. (1979). Nasal polyposis: relationships to allergy and acetylsalicyclic acid intolerance. *Acta Otolaryngol. (Stockh)* **87**, 330–4. [p. 214]
812. Horii, Y., Matsuoka, H., and Owhashi, M. (1986). Chemotactic activity of soluble extract of Schistosoma japonicum eggs for human and monkey eosinophils. *Z. Parasitenkd.* **72**, 557–9. [p. 100]
813. Hornung, M. (1962). Preservation recrystallization and preliminary biochem-

ical characterization of Charcot–Leyden crystals. *Proc. Soc. Exp. Biol. Med.* **110**, 119–24. [p. 64]

814. Horny, H. P. and Horst, H. A. (1986). Frequency distribution of tissue mast cells and eosinophilic granulocytes in tumor-draining axillary and paracolic lymph nodes. *J. Cancer Res. Clin. Oncol.* **112**, 151–5. [p. 170]
815. Horny, H. P. and Horst, H. A. (1987). Lymphoreticular infiltrates in adenocarcinoma of the large intestine. *Pathol. Res. Pract.* **182**, 222–7. [p. 172]
816. Horobin, R. W. and Walter, K. J. (1987). Understanding Romanowsky staining. I: The Romanowsky-Giesma effect in blood smears. *Histochemistry* **86**, 331–6. [p. 37]
817. Horowitz, L. (1975). Atopy as factor in penicillin reactions. *N. Engl. J. Med.* **292**, 1243–4. [p. 310, 311]
818. Houwerzijl, J., de Gast, G. C., Nater, J. P., Esselink, M. T., and Nieweg, H. O. (1977). Lymphocyte-stimulation tests and patch tests in carbamazepine hypersensitivity. *Clin. Exp. Immunol.* **29**, 272–7. [p. 313]
819. Hromas, R. A. and Murray, J. L. (1984). Bone marrow in the acquired immunodeficiency syndrome (letter). *Ann. Intern. Med.* **101**, 877. [p. 135]
820. Hsu, S. Y., Hsu, H. F., Mitros, F. A., Helms, C. M., and Solomon, R. I. (1980). Eosinophils as effector cells in the destruction of Schistosoma mansoni eggs in granulomas. *Ann. Trop. Med. Parasitol.* **74**, 179–83. [p. 114]
821. Huang, C. S., Gomez, G. A., Kohno, S. I., Sokal, J. E., and Sandberg, A. A. (1979). Chromosomes and causation of human cancer and leukemia. XXXIV. A case of 'hypereosinophilic syndrome' with unusual cytogenetic findings in a chloroma, terminating in blastic transformation and CNS leukemia. *Cancer* **44**, 1284–9. [p. 152, 155]
822. Hubscher, T. (1975). Role of the eosinophil in the allergic reactions. I. EDI, an eosinophil-derived inhibitor of histamine release. *J. Immunol.* **114**, 1379–88. [p. 79]
823. Hubscher, T. (1975). Role of the eosinophil in the allergic reactions. II. Release of prostaglandins from human eosinophilic leukocytes. *J. Immunol.* **114**, 1389–93. [p. 71]
824. Hudson, G. and Maxwell, M. H. (1982). Eosinophil leucocytes: granules and cell functions. In *Topical Reviews of Haematology. 2.* (ed. S. Roath), pp. 43–74. Wright PSG, Bristol. [p. 324]
825. Hulliger, L. and Blazkovec, A. A. (1967). A simple and efficient method of separating peripheral-blood leucocytes for in-vitro work. *Lancet* **i**, 1304–5. [p. 32]
826. Humayun, H. M., Ing, T. S., Daugirdas, J. T., Gandhi, V. C., Popli, S., Robinson, J. A., Hano, J. E., and Zayas, I. (1981). Peritoneal fluid eosinophilia in patients undergoing maintenance peritoneal dialysis. *Arch. Intern. Med.* **141**, 1172–3. [p. 221]
827. Humphrey, M. J., Hutter, Jr., and Tom, W. W. (1981). Hypereosinophilia in a monosomy 7 myeloproliferative disorder in childhood. *Am. J. Hematol.* **11**, 107–10. [p. 25, 155, 156]
828. Hunninghake, G. W. and Fauci, A. S. (1979). State of the art: pulmonary involvement in the collagen vascular diseases. *Am. Rev. Respir. Dis.* **119**, 471–503. [p. 210]
829. Hurwitz, N. (1969). Predisposing factors in adverse reactions to drugs. *Br. Med. J.* **i**, 536–9. [p. 311]

830. Hurwitz, N. and Wade, O. L. (1969). The incidence of adverse reactions in relation to the use of drugs in hospital. *Br. Med. J.* **1**, 531–6. [p. 310]
831. Hussain, R. and Ottesen, E. A. (1986). IgE responses in human filariasis. IV. Parallel antigen recognition by IgE and IgG4 subclass antibodies. *J. Immunol.* **136**, 1859–63. [p. 142, 143]
832. Hutt, M. S. (1983). Epidemiology aspects of endomyocardial fibrosis. *Postgrad. Med. J.* **59**, 142–4. [p. 255]
833. Hyder, S. L., Cayer, M. L., and Pettey, C. L. (1983). Cell types in peripheral blood of the nurse shark: an approach to structure and function. *Tissue Cell* **15**, 437–55. [p. 124]
834. Hyman, P. M., Teichberg, S., Starrett, S., Vinciguerra, V., and Degnan, T. J. (1978). Secretion of primary granules from developing human eosinophilic promyelocytes. *Proc. Soc. Exp. Biol. Med.* **159**, 380–5. [p. 57]
835. Ichimaru, K. and Horie, A. (1987). Microangiopathic changes of subepidermal capillaries in end-stage renal failure. *Nephron.* **46**, 144–9. [p. 223]
836. Idell, S., Johnson, M., Beauregard, L., and Learner, N. (1983). Pneumonia associated with rising cytomegalovirus antibody titres in a healthy adult. *Thorax* **38**, 957–8. [p. 212]
837. Iguchi, Y., Inoue, T., Shimono, M., Yamamura, T., Shigematsu, T., and Takahashi, S. (1986). Kimura's disease and its relation to angiolymphoid hyperplasia with eosinophilia: report of three cases and review of the literature. *J. Oral. Pathol.* **15**, 132–7. [p. 167, 168]
838. Ijuhin, N., Rose, G. G., Kobayashi, K., Mahan, C. J., Romsdahl, M. M. (1976). The Lx bodies of an eosinophilic granuloma in vivo and in vitro. *Texas Reports Biol. Med.* **34**, 267–88. [p. 164]
839. Ikaheimo, M. J., Karkola, P. J., and Takkunen, J. T. (1981). Surgical treatment of Löffler's eosinophilic endocarditis. *Br. Heart J.* **45**, 729–32. [p. 243]
840. Inoh, T., Hatani, H., Tsuchiya, G., Matsumoto, K., Kyogoku, M., and Fukuzaki, H. (1980). Clinical features and post-mortem coronary angiograms of several types of myocardial fibrosis in five cases. *Kobe J. Med. Sci.* **26**, 211–22. [p. 252]
841. Inoue, T., Iwasaki, K., Chihara, T., and Torisu, M. (1981). Cervical carcinoma and eosinophil I. Eosinophil chemotactic factor derived from invasive cervical carcinoma with eosinophil infiltration. *Clin. Immunol. Immunopathol.* **21**, 320–31. [p. 101]
842. Iozzo, R. V., MacDonald, G. H., and Wight, T. N. (1982). Immunoelectron microscopic localization of catalase in human eosinophilic leukocytes. *J. Histochem. Cytochem.* **30**, 697–701. [p. 62]
843. Isaacson, N. H. and Rapoport, P. (1946). Eosinophilia in malignant tumors: its significance. *Ann. Intern. Med.* **25**, 893–902. [p. 169]
844. Iscove, N. N., Senn, J. S., Till, J. E., and McCulloch, E. A. (1971). Colony formation by normal and leukemic human marrow cells in culture: effect of conditioned medium from human leukocytes. *Blood* **37**, 1–5. [p. 8, 15]
845. Ishibashi, T., Kimura, H., Abe, R., Matsuda, S., Uchida, T., and Kariyone, S. (1986). Involvement of eosinophils in leukemia: cytogenetic study of eosinophilic colonies from acute myelogenous leukemia associated with translocation (8;21). *Cancer Genet. Cytogenet.* **22**, 189–94. [p. 159]
846. Ishii, T., Koide, O., Hosoda, Y., and Takahashi, R. (1977). Hypereosino-

philic multiple thrombosis: a proposal of a new designation of disseminated eosinophilic 'collagen disease'. *Angiology* **28**, 361–75. [p. 271]

847. Ishii, T., Sternby, N. H., and Hosoda, Y. (1978). Hypereosinophilic multiple thrombosis. *Vasa* **7**, 303–8. [p. 271]

848. Ishikawa, T., Mang, C. Yu, Arbesman, C. E. (1972). Electron microscopic determination of phagocytosis of Candida albicans by human eosinophil leucocytes. *J. Allergy Clin. Immunol.* **50**, 183–7. [p. 89]

849. Ishikawa, T., Wicher, K., and Arbesman, C. E. (1974). In vitro and in vivo studies on uptake of antigen-antibody complexes by eosinophils. *Int. Arch. Allergy Appl. Immunol.* **46**, 230–48. [p. 79, 89]

850. Ishizeki, K., Nawa, T., Tachibana, T., Sakakura, Y., and Iida, S. (1984). Hemopoietic sites and development of eosinophil granulocytes in the loach, Misgurnus anguillicaudatus. *Cell Tissue Res.* **235**, 419–26. [p. 124]

851. Islam, N., Karim, A. K., and Rahman, K. M. (1972). Eosinophilic leukaemia. *Postgrad. Med. J.* **48**, 442–5. [p. 153]

852. Isner, J. M., Michlewitz, H., Clarke, R. H., Estes, N. A., Donaldson, R. F., Salem, D. N., Bahn, L., Payne, D. D., and Cleveland, R. J. (1985). Laser photoablation of pathological endocardium: in vitro findings suggesting a new approach to the surgical treatment of refractory arrhythmias and restrictive cardiomyopathy. *Ann. Thorac. Surg.* **39**, 201–6. [p. 245]

853. Isoda, M. and Yasumoto, S. (1986). Eosinophil chemotactic factor derived from a malignant fibrous histiocytoma. *Clin. Exp. Dermatol.* **11**, 253–9. [p. 101]

854. Ivanick, M. J. and Donohue, J. F. (1986). Chronic eosinophilic pneumonia: a cause of adult respiratory distress syndrome. *South Med. J.* **79**, 686–90. [p. 207]

855. Ive, F. A., Willis, A. J., Ikeme, A. C., and Brockington, I. F. (1967). Endomyocardial fibrosis and filariasis. *Q. J. Med.* **36**, 495–516. [p. 250, 256]

856. Iwasaki, K., Torisu, M., and Fujimura, T. (1986). Malignant tumor and eosinophils. I. Prognostic significance in gastric cancer. *Cancer* **58**, 1321–7. [p. 171]

857. Jacob, H. S., Sidd, J. J., Greenberg, B. H., and Lingley, J. F. (1964). Extreme eosinophilia with iodide hypersensitivity: report of a case with observations on the cellular composition of inflammatory exudates. *N. Engl. J. Med.* **271**, 1138–40. [p. 310]

858. Jacobs, M. B. (1985). Eosinophilic fasciitis, reactive hepatitis, and splenomegaly. *Arch. Intern. Med.* **145**, 162–3. [p. 181]

859. Jacobsen, R., Temple, M., and Sacher, R. (1984). Acute myeloblastic leukaemia and t(8;21) translocation. *Br. J. Haematol.* **57**, 539–41. [p. 156]

860. Jacox, R. F., Waterhouse, C., and Taves, D. R. (1982). Transient painful osteolysis – a metabolic study. *J. Rheumatol.* **9**, 279–83. [p. 176]

861. Jaffe, J. P. and Loprinzi, C. L. (1983). Basophilic-eosinophilic meningitis in an undifferentiated myeloproliferative disorder. *JAMA* **249**, 73–4. [p. 216]

862. Jain, V. K. and Beniwal, O. P. (1984). Unusual presentation of tropical pulmonary eosinophilia. *Thorax* **39**, 634–5. [p. 141]

863. Jaiyesimi, F. (1982). Electrocardiographic abnormalities in Ebstein's anomaly. Deductions based on comparison with endomyocardial fibrosis. *Cardiology* **69**, 61–9. [p. 251]

864. Jaiyesimi, F., Salimonu, L. S., and Antia, A. U. (1984). Serum immunoglob-

ulins in children with cardiomyopathies. *Trans. R. Soc. Trop. Med. Hyg.* **78**, 127–31. [p. 255]

865. Jaliman, H. D., Phelps, R. G., and Fleischmajer, R. (1986). Eosinophilic pustular folliculitis. *J. Am. Acad. Dermatol.* **14**, 479–82. [p. 304]
866. James, S. L. and Colley, D. G. (1975). Eosinophils and immune mechanisms: production of the lymphokine eosinophil stimulation promotor (ESP) in vitro by isolated intact granulomas. *J. Reticuloendothel. Soc.* **18**, 283–93. [p. 18]
867. James, S. L. and Colley, D. G. (1976). Eosinophil-mediated destruction of Schistosoma mansoni eggs. *J. Reticuloendothel. Soc.* **20**, 359–74. [p. 104]
868. James, S. L. and Colley, D. G. (1978). Eosinophil-mediated destruction of Schistosoma mansoni eggs III. Lymphokine involvement in the induction of eosinophil functional abilities. *Cell Immunol.* **38**, 48–58. [p. 105, 120]
869. James, S. L. and Colley, D. G. (1978). Eosinophil-mediated destruction of S. mansoni eggs IV. Effects of several inhibitory substances on eosinophil function. *Cell Immunol.* **38**, 59;-67. [p. 114]
870. James, S. L., Leid, R. W. Jr, and Sher, A. (1979). Purification of rodent eosinophils on discontinuous metrizamide gradients. *J. Immunol. Methods.* **27**, 373–82. [p. 127]
871. Jaski, B. E., Goetzl, E. J., Said, J. W., and Fishbein, M. C. (1978). Endomyocardial disease and eosinophilia: report of a case. *Circiulation* **57**, 824–7. [p. 246]
872. Jeanes, A. L. (1965). Cerebrospinal eosinophilia following Torkildsen's operation. *Guy's Hosp. Rep.* **114**, 28–31. [p. 216]
873. Jelihovsky, T. (1983). The structure of bronchial plugs in mucoid impaction, bronchocentric granulomatosis and asthma. *Histopathology* **7**, 153–67. [p. 133]
874. Jenkins, H. R., Pincott, J. R., Soothill, J. F., Milla, P. J., and Harries, J. T. (1984). Food allergy: the major cause of infantile colitis. *Arch. Dis. Child.* **59**, 326–9. [p. 189]
875. Jensen, R., Alexander, A. F., Dahlgren, R. R., Jolley, W. R., Marquardt, W. C., Flack, D. E., Bennett, B. W., Cox, M. F., Harris, C. W., Hoffmann, G. A., *et al.* (1986). Eosinophilic myositis and muscular sarcocystosis in the carcasses of slaughtered cattle and lambs. *Am. J. Vet. Res.* **47**, 587–93. [p. 180]
876. Jessop, J. D., Dippy, J., Turnbull, A., and Bright, M. (1974). Eosinophilia during gold therapy. *Rheumatol. Rehabil.* **13**, 75–9. [p. 312]
877. Jeunet, F. S. and Good, R. A. (1968). Thymoma, immunological deficiencies and hematological abnormalities. In *Immunologic Deficiency Diseases in Man. Birth Defects. 4.* (eds. R. A. Good and D. Bergsma), pp. 192–206. March of Dimes, National Foundation Press, New York. [p. 315]
878. John, S., Mani, G. K., Muralidharan, S., Krishnaswamy, S., and Cherian, G. (1980). Endomyocardial fibrosis from a surgical standpoint. *J. Thorac Cardiovasc. Surg.* **80**, 437–40. [p. 255]
879. Johnson, G. R. and Metcalf, D. (1980). Detection of a new type of mouse eosinophil colony by Luxol-fast-blue staining. *Exp. Hematol.* **8**, 549–61. [p. 15]
880. Johnson, G. R., Nicholas, W. L., Metcalf, D., McKenzie, I. F., and Mitchell, G. F. (1979). Peritoneal cell population of mice infected with Mesocestoides

corti as a source of eosinophils. *Int. Arch. Allergy Appl. Immunol.* **59**, 315–22. [p. 127]

881. Johnson, K. R., Nauseef, W. M., Care, A., Wheelock, M. J., Shane, S., Hudson, S., Koeffler, H. P., Selsted, M., Miller, C., and Rovera, G. (1987). Characterization of cDNA clones for human myeloperoxidase: predicted amino acid sequence and evidence for multiple mRNA species. *Nucleic Acids Res.* **15**, 2013–28. [p. 259]
882. Johnston, N. W. and Bienenstock, J. (1974). Abolition of non-specific fluorescent stainign of eosinophils. *J. Immunol. Methods* **4**, 189–94. [p. 37]
883. Johnstone, J. M. and Morson, B. C. (1978). Eosinophilic gastroenteritis. *Histopathology* **2**, 335–48. [p. 185]
884. Johnstone, J. M. and Morson, B. C. (1978). Inflammatory fibroid polyp of the gastrointestinal tract. *Histopathology* **2**, 349–61. [p. 186]
885. Jolobe, O. M. and Melnick, S. C. (1983). Asthma, pulmonary eosinophilia, and eosinophilic pericarditis. *Thorax* **38**, 690–1. [p. 229]
886. Jones, D. B., Castleden, M., Smith, J. L., Mepham, B. L., and Wright, D. H. (1978). Immunopathology of angioimmunoblastic lymphadenopathy. *Br. J. Cancer.* **37**, 1053–62. [p. 163]
887. Jones, D. G. and Kay, A. B. (1976). The effect of anti-eosinophil serum on skin histamine replenishment following passive cutaneous anaphylaxis in the guinea-pig. *Immunology* **31**, 333–6. [p. 84]
888. Jones, H. R. Jr., Beetham, W. P. Jr., Silverman, M. L., and Margles, S. W. (1986). Eosinophilic fasciitis and the carpal tunnel syndrome. *J. Neurol Neurosurg. Psychiatry* **49**, 324–7. [p. 181]
889. Jong, E. C., Chi, E. Y., and Klebanoff, S. J. (1984). Human neutrophil-mediated killing of schistosomula of Schistosoma mansoni: augmentation by schistosomal binding of eosinophil peroxidase. *Am. J. Trop. Med. Hyg.* **33**, 104–15. [p. 60]
890. Jong, E. C., Henderson, W. R., and Klebanoff, S. J. (1980). Bactericidal activity of eosinophil peroxidase. *J. Immunol.* **124**, 1378–82. [p. 59, 120]
891. Jong, E. C. and Klebanoff, S. J. (1980). Eosinophil-mediated mammalian tumor cell cytotoxicity: role of the peroxidase system. *J. Immunol.* **124**, 1949–53. [p. 120]
892. Jong, E. C., Mahmoud, A. A., and Klebanoff, S. J. (1981). Peroxidase-mediated toxicity to schistosomula of Schistosoma mansoni. *J. Immunol.* **126**, 468–71. [p. 60, 120]
893. Jorg, A., Henderson, W. R., Murphy, R. C., and Klebanoff, S. J. (1982). Leukotriene generation by eosinophils. *J. Exp. Med.* **155**, 390–402. [p. 70]
894. Jorg, A., Pasquier, J. M., and Klebanoff, S. J. (1982). Purification of horse eosinophil peroxidase. *Biochim. Biophys. Acta* **701**, 185–91. [p. 58]
895. Jorg, A., Portmann, P., Fellay, G., Dreyer, J. L., and Meyer, J. (1978). A rapid and simple method for the isolation of pure eosinophilic leukocytes from horse blood. *Experientia* **34**, 1654–6. [p. 58]
896. Jose, D. G., Gatti, R. A., and Good, R. A. (1971). Eosinophilia with Pneumocystis carinii pneumonia and immune deficiency syndrome. *J. Pediatr.* **79**, 748–54. [p. 315]
897. Joshua, H., Zucker, A., and Presentey, B. (1976). Peroxidase and phospholipid deficiency in eosinophilic granulocytes among Arabs of the Nazareth district. *Isr. J. Med. Sci.* **12**, 71–3. [p. 260]

898. Jouvin-Marche, E., Grzych, J. M., Boullet, C., Capron, M., and Benveniste, J. (1984). Formation of PAF-aceter by human eosinophils (Abstract). *Fed. Proc.* **43**, 1924. [p. 72, 282]
899. Juhlin, L. and Michaelsson, G. (1977). A new syndrome characterised by absence of eosinophils and basophils. *Lancet* **i**, 1233–5. [p. 11, 315]
900. Juhlin, L. and Venge, P. (1987). Total absence of eosinophils in a patient with chronic urticaria and vitiligo. *Eur. J. Haematol.* **40**, 368–70. [p. 316]
901. Kaijser, R. (1937). Zur kenntnis der allergischen affectionen des verdauungskanals vom standpunkt des chirurgen aus. *Arch. Klin. Chir.* **188**, 36–64. [p. 184]
902. Kajita, T., Yui, Y., Mita, H., Taniguchi, N., Saito, H., Mishima, T., and Shida, T. (1985). Release of leukotriene C4 from human eosinophils and its relation to the cell density. *Int. Arch. Allergy Appl. Immunol.* **78**, 406–10. [p. 70]
903. Kamal, K. A., Skelly, R. R., and Ahmed, A. (1986). Granulocyte precursor cell studies in Schistosoma mansoni patients with eosinophilia. *Ann. Clin. Lab. Sci.* **16**, 455–60. [p. 16]
904. Kaneko, Y., Kimpara, H., Kawai, S., and Fumjimoto, T. (1983). 8;21 chromosome translocation in eosinophilic leukemia. *Cancer Genet. Cytogenet.* **9**, 181–3. [p. 25, 153, 156]
905. Kanitakis, J., Schmitt, D., Euvrard, S., and Thivolet, J. (1986). Ultrastructural observation of Charcot–Leyden crystals in mechlorethamine-treated cutaneous lesions of histiocytosis X. *J. Am. Acad. Dermatol.* **14**, 483–6. [p. 64]
906. Kanner, R. E. and Hammar, S. P. (1977). Chronic eosinophilic pneumonia: ultrastructural evidence of marked immunoglobulin production plus macrophagic ingestion of eosinophils and eosinophilic lysosomes leading to intracytoplasmic Charcot–Leyden crystals. *Chest* **71**, 95–8. [p. 64]
907. Kanthack, A. A. and Hardy, W. B. (1895). On the characters and behaviour of wandering (migrating) cells of the frog, especially in relation to microorganisms. *Philos. Trans. R. Soc. Lond. (Biol)* **279**, 1895. [p. 90]
908. Kaplan, A. P. (1984). Angioedema (editorial). *N. Engl. J. Med.* **310**, 1662–4. [p. 273]
909. Kapp, D. S. and LiVolsi, V. A. (1983). Intense eosinophilic stromal infiltratioin in carcinoma of the uterine cervix: a clinicopathologic study of 14 cases. *Gynecol. Oncol.* **16**, 19–30. [p. 175]
910. Karle, H. and Videbaek, A. (1966). Eosinophilic leukaemia or a collagen disease with eosinophilia. *Dan. Med. Bull.* **13**. 41–5. [p. 238, 284]
911. Kartha, C. C., Mathai, A., Balakrishnan, K. G., and Valiathan, M. S. (1984). Immunohistological studies in endomyocardial fibrosis. *Indian Heart J.* **36**, 90–1. [p. 252]
912. Kartha, C. C. and Sandhyamani, S. (1985). An autopsy study of tropical endomyocardial fibrosis in Kerala. *Indian J. Med. Res.* **82**, 439–46. [p. 252]
913. Kashima, T., Nomura, T., Arai, S., Nomura, Y., Tsuchiya, T., and Saito, Y. (1982). A case of myeloid leukaemia (eosinophilic) in swine. *Nippon Juigaku Zasshi* **44**, 529–33. [p. 157]
914. Kasinath, B. S. and Lewis, E. J. (1987). Eosinophilia as a clue to the diagnosis of atheroembolic renal disease (editorial). *Arch. Intern. Med.* **147**, 1384–5. [p. 230]

915. Kass, L. (1981). Staining of granulocytic cells by Chlorazol black E. *Am. J. Clin. Pathol.* **76**, 810–2. [p. 38]

916. Kass, L. (1987). C. I. acid red 52: a new stain for cells of granulocytic origin. *Stain Technol* **62**, 77–84. [p. 38]

917. Kater, L. A., Goetzl, E. J., and Austen, K. F. (1976). Isolation of human eosinophil phospholipase D. *J. Clin. Invest.* **57**, 1173–80. [p. 62]

918. Katz, A. J., Goldman, H., and Grand, R. J. (1977). Gastric mucosal biopsy in eosinophilic (allergic) gastroenteritis. *Gastroenterology* **73**, 705–9. [p. 183]

919. Katzen, D. R., Leiferman, K. M., Weller, P. F., and Leung, D. Y. (1986). Hypereosinophilia and recurrent angioneurotic edema in a 2½-year-old girl. *Am. J. Dis. Child.* **140**, 62–4. [p. 9, 300]

920. Katzenstein, A. L., Sale, S. R., and Greenberger, P. A. (1983). Pathologic findings in allergic aspergillus sinusitis: a newly recognized form of sinusitis. *Am. J. Surg. Pathol.* **7**, 439–43. [p. 214]

921. Kauffman, H. F., van der Belt, B., de Monchy, J. G., Boelens, H., Koeter, G. H., and de Vries, K. (1987). Leukotriene C4 production by normal-density and low-density eosinophils of atopic individuals and other patients with eosinophilia. *J. Allergy Clin. Immunol.* **79**, 611–9. [p. 70, 198]

922. Kauffmann, F., Neukirch, F., Korobaeff, M., Marne, M. J., Claude, J. R., and Lellouch, J. (1986). Eosinophils, smoking, and lung function: an epidemiologic survey among 912 working men. *Am. Rev. Respir. Dis.* **134**, 1172–5. [p. 194]

923. Kawamura, J., Kohri, Y., and Oka, N. (1983). Eosinophilic meningoradiculomyelitis caused by Gnathostoma spinigerum: a case report. *Arch. Neurol.* **40**, 583–5. [p. 146]

924. Kay, A. B. (1970). Studies on eosinophil leukocyte migration. I. Eosinophil and neutrophil accumulation following antigen-antibody reactions in guinea pig skin. *Clin. Exp. Immunol.* **6**, 75–86. [p. 97]

925. Kay, A. B. (1977). Eosinophil leucocytes: recruitment, localization and function in immediate-type hypersensitivity. *Monogr. Allergy* **12**, 222–30. [p. 323]

926. Kay, A. B. (1979). The role of the eosinophil. *J. Allergy Clin. Immunol.* **64**, 90–104. [p. 323]

927. Kay, A. B. (1982). Complement receptor enhancement by chemotactic factors. *Mol. Immunol.* **19**, 1307–11. [p. 324]

928. Kay, A. B. (1984). Eosinophils. In *Immunology of the Lung and Upper Respiratory Tract* (ed. J. Bienenstock), pp. 139–56. McGraw Hill, Maidenhead. [p. 325]

929. Kay, A. B. (1985). Eosinophils as effector cells in immunity and hypersensitivity disorders. *Clin. Exp. Immunol.* **62**, 1–12. [p. 325]

930. Kay, A. B., Glass, E. J., and Salter, D. M. (1979). Leucoattractants enhance complement receptors on human phagocytic cells. *Clin. Exp. Immunol.* **38**, 294–9. [p. 82]

931. Kay, A. B., McVie, J. G., Stuart, A. E., Krajewski, A., and Turnbull, L. W. (1975). Eosinophil chemotaxis of supernatants from cultured Hodgkin's lymph node cells. *J. Clin. Pathol.* **28**, 502–5. [p. 101]

932. Kay, A. B., Roberts, E. M., and Jones, D. G. (1976). Tissue inactivation of slow reacting substance of anaphylaxis. *Immunology 30*, 83–7. [p. 61]

933. Kay, A. B., Stechschulte, D. J., and Austen, K. F. (1971). An eosinophil

leukocyte chemotactic factor of anaphylaxis. *J. Exp. Med.* **133**, 602–19. [p. 7, 99]

934. Kay, A. B., Walsh, G. M., Moqbel, R., Macdonald, A. J., Nagakura, T., Carroll, M. P., and Richerson, H. B. (1987). Disodium cromoglycate inhibits activation of human inflammatory cells in vitro. *J. Allergy Clin. Immunol.* **80**, 1–8. [p. 82, 120]
935. Kay, A. G. (1976). Myelotoxicity of gold. *Br. Med. J.* **i**, 1266–8. [p. 312]
936. Kazi, J. I., Alam, S. M., Khan, A. A., and Ara, J. (1987). Eosinophilic gastritis. *JPMA* **37**, 9–13. [p. 185]
937. Kazmierowski, J. A., Chusid, M. J., Parrillo, J. E., Fauci, A. S., and Wolff, S. M. (1978). Dermatologic manifestations of hypereosinophilic syndrome. *Arch. Dermatol.* **114**, 531–5. [p. 273]
938. Kazura, J. W. (1981). Host defense mechanisms against nematode parasites: destruction of newborn Trichinella spiralis larvae by human antibodies and granulocytes. *J. Infect. Dis.* **143**, 712–8. [p. 115]
939. Kazura, J. W. and Aikawa, M. (1980). Host defense mechanisms against Trichinella spiralis infection in the mouse: eosinophil-mediated destruction of newborn larvae in vitro. *J. Immunol.* **124**, 355–61. [p. 115]
940. Kazura, J. W., Fanning, M., and Mahmoud, A. A. (1980). Granulocyte cytotoxicity to multicellular organisms is mediated by peroxidative mechanisms. *Trans. Assoc. Am. Physicians* **93**, 336–40. [p. 120]
941. Kazura, J. W., Fanning, M. M., Blumer, J. L., and Mahmoud, A. A. (1981). Role of cell-generated hydrogen peroxide in granulocyte-mediated killing of schistosomula of Schistosoma mansoni in vitro. *J. Clin. Invest.* **67**, 93–102. [p. 119]
942. Kazura, J. W. and Grove, D. I. (1978). Stage-specific antibody-dependent eosinophil-mediated destruction of Trichinella spiralis. *Nature* **274**, 588–9. [p. 115]
943. Keene, P., Mendelow, B., Pinto, M. R., Bezwoda, W., MacDougall, L., Falkson, G., Ruff, P., and Bernstein, R. (1987). Abnormalities of chromosome 12p13 and malignant proliferation of eosinophils: a nonrandom association. *Br. J. Haematol.* **67**, 25–31. [p. 12, 25, 155, 266]
944. Keeping, H. S. and Lyttle, C. R. (1984). Monoclonal antibody to rat uterine peroxidase and its use in identification of the peroxidase as being of eosinophil origin. *Biochim. Biophys. Acta.* **802**, 399–406. [p. 59]
945. Keidan, A. J., Catovsky, D., Tavares de Castro, J., and Spry, C. J. (1985). Hypereosinophilic syndrome preceding T-cell lymphoblastic lymphoma. *Clin. Lab. Haematol.* **7**, 83–8. [p. 19, 161]
946. Keith, R. G., Keshavjee, S. H., and Kerenyi, N. R. (1985) Neuropathology of chronic pancreatitis in humans. *Can. J. Surg.* **28**, 207–11. [p. 191]
947. Kelenyi, G. (1968). Degranulation of tissue eosinophil leukocytes. *Acta Morphol. Acad. Sci. Hung.* **16**, 265–9. [p. 91]
948. Kelenyi, G. and Nemeth, A. (1969). Comparative histochemistry and electron microscopy of the eosinophil leucocytes of vertebrates. I. A study of avian, reptile, amphibian and fish leucocytes. *Acta. Biol. Acad. Sci. Hung.* **20**, 405–22. [p. 124, 127]
949. Kelenyi, G., Zombai, E., and Nemeth, A. (1965). Histochemische and elektronenmikroskopische beobachtungen an der spezifischen granulation der eosinophilen granulozyten. *Acta Histochem. (Jena)* **22**, 77–89. [p. 59]

950. Kelso, A., Metcalf, D., and Gough, N. M. (1986). Independent regulation of granulocyte-macrophage colony-stimulating factor and multi-lineage colony-stimulating factor production in T-lymphocyte clones. *J. Immunol.* **136**, 1718–25. [p. 20]

951. Kephart, G. M., Gleich, G. J., Connor, D. H., Gibson, D. W., and Ackerman, S. J. (1984). Deposition of eosinophil granule major basic protein onto microfilariae of Onchocerca volvulus in the skin of patients treated with diethylcarbamazine. *Lab. Invest.* **50**, 51–61. [p. 113, 143]

952. Kern, P. and Dietrich M. (1984). In vitro differentiation of myeloid progenitor cells in patients with eosinophilia. *Br. J. Haematol.* **57**, 81–8. [p. 16]

953. Kern, P. and Dietrich, M. (1986). Eosinophil differentiating activity in sera of patients with AIDS under recombinant IL–2 substitution. *Blut* **52**, 249–54. [p. 23]

954. Kern, P., Horstmann, R. D., and Dietrich, M. (1987). Eosinophil production in human bone-marrow cultures induced by 80–85 kDa serum component(s) of patients with eosinophilia. *Br. J. Haematol.* **66**, 165–72. [p. 21, 24, 284]

955. Keshavarzian, A., Saverymuttu, S. H., Tai, P.-C., Thompson, M., Barter, S., Spry, C. J., and Chadwick, V. S. (1985). Activated eosinophils in familial eosinophilic gastroenteritis. *Gastroenterology* **88**, 1041–9. [p. 183, 185]

956. Keslin, M. H., McCoy, E. L., McCusker, J. J., and Lutch, J. S. (1979). Corynebacterium pseudotuberculosis: a new cause of infectious and eosinophilic pneumonia. *Am. J. Med.* **67**, 228–31. [p. 131]

957. Khalife, J., Capron, M., Cesbron, J. Y., Tai, P.-C., Taelman, H., Prin, L., and Capron, A. (1986). Role of specific IgE antibodies in peroxidase (EPO) release from human eosinophils. *J. Immunol.* **137**, 1659–64. [p. 81, 91]

958. Khansur, T., Little, D., and Tavassoli, M. (1984). Fulminant and fatal angioedema caused by bleomycin treatment. *Arch. Intern. Med.* **144**, 2267. [p. 309]

959. Kien, C. L. and Chusid, M. J. (1979). Eosinophilia in children receiving parenteral nutrition support. *JPEN* **3**, 468–9. [p. 294]

960. Kierszenbaum, F., Ackerman, S. J., and Gleich, G. J. (1981). Destruction of bloodstream forms of Trypanosoma cruzi by eosinophil granule major basic protein. *Am. J. Trop. Med. Hyg.* **30**, 775–9. [p. 116]

961. Kierszenbaum, F., Ackerman, S. J., and Gleich, G. J. (1982). Inhibition of antibody-dependent eosinophil-mediated cytotoxicity by heparin. *J. Immunol.* **128**, 515–17. [p. 116]

962. Kierszenbaum, F., Villalta, F., and Tai, P.-C. (1986). Role of inflammatory cells in Chagas' disease. III. Kinetics of human eosinophil activation upon interaction with parasites (Trypanosoma cruzi). *J. Immunol.* **136**, 662–6. [p. 89, 94]

963. Kim, C. H., Vlietstra, R. E., Edwards, W. D., Reeder, G. S., and Gleich, G. J. (1984). Steroid-responsive eosinophilic myocarditis: diagnosis by endomyocardial biopsy. *Am. J. Cardiol.* **53**, 1472–3. [p. 243]

964. Kimura, H., Abe, R., Shiga, Y., Sato, T., Kawaguchi, M., Matsuda, S., Uchida, T., and Kariyone, S. (1987). A case of acute myelogenous leukaemia associated with eosinophilia: cytogenetic study of eosinophilic colonies showing the origin of the normal clone. *Acta Haematol. (Basel)* **77**, 15–19. [p. 150, 158]

965. Kimura, T., Yoshima, S., and Ishikawa, E. (1948). Unusual granulation

combined with hyperplastic change of lymphoid tissue. *Trans. Jpn. Path. Soc.* **37**, 179. [p. 167]

966. Kinashi, T., Harada, N., Severinson, E., Tanabe, T., Sideras, P., Konishi, M., Azuma, C., Tominaga, A., Bergstedt Lindqvist, S., Takahashi, M., Matsuda, F., Yaoita, Y., and Honjo, T. (1986). Cloning of complementary DNA encoding T-cell replacing factor and identity with B-cell growth factor II. *Nature* **324**, 70–3. [p. 19]
967. King, D. H., Loh, K. K., Ayala, A. G., and Gamble, J. F. (1975). Letter: Eosinophilic meningitis and lymphomatous meningitis. *Ann. Intern. Med.* **82**, 228. [p. 216]
968. King, L. S. (1939). Encephalopathy following injections of bone marrow extract. *J. Exp. Med.* **70**, 303–14. [p. 53]
969. Kingston, D. and Pearson, J. R. (1981). The use of the peroxidase reaction to obliterate staining of eosinophils by fluorescein-labelled conjugates. *J. Immunol. Methods* **44**, 191–8. [p. 37]
970. Kirber, W. M., Nichols, C. W., and Braunstein, S. N. (1979). Unusual presentation of ocular toxocariasis in friends. *Ann. Opthalmol.* **11**, 573–6. [p. 140]
971. Kirby, J. G., Hargreave, F. E., Gleich, G. J., and O'Byrne, P. M. (1987). Bronchoalveolar cell profiles of asthmatic and nonasthmatic subjects. *Am. Rev. Respir. Dis.* **136**, 379–83. [p. 199, 200]
972. Kirshner, J. J. and Goldberg, J. (1980). Types of colonies formed by normal human bone marrow, peripheral blood and umbilical cord blood CFUc. *Exp. Hematol.* **8**, 1202–7. [p. 15]
973. Kishimoto, C., Spry, C. J., Tai, P.-C., Tomioka, N., and Kawai, C. (1986). The in vivo cardiotoxic effect of eosinophilic cationic protein in an animal preparation. *Jpn. Circ. J.* **50**, 1264–7. [p. 118]
974. Klebanoff, S. J. (1967). Iodination of bacteria: a bactericidal mechanism. *J. Exp. Med.* **126**, 1063–78. [p. 120]
975. Klebanoff, S. J., Durack, D. T., Rosen, H., and Clark, R. A. (1977). Functional studies on human peritoneal eosinophils. *Infect. Immun.* **17**, 167–73. [p. 59, 67, 82, 120]
976. Klebanoff, S. J., Henderson, W. R. Jr, Jong, E. C., Jorg, A., and Locksley, R. M. (1983). Role of peroxidase in eosinophil function. In *Immunobiology of the eosinophil* (eds. T. Yoshida and M. Torisu, pp 261–82. Elsevier Biomedical, New York. [p. 58, 325]
977. Klebanoff, S. J., Jong, E. C., and Henderson, W. R. Jr. (1980). The eosinophil peroxidase: purification and biological properties. In *The Eosinophil in Health and Disease* (eds. A. A. Mahmoud and K. F. Austen), pp. 99–114. Grune and Stratton, New York. [p. 59]
978. Klebanoff, S. J. and Shepard, C. C. (1984). Toxic effect of the peroxidase-hydrogen peroxide-halide antimicrobial system on Mycobacterium leprae. *Infect. Immun.* **44**, 534–6. [p. 120]
979. Klein, N. C., Hargrove, R. L., Sheisenger, M. H., Jeffries, G. H. (1970). Eosinophilic gastroenteritis. *Medicine (Baltimore)* **49**, 299–319. [p. 186]
980. Kliks, M. M., Kroenke, K., and Hardman, J. M. (1982). Eosinophilic radiculomyeloencephalitis: an angiostrongyliasis outbreak in American Samoa related to ingestion of Achatina fulica snails. *Am. J. Trop. Med. Hyg.* **31**, 1114–22. [p. 139]

981. Klofkorn, R. W. and Lehman, T. J. (1982). Eosinophilic synovial effusions complicating chronic urticaria and angioedema. *Arthritis Rheum.* **25**, 708–9. [p. 178]

982. Knorr D. and Scheppe, K. J. (1958). (Loffler's fibroplastic parietal endocarditis with eosinophilia in a seven-year-old child.) *Z. Kinderheilkd.* **81**, 102–12. [p. 236, 269]

983. Knox, A. J., Johnson, C. E., and Page, R. L. (1986). Eosinophilia associated with thoracic malignancy. *Br. J. Dis. Chest.* **80**, 92–5. [p. 174]

984. Knox-Macaulay, H. H. (1981). Transient hypereosinophilia in Necator americanus and Schistosoma mansoni infections (letter). *Trans. R. Soc. Trop. Med. Hyg.* **75**, 906–7. [p. 143, 147]

985. Kociecka, W., Nowosielski, J., Stefaniak, J., and Budzynska, L. (1985). Blood eosinophils in patients with Taenia saginata taeniasis. *Wiad Parazytol* **31**, 139–45. [p. 138]

986. Kodama, T., Takada, K., Kameya, T., Shimosato, Y., Tsuchiya, R., and Okabe, T. (1984). Large cell carcinoma of the lung associated wtih marked eosinophilia: a case report. *Cancer* **54**, 2313–7. [p. 22, 101]

987. Koeffler, H. P. (1987). Syndromes of acute nonlymphocytic leukemia. *Ann. Intern. Med.* **107**, 748–58. [p. 158, 326]

988. Koeffler, H. P., Billing, R., Levine, A. M., and Golde, D. W. (1980). Ia antigen is a differentiation marker on human eosinophils. *Blood* **56**, 11–4. [p. 75]

989. Koeffler, H. P., Levine, A. M., Sparkes, M., and Sparkes, R. S. (1980). Chronic myelocytic leukemia: eosinophils involved in the malignant clone. *Blood* **55**, 1063–5. [p. 159]

990. Kojima, S., Niimura, M., and Kanazawa, T. (1987). Production and properties of a mouse monoclonal IgE antibody to Schistosoma japonicum. *J. Immunol.* **139**, 2044–9. [p. 80]

991. Kojima, S., Yamamoto, N., Kanazawa, T., and Ovary, Z. (1985). Monoclonal IgE-dependent eosinophil cytotoxicity to haptenated schistosomula of Schistosoma japonicum: enhancement of the cytotoxicity and expression of Fc receptors for IgE by Nippostrongylus brasiliensis infection. *J. Immunol.* **134**, 2719–22. [p. 80]

992. Kojima, S., Yamamoto, N., Kanazawa, T., Shigematsu, H., and Ovary, Z. (1985). Enhancement of IgE-dependent eosinophil cytotoxicity to dinitrophenylated schistosomula by a nematode infection. *Int. Arch. Allergy Appl. Immunol.* **76**, 91–4. [p. 80]

993. Kokkola, K. and Valta, R. (1974). Aetiology and findings in eosinophilic pleural effusion. *Scand. J. Respir. Dis. (Suppl)* **89**, 159–65. [p. 212]

994. Kolb, E. and Muller, E. (1979). Local responses in primary and secondary human lung cancers. II. Clinical correlations. *Br. J. Cancer* **40**, 410–16. [p. 174]

995. Kollegger, H., Preis, P., Maida, E., Zielinski, C. C., Linkesch, W., Bettelheim, P., and Aiginger, P. (1986). CSF cytology of a patient with conversion of an acute lymphatic leukemia to an acute eosinophilic leukemia. *Eur. Neurol.* **25**, 320–6. [p. 12, 152, 153, 216]

996. Komiyama, A. K. and Spicer, S. S. (1975). Microendocytosis in eosinophil leukocytes. *J. Cell. Biol.* **64**, 622–35. [p. 44, 90]

997. Konig, W. (1978). (Structure and function of the eosinophil leucocytes). *Immun. Infekt.* **6**, 97–105. [p. 323]

998. Konig, W., Kroegel, C., Pfeiffer, P., and Tesch, H. (1981). Modulation of the eosinophil chemotactic factor (ECF) release from various cells and their subcellular components by phospholipids. *Int. Arch. Allergy Appl. Immunol.* **65**, 417–31. [p. 119]

999. Kornfeld, S. (1987). Trafficking of lysosomal enzymes. *Faseb. J.* **1**, 462–8. [p. 13]

1000. Kosnai, I., Kuitunen, P., Savilahti, E., and Sipponen, P. (1984). Mast cells and eosinophils in the jejunal mucosa of patients with intestinal cow's milk allergy and celiac disease in childhood. *J. Pediatr. Gastroenterol. Nutr.* **3**, 368–72. [p. 188]

1001. Kovach, J. S. and Gleich, G. J. (1986). Eosinophilia and fluid retention in systemic administration of interleukin-2 (letter). *J. Clin. Oncol.* **4**, 815–16. [p. 301]

1002. Kozlowski, K., Diard, F., Padovani, J., Sprague, P., and Pietron, K. (1986). Unilateral mid-femoral periosteal newbone of varying aetiology in children: radiographic analysis of 25 cases. *Pediatr. Radiol.* **16**, 475–82. [p. 165]

1003. Krause, J. R. and Boggs, D. R. (1987). Search for eosinophilia in hospitalized patients with normal blood leukocyte concentration. *Am. J. Hematol.* **24**, 55–63. [p. 31, 315]

1004. Kreipe, H., Radzun, H. J., Heidorn, K., Mader, C., and Parwaresch, M. R. (1987). Human neutrophilic and eosinophilic granulocytes display different levels of c-fos proto-oncogene expression: an in situ hybridization study. *J. Histochem. Cytochem.* **35**, 837–42. [p. 26]

1005. Krishnaswami, H., Date, A., Bhaktaviziam, A., Krishnaswami, S., and Cherian, G. (1984). Electron microscopic changes in tropical endomyocardial fibrosis. *Trans. R. Soc. Trop. Med. Hyg.* **78**, 205–8. [p. 253]

1006. Kroegel, C., Costabel, U., and Matthys, H. (1987). Mechanism of membrane damage mediated by eosinophil major basic protein (letter). *Lancet* **i**, 1380–1. [p. 119]

1007. Kuberski, T. (1979). Eosinophils in the cerebrospinal fluid. *Ann. Intern. Med.* **91**, 70–5. [p. 216]

1008. Kuberski, T. (1981). Eosinophils in cerebrospinal fluid criteria for eosinophilic meningitis. *Hawaii Med. J.* **40**, 97–8. [p. 216]

1009. Kudenchuk, P. J., Hosenpud, J. D., and Fletcher, S. (1986). Eosinophilic endomyocardiopathy. *Clin. Cardiol.* **9**, 344–8. [p. 239, 278]

1010. Kueh Y. K. and Teo C. G. (1986). Eosinophilic purpura – the syndrome of acquired platelet dysfunction with eosinophilia – a tropical phenomenon. *Ann. Acad. Med. Singapore* **15**, 262–7. [p. 262]

1011. Kuehl, F. A. Jr., Zanetti, M. E., Soderman, D. D., Miller, D. K., and Ham, E. A. (1987). Cyclic AMP-dependent regulation of lipid mediators in white cells: a unifying concept for explaining the efficacy of theophylline in asthma. *Am. Rev. Respir. Dis.* **136**, 210–13. [p. 71]

1012. Kuipers, F. C., Thiel, P. H. von., Rodenberg, W., Wielinga, W. J., and Roskam, R. T. (1960). Eosinophilic phlegmon of the alimentary canal caused by a worm. *Lancet* **2**, 1171–3. [p. 187]

1013. Kulczycki, A. Jr. (1984). Human neutrophils and eosinophils have structurally distinct Fc receptors. *J. Immunol.* **133**, 849–54. [p. 77]

1014. Kullberg, F. C., Funahashi, A., and Siegesmund, K. A. (1982). Pulmonary eosinophilic granuloma: electron microscopic detection of X-bodies on lung lavage cells and transbronchoscopic lung biopsy in one patient. *Ann. Intern. Med.* **96**, 188–9. [p. 211]

1015. Kung, I. T., Gibson, J. B., and Bannatyne, P. M. (1984). Kimura's disease: a clinico-pathological study of 21 cases and its distinction from angiolymphoid hyperplasia with eosinophilia. *Pathology* **16**, 39–44. [p. 167]

1016. Kuo, T. T., Chen, S. Y., and Chan, H. L. (1986). Tinea infection histologically simulating eosinophilic pustular folliculitis. *J. Cutan. Pathol.* **13**, 118–22. [p. 132, 304]

1017. Kuo, T. T., Hsueh, S., Su, I. J., Gonzalez Crussi, F., and Chen, J. S. (1985). Histiocytoid hemangioma of the heart with peripheral eosinophilia. *Cancer* **55**, 2854–61. [p. 166, 170]

1018. Kuo, T. T. and Wang, C. N. (1986). Charcot–Leyden crystals in pemphigus vegetans. *J. Cutan. Pathol.* **13**, 242–5. [p. 64]

1019. Kurachi, K., Davie, E. W., Strydom, D. J., Riordan, J. F., and Vallee, B. L. (1985). Sequence of the cDNA and gene for angiogenin, a human angiogenesis factor. *Biochemistry* **24**, 5494–9. [p. 51]

1020. Kurner, T., Burkart, V., and Kolb, H. (1986). Large increase of cytotoxic/suppressor T-lymphoblasts and eosinophils around manifestation of diabetes in BB rats. *Diabetes Res.* **3**, 349–53. [p. 306]

1021. Laitinen, L. A., Heino, M., Laitinen, A., Kava, T., and Haahtela, T. (1985). Damage of the airway epithelium and bronchial reactivity in patients with asthma. *Am. Rev. Respir. Dis.* **131**, 599–606. [p. 197]

1022. Lam, S., LeRiche, J., Phillips, D., Chan Yeung, M. (1987). Cellular and protein changes in bronchial lavage fluid after late asthmatic reaction in patients with red cedar asthma. *J. Allergy Clin. Immunol.* **80**, 44–50. [p. 201]

1023. Lambertenghi-Deliliers, G., Pozzoli, E., Benazzi, E., Maiolo, A. T., Foa, P., and Polli, E. (1986). Bone marrow biopsy in chronic myeloid leukemia: significance of some histological parameters. *Haematologica (Pavia)* **71**, 113–6. [p. 159]

1024. Lamotte-Barrillon, S., Carbon, C., Bernard, J. F., Gaudin, H., Teilet, F., and Barge, J. (1976). Leucemie avec eosinophiles et coagulation intravasculaire disseminee. *Sem. Hop. Paris* **52**, 987–8. [p. 270, 284]

1025. Landais, P., Goldfarb, B., and Kleinknecht, D. (1987). Eosinophiluria and drug-induced acute interstitial nephritis (letter). *N. Engl. J. Med.* **316**, 1664. [p. 220]

1026. Landres, R. T., Kuster, G. G., and Strum, W. B. (1978). Eosinophilic esophagitis in a patient with vigorous achalasia. *Gastroenterology* **74**, 1298–1301. [p. 183]

1027. Lang, P. G. Jr. (1979). Severe hypersensitivity reactions to allopurinol. *South Med. J.* **72**, 1361–8. [p. 308]

1028. Lange, R. D. (1983). Cyclic hematopoiesis: human cyclic neutropenia. *Exp. Hematol.* **11**, 435–51. [p. 261]

1029. Lanham, J. G., Cooke, S., Davies, J., and Hughes, G. R. (1985). Endomyocardial complications of the Churg-Strauss syndrome. *Postgrad. Med. J.* **61**, 341–4. [p. 237]

1030. Lanham, J. G., Elkon, K. B., Pusey, C. D., Hughes, G. R. (1984). Systemic vasculitis with asthma and eosinophilia: a clinical approach to the Churg-Strauss syndrome. *Medicine (Baltimore)* **63**, 65–81. [p. 203]

1031. Larrey, D., Hadengue, A., Pessayre, D., Choudat, L., DeGott, C., and Benhamou, J. P. (1987). Carbamazepine-induced acute cholangitis. *Dig. Dis. Sci.* **32**, 554–7. [p. 310]

1032. Larsen, G. L., Wilson, M. C., Clark, R. A., and Behrens, B. L. (1987). The inflammatory reaction in the airways in an animal model of the late asthmatic response. *Fed. Proc.* **46**, 105–12. [p. 197]

1033. Larson, R. A., Williams, S. F., Le Beau, M. M., Bitter, M. A., Vardiman, J. W., and Rowley, J. D. (1986). Acute myelomonocytic leukemia with abnormal eosinophils and inv(16) or t(16;16) has a favorable prognosis. *Blood* **68**, 1242–9. [p. 158]

1034. Laubry, C. (1912). Actions des rayons X sur les eosinophiles. *Arch. Mal Coeur Vaiss Sang* **5**, 806–8. [p. 289]

1035. Laufer, P., Cryssanthopoulos, C., Laufer, R., and Hause, L. L. (1987). The determination of the eosinophil count: comparison of two techniques. *J. Allergy Clin. Immunol.* **79**, 438–41. [p. 30]

1036. Lautenschlager, I., von Willebrand, E., and Hayry, P. (1985). Blood eosinophilia, steroids, and rejection. *Transplantation* **40**, 354–7. [p. 225]

1037. Laviolette, M., Picard, S., Braquet, P., and Borgeat, P. (1986). Comparison of 5- and 15-lipoxygenase activities in blood and alveolar leukocyte preparations from normal subjects and patients with eosinophilia. *Prostaglandins Leukotrienes Med.* **23**, 191–1. [p. 199]

1038. Lawrence, R. Jr, Church, J. A., Richards, W., Lipsey, A. I. (1980). Eosinophilia in the hospitalized neonate. *Ann. Allergy* **44**, 349–52. [p. 294]

1039. Layzer, R. B., Shearn, M. A., and Satya Murti, S. (1977). Eosinophilic polymyositis. *Ann. Neurol.* **1**, 65–71. [p. 179]

1040. Le Beau, M. M., Larson, R. A., Bitter, M. A., Vardiman, J. W., Golomb, H. M., and Rowley, J. D. (1983). Association of an inversion of chromosome 16 with abnormal marrow eosinophils in acute myelomonocytic leukemia: unique cytogenetic-clinicopathological association. *N. Engl. J. Med.* **309**, 630–6. [p. 156, 158]

1041. Learn, D. B. and Brestel, E. P. (1982). A comparison of superoxide production by human eosinophils and neutrophils. *Agents Actions* **12**, 485–8. [p. 69]

1042. Leary, A. G. and Ogawa, M. (1984). Identification of pure and mixed basophil colonies in culture of human peripheral blood and marrow cells. *Blood* **64**, 78–83. [p. 12]

1043. Leary, A. G., Ogawa, M., Strauss, L. C., and Civin, C. I. (1984). Single cell origin of multilineage colonies in culture: evidence that differentiation of multipotent progenitors and restriction of proliferative potential of monopotent progenitors are stochastic processes. *J. Clin. Invest.* **74**, 2193–7. [p. 15]

1044. Leary, A. G., Strauss, L. C., Civin, C. I., and Ogawa, M. (1985)., Disparate differentiation in hemopoietic colonies derived from human paired progenitors. *Blood* **66**, 327–32. [p. 11]

1045. Leder, L. D., Stutte, H. J., and Pape, B. (1970). Zur selektiven Darstellung von eosinophilen Granulozyten und ihren Vorstufen in Ausstrichen und Schnitten. *Klin. Wochenschr.* **48**, 191–2. [p. 38]

1046. Lederman, J., Hasselbalch, H., and Hippe, E. (1988). Alcohol intolerance in the hypereosinophilic syndrome. *Alcoholism (NY)* **12**, 147–8. [p. 271]

1047. Lee, M. C., Turcinov, D., and Damjanov, I. (1987). Lectins as markers for eosinophilic leukocytes. *Histochemistry* **86**, 269–73. [p. 38]

1048. Lee, R. G. (1985). Marked eosinophilia in esophageal mucosal biopsies. *Am. J. Surg. Pathol.* **9**, 475–9. [p. 183, 184]

1049. Lee, T., Lenihan, D. J., Malone, B., Roddy, L. L., and Wasserman, S. I. (1984). Increased biosynthesis of platelet-activating factor in activated human eosinophils. *J. Biol. Chem.* **259**, 5526–30. [p. 72, 247]

1050. Leegaard, M. (1980). Eosinophilic cholecystitis. *Acta Chir. Scand.* **146**, 295–6. [p. 191]

1051. Lefor, A. T. and Miller, M. (1985). Factitious hypoglycemia associated with eosinophilic leukemoid reaction. *NY State J. Med.* **85**, 34–5. [p. 66, 172]

1052. Leiferman, K. M., Ackerman, S. J., Sampson, H. A., Haugen, H. S., Venencie, P. Y., and Gleich, G. J., (1985). Dermal deposition of eosinophil-granule major basic protein in atopic dermatitis. Comparison with onchocerciasis. *N. Engl. J. Med.* **313**, 282–5. [p. 298]

1053. Leiferman, K. M., Gleich, G. J., Kephart, G. M., Haugen, H. S., Hisamatsu, K., Proud, D., Lichtenstein, L. M., and Ackerman, S. J. (1986). Differences between basophils and mast cells: failure to detect Charcot–Leyden crystal protein (lysophospholipase) and eosinophil granule major basic protein in human mast cells. *J. Immunol.* **136**, 852–5. [p. 45]

1054. Leiferman, K. M., O'Duffy, J. D., Perry, H. O., Greipp, P. R., Giuliani, E. R., and Gleich, G. J. (1982). Recurrent incapacitating mucosal ulcerations: a prodrome of the hypereosinophilic syndrome. *JAMA* **247**, 1018–20. [p. 272]

1055. Leiferman, K. M., Peters, M. S., and Gleich, G. J. (1986). The eosinophil and cutaneous edema. *J. Am. Acad. Dermatol.* **15**, 513–17. [p. 297]

1056. Lendrum, A. C. (1944). The staining of eosinophil polymorphs and enterochromaffin cells in histological sections. *J. Path. Bact.* **56**, 441. [p. 37]

1057. Lengyel, M., Arvay, A., and Palik, I. (1985). Massive endocardial calcification associated with endomyocardial fibrosis. *Am. J. Cardiol.* **56**, 815–16. [p. 238]

1058. Lengyel, M. and Dekov, E. (1982). Two-dimensional echocardiographic features of Löffler's endocarditis. *Acta Cardiol. (Brux)* **37**, 59–69. [p. 240]

1059. Lennox, B. (1948). Acute parietal endocarditis in a case of status asthmaticus: a possible early stage of Löffler's endocarditis parietalis fibroplastica with eosinophilia. *J. Path. Bact.* **60**, 621–8. [p. 232]

1060. Lepelley, P., Zandecki, M., Paquet, S., Lerche, B., Estienne, M. H., Fennaux, P., Torpier, G., and Cosson, A. (1987). Total peroxidase deficiency in eosinophils: a report on twin sisters, one with a refractory anaemia. *Eur. J. Haematol.* **39**, 77–81. [p. 59, 260]

1061. Leung, A. C., McLay, A., Dobbie, J. W., and Jones, J. M. (1985). Phenylbutazone-induced systemic vasculitis with crescentic glomerulonephritis. *Arch. Intern. Med.* **145**, 685–7. [p. 309]

1062. Levinson, J. D., Ramanathan, V. R., and Nozick, J. H. (1977). Eosinophilic gastroenteritis with ascites and colon involvement. *Am. J. Gastroenterol.* **68**, 603–7. [p. 186]

1063. Lewinsohn, D. M., Bargatze, R. F., and Butcher, E. C. (1987). Leukocyte-endothelial cell recognition: evidence of a common molecular mechanism shared by neutrophils, lymphocytes, and other leukocytes. *J. Immunol.* **138**, 4313–21. [p. 98]

1064. Lewis, D. M., Lewis, J. C., Loegering, D. A., and Gleich, G. J. (1978). Localization of the guinea pig eosinophil major basic protein to the core of the granule. *J. Cell. Biol.* **77**, 702–13. [p. 46]

1065. Lewis, D. M., Loegering, D. A., and Gleich, G. J. (1976). Antiserum to the major basic protein of guinea pig eosinophil granules. *Immunochemistry* **13**, 743–6. [p. 46]

1066. Lewis, D. M., Loegering, D. A., and Gleich, G. J. (1976). Isolation and partial characterization of the major basic protein from rat eosinophil granules. *Proc. Soc. Exp. Biol. Med.* **152**, 512–5. [p. 46]

1067. Lewis, F. A., Carter, C. E., and Colley, D. G. (1977). Eosinophils and immune mechanisms. V. Demonstration of mouse spleen cell-derived chemotactic activities for eosinophils and mononuclear cells and comparisons with eosinophil stimulation promoter. *Cell Immunol.* **32**, 86–96. [p. 100]

1068. Lewis, J. G. (1964). Eosinophilic granuloma and its variants with special reference to lung involvement. *Q. J. Med.* **33**, 337–59. [p. 211]

1069. Lewis, M. G., Kociba, G. J., Rojko, J. L., Stiff, M. I., Haberman, A. B., Velicer, L. F., and Olsen, R. G. (1985). Retroviral-associated eosinophilic leukemia in the cat. *Am. J. Vet. Res.* **46**, 1066–70. [p. 157]

1070. Lewis, R. E. and Granger, H. J. (1986). Neutrophil-dependent mediation of microvascular permeability. *Fed. Proc.* **45**, 109–13. [p. 122]

1071. Lewis, S. I., Van Epps, D. E., and Chenoweth, D. E. (1986). Density changes in leukocytes following hemodialysis or exposure to chemotactic factors. *Am. J. Nephrol.* **6**, 34–41. [p. 220]

1072. Leyden, E. (1872). Zur Kenntniss des Bronchial Asthma. *Virchows Arch. (Pathol. Anat.)* **54**, 324–44. [p. 64]

1073. Leys, A., Tackeon, E., Jansen, J., and Missotten, L. (1980). Case reports: axoplasma transport obstruction in eosinophilia and in Coats disease. *Bull. Soc. Belge Ophtalmol.* **191**, 1–4. [p. 275]

1074. Li, H. L. and Glick, A. D. (1987). Ultrastructural localization of 2-naphthylthiol acetate nonspecific esterase in human blood cells and leukemic cells. *Exp. Mol. Pathol.* **46**, 321–30. [p. 62]

1075. Libanoff A. F. and McMahon N. J. (1976). Eosinophilia and endomyocardial fibrosis. *Am. J. Cardiol.* **37**, 438–41. [p. 236]

1076. Libby, D. M. (1987). The eosinophil in idiopathic pulmonary fibrosis (editorial). *Chest* **92**, 7–8. [p. 209]

1077. Lichenstein, A., Ganz, T., Selsted, M. E., and Lehrer, R. I. (1986). In vitro tumor cell cytolysis mediated by peptide defensins of human and rabbit granulocytes. *Blood* **68**, 1407–10. [p. 119]

1078. Liebow, A. A. and Carrington, C. B. (1969). The eosinophilic pneumonias. *Medicine (Baltimore)* **48**, 251–85. [p. 208]

1079. Liebow, A. A., Carrington, C. R. B., and Friedman, P. J. (1972). Lumphomatoid granulomatosis. *Hum. Pathol.* **3**, 457–558. [p. 210]

1080. Limberg, M. B., Margo, C. E., and Lyman, G. H. (1986). Eosinophils in corneas removed by penetrating keratoplasty. *Br. J. Ophthalmol* **70**, 343–6. [p. 219]

1081. Lindor, L. J., Loegering, D. A., Wassom, D. L., and Gleich, G. J. (1981).

Recovery of eosinophils from the peritoneal cavity of the guinea pig. *J. Immunol. Methods* **41**, 125–34. [p. 126]
1082. Linthicum, D. S. (1975). Ultrastructure of Hagfish blood leukocytes. *Adv. Exp. Med. Biol.* **64**, 241–50. [p. 124]
1083. Linton, A. L., Clark, W. F., Driedger, A. A., Turnbull, D. I., and Lindsay, R. M. (1980). Acute interstitial nephritis due to drugs: review of the literature with a report of nine cases. *Ann. Intern. Med.* **93**, 735–41. [p. 309]
1084. Liso, V., Troccoli, G., Specchia, G., and Magno, M. (1977). Cytochemical 'normal' and 'abnormal' eosinophils in acute leukemias. *Am. J. Hematol.* **2**, 123–31. [p. 159]
1085. Litt, M. (1964). Eosinophils and antigen-antibody reactions. *Ann. NY Acad. Sci.* **116**, 964–85. [p. 6]
1086. Litt, M. (1964). Studies in experimental eosinophilia VI. Uptake of immune complexes by eosinophils. *J. Cell. Biol.* **23**. 355–61. [p. 6]
1087. Littleton, R. H., Farah, R. N., and Cerny, J. C. (1982). Eosinophilic cystitis: an uncommon form of cystitis. *J. Urol.* **127**, 132–3. [p. 223]
1088. Liu, Y. Q., Wang, Z. L. and Wei, E. Y. (1983). Radiological study of 4 cases of endomyocardial fibrosis. *Chin. Med. J. (Engl)* **96**, 569–74. [p. 252]
1089. Locksley, R. M., Wilson, C. B., and Klebanoff, S. J. (1982). Role for endogenous and acquired peroxidase in the toxoplasmacidal activity of murine and human mononuclear phagocytes. *J. Clin. Invest.* **69**, 1099–111. [p. 60, 120]
1090. Loeliger, E. A. (1972). Drugs affecting blood clotting and fibrinolysis. In *Side effects of drugs. 7. A survey of unwanted effects of drugs reported in 1968–71.* (eds. L. Meyler and A. Herxhimer), p. 488. Excepta Medica, Amsterdam. [p. 310]
1091. Löffler, W. (1932). Zur Differential-Diagnose der Lungeninfiltrierugen. I. Fruhinfiltrate unter besonderer Beruchsichtigung der Ruckbildungzeiten. II. Uber fluchtige succedan-Infiltrate (mit Eosinophilie). *Beitrage zur Klinik der Tuberkulose und spezifischen Tuberkulose Forschung.* **79**, 338–82. [p. 206]
1092. Löffler, W. (1936). Endocarditis parietalis fibroplastica mit Bluteosinophilie, in eigenartiger Krankheitsbild. *Schweiz Med. Wochenschr.* **17**, 817–20. [p. 232]
1093. Löffler, W. (1947). The pathogenetic significance of the so-called endocarditis parietalis fibroplastica. *Bull. Schweiz Akad. Med. Wiss.* **2**, 287. [p. 237]
1094. Loftin, E. B. (1987). Eosinophilic fasciitis: 171 cases reviewed. *IMJ* **171**, 289–93. [p. 181]
1095. Lohr, K. and Jahnecke, J. (1965). Ueber einer fall von Endocarditis parietalis fibroplastica mit Bluteosinophilie (Löffler) mit dem klinischer bild einer 'eosinophilen leukamie'. *Dtsch. Arch. Klin. Med.* **210**, 110. [p. 246]
1096. Lombard, C. M., Tazelaar, H. D., and Krasne, D. L. (1987). Pulmonary eosinophilia in coccidioidal infections. *Chest* **91**, 734–6. [p. 133]
1097. Lonnqvist, B., Gahrton, G., Eriksson, P., Friberg, K., and Zech, L. (1979). Isochromosome 17 in a patient with a myeloproliferative disorders terminating in eosinophilic leukemia. *Acta Med. Scand.* **206**, 321–5. [p. 155]
1098. Looi, L. M. (1987). Tumor-associated tissue eosinophilia in nasopharyngeal carcinoma: a pathologic study of 422 primary and 138 metastatic tumors. *Cancer* **59**, 466–70. [p. 173]
1099. Looney, R. J., Ryan, D. H., Takahashi, K., Fleit, H. B., Cohen, H. J.,

Abraham, G. N., and Anderson, C. L. (1986). Identification of a second class of IgG Fc receptors on human neutrophils. A 40 kilodalton molecule also found on eosinophils. *J. Exp. Med.* **163**, 826–36. [p. 77]

1100. Lopes-Pontes, E., Piris, J., Jewell, D., and Truelove, S. C. (1981). Changes in the populations of mucosal immunoglobulin-containing cells preceding a relapse in ulcerative colitis. *Gut* **22**, A421–2. [p. 190]

1101. Lopez, A. F., Begley, C. G., Williamson, D. J., Warren, D. J., Vadas, M. A., and Sanderson, C. J. (1986). Murine eosinophil differentiation factor: an eosinophil-specific colony-stimulating factor with activity for human cells. *J. Exp. Med.* **163**, 1085–99. [p. 19, 137]

1102. Lopez, A. F., Begley, G., Andrews, P., Butterworth, A. E., and Vadas, M. A. (1985). Identification of a human granulocyte functional antigen (GFA–2) involved in antibody-dependent cell-mediated cytotoxicity and phagocytosis. *J. Immunol.* **134**, 3969–77. [p. 87]

1103. Lopez, A. F., To, L. B., Yang, Y. C., Gamble, J. R., Shannon, M. F., Burns, G. F., Dyson, P. G., Juttner, C. A., Clark, S., and Vadas, M. A. (1987). Stimulation of proliferation, differentiation, and function of human cells by primate interleukin 3. *Proc. Natl. Acad. Sci. USA* **84**, 2761–5. [p. 22, 110, 120]

1104. Lopez, A. F. and Vadas, M. A. (1984). Stimulation of human granulocyte function by monoclonal antibody WEM-G1. *Proc. Natl. Acad. Sci. USA* **81**, 1818–21. [p. 87]

1105. Lopez, A. F., Williamson, D. J., Gamble, J. R., Begley, C. G., Harlan, J. M., Klebanoff, S. J., Waltersdorph, A., Wong, G., Clark, S. C., and Vadas, M. A. (1986). Recombinant human granulocyte-macrophage colony-stimulating factor stimulates *in vitro* mature human neutrophil and eosinophil function, surface receptor expression, and survival. *J. Clin. Invest.* **78**, 1220–8. [p. 35]

1106. Loria Cortes, R. and Lobo Sanahuja, J. F. (1980). Clinical abdominal angiostronglylosis: a study of 116 children with intestinal eosinophilic granuloma caused by Angiostrongylus costaricensis. *Am. J. Trop. Med. Hyg.* **29**, 538–44. [p. 138]

1107. Losco, P. E. (1986). Local and peripheral eosinophilia in a dog with anaplastic mammary carcinoma. *Vet. Pathol.* **23**, 536–8. [p. 175]

1108. Loughnan, M. S., Takatsu, K., Harada, N., and Nossal, G. J. (1987). T-cell-replacing factor (interleukin 5) induces expression of interleukin 2 receptors on murine splenic B cells., *Proc. Natl. Acad. Sci. USA* **84**, 5399–403. [p. 20]

1109. Lowe, D. and Fletcher, C. D. (1984). Eosinophilia in squamous cell carcinoma of the oral cavity, external genitalia and anus – clinical correlations. *Histopathology* **8**, 627–32. [p. 150, 173]

1110. Lowe, D., Fletcher, C. D., and Carpenter, G. (1985). Urine eosinophilia in bladder cancer (letter). *Acta Cytol. (Baltimore)* **29**, 187. [p. 175]

1111. Lowe, D., Fletcher, C. D., and Gower, R. L. (1984). Tumour-associated eosinophilia in the bladder. *J. Clin. Pathol* **37**, 500–2. [p. 175]

1112. Lowe, D., Fletcher, C. D., Shaw, M. P., and McKee, P. H. (1984). Eosinophil infiltration in keratoacanthoma and squamous cell carinoma of the skin. *Histopathology* **8**, 619–25. [p. 173]

1113. Lowe, D., Jorio, J., and Hutt, M. S. (1981). Tumour-associated eosinophilia: a review. *J. Clin. Pathol.* **34**, 1343–8. [p. 169, 170, 173, 174]

1114. Lowe, D., Jorizzo, J., Chiphangwi, J., and Hutt, M. S. (1981). Cervical carcinoma in Malawi: a histopathologic study of 260 cases. *Cancer* **47**, 2493–5. [p. 170, 174]

1115. Lowe, D., Tai, P.-C., and Spry, C. J. (1986). Electron microscopic localisation of human eosinophil cationic protein in activated eosinophils (abstract). *J. Pathol.* **148**, 86A. [p. 50]

1116. Lu, L., Broxmeyer, H. E., Pelus, L. M., Andreeff, M., and Moore, M. A. (1981). Detection of luxol-fast-blue positive cells in human promyelocytic leukemia cell line HL–60. *Exp. Hematol.* **9**, 887–92. [p. 26]

1117. Lucisano, Y. M. and Mantovani, B. (1984). Lysosomal enzyme release from polymorphonuclear leukocytes induced by immune complexes of IgM and of IgG. *J. Immunol.* **132**, 2015–20. [p. 78]

1118. Lucky, A. W., Esterly, N. B., Heskel, N., Krafchik, B. R., and Solomon, L. M. (1984). Eosinophilic pustular folliculitis in infancy. *Pediatr. Dermatol* **1**, 202–6. [p. 304]

1119. Lucky, A. W. and McGuire, J. S. (1982). Infatile acropustulosis with eosinophilic pustules. *J. Pediatr.* **100**, 428–9. [p. 302]

1120. Luzar, M. J. and Friedman, B. M. (1982). Acute synovial fluid eosinophilia. *J. Rheumatol.* **9**, 961–2. [p. 178]

1121. Lynes, W. L., Flynn, S. D., Shortliffe, L. D., Lemmers, M., Zipser, R., Roberts, L. J., and Stamey, T. A. (1987). Mast cell involvement in interstitial cystitis. *J. Urol.* **138**, 746–52. [p. 223]

1122. MacFadyen, R., Tron, V., Keshmiri, M., and Road, J. D. (1987). Allergic angiitis of Churg and Strauss syndrome: response to pulse methylprednisolone. *Chest* **91**, 629–31. [p. 203]

1123. Macintyre, E. A., Vaughan Hudson, B., Vaughan Hudson, G., Jelliffe, A. M., and Linch, D. C. (1987). Incidence and clinical importance of bone marrow eosinophilia in Hodgkin's disease (BNLI Report No 29). British National Lymphoma Investigation. *J. Clin. Pathol.* **40**, 245–6. [p. 162]

1124. Mackenzie, C. D., Jungery, M., Taylor, P. M., and Ogilvie, B. M. (1981). The in vitro interaction of eosinophils, neutrophils, macrophages and mast cells with nematode surfaces in the presence of complement or antibodies. *J. Pathol.* **133**, 161–75. [p. 127]

1125. Mackenzie, C. D., Williams, J. F., Sisley, B. M., Steward, M. W., and O'Day, J. (1985). Variations in host responses and the pathogenesis of human onchocerciasis. *Rev. Infect. Dis.* **7**, 802–8. [p. 143]

1126. Mackowiak, P. A. and LeMaistre, C. F. (1987). Drug fever: a critical appraisal of conventional concepts; an analysis of 51 episodes in two Dallas hospitals and 97 episodes reported in the English literature. *Ann. Intern. Med.* **106**, 728–33. [p. 308]

1127. MacMillan, R. H., Cooper, P. H., Body, B. A., and Mills, A. S. (1987). Allergic fungal sinusitis due to Curvularia lunata. *Hum. Pathol.* **18**, 960–4. [p. 214]

1128. Maddox, D. E., Butterfield, J. H., Ackerman, S. J., Coulam, C. B., and Gleich, G. J. (1983). Elevated serum levels in human pregnancy of a molecule immunochemically similar to eosinophil granule major basic protein. *J. Exp. Med.* **158**, 1211–26. [p. 227]

1129. Maddox, D. E., Kephart, G. M., Coulam, C. B., Butterfield, J. H., Benirschke, K., and Gleich, G. J. (1984). Localization of a molecule immunochemically similar to eosinophil major basic protein in human placenta. *J. Exp. Med.* **160**, 29–41. [p. 227]

1130. Maeda, K., VanSlyck, E. J., and VanDyke, D. L. (1985). Multiple myeloma terminating in acute eosinophilic leukemia. *Cancer Genet. Cytogenet.* **16**, 81–9. [p. 152]

1131. Magee, F., Wright, J. L., Chan, N., Currie, W., Karr, G., Hogg, J., and Thurlbeck, W. M. (1986). Two unusual pathological reactions to nitrofurantoin: case reports. *Histopathology* **10**, 701–6. [p. 185, 309]

1132. Magnani, J. L., Ball, E. D., Fanger, M. W., Hakomori, S. I., and Ginsburg, V. (1984). Monoclonal antibodies PMN 6, PMN 29, and PM–81 bind differently to glycolipids containing a sugar sequence occurring in lacto-N-fucopentaose III. *Arch. Biochem. Biophys.* **233**, 501–6. [p. 87]

1133. Mahmoud, A. A. (1980). Eosinophilopoiesis. In *The eosinophil in health and disease* (eds. A. A. Mahmoud, K. F. Austen, and A. S. Simon), pp. 61–75. Grune and Stratton, New York. [p. 17]

1134. Mahmoud, A. A., Austen, K. F., and Simon, A. S., eds. (1980). *The eosinophil in health and disease.* Grune and Stratton, New York. [p. 322]

1135. Mahmoud, A. A., Billings, F. T. III, Stone, M. K., and Kellermeyer, R. W. (1978). Human eosinophilopoietin (abstract). *Clin. Res.* **26**, 555A. [p. 17]

1136. Mahmoud, A. A., Kellermeyer, R. W., and Warren, K. S. (1977). Monospecific antigranulocyte sera against human neutrophils, eosinophils, basophils, and myeloblasts. *Lancet* **ii**, 1163–6. [p. 85]

1137. Mahmoud, A. A., Kellermeyer, R. W., and Warren, K. S. (1974). Production of monospecific rabbit antihuman eosinophil serums and demonstration of a blocking phenomenon. *N. Engl. J. Med.* **290**, 417–20. [p. 85]

1138 Mahmoud, A. A., Stone, M. K., and Kellermeyer, R. W. (1977). Eosinophilopoietin: a circulating low molecular weight peptide-like substance which stimulates the production of eosinophils in mice. *J. Clin. Invest.* **60**, 675–82. [p. 16, 17, 18]

1139. Mahmoud, A. A., Stone, M. K., and Kellermeyer, R. W. (1977). Eosinophilopoietin: a low molecular weight peptide stimulating eosinophil production in mice. *Trans. Assoc. Am. Physicians.* **90**, 127–34. [p. 17]

1140. Mahmoud, A. A., Stone, M. K., and Tracy, J. W. (1979). Eosinophilopoietin production: relationship to eosinophilia of infection and thymus function. *Assoc. Am. Physicians* **92**, 355–9. [p. 16, 17, 18]

1141. Mahmoud, A. A., Warren, K. S., and Boros, D. L. (1973). Production of a rabbit antimouse eosinophil serum with no cross-reactivity to neutrophils. *J. Exp. Med.* **137**, 1526–31. [p. 84]

1142. Mahmoud, A. A., Warren, K. S., and Peters, P. A. (1975). A role for the eosinophil in acquired resistance to Schistosoma mansoni infection as determined by antieosinophil serum. *J. Exp. Med.* **142**, 805–13. [p. 84]

1143. Mainwaring, G. and Rowley, A. F. (1985). Separation of leucocytes in the dogfish (Scyliorhinus canicula) using density gradient centrifugation and differential adhesion to glass coverslips. *Cell Tissue Res.* **241**, 283–90. [p. 124]

1144. Major, R. H. and Leger, L. H. (1939). Marked eosinophilia in Hodgkin's disease. *JAMA* **112**, 2601–2. [p. 162]

1145. Male, P. J., de Toledo, F., Widgren, S., de Peyer, R., and Berthoud, S. (1983). Pseudotumoral enterocolitis and massive eosinophilia. *Gut* **24**, 345–50. [p. 187]

1146. Male, P. J., Schaer, B., and Posternak, F. (1978). Reaction d'hypersensibilite a l'allopurinol. *Schweiz Med. Wochenschr.* **108**, 681–8. [p. 313]

1147. Malech, H. L. and Gallin, J. I. (1987). Current concepts in immunology: neutrophils in human disease. *N. Engl. J. Med.* **137**, 687–94. [p. 45, 82, 91, 119, 259, 261]

1148. Malklewicz, B., Pajdak, W., Okulski, J., and Lisiewicz, J. (1971). Recherches sur l'activite thromboplastique des eosinophiles d'un malade atteint de leucemie eosinophilique. *Haematologica (Pavia)* **5**, 439–46. [p. 247]

1149. Malmsten, C. L. (1984). Leukotrienes: mediators of inflammation and immediate hypersensitivity reactions. *CRC Crit. Rev. Immunol.* **4**, 307–34. [p. 325]

1150. Mansouri, A., Perry, C. A., Boyd, C. M., and Hsu, S. D. (1983). Eosinophilic granulocytes as a possible source of vitamin B12-binding protein. *Scand. J. Haematol.* **341**, 507–9. [p. 62]

1151. Manthorpe, R., Egeberg, J., Hesselvik, M., and Videbaek, A. (1977). Unique eosinophil granules in a case of T-cell lymphoma. *Scand. J. Haematol.* **19**, 129–44. [p. 12]

1152. Margolis, H. S., Middaugh, J. P., and Burgess, R. D. (1979). Arctic trichinosis: two Alaskan outbreaks from walrus meat. *J. Infect. Dis.* **139**, 102–5. [p. 145]

1153. Marinone, G., Rossi, G., and Verzura, P. (1983). Eosinophilic blast crisis in a case of chronic myeloid leukaemia. *Br. J. Haematol.* **55**, 251–6. [p. 261]1154. Markowitz, S. M., Martinez, A. J., Duma, R. J., and Shiel, F. O. (1974). Myocarditis associated with primary amebic (Naegleria) meningoencephalitis. *Am. J. Clin. Pathol.* **62**, 619–28. [p. 148]

1155. Marks, P. (1981). Bronchial neoplasm with eosinophilia. *Br. J. Clin. Pract.* **35**, 418–20. [p. 174, 295]

1156. Marmor, M., Glickman, L., Schofer, F., Faich, L. A., Rosenberg, C., Cornblatt, B., and Friedman, S. (1987). Toxocara canis infection of children: epidemiologic and neuropsychologic findings. *Am. J. Public Health.* **77**, 554–9. [p. 139]

1157. Marom, Z., Shelhamer, J. H., Bach, M. K., Morton, D. R., and Kaliner, M. (1982). Slow-reacting substances, leukotrienes C4 and D4, increase the release of mucus from human airway in vitro. *A. Rev. Respir. Dis.* **126**, 449–51. [p. 70]

1158. Marshak, R. H., Lindner, A., Maklansky, D., and Gelb, A. (1981). Eosinophilic gastroenteritis. *JAMA* **245**, 1677–80. [p. 185]

1159. Martensson, G., Pettersson, K., and Thiringer, G. (1985). Differentiation between malignant and non-malignant pleural effusion. *Eur. J. Respir. Dis.* **67**, 326–34. [p. 212]

1160. Marti, G. E., Chiang, J. L., and Patterson, R. (1980). The syndrome of hypergammaglobulinemia M., eosinophilia, edema, and fatigue: immunologic studies and long-term evaluation of two patients. *Int. Arch. Allergy Appl. Immunol.* **63**, 83–7. [p. 302]

1161. Martin, D. M., Goldman, J. A., Gilliam, J., and Nasrallah, S. M. (1981).

Gold-induced eosinophilic enterocolitis: response to oral cromolyn sodium. *Gastroenterology* **80**, 1567–70. [p. 183]

1162. Martin Gonzalez, E., Yebra, M., Garcia Merino, A., and Liano, H. (1986). Neurologic dysfunction in the idiopathic hypereosinophilic syndrome (letter). *Ann. Intern. Med.* **104**, 448–9. [p. 276]

1163. Mateo, M. R., Roberts, E. D., and Enright, F. M. (1984). Morphologic, cytochemical, and functional studies of peripheral blood cells of young healthy American alligators (Alligator mississippiensis). *Am. J. Vet. Res.* **45**, 1046–53. [p. 127]

1164. Maubach, P. A., Bauchinger, M., Emmerich, B., and Rastetter, J. (1985). Trisomy 7 and 8 in Ph-negative chronic eosinophilic leukemia. *Cancer Genet. Cytogenet.* **17**, 159–64. [p. 156]

1165. Maxwell, C., Hussain, R., Nutman, T. B., Poindexter, R. W., Little, M. D., Schad, G. A., and Ottesen, E. A. (1987). The clinical and immunologic responses of normal human volunteers to low dose hookworm (Necator americanus) infection. *Am. J. Trop. Med. Hyg.* **37**, 126–34. [p. 144]

1166. Maxwell, M. H. (1978). The fine structure of granules in eosinophil leucocytes from aquatic and terrestrial birds. *Tissue Cell.* **10**, 303–17. [p. 124]

1167. Maxwell, M. H. (1979) The ultrastructure of eosinophil granules of the black-necked crowned crane. *J. Anat.* **128**, 53–63. [p. 124]

1168. Maxwell, M. H. and Burns, R. B. (1986). Experimental stimulation of eosinophil production in the domestic fowl. (Gallus gallus domesticus). *Res. Vet. Sci.* **41**, 114–23. [p. 124]

1169. Mayer, D. and Bannasch, P. (1983). Endomyocardial fibrosis in rats treated with N-nitrosomorpholine. *Virchows Arch. (A)* **401**, 129–35. [p. 257]

1170. McCarthy, D. S. and Pepys, J. (1973). Cryptogenic pulmonary eosinophilia. *Clin. Allergy* **3**, 339–51. [p. 206, 207]

1171. McCarthy, L. J., Aguilar, J. C., and Ransburg, R. (1979). Fatal benign phenytoin lymphadenopathy. *Arch. Intern. Med.* **139**, 367–8. [p. 309]

1172. McDonald, S. and Shaw, A. F. (1922). Persistent eosinophilia and splenomegaly. *Br. Med. J.* **ii**, 966–71. [p. 64, 263, 289]

1173. McEwen, S. A., Valli, V. E., and Hulland, T. J. (1985). Hypereosinophilic syndrome in cats: a report of three cases. *Can. J. Comp. Med.* **49**, 248–53. [p. 268]

1174. McGrath, C. R., Hitchcock, D. C., and van Assendelft, O. W. (1982). Total white blood cell counts for persons ages 1–74 years with differential leukocyte counts for adults ages 25–74 years: United States, 1971–75. *Vital Health Stat* **11**, 1–36. [p. 31]

1175. McKelvey, E. M., Luce, J. K., Talley, R. W., Hersh, E. M., Hewlett, J. S., and Moon, T. E. (1977). Combination chemotherapy with bis chloroethyl nitrosourea (BCNU), vincristine and dimethyl triazeno imidazole carboxamide (DTIC) in disseminated malignant melanoma. *Cancer* **39**, 1–4. [p. 173]

1176. McKusick, V. A. and Cochrane, T. H. (1952). Constrictive endocarditis: report of case. *Bull. Johns Hopkins Hosp.* **90**, 90–7. [p. 237]

1177. McLaren, D. J., Mackenzie, C. D., and Ramalho. Pinto, F. J. (1977). Ultrastructural observations on the in vitro interaction between rat eosinophils and some parasitic helminths (Schistosoma mansoni, Trichinella spiralis and Nippostrongylus brasiliensis). *Clin. Exp. Immunol.* **30**, 105–18. [p. 113]

1178. McLaren, D. J., McKean, J. R., Olsson, I., Venges, P., and Kay, A. B. (1981). Morphological studies on the killing of schistosomula of Schistosoma mansoni by human eosinophil and neutrophil cationic proteins in vitro. *Parasite Immunol.* **3**, 359–73. [p. 51, 52]

1179. McLaren, D. J., Peterson, C. G., and Venge, P. (1984). Schistosoma mansoni: further studies of the interaction between schistosomula and granulocyte-derived cationic proteins in vitro. *Parasitology* **88**, 491–503. [p. 52, 55]

1180. McLaren, D. J., Ramalho Pinto, F. J., and Smithers, S. R. (1978). Ultrastructural evidence for complement and antibody-dependent damage to schistosomula of Schistosoma mansoni by rat eosinophils in vitro. *Parasitology* **77**, 313–24. [p. 114]

1181. McLeod, W. A. and Winkelmann, R. K. (1985). Eosinophilic histiocytosis: a variant form of lymphomatoid papulosis or a disease sui generis? *J. Am. Acad. Dermatol.* **13**, 952–8. [p. 304]

1182. McMaster, K. R. and Hennigar, G. R. (1981). Drug-induced granulomatous hepatitis. *Lab. Invest.* **44**, 61–73. [p. 310]

1183. McMenanmin, R. A., Davies, L. M., and Craswell, P. W. (1976). Drug induced interstitial nephritis, hepatitis and exfoliative dermatitis. *Aust. NZ J. Med.* **6**, 583–7. [p. 309]

1184. McNabb, P. C., Fleming, C. R., Higgins, J. A., and Davis, G. L. (1979). Transmural eosinophilic gastroenteritis with ascites. *Mayo Clin. Proc.* **54**, 119–22. [p. 186]

1185. McRury, J., De Messias, I. T., Walzer, P. D., Huitger, T., and Genta, R. M. (1986). Specific IgE responses in human strongyloidiasis. *Clin. Exp. Immunol.* **65**, 631–8. [p. 146]

1186. Mecucci, C., Bosly, A., Michaux, J. L., Broeckaert Van Orshoven, A., and Van den Berghe, H. (1985). Acute nonlymphoblastic leukemia with bone marrow eosinophilia and structural anomaly of chromosome 16. *Cancer Genet. Cytogenet.* **17**, 359–63. [p. 158]

1187. Meisel, S., and North, C. Q. (1984). Carbamazepine-associated erythema multiforme with extreme eosinophilia (letter). Clin. Pharm. **3**, 15, 18–19. [p. 309]

1188. Menard, H. A., de Medicis, R., Lessier, A., and Brown, J. (1981). Charcot–Leyden crystals in synovial fluid (letter). *Arthritis Rheum.* **24**, 1591–3. [p. 178]

1189. Menegazzi, R., Zabucchi, G., and Patriarca, P. (1986). A simple procedure for the purification of eosinophil peroxidase from normal human blood. *J. Immunol. Methods* **91**, 283–8. [p. 58]

1190. Meseguer, J., Lozano, M. T., and Agulleiro, B. (1985). Ultrastructure of the renal granulopoietic tissue of the Rana ridibunda tadpole. *J. Submicrosc. Cytol.* **17**, 391–401. [p. 124]

1191. Metcalf, D. (1983). Clonal analysis of the response of HL60 human myeloid leukemia cells to biological regulators. *Leuk. Res.* **7**, 117–32. [p. 26]

1192. Metcalf, D. (1984). *The hemopoietic colony stimulating factors.* Elsevier, Amsterdam. [p. 20]

1193. Metcalf, D., Begley, C. G., Johnson, G. R., Nicola, N. A., Vadas, M. A., Lopez, A. F., Williamson, D. J., Wong, G. G., Clark, S. C., and Wang, E.

A., (1986). Biologic properties in vitro of a recombinant human granulocyte-macrophage colony-stimulating factor. *Blood* **67**, 37–45. [p. 21]

1194. Metcalf, D., Begley, C. G., Nicola, N. A., and Johnson, G. R. (1987). Quantitative responsiveness of murine hemopoietic populations in vitro and in vivo to recombinant multi-CSF (IL–3). *Exp. Hematol.* **15**, 288–95. [p. 22]

1195. Metcalf, D., Burgess, A. W., Johnson, G. R., Nicola, N. A., Nice, E. C., De Lamarter, J., Thatcher, D. R., and Mermod, J. J. (1986). In vitro actions on hemopoietic cells of recombinant murine GM-CSF purified after production in Escherichia coli: comparison with purified native GM-CSF. *J. Cell. Physiol.* **128**, 421–31. [p. 21]

1196. Metcalf, D., Parker, J., Chester, H. M., and Kincade, P. W. (1974). Formation of eosinophilic-like granulocytic colonies by mouse bone marrow cells in vitro. *J. Cell. Physiol.* **84**, 275–90. [p. 20]

1197. Metcalf, D. D., Gadek, J. E., Raphael, G. D., Frank, M. M., Kaplan, A. P., and Kaliner, M. (1977). Human eosinophil adherence to serum-treated sepharose: granule-associated enzyme release and requirement for activation of the alternative complement pathway. *J. Immunol.* **119**, 1744–50. [p. 82, 114]

1198. Metcalfe, D. D., Litvin, J., and Wasserman, S. I. (1982). The isolation, identification and characterization of sulfated glycosaminoglycans synthesized in vitro by human eosinophils. *Biochim, Biophys. Acta* **715**, 196–204. [p. 73]

1199. Metras, D., Coulibaly, A. O., and Ouattara, K. (1985). The surgical treatment of endomyocardial fibrosis: results in 55 patients. *Circulation* **72**, 274–9. [p. 254]

1200. Metras, D., Coulibaly, A. O., Ouattara, K., Chauvet, J., Ekra, A., Longechaud, A., and Bertrand, E. (1982). Endomyocardial fribrosis: early and late results of surgery in 20 patients. *J. Thorac. Cardiovasc. Surg.* **83**, 52–64. [p. 254]

1201. Metras, D., Ouattara, K., Coulibaly, A. O., and Touze, J. E. (1983). Left endomyocardial fibrosis with severe mitral insufficiency; the case for mitral valve repair: a report of 4 cases. *Thorac. Cardiovasc. Surg.* **31**, 297–300. [p. 254]

1202. Metras, D., Ouezzin Coulibaly, A., Ouattara, K., Bertrand, E., and Chauvet, J. (1983). Endomyocardial fibrosis masquerading as rheumatic mitral incompetence: a report of six surgical cases. *J. Thorac. Cardiovasc. Surg.* **86**, 753–6. [p. 254]

1203. Metzger, W. J., Nugent, K., Richerson, H. B., Moseley, P., Lakin, R., Zavala, D., and Hunninghake, G. W. (1985). Methods for bronchoalveolar lavage in asthmatic patients following bronchoprovocation and local antigen challenge. *Chest* **87** (1 Suppl), 16S–19S. [p. 195]

1204. Metzger, W. J., Richerson, H. B., and Wasserman, S. I. (1986). Generation and partial characterization of eosinophil chemotactic activity and neutrophil chemotactic activity during early and late-phase asthmatic response. *J. Allergy Clin. Immunol.* **78**, 282–90. [p. 200]

1205. Metzger, W. J., Richerson, H. B., Worden, K., Monick, M., and Hunninghake, G. W. (1986). Bronchoalveolar lavage of allergic asthmatic patients following allergen bronchoprovocation. *Chest* **89**, 477–83. [p. 200]

1206. Metzger, W. J., Zavala, D., Richerson, H. B:, Moseley, P., Iwamota, P.,

Monick, M., Sjoersdsma, K., Hunninghake, G. W. (1987). Local allergen challenge and bronchoalveolar lavage of allergic asthmatic lungs. Description of the model and local airway inflammation. *Am. Rev. Respir. Dis.* **135**, 433–40. [p. 201]

1207. Mickenberg, I. D., Root, R. K., and Wolff, S. M. (1972). Bactericidal and metabolic properties of human eosinophils. *Blood* **39**, 67–80. [p. 67, 270, 282]

1208. Middleton, W. G., Paterson, I. C., Grant, I. W., and Douglas, A. C. (1977). Asthmatic pulmonary eosinophilia: a review of 65 cases. *Br. J. Dis. Chest.* **71**, 115–22. [p. 133]

1209. Migler, R., De Chatelet, L. R., and Bass, D. A. (1978). Human eosinophilic peroxidase: role in bacterial activity. *Blood* **51**, 445–56. [p. 59, 120]

1210. Mihailescu, E. and Micu, D. (1985). Eosinophilia in the pleural and peritoneal effusions. *Med. Interne* **23**, 191–4. [p. 212]

1211. Millar, D. S., Davis, L. R., Rodeck, C. H., Nicolaides, K. H., and Mibashan, R. S. (1985). Normal blood cell values in the early mid-trimester fetus. *Prenat. Diagn.* **5**, 367–73. [p. 10]

1212. Miller, A. M. and McGarry, M. P. (1976). A diffusible stimulator of eosinophilopoiesis produced by lymphoid cells as demonstrated with diffusion chambers. *Blood* **48**, 293–300. [p. 19]

1213. Miller, F., de Harven, E., and Palade, G. E. (1966). The structure of eosinophil leukocyte granules in rodents and man. *J. Cell. Biol.* **31**, 349–62. [p. 38]

1214. Miller, W., Walsh, R., and McCall, D. (1987). Eosinophilic heart disease presenting with features suggesting hypertrophic obstructive cardiomyopathy. *Cathet. Cardiovasc. Diagn.* **13**, 185–8. [p. 241]

1215. Miller, W. M., Adcook, K. J., Moniot, A. L., Raymond, L. W., Hutcheson, J., and Elliott, R. C. (1977). Progressive hypereosinophilia with lung nodules due to thyroid carcinoma. *Chest* **71**, 789–91. [p. 172]

1216. Mine, S., Sato, A., Yamaura, A., Tamachi, S., Makino, H., and Tomioka, H. (1986). Eosinophilia of the cerebrospinal fluid in a case of shunt infection: case report. *Neurosurgery* **19**, 835–6. [p. 217]

1217. Miossec, P., Sullivan, T. J., Tharp, M. D., Volant, A., and Le Goff, P. (1987). Acute synovial fluid eosinophilia associated with delayed pressure urticaria: a role for mast cells? *J. Rheumatol.* **14**, 372–4. [p. 178]

1218. Mir Madjlessi, S. H., Sivak, M. V. Jr., and Farmer, R. G. (1986). Hypereosinophilia, ulcerative colitis, sclerosing cholangitis, and bile duct carcinoma. *Am. J. Gastroenterol.* **81**, 483–5. [p. 172]

1219. Mitas, J. A. and Thompson, T. (1985). Ureteral involvement complicating eosinophilic cystitis. *Urology* **26**, 67–70. [p. 223]

1220. Mitchell, E. B., Platts Mills, T. A., Pereira, R. S., Malkovska, V., and Webster, A. D. (1983). Basophil and eosinophil deficiency in a patient with hypogammaglobulinemia associated with thymoma. *Birth Defects* **19**, 331. [p. 24, 316]

1221. Mitchell, E. B., Platts Mills, T. A., Pereira, R. S., Malkovska, V., and Webster, A. D. (1983). Acquired basophil and eosinophil deficiency in a patient with hypogammaglobulinaemia associated with thymoma. *Clin. Lab. Haematol.* **5**, 253–7. [p. 316]

1222. Mitelman, F., Panani, A., and Brandt, L. (1975). Isochromosome 17 in a case of eosinophilic leukaemia: an abnormality common to eosinophilic and neutrophilic cells. *Scand. J. Haematol.* **14**, 308–12. [p. 155]

1223. Mitrakul, C. (1975). Transient spontaneous bruising with long bleeding time and normal platelet count. *Am. J. Clin. Pathol.* **63**, 81–6. [p. 262]

1224. Mitter, N. S. and Weiskopf, R. W. (1987). Unusual chromosome 7 aberrations in a case of eosinophilic myeloproliferative syndrome. *Cancer Genet. Cytogenet.* **26**, 209–12. [p. 25, 159]

1225. Mlynek, M. L. (1985). Comparative investigations on the specificity of Adams' reaction and the Biebrich scarlet stain for the demonstration of eosinophilic granules. *Klin. Wochenschr.* **63**, 646–7. [p. 38]

1226. Mlynek, M. L. and Leder, L. D. (1985). The cytochemical demonstration of cyanide resistant peroxidase does not identify eosinophils selectively. *Blut* **51**, 347–53. [p. 59, 260]

1227. Mlynek, M. L. and Leder, L. D. (1986). Lineage infidelity in chronic myeloid leukemia: demonstration and significance of hybridoid leukocytes. *Virchows Arch. (Cell. Pathol.)* **51**, 107–14. [p. 11]

1228. Modig, J., Samuelsson, T., and Hallgren, R. (1986). The predictive and discriminative value of biologically active products of eosinophils, neutrophils and complement in bronchoalveolar lavage and blood in patients with adult respiratory distress syndrome. *Resuscitation* **14**, 121–34. [p. 211]

1229. Mogensen, K., Pahle, E., and Kowalski, K. (1985). Enterobius vermicularis and acute appendicitis. *Acta Chir. Scand.* **151**, 705–7. [p. 146]

1230. Mohamed, A. E. (1985). The Katayama syndrome in Saudis. *J. Trop. Med. Hyg.* **88**, 319–22. [p. 147]

1231. Moir, D. J., Pearson, J., and Buckle, V. J. (1984). Acute promyelocytic transformation in a case of acute myelomonocytic leukemia. *Cancer Genet. Cytogenet.* **12**, 359–64. [p. 156]

1232. Monahan, R. A., Dvorak, H. F., and Dvorak, A. M. (1981). Ultrastructural localization of non-specific esterase activity in guinea pig and human monocytes, macrophages, and lymphocytes. *Blood* **58**, 1089–99. [p. 62]

1233. Moore, P. M., Harley, J. B., and Fauci, A. S., (1985). Neurologic dysfunction in the idiopathic hypereosinophilic syndrome. *Ann. Intern. Med.* **102**, 109–14. [p. 275, 276]

1234. Moqbel, R., MacDonald, A. J., and Kay, A. B. (1985). Enhancement of human eosinophil- and neutrophil-mediated killing of schistosomula of Schistosoma mansoni by reversed type (IgE-mediated) anaphylaxis, in vitro. *Clin. Exp. Immunol.* **59**, 577–86. [p. 108]

1235. Moqbel, R., MacDonald, and A. J., Kay, A. B. (1986). Enhanced granulocyte cytotoxicity by mediators derived from anti-IgE-stimulated human leucocytes. *Immunology* **59**, 87–93. [p. 120]

1236. Moqbel, R., MacDonald, A. J., and Kay, A. B. Platelet activating factor (PAF-acether) enhances eosinophil cytotoxicity in vitro. Presented to the 6th International Congress of Immunology, Toronto, Canada, 1986. [p. 109]

1237. Moqbel, R., Sass Kuhn, S. P., Goetzl, E. J., and Kay, A. B. (1983). Enhancement of neutrophil- and eosinophil-mediated complement-dependent killing of schistosomula of Schistosoma mansoni in vitro by leukotriene B4. *Clin. Exp. Immunol.* **52**, 519–27. [p. 120]

1238. Moraes, C. R., Buffolo, E., Lima, R., Victor, E., Lira, V., Escobar, M.,

Rodrigues, J., Saraiva, L., and Andrade, J. C. (1983). Surgical treatment of endomyocardial fibrosis. *J. Thorac. Cardiovasc. Surg.* **85**, 738–45. [p. 255]

1239. Moreau, J. F., Bonneville, M., Godard, A., Gascan, H., Gruart, V., Moore, M. A., and Soulillou, J. P. (1987). Characterization of a factor produced by human T cell clones exhibiting eosinophil-activating and burst-promoting activities. *J. Immunol.* **138**, 3844–9. [p. 107]

1240. Moreland, M. E. and Johnson, W. T. (1981). Lymphomatoid papulosis with eosinophilia. *Arch. Dermatol.* **117**, 181–2. [p. 304]

1241. Moreno, A., Noguera, J., and de Moragas, J. M. (1985). Polymorphic eruption of pregnancy: histopathologic study. *Acta Derm. Venereol. (Stockh.)* **65**, 313–18. [p. 302]

1242. Morley, J., Bray, M. A., Jones, R. W., Nugteren, D. H., and van Dorp, D. A. (1979). Prostaglandin and thromboxane production by human and guinea-pig macrophages and leucocytes. *Prostaglandins* **17**, 729–46. [p. 71]

1243. Morris, D. D., Bloom, J. C., Roby, K. A., Woods, K., and Tablin, F. (1984). Eosinophilic myeloproliferative disorder in a horse. *J. Am. Vet. Med. Assoc.* **185**, 993–6. [p. 157]

1244. Morris P. D. and Katerndahl, D. A. (1987). Human toxocariasis: review with report of a probable case. *Postgrad. Med.* **81**, 263–7. [p. 140]

1245. Morrissey, W. L., Gaensler, E. A., Carrington, C. B., and Turner, H. G. (1975). Chronic eosinophilic pneumonia. *Respiration* **32**, 453–68. [p. 207]

1246. Mortensen, S. A., Hansen, B. F., and Bundgaard, A. (1983). Eosinophilia and myocardial ischemia secondary to polyarteritis: a discussion of pathogenesis on the basis of a case history. *Acta Cardiol. (Brux)* **38**, 237–45. [p. 231]

1247. Motojima, S., Loegering, D. A., Frigas, E., and Gleich, G. J. (1986). Toxic effects of eosinophil granule cationic proteins on respiratory epithelium (abstract). *Fed. Proc.* **45**, 994. [p. 199]

1248. Mullarkey, M. F., Hill, J. S., and Webb, D. R. (1980). Allergic and nonallergic rhinitis: their characterization with attention to the meaning of nasal eosinophilia. *J. Allergy Clin. Immunol.* **65**, 122–6. [p. 214]

1249. Muller, E. and Kolb, E. (1979). Local responses in primary and secondary human lung cancers. I. Patterns of cellular (eosinophils and macrophages) and extracellular (acid mucopolysaccharide) reactions. *Br. J. Cancer* **40**, 403–9. [p. 174]

1250. Muller, W., Schorre, W., Suchenwirth, R., Zitz, H. M., and Konorza, G. (1978). A case of fatal cryptococcus meningitis with intraventricular granuloma. *Acta Neurochir. (Wien)* **44**, 223–35. [p. 134]

1251. Mullick, F. G., McAllister, H. A. Jr., Wagner, B. M., and Fenoglio, J. J. Jr. (1979). Drug related vasculitis: clinicopathologic correlations in 30 patients. *Hum. Pathol.* **10**, 313–25. [p. 312]

1252. Mullin, G. T., Caperton, E. M. Jr., Crespin, S. R., and Williams, R. C. Jr. (1968). Arthritis and skin lesions resembling erythema nodosum in pancreatic disease. *Ann. Intern. Med.* **68**, 75–87. [p. 191]

1253. Munker, R., Gasson, J., Ogawa, M., and Koeffler, H. P. (1986). Recombinant human TNF induces production of granulocyte-monocyte colony-stimulating factor. *Nature* **323**, 79–82. [p. 109]

1254. Murray, S. M. and Woods, C. J. (1981). Disseminated eosinophilic infiltration of a newborn infant, with perforation of the terminal ileum and bile duct obstruction. *Arch. Dis. Child.* **56**, 66–71. [p. 270]

1255. Muthiah, M. M., Mitchell, T. R., and Thorn, C. T. (1984). Acquired platelet dysfunction with eosinophilia. *Br. Med. J. (Clin. Res.).* **289**, 1044. [p. 262]
1256. Nagato, Y., Mitsui, T., Kushida, T., and Kushida, H. (1986). PAS staining of eosinophils in semi-thin sections of bone marrow embedded in glycol methacrylate. *Tokai J. Exp. Clin. Med.* **11**, 171–7. [p. 63]
1257. Nagy, L., Lee, T. H., Goetzl, E. J., Pickett, W. C., and Kay, A. B. (1982). Complement receptor enhancement and chemotaxis of human neutrophils and eosinophils by leukotrienes and other lipoxygenase products. *Clin. Exp. Immunol.* **47**, 541–7. [p. 82, 101]
1258. Nair, D. V. and Thankam, S. (1980). Unusual case of right ventricular and right atrial endomyocardial fibrosis with gross calcification of endocardium and myocardium. *J. Assoc. Physicians India* **28**, 389–92. [p. 251]
1259. Nair, U., Evans, T., and Oakley, D. (1980). Surgical treatment of endomyocardial fibrosis with preservation of mitral valve. *Br. Heart J.* **43**, 357–9. [p. 254]
1260. Najfeld, V., Seremetis, S., Troy, K., Uehlinger, J., Schwartz, P., and Cuttner, J. (1986). Trisomy 22 – a new abnormality found in acute leukemia characterized by eosinophilia and monocytoid blasts expressing immature differentiation antigens. *Cancer Genet. Cytogenet.* **23**, 105–14. [p. 156]
1261. Nakada, T., Ishikawa, S., Sakamota, M., Katayama, T., Igarashi, T., Mizumura, Y., Koizumi, F., Shigematsu, H., and Fukuda, T. (1986). N–(3′, 4′–dimethoxycinnamoyl) anthranillic acid, an antiallergic compound, induced eosinophilic cystitis. *Urol. Int.* **41**, 457–64. [p. 309]
1262. Nakahata, T., Spicer, S. S., Leary, A. G., Ogawa, M., Franklin, W., and Goetzl, E. J. (1984). Circulating eosinophil colony-forming cells in pure eosinophil aplasia. *Ann. Intern. Med.* **101**, 321–4. [p. 316]
1263. Nakahata, T., Tsuji, K., Ishiguro, A., Ando, O., Norose, N., Koike, K., and Akabane, T. (1985). Single-cell origin of human mixed hemopoietic colonies expressing various combinations of cell lineages. *Blood* **65**, 1010–16. [p. 11]
1264. Nakayama, Y., Kohriyama, T., Yamamoto, S., Deguchi, H., Suwa, M., Kino, M., Hirota, Y., Imamura, K., Kitaura, Y., Kawamura, K., and Spry, C. J. (1985). Electronmicroscopic and immunohistochemical studies on endomyocardial biopsies from a patient with eosinophilic endomyocardial disease. *Heart Vessels Suppl.* **1**, 250–5. [p. 242, 247]
1265. Nassberger, L. and Arbin, A. (1987). Eosinophilic peritonitis – hypothesis. *Nephron.* **46**, 103–4. [p. 221]
1266. Nathan, C. F. and Klebanoff, S. J. (1982). Augmentation of spontaneous macrophage-mediated cytolysis by eosinophil peroxidase. *J. Exp. Med.* **155**, 1291–308. [p. 60]
1267. Naylor, A. R. and Pollet, J. E. (1985). Eosinophilic colitis. *Dis. Colon Rectum* **28**, 615–18. [p. 185]
1268. Naylor, B. and Novak, P. M. (1985). Charcot–Leyden crystals in pleural fluids. *Acta Cytol. (Baltimore)* **29**, 781–4. [p. 64]
1269. Neeman, A. and Kadish, U. (1987). Marked eosinophilia in a patient with primary sclerosing cholangitis (letter). *Am. J. Med.* **83**, 378–9. [p. 191]
1270. Nelkan, R. P. and Stockman, J. A. III. (1976). The hypereosinophilic

syndrome in association with acute lymphoblastic leukemia. *J. Pediatr.* **89**, 771–3. [p. 161]

1271. Nelson, D. A. and Jarratt, M. (1984). Angiolymphoid hyperplasia with eosinophilia. *Pediatr. Dermatol.* **1**, 210–4. [p. 168]

1272. Neusser, E. (1892). Klinisch-haematologische mittheilungen. *Wien Klin. Wochenschr.* **5**, 41–46, 64–68. [p. 5]

1273. Neva, F. A. and Ottesen, E. A. (1978). Tropical (filarial) eosinophilia. *N. Engl. J. Med.* **298**, 1129–31. [p. 141]

1274. Newinger, G., Fournier, E., Hatron, P. Y., Lafitte, J., Servais, B., Tonnel, A. B., Devulder, B., and Voisin, C. (1984). (Systemic manifestations of angiitis with asthma and hypereosinophilia. Study of 10 cases). *Rev. Med. Interne* **5**, 165–171. [p. 203]

1275. Newsome, F. V. (1987). Suramin and eosinophil degranulation and vacuolation in onchocerciasis (letter). *Lancet* **i**, 1381–2. [p. 95]

1276. Nguyen, M. T., Patterson, K., and Sly, R. M. (1985). Causes of death from asthma in children. *Ann. Allergy* **55**, 448–53. [p. 195]

1277. Nicola, N. A. and Metcalf, D. (1986). Binding of iodinated multipotential colony-stimulating factor (interleukin-3) to murine bone marrow cells. *J. Cell Physiol.* **128**, 180–8. [p. 22]

1278. Nippoldt, T. B., Edwards, W. D., Holmes, D. R. Jr., Reeder G. S., Hartzler, G. O., and Smith, H. C. (1982). Right ventricular endomyocardial biopsy: clinicopathologic correlates in 100 consecutive patients. *Mayo Clin. Proc.* **57**, 407–18. [p. 241]

1279. Nir, M. A. and Westfried, M. (1981). Hypereosinophilic dermatitis: a distinct manifestation of the hypereosinophilic syndrome with response to dapsone. *Dermatologica* **162**, 444–50. [p. 273]

1280. Nissen Druey, C. and Speck, B. (1978). Differential counts of neutrophil, eosinophil, and macrophage colonies in cultures from human bone marrow and peripheral blood. *Blut* **37**, 241–8. [p. 16]

1281. Nissenblatt, M. J. (1980). Basophilic transformation of chronic myelogenous leukemia. *South. Med. J.* **73**, 1316–19. [p. 12]

1282. Nix, M. (1984). Angiolymphoid hyperplasia with eosinophilia in association with a vascular malformation. *J. Dermatol. Surg. Oncol.* **10**, 632–6. [p. 168]

1283. Nogueira, N. M., Klebanoff, S. J., and Cohn, Z. A. (1982). T. cruzi: sensitization to macrophage killing by eosinophil peroxidase. *J. Immunol.* **128**, 1705–8. [p. 60, 120]

1284. Nolan, C. R., Anger, M. S., and Kelleher, S. P. (1986). Eosinophiluria – a new method of detection and definition of the clinical spectrum. *N. Engl. J. Med.* **315**, 1516–19. [p. 37, 224]

1285. Norlander, N. B. (1951). Eosinophilic leukemia infiltrating the Gasserian ganglion. *Acta Med. Scand.* **139**, 146–52. [p. 152]

1286. Novack, S. N., Kun, T. L., and Goldberg, L. S. (1971). Arterial calcification associated with hypereosinophilic syndrome. *Ann. Intern. Med.* **74**, 99–101. [p. 271, 272, 289]

1287. Novato Silva, E., Nogueira Machado, J. A., and Gazzinelli, G. (1980). Schistosoma mansoni: comparison of the killing effect of granulocytes and complement with or without antibody on fresh and cultured schistosomula in vitro. *Am. J. Trop. Med. Hyg.* **29**, 1263–7. [p. 114]

1288. Novello, A. C. and Port, F. K. (1982). Hemodialysis eosinophilia. *Int. J. Artif. Organs* **5**, 5–7. [p. 222]

1289. Nunzi, E., Parodi, A., and Rebora, A. (1985). Ofuji's disease: high circulating titers of IgG and IgM directed to basal cell cytoplasm. *J. Am. Acad. Dermatol.* **12**, 268–73. [p. 304]

1290. Nutman, T. B., Miller, K. D., Mulligan, M., and Ottesen, E. A. (1986). Loa loa infection in temporary residents of endemic regions: recognition of a hyperresponsive syndrome with characteristic clinical manifestations. *J. Infect. Dis.* **154**, 10–18. [p. 143]

1291. Nutman, T. B., Ottesen, E. A., Ieng, S., Samuels, J., Kimball, E., Lutkoski, M., Zierdt, W. S., Gam, A., and Neva, F. A. (1987). Eosinophilia in Southeast Asian refugees: evaluation at a referral center. *J. Infect. Dis.* **155**, 309–13. [p. 136]

1292. O'Boyle, C. P., Dempsey, J., Otridge, B., and Barniville, H. (1981). Malignant islet-cell tumour of the pancreas presenting with non-bacterial thrombotic endocarditis and eosinophilia. *Postgrad. Med. J.* **57**, 457–8. [p. 172]

1293. Odeberg, B. (1965). Eosinophilic leukemia and disseminated eosinophilic collagen disease: a disease entity? *Acta Med. Scand.* **177**, 129–44. [p. 276]

1294. O'Donnell, M. C., Ackerman, S. J. Gleich, G. J., and Thomas, L. L. (1983). Activation of basophil and mast cell histamine release by eosinophil granule major basic protein. *J. Exp. Med.* **157**, 1981–91. [p. 48]

1295. O'Driscoll, B. R., Cromwell, O., and Kay, A. B. (1984). Sputum leukotrienes in obstructive airways diseases. *Clin. Exp. Immunol.* **55**, 397–404. [p. 199]

1296. Oetgen, W. J. (1977). Pertussoid eosinophilic pneumonia: pulmonary infiltrates with eosinophilia in very young infants. *Chest* **71**, 492–6. [p.296]

1297. Ofuji, S. (1987). Eosinophilic pustular folliculitis. *Dermatologica* **174**, 53–6. [p. 304]

1298. Ogawa, H. (1986). Atopic aspect of eosinophilic nasal polyposis and a possible mechanism of eosinophil accumulation. *Acta Otolaryngol. (Suppl) Stockh)* **430**, 12–7. [p. 214]

1299. Ogawa, H., Kunkel, S. L., Fantone, J. C., and Ward, P. A. (1981). Digestion of the fifth component of complement by eosinophil lysosomal enzymes: production of eosinophil specific chemotactic activity. *Virchows Arch. (Cell Pathol.)* **38**, 149–57. [p. 101]

1300. Ogilvie, B. M., Askenase, P. W., and Rose, M. E. (1980). Basophils and eosinophils in three strain of rats and in athymic (nude) rats following infection with the nematodes Nippostrongylus brasiliensis or Trichinella spiralis. *Immunology* **39**, 385–9. [p. 313]

1301. Ogino, S., Harada, T., Okawachi, I., Irifune, M., Matsunaga, T., and Nagano, T. (1986). Aspirin-induced asthma and nasal polyps. *Acta Otolaryngol. (Suppl) (Stockh)* **430**, 21–7. [p. 202, 214]

1302. Ogushi, F., Ozaki, T., Kawano, T., and Yasouka, S. (1987). PGE2 and PGF2 alpha content in bronchoalveolar lavage fluid obtained from patients with eosinophilic pneumonia. *Chest* **91**, 204–6. [p. 207]

1303. Oh, S. J., Herrara, G. A., and Spalding, D. M. (1986). Eosinophilic vasculitic neuropathy in the Churg-Strauss syndrome (letter). *Arthritis Rheum.* **29**, 1173–5. [p. 203]

1304. Ohga, S., Ishii, E., Fujioka, K., and Ueda, K. (1987). Inversion of chromosome 16 with abnormal marrow eosinophils in acute myelomonocytic leukemia: a case report of a 9-month-old infant. *Acta Haematol. Jap.* **50**, 114–18. [p. 158]

1305. Ohto, H., Shibata, Y., Takeuchi, A., Chen, R. F., and Maaeda, H. (1985). Expression of the platelet-common acute lymphoblastic leukemia associated antigen on normal eosinophils. *Scand. J. Haematol.* **34**, 281–7. [p. 86]

1306. Ojala, K., Sipila, P., Sorri, M., and Karma, P. (1982). Role of atopic allergy in chronic otitis media: evaluation based on serum IgE and nasal/aural cytologic findings in patients with operated chronic ears. *Acta Otolaryngol. (Stockh)* **93**, 55–60. [p. 213]

1307. Okada, M., Yamada, O., Mizoguchi, H., Kubota, K., and Nomura, Y. (1985). Inv(16) abnormality and eosinophilia in a patient with acute nonlymphocytic leukemia. *Cancer Genet. Cytogenet.* **14**, 185–7. [p. 158]

1308. Okafo, B. A., Jones, H. W., Dow, D., and Kiruluta, H. G. (1985). Eosinophilic cystitis: pleomorphic manifestations. *Can. J. Surg.* **28**, 17–8. [p. 223]

1309. Okelo, G. B., Mukiibi, J. M., and Kyobe, J. (1979). Eosinophilia in intestinal parasitic infestations in Kenyan africans. *East Afr. Med. J.* **56**, 266–9. [p. 31]

1310. Okuda, M. and Sakaguchi, Y. Extracellular transport of eosinophil peroxidase (EPO) (abstract). Presented to the 6th International Congress of Immunology, Toronto, Canada, 1986. [p. 93]

1311. Okuda, M., Takenaka, T., Kawabori, S., and Ogami, Y. (1981). Ultastructural study of the specific granule of the human eosinophil. *J. Submicrosc. Cytol.* **13**, 465–71. [p. 78]

1312. Olofsson, T., Gartner, I., and Olsson, I. (1980). Separation of human bone marrow cells in density gradients of polyvinylpyrrolidone coated silica gel (Percoll). *Scand. J. Haematol.* **24**, 254–62. [p. 16]

1313. Olsen, E. G. (1977). Endomyocardial fibrosis and Löffler's endocarditis parietalis fibroplastica. *Postgrad. Med. J.* **53**, 538–40. [p. 252]

1314. Olsen, E. G. (1982). The pathology of cardiomyopathy: present state of knowledge. *Arq. Bras. Cardiol.* **38**, 325–9. [p. 242]

1315. Olsen, E. G. (1983). Pathological aspects of endomyocardial fibrosis. *Postgrad. Med. J.* **59**, 135–39. [p. 257]

1316. Olsen, E. G. (1983). Eosinophilic heart disease. *Trans. R. Soc. Trop. Med. Hyg.* **77**, 2–4. [p. 257]

1317. Olsen, E. G. and Spry, C. J. (1979). The pathogenesis of Löffler's endomyocardial disease and its relationship to endomyocardial fibrosis. *Prog. Cardiol.* **8**, 281–303. [p. 246, 323]

1318. Olsen, E. G. and Spry, C. J. (1982). The pathophysiology of endomyocardial fibrosis. *Arq. Bras. Cardiol.* **38**, 319–23. [p. 234]

1319. Olsen, E. G., and Spry, C. J. (1985). Relation between eosinophilia and endomyocardial disease. *Prog. Cardiovasc. Dis.* **27**, 241–54. [p. 234, 325]

1320. Olsen, E. G. J. and Richardson, P. J., Eds. (1983). Endomyocardial disease. *Postgrad. Med. J.* **59**, 133–190. [p. 250]

1321. Olsen, R. L. and Little, C. (1983). Purification and some properties of myeloperoxidase and eosinophil peroxidase from human blood. *Biochem. J.* **209**, 781–7. [p. 58]

1322. Olsen, R. L., Syse, K., Little, C., and Christensen, T. B. (1985). Further characterization of human eosinophil peroxidase. *Biochem. J.* **229**, 779–84. [p. 58]

1323. Olsen, T. G. and Helwig, E. B. (1985). Angiolymphoid hyperplasia with eosinophilia: a clinicopathologic study of 116 patients. *J. Am. Acad. Dermatol.* **12**, 781–96. [p. 167]

1324. Olson, T. A., Virmani, R., Ansinelli, R. A., Lee, D. H., Mosijczuk, A. D., Marsella, R. C., and Ruymann, F. B. (1982). Cardiomyopathy in a child with hypereosinophilic syndrome. *Pediatr. Cardiol.* **3**, 161–9. [p. 236]

1325. Olsson, I., Egesten, A., Gullberg, U., Lantz, M., Stromberg, K., and Winqvist, I. (1986). The biosynthesis of neutrophil and eosinophil granule proteins. *Folia Histochem. Cytobiol.* **24**, 89–97. [p. 48]

1326. Olsson, I., Persson, A. M., Stromberg, K., Winqvist, I., Tai, P.-C. and Spry, C. J. (1985). Purification of eosinophil peroxidase and studies of biosynthesis and processing in human marrow cells. *Blood* **66**, 1143–8. [p. 57, 58]

1327. Olsson, I., Persson, A. M., and Winqvist, I. (1986). Biochemical properties of the eosinophil cationic protein and demonstration of its biosynthesis *in vitro* in marrow cells from patients with an eosinophilia. *Blood* **67**, 498–503. [p. 48, 49]

1328. Olsson, I. and Venge, P. (1972). Cationic proteins of human granulocytes. 1. Isolation of the cationic proteins from the granules of leukaemic myeloid cells. *Scand. J. Haematol.* **9**, 204–14. [p. 7]

1329. Olsson, I. and Venge, P. (1974). Cationic proteins of human granulocytes. II. Separation of the cationic proteins of the granules of leukaemic myeloid cells. *Blood* **44**, 235–46. [p. 48]

1330. Olsson, I. and Venge, P. (1979). The role of the eosinophil granulocyte in the inflammatory reaction. *Allergy* **34**, 353–67. [p. 323]

1331. Olsson, I., Venge, P., Spitznagel, J. K., and Lehrer, R. I. (1977). Arginine-rich cationic proteins of human eosinophil granules: comparison of the constituents of eosinophilic and neutrophilic leukocytes. *Lab. Invest.* **36**, 493–500. [p. 48, 49, 51]

1332. Oneson, R., Sabio, H., and Innes, D. J. Jr. (1987). Acute lymphoblastic leukaemia in a child with familial Pelger-Hüet anomaly. *Br. J. Haematol.* **66**, 193–7. [p. 261]

1333. Oppenheim, S., Rogell, G., and Peyser, R. (1985). Diffuse unilateral subacute neuroretinitis. *Ann. Ophthalmol.* **17**, 336–8. [p. 219]

1334. Orange, R. P., Murphy, R. C., and Austen, K. F. (1974). Inactivation of slow reacting substance of anaphylaxis (SRS-A) by arylsulfatases. *J. Immunol.* **113**, 316–22. [p. 61]

1335. Organick, A. B. and Wilson, E. M. (1968). Multiple drugs in retreatment of chronic pulmonary tuberculosis: results with capreomycin and ethambutol. *Dis. Chest* **53**, 560–4. [p. 309]

1336. Ortega Pierres, G., Mackenzie, C. D., and Parkhouse, R. M. (1984). Protection against Trichinella spiralis induced by a monoclonal antibody that promotes killing of newborn larvae by granulocytes. *Parasite Immunol.* **6**, 275–84. [p. 116]

1337. O'Shea, J. J., Jaffe, E. S., Lane, H. C., MacDermott, R. P., and Fauci, A. S. (1987). Peripheral T-cell lymphoma presenting as hypereosinophilia with vasculitis: clinical, pathologic, and immunologic features. *Am. J. Med.* **82**, 539–45. [p. 163]

1338. Ottesen, E. A. (1987). Description, mechanisms and control of reactions to treatment in the human filariases. *Ciba Found. Symp.* **127**, 265–83. [p. 142]

1339. Ottesen, E. A., Skvaril, F., Tripathy, S. P., Poindexter, R. W., and Hussain, R. (1985). Prominence of IgG4 in the IgG antibody response to human filariasis. *J. Immunol.* **134**, 2707–12. [p. 142]

1340. Ottesen, E. A., Stanley, A. M., Gelfand, J. A., Gadek, J. E., Frank, M. M., Nash, T. E., and Cheever, A. W. (1977). Immunoglobulin and complement receptors on human eosinophils and their role in cellular adherence to schistosomules. *Am. J. Trop. Med. Hyg.* **26**, 134–41. [p. 76, 77]

1341. Otto, G. F., Berthrong, M., Appleby, R. E., Rawlins, J. C., and Wilbur, O. (1954). Eosinophilia and hepatomegaly due to Capillaria hepatica infection. *Bull. Johns Hopkins Hosp.* **94**, 319–36. [p. 144]

1342. Ottolenghi, A. (1970). The relationship between eosinophilic leukocytes and phospholipase B: activity in some rat tissues. *Lipids* **5**, 531–8. [p. 29]

1343. Ottolenghi, A. (1986). Eosinophilic leucocytes and phospholipase B of rat tissues. *Cell Tissue Kinet.* **19**, 391–406. [p. 29]

1344. Ottolenghi, A., Pickett, J. P., and Greene, W. B. (1967). Histochemical demonstration of phospholipase B (lysolecithinase) activity in rat tissues. *J. Histochem. Cytochem.* **14**, 907–14. [p. 29]

1345. Owen, J. and Scott, J. G. (1979). Transition of the hypereosinophilic syndrome to myelomonocytic leukemia. *Can. Med. Assoc. J.* **121**, 1489–91. [p. 265]

1346. Owen, W. F. Jr, Rothenberg, M. E., Silberstein, D. S., Gasson, J. C., Stevens, R. L., Austen, K. F., and Soberman, R. J. (1987). Regulation of human eosinophil viability, density, and function by granulocyte/macrophage colony-stimulating factor in the presence of 3T3 fibroblasts. *J. Exp. Med.* **166**, 129–41. [p. 36, 108]

1347. Owen, W. F. Jr, Soberman, R. J., Yoshimoto, T., Sheffer, A. L., Lewis, R. A., and Austen, K. F. (1987). Synthesis and release of leukotriene C4 by human eosinophils. *J. Immunol.* **138**, 532–8. [p. 70]

1348. Owhashi, M. and Nawa, Y. (1987). Eosinophil chemotactic lymphokine produced by spleen cells of Schistosoma japonicum-infected mice. *Int. Arch. Allergy Appl. Immunol.* **82**, 20–5. [p. 100]

1349. Ownby, H. E., Roi, L. D., Isenberg, R. R., and Brennan, M. J. (1983). Peripheral lymphocyte and eosinophil counts as indicators of prognosis in primary breast cancer. *Cancer* **52**. 126–30. [p. 170]

1350. Oyaizu, N., Uemura, Y., Izumi, H., Morii, S., Nishi, M., and Hioki, K. (1985). Eosinophilic gastroenteritis: immunohistochemical evidence for IgE mast cell-mediated allergy. *Acta Pathol. Jpn.* **35**, 759–66. [p. 185]

1351. Packe, G. E., Stentiford, N. H., and Richardson, S. G. (1984). Eosinophilic leukaemia presenting with intolerance of alcohol. *Br. Med. J. (Clin. Res.)* **288**, 1123–4. [p. 154, 271, 277]

1352. Page, C. P. (1987). A role for platelet activating factor and platelets in the induction of bronchial hyperreactivity. *Int. J. Tissue. React.* **9**, 27–32. [p. 195]

1353. Paleologo, F. P., Neafie, R. C., and Connor, D. H. (1984). Lymphadenitis caused by Loa loa. *Am. J. Trop. Med. Hyg.* **33**, 395–402. [p. 143]

1354. Palermo, A., Moretti, S., Difonzo, E. M., and Fattorossi, A. (1984). Mycosis fungoides with monoclonal gammopathy, hypereosinophilia, and hyper-IgE. *Dermatologica* **169**, 194–6. [p. 164]

1355. Palmblad, J., Gyllenhammar, H., Lindgren, J. A., and Malmsten, C. L. (1984). Effects of leukotrienes and f-Met-Leu-Phe on oxidative metabolism of neutrophils and eosinophils. *J. Immunol.* **132**, 3041–5. [p. 68]

1356. Panush, R. S., Franco, A. E., and Schur, P. H. (1971). Rheumatoid arthritis associated with eosinophilia. *Ann. Intern. Med.* **76**, 199–205. [p. 177]

1357. Panush, R. S., Wilkinson, L. S., and Fagin, R. R. (1973). Chronic active hepatitis associated with eosinophilia and Coombs'-positive hemolytic anemia. *Gastroenterology* **64**, 1015–9. [p. 190]

1358. Parish, W. E. and Luckhurst, E. (1982). Eosinophilia VI, spontaneous synthesis of chemokinetics, chemotactic, complement receptor-inducing activities for eosinophils by bronchial T-lymphocytes of asthmatic-bronchitic patients. *Clin. Allergy* **12**, 475–88. [p. 100]

1359. Parker, C. W., Koch, D. A., Huber, M. M., and Falkenhein, S. F. (1980). Arylsulfatase inactivation of slow reacting substance. Evidence for proteolysis as a major mechanism when ordinary commercial preparations of the enzyme are used. *Prostaglandins* **20**, 887–908. [p. 61]

1360. Parker, D., Graham Pole, J., Malpas, J. S., and Paxton, A. (1979). Acute lymphoblastic leukemia with eosinophilia and basophilia. *Am. J. Pediatr. Hematol. Oncol.* **1**, 195–9. [p. 12, 161, 216]

1361. Parmley, R. T., Crist, W. M., Roper, M., Takagi, M., and Austin, R. L. (1981). Intranuclear crystalloids associated witih abnormal granules in eosinophilic leukocytes. *Blood* **58**, 1134–40. [p. 261]

1362. Parmley, R. T. and Spicer, S. S. (1974). Cytochemical and ultrastructural identification of a small type granule in human late eosinophils. *Lab. Invest.* **30**, 557–67. [p. 43, 50]

1363. Parmley, R. T. and Spicer, S. S. (1975). Altered tissue eosinophils in Hodgkin's disease. *Exp. Mol. Pathol.* **23**, 70–82. [p. 44]

1364. Parmley, R. T., Takagi, M., Spicer, S. S., Thrasher, A., and Denys, F. R. (1982). Ultrastructural visualization of complex carbohydrates in eosinophilic leukocytes. *Am. J. Anat.* **165**, 53–67. [p. 72]

1365. Parreira, L., Taveres de Castro, J., Hibbin, J. A., Marsh, J. C., Marcus, R. E., Babapulle, V. B., Spry, C. J., Goldman, J. M., and Catovsky, D. (1986). Chromosome and cell culture studies in eosinophilic leukaemia. *Br. J. Haematol.* **62**, 659–69. [p. 25, 155, 156]

1366. Parrillo, J. E., Borer, J. S., Henry, W. L., Wolff, S. M., and Fauci, A. S. (1979). The cardiovascular manifestations of the hypereosinophilic syndrome: prospective study of 26 patients, with review of the literature. *Am. J. Med.* **67**, 572–82. [p. 234, 239]

1367. Parrillo, J. E., and Fauci, A. S. (1978). Human eosinophils: purification and cytotoxic capability of eosinophils from patients with the hypereosinophilic syndrome. *Blood* **51**, 457–73. [p. 76, 118, 191, 246, 283]

1368. Parrillo, J. E., Fauci, A. S., and Wolff, S. M. (1977). The hypereosinophilic syndrome: dramatic response to therapeutic intervention. *Trans. Assoc. Am. Physicians* **90**, 135–44. [p. 290]

1369. Parrillo, J. E., Lawley, T. J., Frank, M. M., Kaplan, A. P., and Fauci, A. S. (1979). Immunologic reactivity in the hypereosinophilic syndrome. *J. Allergy Clin. Immunol.* **64**, 113–21. [p. 53, 286]

1370. Parry, E. H. and Abrahams, D. G. (1965). The natural history of endomyocardial fibrosis. *Q. J. Med.* **34**, 383–408. [p. 255]

1371. Parwaresch, M. R., Walle, A. J., and Arndt, D. (1976). The peripheral kinetics of human radiolabelled eosinophils. *Virchows Arch. (Cell Pathol.)* **21**, 57–66. [p. 27]

1372. Paschke, R. and Heine, M. (1985). Pathophysiological aspects of dacarbazine-induced human liver damage. *Hepatogastroenterology* **32**, 273–5. [p. 310]

1373. Passerini, C. G., Donati, M. B., Semeraro, N., Cofrancesco, E., and Cortellaro, M. (1983). Monocyte procoagulant activity in hypereosinophilic syndrome (letter). *Lancet* **ii**, 460–1. [p. 286]

1374. Pastrnak, A. and Jansa, P. (1984). Local eosinophilia in stroma of tumors related to prognosis. *Neoplasma* **31**, 323–6. [p. 175]

1375. Patchell, R. and Perry, M. C. (1981). Eosinophilic meningitis in Hodgkin disease. *Neurology (NY)* **31**, 887–8. [p. 216]

1376. Patel, A. K., D'Arbela, P. G., and Somers, K. (1977). Endomyocardial fibrosis and eosinophilia. *Br. Heart. J.* **39**, 238–41. [p. 256]

1377. Patterson, N. W., Brenbridge, A. N., and Paling, M. R. (1984). Computed tomography of mural thrombosis in the hypereosinophilic syndrome. *J. Comput. Tomogr.* **8**, 129–32. [p. 239]

1378. Patterson, R., Lerner, C., Roberts, M., Moel, D., and Grammer, L. C. (1986). Ethylene oxide (ETO) as a possible cause of an allergic reaction during peritoneal dialysis and immunologic detection of ETO from dialysis tubing. *Am. J. Kidney Dis.* **8**, 64–6. [p. 221]

1379. Patterson, R., Oh, S. H., Roberts, M., and Hsu, C. C. (1975). Massive polyclonal hyperimmunoglobulinemia E, eosinophilia and increased IgE-bearing lymphocytes. *Am. J. Med.* **58**, 553–8. [p. 317]

1380. Pattison, N., Wright, T., and Herrod, H. G. (1987). Pneumocystis carinii pneumonitis, eosinophilia and hypogammaglobulinemia. *Pediatr. Infect Dis. J.* **6**, 293–4. [p. 148, 315]

1381. Pearlman, D. S. (1984). Chronic rhinitis in children. *Clin. Rev. Allergy* **2**, 197–211. [p. 213]

1382. Pearson, D. L. and Rosenow, E. C. (1978). Chronic eosinophilic pneumonia (Carrington's): a follow-up study. *Mayo Clin. Proc.* **53**, 73–8. [p. 206, 207, 208]

1383. Pedersen, H. (1964). Endocarditis parietalis fibroplastica (Löffler) med overvejende cerebrale initialsymptomer. *Ugeskr Laeger* **126**, 274–9. [p. 275]

1384. Peer, A., Witz, E., Yona, E., Manor, H., and Reif, R. (1985). Solitary eosinophilic granuloma of sternum: case report with review of the literature. *Br. J. Radiol.* **58**, 1173–6. [p. 165]

1385. Peison, B. and Benisch, B. (1980). Hypereosinophilic syndrome. *NY State J. Med.* **80**, 89–92. [p. 246]

1386. Pelikan, Z. and Pelikan Filipek, M. (1986). The late asthmatic response to allergen challenge – Part I. *Ann. Allergy* **56**, 414–20. [p. 200]

1387. Pereira, F., Moreno, H., Crist, W., and Ermocilla, R. (1977). Löffler's endomyocardial fibrosis, eosinophilia, and acute lymphoblastic leukemia. *Pediatrics* **59**, 950–1. [p. 161]

1388. Pesci, A., Bertorelli, G., Manganelli, P., and Ambanelli, U. (1986). Bronchoalveolar lavage analysis of interstitial lung disease in CREST syndrome. *Clin. Exp. Rheumatol.* **4**, 121–4. [p. 209]

1389. Peters, M. S., Gleich, G. J., Dunnette, S. L., and Fukuda, T. (1988). Ultrastructural study of eosinophils from patients with the hypereosinophilic syndrome: a morphological basis of hypodense eosinophils. *Blood* **71**, 780–5. [p. 34, 46, 47, 279, 281, 282, 284, 301]

1390. Peters, M. S., Rodriguez, M., and Gleich, G. J. (1986). Localization of human eosinophil granule major basic protein, eosinophil cationic protein, and eosinophil-derived neurotoxin by immunoelectron microscopy, *Lab. Invest.* **54**, 656–62. [p. 46, 50, 55]

1391. Peters, M. S., Schroeter, A. L., and Gleich, G. J. (1983). Immunofluorescence identification of eosinophil granule major basic protein in the flame figures of Wells' syndrome. *Br. J. Dermatol.* **109**, 141–8. [p. 168]

1392. Peters, M. S., Schroeter, A. L., Kephart, G. M., and Gleich, G. J. (1983). Localization of eosinophil granule major basic protein in chronic urticaria. *J. Invest. Dermatol.* **81**, 39–43. [p. 299]

1393. Peters, M. S., Winkelmann, R. K., Greaves, M. W., Kephart, G. M., and Gleich, G. J. (1987). Extracellular deposition of eosinophil granule major basic protein in pressure urticaria. *J. Am. Acad. Dermatol.* **16**, 513–7. [p. 299]

1394. Peterson, A. P., Altman, L. C., Hill, J. S., Gosney, K., and Kadin, M. E. (1981). Glucocorticoid receptors in normal human eosinophils: comparison with neutrophils. *J. Allergy Clin. Immunol.* **68**, 212–17. [p. 82]

1395. Peterson, C. (1987). Eosinophil granule proteins. Biochemical and functional studies. Doctoral Thesis at Uppsala University, Sweden. [p. 49, 50, 51, 54, 55, 91]

1396. Peterson, C. G., Skoog, V., and Venge, P. (1986). Human eosinophil cationic proteins (ECP and EPX) and their suppressive effects on lymphocyte proliferation. *Immunobiology* **171**, 1–13. [p. 52, 56, 57]

1397. Peterson, C. G. and Venge, P. (1983). Purification and characterization of a new cationic protein – eosinophil protein-X (EPX) – from granules of human eosinophils. *Immunology* **50**, 19–26. [p. 53, 54]

1398. Peterson, C. G. and Venge, P. (1987). Interaction and complex-formation between the eosinophil cationic protein and alpha 2-macroglobulin. *Biochem. J.* **245**, 781–7. [p. 51, 284]

1399. Peterson, M. W., Monick, M., and Hunninghake, G. W. (1987). Prognostic role of eosinophils in pulmonary fibrosis. *Chest* **92**, 51–6. [p. 209]

1400. Petreccia, D. C., Nauseef, W. M., and Clark, R. A. (1987). Respiratory burst of normal human eosinophils. *J. Leukocyte Biol.* **41**, 283–8. [p. 68]

1401. Pettersson, T. and Riska, H. (1981). Diagnostic value of total and differential leukocyte counts in pleural effusions. *Acta Med. Scand.* **210**, 129–35. [p. 212]

1402. Phanuphak, P. and Kohler, P. F. (1980). Onset of polyarteritis nodosa during allergic hyposensitization treatment. *Am. J. Med.* **68**, 479–85. [p. 203]

1403. Pier, S. A. and Gallagher, J. E. (1978). A method for locating individual leukocytes for comparative study by light and scanning electron microscopy. *Am. J. Vet. Res.* **39**, 189–91. [p. 74]

1404. Pierce, L. E., Husseinian, A. H., and Constantine, A. B. (1967). Disseminated eosinophilic collagen disease. *Blood* **29**, 540–9. [p. 276]

1405. Pihl, E., Gustafson, G. T., Joseffson, B., and Paul, K. G. (1967). Heavy metals in granules of eosinophilic granulocytes. *Scand. J. Haematol.* **4**, 371–9. [p. 63]

1406. Pimenta, P. F. and De Souza, W. (1982). Surface charge of eosinophils: binding of cationic particles and measurement of cellular electrophoretic mobility. *Histochemistry* **74**, 569–76. [p. 271]

1407. Pimenta, P. F. and De Souza, W. (1982). Ultrastructure and cytochemistry of the cell surface of eosinophils. *J. Submicrosc. Cytol.* **14**, 227–37. [p. 74, 75, 83, 127]

1408. Pimenta, P. F., Dos Santos, M. A., and De Souza, W. (1987). Fine structure and cytochemistry of the interaction between Leishmania mexicana amazonensis and rat neutrophils and eosinophils. *J. Submicrosc. Cytol.* **19**, 387–95. [p. 117]

1409. Pimenta, P. F., Loures, M. A., and De Souza, W. (1980). Ultrastructural localization of basic proteins in cytoplasmic granules of rat eosinophils and mast cells. *J. Histochem. Cytochem.* **28**, 238–44. [p. 43]

1410. Pincus, S. H. (1978). Production of eosinophil-rich guinea pig peritoneal exudates. *Blood* **52**, 127–34. [p. 126]

1411. Pincus, S. H. (1980). Peroxidase-mediated iodination by guinea pig peritoneal exudate eosinophils. *Inflammation* **4**, 89–106. [p. 59]

1412. Pincus, S. H. (1983). Hydrogen peroxide release from eosinophils: quantitative, comparative studies of human and guinea pig eosinophils. *J. Invest. Dermatol.* **80**, 278–81. [p. 69]

1413. Pincus, S. H. (1986). Lectin binding by eosinophils. *Proc. Soc. Exp. Biol. Med.* **182**, 344–9. [p. 84]

1414. Pincus, S. H., Butterworth, A. E., David, J. R., Robbins, M., and Vadas, M. A. (1981). Antibody-dependent eosinophil-mediated damage to schistosomula of Schistosoma mansoni: lack of requirement for oxidative metabolism. *J. Immunol.* **126**, 1794–9. [p. 119]

1415. Pincus, S. H., Dessein, A., Lenzi, H., Vadas, M. A., and David, J. (1984). Eosinophil-mediated killing of schistosomula of Schistosoma mansoni: oxidative requirement for enhancement by eosinophil colony stimulating factor (CSF-alpha) and supernatants with eosinophil cytotoxicity enhancing activity (E-CEA). *Cell Immunol.* **87**, 424–33. [p. 119]

1416. Pincus, S. H., DiNapoli, A. M., and Schooley, W. R. (1982). Superoxide production by eosinophils: activation by histamine. *J. Invest. Dermatol.* **79**, 53–7. [p. 100]

1417. Pincus, S. H., Ramesh, K. S., and Wyler, D. J. (1987). Eosinophils stimulate fibroblast DNA synthesis. *Blood* **70**, 572–4. [p. 63]

1418. Pincus, S. H., Schooley, W. R., DiNapoli, A. M., and Broder, S. (1981). Metabolic heterogeneity of eosinophils from normal and hypereosinophilic patients. *Blood* **58**, 1175–81. [p. 282]

1419. Pincus, S. H. and Whitcomb, E. Intracellular Ca^{++} in eosinophils and neutrophils (abstract). Presented to the 6th International Congress of Immunology, Toronto, Canada, 1986. [p. 95]

1420. Pincus, S. H., Whitcomb, E. A., and Dinarello, C. A. (1986). Interaction of IL 1 and TPA in modulation of eosinophil function. *J. Immunol.* **137**, 3509–14. [p. 109]

1421. Pineda, A. A., Brzica, S. M. Jr., and Taswell, H. F. (1977). Continuous- and semicontinuous-flow blood centrifugation systems: therapeutic applications, with plasma-, platelet, lympha-, and eosinapheresis. *Transfusion* **17**, 407–16. [p. 292]
1422. Pinkston, P., Vijayan., V. K., Nutman, T. B., Rom, W. N., O'Donnell, K. M., Cornelius, M. J., Kumaraswami, V., Ferrans, V. J., Takemura, T., and Yenokida, G., *et al.* (1987). Acute tropical pulmonary eosinophilia: characterization of the lower respiratory tract inflammation and its response to therapy. *J. Clin. Invest.* **80**, 216–25. [p. 141]
1423. Piraino, B. M., Silver, M. R., Dominquez, J. H., and Puschett, J. B. (1984). Peritoneal eosinophils during intermittent peritoneal dialysis. *Am. J. Nephrol.* **4**, 152–7. [p. 221]
1424. Pitkin, R. M. and Witte, D. L. (1979). Platelet and leukocyte counts in pregnancy. *JAMA* **242**, 2696–8. [p. 227]
1425. Plavsic, B., Kuzmanic, D., and Rotkvic, I. (1983). Eosinophilia caused by iodinated radiographic contrast media. *Clin. Radiol.* **34**, 639–42. [p. 310]
1426. Pober, J. S., Brock, T. A., Lapierre, L. A., Mendrick, D. L., Fiers, W., and Gimbrone, M. A. Jr. (1986). Mechanisms of tumor necrosis factor (TNF)-dependent antigen induction in vascular endothelium (abstract). *Fed. Proc.* **45**, 941. [p. 98]
1427. Podell, T. E., Ault, M., Sullman, P., and Klinenberg, J. R. (1980). Synovial fluid eosinophilia. *Arthritis Rheum.* **23**, 1060–1. [p. 178]
1428. Polliack, A., and Douglas, S. D. (1975). Surface features of human eosinophils: a scanning and transmission electron microscopic study of a case of eosinophilia. *Br. J. Haematol.* **30**, 303–6. [p. 74]
1429. Popper, H. (1984). Experimental monoarthritis. Modulatory effect of injected eosinophils on influx of various types of inflammatory cells. *Inflammation* **8**, 301–12. [p. 163]
1430. Port, C. D. and Richter, W. R. (1977). Eosinophilic leukemia in a Syrian hamster. *Vet. Pathol.* **14**, 283–6. [p. 157]
1431. Porter, J. and Jick, H. (1980). Amoxicillin and ampicillin: rashes equally likely. *Lancet* **i**, 1037. [p. 310]
1432. Portner, M. M. and Gracie, W. A. Jr. (1966). Rheumatoid lung disease with cavitary nodules, pneumothorax and eosinophilia. *N. Engl. J. Med.* **275**, 697–700. [p. 177]
1433. Pospisil, J., Kase, F., and Vahala, J. (1985). Basic haematological values in the African buffalo (Syncerus caffer caffer) and in the red buffalo (Syncerus caffer nanus). *Comp. Biochem. Physiol. (A)* **82**, 495–8. [p. 125]
1434. Potier, J. C., Khayat, A., and Foucault, J. P. (1978). (Distomatosis and cardiac disease. Apropos of 2 new cases. Trials of classification and pathogenetic hypotheses). *Arch. Mal Coeur* **71**, 1299–1306. [p. 236]
1435. Powers, N. G. and Carson, S. H. (1987). Idiosyncratic reactions to phenytoin. *Clin. Pediatr. (Phila)* **26**, 120–4. [p. 308]
1436. Prata, M. M., Pinto, J. L., de Oliveira, J. B., and Nunes, M. A. (1984). Eosinophilia in chronic dialysis patients. *Acta Med. Port.* **5**, 209–10. [p. 222]
1437. Presentey, B. (1968). A new anomaly of eosinophilic granulocytes. *Am. J. Clin. Pathol.* **49**, 887–90. [p. 36, 260, 280]

1438. Presentey, B. (1969). Cytochemical characterization of eosinophils with respect to a newly discovered anomaly. *Am. J. Clin. Pathol.* **51**, 451–7. [p. 260]

1439. Presentey, B. (1969). Morphologic observations and genetic follow-up of a familial anomaly of eosinophils. *Am. J. Clin. Pathol.* **51**, 458–62. [p. 260]

1440. Presentey, B. (1970). Partial and severe peroxidase and phospholipid deficiency in eosinophils: cytochemical and genetic considerations. *Acta Haematol. (Basel)* **44**, 345–54. [p. 260]

1441. Presentey, B. (1984). Ultrastructure of human eosinophils genetically lacking peroxidase. *Acta Haematol. (Basel)* **71**, 334–40. [p. 260]

1442. Presentey, B., Jerushalmy, Z., Ben Bassat, M., and Perk, K. (1980). Genesis, ultrastructure and cytochemical study of the cat eosinophil. *Anat. Rec.* **196**, 119–27. [p. 125]

1443. Presentey, B., Jerushalmy, Z., de Vries, A., Rosin, A. J., and Perk, K. (1973). Selective degeneration of specific granules of eosinophils: report of a case. *Am. J. Clin. Pathol.* **60**, 927–31. [p. 314]

1444. Presentey, B. and Joshua, H. (1982). Peroxidase and phospholipid deficiency in human eosinophilic granulocytes – a marker in population genetics. *Experientia* **38**, 628–9. [p. 260]

1445. Press, M. F. and King, W. J. (1986). Distribution of peroxidase and granulocytes in the human uterus. *Lab. Invest.* **54**, 188–203. [p. 226]

1446. Presti, C., Ryan, T., and Armstrong, W. F. (1987). Two-dimensional and Doppler echocardiographic findings in hypereosinophilic syndrome. *Am. Heart J.* **114**, 172–5. [p. 239]

1447. Pretlow, T. P., Boohaker, E. A., Pitts, A. M., Macfadyen, A. J., Bradley, E. L. Jr., and Pretlow, T. G. (1984). Heterogeneity and subcompartmentalization in the distribution of eosinophils in human colonic carcinomas. *Am. J. Pathol.* **116**, 207–13. [p. 171]

1448. Pretlow, T. P., Keith, E. F., Cryar, A. K., Bartolucci, A. A., Pitts, A. M., Pretlow, T. G., Kimball, P. M., and Boohaker, E. A. (1983). Eosinophil infiltration of human colonic carcinomas as a prognostic indicator. *Cancer Res.* **43**, 2997–3171. [p. 171]

1449. Price, H. I. and Batnikszky, S. (1985). The computed tomographic findings in benign diseases of the vertebral column. *CRC Crit. Rev. Diagn. Imaging* **24**, 39–89. [p. 165]

1450. Prigent, C. P., Baculard, P., Carpentier, A., Passelecq, J., and Dubost, C. (1973). Endocardite fibreuse du ventricle gauche chez un filarien: cure chirurgicale. *Arch. Mal Coeur* **66**, 1101–10. [p. 254]

1451. Prin, L., Capron, M., Gosset, P., Wallaert, B., Kusnierz, J. P., Bletry, O., Tonnel, A. B., and Capron, A. (1986). Eosinophilic lung disease: immunological studies of blood and aveolar eosinophils. *Clin. Exp. Immunol.* **63**, 249–57. [p. 208]

1452. Prin, L., Capron, M., Tonnel, A. B., Bletry, O., and Capron, A. (1983). Heterogeneity of human peripheral blood eosinophils: variability in cell density and cytotoxic ability in relation to the level and the origin of hypereosinophilia. *Int. Arch. Allergy Appl. Immunol.* **72**, 336–46. [p. 34]

1453. Prin, L., Charon, J., Capron, M., Gosset, P., Taelman, H., Tonnel, A. B., and Capron, A. (1984). Heterogeneity of human eosinophils. II. Variability of respiratory burst activity related to cell density. *Clin. Exp. Immunol.* **57**, 735–42. [p. 34, 68]

1454. Proujansky, R., Center, D. M., and Weller, P. F. Histamine elicits human eosinophil-active lymphokines. Presented to the 6th International Congress of Immunology, Toronto, Canada, 1986. [p. 102, 110]

1455. Pryzwansky, K. B. (1987). Human leukocytes as viewed by stereo high-voltage electronmicroscopy. *Blood Cells* **12**, 505–30. [p. 41]

1456. Przybojewski, J. Z. (1985). Endomyocardial biopsy: a review of the literature. *Cathet. Cardiovasc. Diagn.* **11**, 287–330. [p. 241]

1457. Puigbo, J. J., Combellas, L., Acquatella, H., Marsiglia, I., Tortoledo, F., Casal, H., and Suarez, J. A. (1983). Endomyocardial disease in South America – report on 23 cases in Venezuela. *Postgrad. Med. J.* **59**, 162–9. [p. 234]

1458. Punch, A. L. and Close, H. G. (1938). A case of unexplained eosinophilia. *Guy's Hosp. Rep.* **88**, 143–9. [p. 263]

1459. Punyagupta, S., Juttijudata, P., and Bunnag, T. (1975). Eosinophilic meningitis in Thailand: clinical studies of 484 typical cases probably caused by Angiostrongylus cantonensis. *Am. J. Trop. Med. Hyg.* **24**, 921–31. [p. 139]

1460. Purdie, G. H., Kotasek, D., and Rischbieth, R. H. (1983). The hypereosinophilic syndrome. *Clin. Exp. Neurol.* **19**, 60–6. [p. 271]

1461. Quinlan, C. D., and Mitchell, D. M. (1970). The hypereosinophilic syndrome. *J. Ir. Med. Assoc.* **63**, 186. [p. 270, 284]

1462. Quinn, J. P., Weinstein, R. A., and Caplan, L. R. (1984). Eosinophilic meningitis and ibuprofen therapy. *Neurology* **34**, 108–9. [p. 217]

1463. Quinonez, G. E., Simon, G. T, and Kay, J. M. (1986). Electron microscopy of chronic eosinophilic pneumonia. *Clin. Invest. Med.* **9**, 238–43. [p. 208]

1464. Rackemann, F. M. and Greene, J. E. (1936). Periarteritis nodosa and asthma. *Trans. Assoc. Am. Physicians* **54**, 112–18. [p. 231]

1465. Racz, P., Tenner Racz, K., Buttner, D. W., and Albiez, E. J. (1982). Ultrastructural evidence for eosinophil-parasite adherence (EPA) reaction in human onchocercal lymphadenitis in the early period following diethylcarbamazine treatment. *Tropenmed. Parasitol.* **33**, 213–8. [p. 116]

1466. Racz, P., Tenner Racz, K., Luther, B., Buttner, D. W., and Albiez, E. J. (1983). Immunopathologic aspects in human onchocercal lymphadenitis. *Bull. Soc. Pathol. Exot. Filiales* **76**, 676–80. [p. 143]

1467. Raizner, A. E., Silverman, M. E., and Waters, W. C. III. (1972). Conduction disturbances and pacemaker failure in Löffler's endomyocarditis. *Am. J. Med.* **53**, 343–7. [p. 238]

1468. Rak, S., Hakansson, L., and Venge, P. (1987). Eosinophil chemotactic activity in allergic patients during the birch pollen season: the effect of immunotherapy. *Int. Arch. Allergy Appl. Immunol.* **82**, 349–50. [p. 102]

1469. Ramakrishnan, T. S., Wolfe, L. W., and Dhand, V. P. (1985). A case of acute hypereosinophilic syndrome with post-mortem findings. *Indian Heart J.* **37**, 399–401. [p. 243, 270]

1470. Ramalho Pinto, F. J., McLaren, D. J., and Smithers, S. R. (1978). Complement-mediated killing of schistosomula of Schistosoma mansoni by rat eosinophils in vitro. *J. Exp. Med.* **147**, 147–56. [p. 114]

1471. Ramesh, K. S., Pincus, S. H., and Rocklin, R. E. (1985). Human lymphocyte-eosinophil interactions. I. Modulation of phytohemagglutinin-induced lymphocyte proliferation by eosinophils. *Cell Immunol.* **92**, 366–75. [p. 53]

1472. Ramesh, K. S., Rocklin, R. E., and Pincus, S. H. (1987). Activated human eosinophils synthesize new proteins. *Biochim. Biophys. Acta* **923**, 241–9. [p. 72]

1473. Ramesh, K. S., Rocklin, R. E., and Pincus, S. H. (1987). Phosphorylation and dephosphorylation of soluble proteins in human eosinophils. *J. Cell Biochem.* **34**, 203–11. [p. 110]

1474. Ramos, A. J. (1956). Diagnostic problems: presentation of a case. *JAMA* **160**, 1317–9. [p. 315]

1475. Ramsey, P. G., Martin, T., Chi, E. and Klebanoff, S. J. (1982). Arming of mononuclear phagocytes by eosinophil peroxidase bound to Staphylococcus aureus. *J. Immunol.* **128**, 415–20. [p. 60]

1476. Randolph, T. G. (1944). Blood studies in allergy. I. The direct counting chamber determination of eosinophils by propylene glycol aqueous stains. *J. Allergy* **15**, 89–96. [p. 30]

1477. Randolph, T. G. (1949). Differentiation and enumeration of eosinophils in the counting chamber with a glycol stain; a valuable technique in appraising ACTH dosage. *J. Lab. Clin. Med.* **34**, 1696–701. [p. 30]

1478. Rao, C. K. and Kumar, S. (1982). Role of filariasis in endomyocardial fibrosis. *J. Commun. Dis.* **14**, 91–5. [p. 256]

1479. Rasche, R. F., Kelsch, R. D., and Weaver, D. K. (1973). Löffler's endocarditis in childhood. *Br. Heart J.* **35**, 774–6. [p. 236, 268]

1480. Rawlings, C. E. 3d and Wilkins, R. H. (1984). Solitary eosinophilic granuloma of the skull. *Neurosurgery* **15**, 155–61. [p. 165]

1481. Redman, J. F. and Downs, R. A. (1984). Simple eosinophilic granulomatous prostatitis. *J. Urol.* **132**. 358. [p. 224]

1482. Reid, H., Fox, H. and Whittaker, J. S. (1977). Eosinophilic granuloma of lymph nodes. *Histopathology* **1**, 31–7. [p. 165, 186]

1483. Reid, I. R. and Wallis, W. E. (1984). The chronic and severe forms of eosinophilic meningitis. *Aust. NZ J. Med.* **14**, 163–5. [p. 139]

1484. Reidenberg, M. M. and Caccese, R. W. (1975). Lymphocyte transformation tests and suspected drug allergy. *J. Lab. Clin. Med.* **86**, 997–1002. [p. 313]

1485. Reinbach, G. (1893). Ueber das Verhalten der Leukocyten bei malignen Tumoren. *Arch. Klin. Chir.* **46**, 486–562. [p. 5, 150, 232]

1486. Remmele, W. and Sessner, H. H. (1959). Zur morphologischen Patholgie und Klinik der Endocarditis parietalis fibroplastica sit Bluteosinophilie (Loffler). *Klin. Wochenschr.* **37**, 374–85. [p. 236]

1487. Resnick, M. and Myerson, R. M. (1971). Hypereosinophilic syndrome. Report of two cases, with prolonged courses. *Am. J. Med.* **51**, 560–4. [p. 288]

1488. Reynolds, H. Y. (1987). Bronchoalveolar lavage. *Am. Rev. Respir. Dis.* **135**, 250–63. [p. 326]

1489. Rich, R. R. and Johnson, J. S. (1973). Salicylate hepatotoxicity in patients with juvenile rheumatoid arthritis. *Arthritis Rheum.* **16**, 1–9. [p. 310]

1490. Rickles, F. R. and Miller, D. R. (1972). Eosinophilic leukemoid reaction: report of a case, its relationship to eosinophilic leukemia and review of the pediatric literature. *J. Pediatr.* **80**, 418–28. [p. 152]

1491. Ricoy, J. R., Cabello, A., Rodriguez, J., and Tellez, I. (1983). Neuropathological studies on the toxic syndrome related to adulterated rapeseed oil in Spain. *Brain* **106**, 817–35. [p. 182]

1492. Rigau Perez, J. G., Perez Alvarez, L., Duenas Castro, S., Choi, K., Thacker, S. B., Germain, J. L., Gonzalez de Andres, G., Canada Royo, L., and Perez Gallardo, F. (1984). Epidemiologic investigation of an oil-associated pneumonic paralytic eosinophilic syndrome in Spain. *Am. J. Epidemiol.* **119**, 250–60. [p. 182]

1493. Ringden, O., Ahstrom, L., Lonnqvist, B., Baryd, I., Svedmyr, E., and Gahrton, G. (1987). Allogeneic bone marrow transplantation in a patient with chemotherapy-resistant progressive histiocytosis X. *N. Engl. J. Med.* **316**, 733–5. [p. 165]

1494. Ringden, O., Persson, U., Johansson, S. G., Wilczek, H., Gahrton, G., Groth, C. G., Lundgren, G., Lonnqvist, B., and Moller, E. (1983). Markedly elevated serum IgE levels following allogeneic and syngeneic bone marrow transplantation. *Blood* **61**, 1190–5. [p. 314]

1495. Rivera, J. V. and Bermudez, R. H. (1984). Radionuclide imaging of the liver in human fascioliasis. *Clin. Nucl. Med.* **9**, 450–3. [p. 147]

1496. Roberts, P. F. and McCann, B. G. (1985). Eosinophilic angiocentric fibrosis of the upper respiratory tract: a mucosal variant of granuloma faciale? A report of three cases. *Histopathology* **9**, 1217–25. [p. 215]

1497. Roberts, R. L. and Gallin, J. I. (1985). Rapid method for isolation of normal human peripheral blood eosinophils on discontinuous Percoll gradients and comparison with neutrophils. *Blood* **65**, 433–40. [p. 34]

1498. Roberts, R. L., Ohno, Y., and Gallin, J. I. (1986). Staining of eosinophils with nitroblue tetrazolium in patients with chronic granulomatous disease. *Pediatr. Res.* **20**, 378–80. [p. 261]

1499. Roberts, W. C., Buja, L. M., Buckley, B. H., O'Connell, J. P., Ferrans, V. J. (1974). Endomyocardial disease and eosinophilia (Loeffler's disease). *Am. J. Cardiol.* **33**, 166–9. [p. 235]

1500. Roberts, W. C., Buja, L. M., and Ferrans, V. J. (1970). Löffler's fibroplastic parietal endocarditis, eosinophilic leukemia, and Davies' endomyocardial fibrosis. The same disease at different stages? *Path. Microbiol. (Basel)* **35**, 90–5. [p. 232]

1501. Roberts, W. C. and Ferrans, V. J. (1975). Pathologic anatomy of the cardiomyopathies: idiopathic dilated and hypertrophic types, infiltrative types, and endomyocardial disease with and without eosinophilia. *Hum. Pathol.* **6**, 287–342. [p. 252]

1502. Roberts, W. C., Liegler, D. G., and Carbone, P. P. (1969). Endomyocardial disease and eosinophilia: a clinical and pathologic spectrum. *Am. J. Med.* **46**, 28–42. [p. 277]

1503. Robertson, J. C. and Eeles, G. H. (1970). Syndrome associated with pancreatic acinar cell carcinoma. *Br. Med. J.* **ii**, 708–9. [p. 172]

1504. Robin, J. B., Schanzlin, D. J., Meisler, D. M., deLuise, V. P., and Clough, J. D. (1985). Ocular involvement in the respiratory vasculitides. *Surv. Ophthalmol.* **30**, 127–40. [p. 231]

1505. Robinowitz, M., Virmani, R., and McAllister, H. A. Jr. (1982). Spontaneous coronary artery dissection and eosinophilic inflammation: a cause and effect relationship? *Am. J. Med.* **72**, 923–8. [p. 231]

1506. Robinson, B. W., Rose, A. H., James, A., Whitaker, D., and Musk, A. W. (1986). Alveolitis of pulmonary asbestosis. Bronchoalveolar lavage studies in crocidolite- and chrysotile-exposed individuals. *Chest* **90**, 396–402. [p. 194]

1507. Rocco, V. K. and Hurd, E. R. (1986). Scleroderma and scleroderma-like disorders. *Semin. Arthritis Rheum.* **16**, 22–69. [p. 325]

1508. Rockey, J. H., Donnelly, J. J., Stromberg, B. E., and Soulsby, E. J. (1979). Immunopathology of Toxocara canis and Ascaris suum infections of the eye: the role of the eosinophil. *Invest. Ophthalmol. Vis. Sci.* **18**, 1172–84. [p. 140]

1509. Rodger, J. C., Irvine, K. G., and Lerski, R. A. (1981). Echocardiography in Löffler's endocarditis. *Br. Heart J.* **46**, 110–2. [p. 239]

1510. Rodnan, G. P., DiBartolomeo, A. G., and Medsger, T. A. Jr. (1975). Eosinophilic fasciitis: report of six cases of newly recognised scleroderma-like syndrome. *Arthritis Rheum.* **18**, 525–30. [p. 181]

1511. Roos, D. and de Boer, M. (1986). Purification and cryopreservation of phagocytes from human blood. *Methods Enzymol.* **132**, 225–43. [p. 32, 35]

1512. Roos, D. and Loos, J. A. (1970). Changes in the carbohydrate metabolism of mitogenicaly stimulated human peripheral lymphocytes. I. Stimulation by phytohaemagglutinin. *Biochim. Biophys. Acta* **222**, 565–82. [p. 32]

1513. Root, R. K. and Cohen, M. S. (1981). The microbicidal mechanisms of human neutrophils and eosinophils. *Rev. Infect. Dis.* **3**, 565–98. [p. 324]

1514. Rosai, J. (1982). Angiolymphoid hyperplasia with eosinophilia of the skin: its nosological position in the spectrum of histiocytoid hemangioma. *Am. J. Dermatopathol.* **4**, 175–84. [p. 168]

1515. Rosario Filho, N. A. (1982). Total serum IgE levels and eosinophil counts in trichiuriasis. *Rev. Inst. Med. Trop. Sao Paulo* **24**, 16–20. [p. 145]

1516. Rose, G. A. and Spencer, H. (1957). Polyarteritis nodosa. *Q. J. Med.* **26**, 43–81. [p. 209]

1517. Rosenberg, J. N., Johnson, G. D., Holborow, E. J., and Bywaters, E. G. (1975). Eosinophil-specific and other granulocyte-specific antinuclear antibodies in juvenile chronic polyarthritis and adult rheumatoid arthritis. *Ann. Rheum. Dis.* **34**. 350–3. [p. 41, 177]

1518. Rosenberg, S. A., Lotze, M. T., Muul, L. M., Leitman, S., Chang, A. E, Ettinghausen, S. E., Matory, Y. L., Skibber, J. M., Shiloni, E., and Vetto, J. T., *et al.* (1985). Observations on the systemic administration of autologous lymphokine-activated killer cells and recombinant interleukin-2 to patients with metastatic cancer. *N. Engl. J. Med.* **313**, 1485–92. [p. 301]

1519. Rosenow, E. C. III. (1972). The spectrum of drug-induced pulmonary disease. *Ann. Intern. Med.* **77**, 977–91. [p. 309]

1520. Rossi, C. R., Campos, M., Ghanekar, S. V., and Panangala, V. S. (1986). A monoclonal antibody that identifies mature T-lymphocytes of cattle. *Vet. Immunol. Immunopathol.* **11**, 319–24. [p. 87]

1521. Rothberg, A. D., Cohn, R. J., Argent, A. C., Sher, R., and Joffe, M. (1983). Eosinophilia in premature neonates: phase 2 of a biphasic granulopoietic response. *S. Afr. Med. J.* **64**, 539–41. [p. 294]

1522. Rothenberg, M. E., Owen, W. F. Jr, Silberstein, D. S., Soberman, R. J., Austen, K. F., and Stevens, R. L. (1987). Eosinophils cocultured with endothelial cells have increased survival and functional properties. *Science* **237**, 645–7. [p. 28, 35, 109, 168, 279]

1523. Rothstein, I., Spring, M., and Berley, B. S. (1953). Effect of ACTH in a case of eosinophilic leukemia. *NY State J. Med.* **53**, 1461–3. [p. 289]

1524. Rotstein, S., Blomgren, H., Nilsson, B., Petrini, B., Wasserman, J., and Baral, E. (1984). Prognostic value of various immunological tests in breast cancer patients treated with adjuvant postoperative chemotherapy. *Chemioterapia* **3**, 227–31. [p. 170]

1525. Rowland, M., Brown, R. B., and Goldman, M. (1985). Eosinophilic peritonitis: an unusual manifestation of spontaneous bacterial peritonitis. *J. Clin. Gastroenterol.* **7**, 369–71. [p. 186]

1526. Rowley, J. D. (1973). A new consistent chromosome abnormality in chronic myelogenous leukaemia identified by quinacrine fluorescence and Giemsa staining. *Nature* **243**, 290–3. [p. 157]

1527. Rozboril, M. B., Maricq, H. R., Rodnan, G. P., Jablonska, S., and Bole, G. G. (1983). Capillary microscopy in eosinophilic fasciitis: a comparison with systemic sclerosis. *Arthritis Rheum.* **26**, 617–22. [p. 181]

1528. Rumans, M. C. and Lieberman, D. A. (1987). Eosinophilic gastroenteritis presenting with biliary and duodenal obstruction. *Am. J. Gastroenterol.* **82**, 775–8. [p. 184]

1529. Rupp, G. H. and Friedman, R. A. (1982). Eosinophilic nonallergic rhinitis in children. *Pediatrics* **70**, 437–9. [p. 214]

1530. Ruscetti, F. W., Cypess, R. H., and Chervenick, P. A. (1976). Specific release of neutrophilic- and eosinophilic-stimulating factors from sensitized lymphocytes. *Blood* **47**, 757–65. [p. 16, 18, 19]

1531. Russell, C. O., Dowling, J. P., and Marshall, R. D. (1979). Acute eosinophilic cholecystitis in association with hepatic echinococcosis. *Gastroenterology* **77**, 758–60. [p. 191]

1532. Russell-Jones, R., Tai, P.-C., Spry, C. J., Eady, R. A., Black, A. K., and Greaves, M. W. (1985). Criteria for the diagnosis of vasculitis and identification of activated eosinophils. In *The urticarias* (eds. R. H. Champion, M. W. Greaves, A. Kobza Black, and R. J. Pye) pp. 149–55. Churchill Livingstone, Edinburgh. [p. 299]

1533. Russo, P. A., Wright, J. E., Ho, S. Y., Maneksa, J. R., and Clitsakis, D. (1985). Endocardectomy for the surgical treatment of endocardial fibrosis of the left ventricle. *Thorax* **40**, 621–5. [p. 242]

1534. Rutgeerts, P., Geboes, K., Vantrappen, G., Kerremans, R., Coenegrachts, J. L., and Coremans, G. (1984). Natural history of recurrent Crohn's disease at the ileocolonic anastomosis after curative surgery. *Gut* **25**, 665–72. [p. 189]

1535. Ryczak, M., Sorber, W. A., Kandora, T. F., Camp, C. J., and Rose, F. B. (1987). Difficulties in diagnosing trichinella encephalitis. *Am. J. Trop. Med. Hyg.* **36**, 573–5. [p. 145]

1536. Sabesin, S. M. (1963). A function of the eosinophil: phagocytosis of antigen-antibody complexes. *Proc. Soc. Exp. Biol. Med.* **112**, 667–71. [p. 6]

1537. Saito, H., Bourinbaiar, A., Ginsburg, M., Minato, K., Ceresi, E., Yamada, K., Machover, D., Breard, J., and Mathe, G. (1985). Establishment and characterization of a new human eosinophilic leukemia cell line. *Blood* **66**, 1233–40. [p. 25, 27]

1538. Saito, H., Hayakawa, T., Yui, Y., and Shida, T. (1987). Effect of human interferon on different functions of human neutrophils and eosinophils. *Int. Arch. Allergy Appl. Immunol.* **82**, 133–40. [p. 109]

1539. Saito, H., Yamada, K., Breard, J., Yoshie, O., and Mathe, G. (1986). A monoclonal antibody reactive with human eosinophils. *Blood* **67**, 50–5. [p. 33, 85]

1540. Sakaguchi, Y. (1984). The response of human eosinophils to calcium ionophore A23187 calcimycan. *J. Nippon. Med. Sch.* **51**. 581–9. [p. 93]

1541. Sakai, N., Johnstone, C., and Weiss, L. (1981). Bone marrow cells associated with heightened eosinophilopoiesis: an electron microscope study of murine bone marrow stimulated by Ascaris suum. *Am. J. Anat.* **161**, 11–32. [p. 10, 12]

1542. Sala, A. M. and Stein, R. J. (1937). A case of carcinoma of the cervix with a blood picture simulating chronic aleukemic eosinophilic leukemia. *Am. J. Cancer* **29**, 125–7. [p. 174]

1543. Salahuddin, S. Z., Markham, P. D., Lindner, S. G., Gootenberg, J., Popovic, M., Hemmi, H., Sarin, P. S., and Gallo, R. C. (1984). Lymphokine production by cultured human T-cells transformed by human T-cell leukemia-lymphoma virus-I. *Science* **223**, 703–7. [p. 22, 135]

1544. Salmon, P. R. and Paulley, J. W. (1967). Eosinophilic granuloma of the gastro-intestinal tract. *Gut* **8**, 8–14. [p. 184, 186]

1545. Samoszuk, M., Sholly, S., and Epstein, A. L. (1987). Eosinophil peroxidase is detectable with a monoclonal antibody in collagen bands of nodular sclerosis Hodgkin's disease. *Lab. Invest.* **56**, 394–400. [p. 59, 163]

1546. Samoszuk, M. K. and Espinoza, F. P. (1987). Deposition of autofluorescent eosinophil granules in pathologic bone marrow biopsies. *Blood* **70**, 597–9. [p. 37]

1547. Samoszuk, M. K., Nathwani, B. N., and Lukes, R. J. (1986). Extensive deposition of eosinophil peroxidase in Hodgkin's and non-Hodgkin's lymphomas. *Am. J. Pathol.* **125**, 426–9. [p. 163]

1548. Sams, W. M. Jr. and Gammon, W. R. (1982). Mechanism of lesion production in pemphigus and pemphigoid. *J. Am. Acad. Dermatol.* **6**, 431–52. [p. 303]

1549. Samter, M., Kofoed, M. A., and Pieper, W. (1953). A factor in the lungs of anaphylactically shocked guinea pigs which can induce eosinophilia in normal animals. *Blood* **8**, 1078–90. [p. 17]

1550. Sanchez, J. L. and Padilla, M. A. (1982). Hypereosinophilic syndrome. *Cutis.* **29**, 490–2, 494. [p. 273]

1551. Sanchez Palacios, A., Quintero de Juana, A., Martinez Sagarra, J., and Aparicio Duque, R. (1984). Eosinophilic food-induced cystitis. *Allergol. Immunopathol. (Madr.)* **12**, 463–9. [p. 224]

1552. Sanderson, C. J., O'Garra, A., Warren, D. J., and Klaus, G. G. (1986). Eosinophil differentiation factor also has B-cell growth factor activity: proposed name interleukin 4. *Proc. Natl. Acad. Sci. USA* **83**, 437–40. [p. 19]

1553. Sanderson, C. J., Strath, M., Warren, D. J., O'Garra, A., and Kirkwood, T. B. (1985). The production of lymphokines by primary alloreactive T-cell clones: a co-ordinate analysis of 233 clones in seven lymphokine assays. *Immunology* **56**, 575–84. [p. 19]

1554. Sanderson, C. J. and Thomas, J. A. (1978). A comparison of the cytotoxic activity of eosinophils and other cells by 51 chromium release and time lapse microcinematography. *Immunology* **34**, 771–80. [p. 112]

1555. Sanderson, C. J., Warren, D. J., and Strath, M. (1985). Identification of a lymphokine that stimulates eosinophil differentiation in vitro: its relationship to interleukin 3, and functional properties of eosinophils produced in cultures. *J. Exp. Med.* **162**, 60–74. [p. 19]

1556. Santoro, A., Zucchelli, P., Trombetti, E., Degli Esposti, E., Sturani, A., Zuccala, A., Chiarini, C., Casadei Maldini, M., and Mazzuca, A. (1985). Effect of eosinophilia on the heterogeneity of the anticoagulant response to heparin in haemodialysis patients. *Proc. Eur. Dial. Transplant Assoc. Eur. Ren. Assoc.* **21**, 143–9. [p. 223]
1557. Saran, R. and Sanyal, R. K. (1973). Diurnal varations in eosinophil count and vacuolisation of eosinophil cells in tropical eosinophilia. *Indian J. Chest Dis. Allied Sci.* **15**, 209–13. [p. 142]
1558. Sarin, S. K., Malhotra, V., Sen Gupta, S., Karol, A., Gaur, S. K., and Anand, B. S. (1987). Significance of eosinophil and mast cell counts in rectal mucosa in ulcerative colitis: a prospective controlled study. *Dig. Dis. Sci.* **32**, 363–7. [p. 190]
1559. Sasidharan, K., Kartha, C. C., Balakrishnan, K. G., and Valiathan, M. S. (1983). Early angiographic features of right ventricular endomyocardial fibrosis. *Cardiology* **70**, 127–31. [p. 252]
1560. Sato, M., Yoshida, H., Yanagawa, T., Yura, Y., Sugi, M., Hamada, S., and Miyazaki, T. (1981). Carcinoma of the maxillary sinus with eosinophilia: report of a case. *Int. J. Oral Surg.* **10**, 62–7. [p. 173]
1561. Sato, N., Asano, S., Ueyama, Y., Mori, M., Okabe, T., Kondo, Y., Ohsawa, N., and Kosaka, K. (1979). Granulocytosis and colony-stimulating activity (CSA) produced by a human squamous cell carcinoma. *Cancer* **43**, 605–10. [p. 101]
1562. Scadding, J. G. (1971). Eosinophilic infiltrations of the lungs in asthmatics. *Proc. R. Soc. Med.* **64**, 381–92. [p. 207]
1563. Schaad, U. B. and Rossi, E. (1982). Infantile chlamydial pneumonia – a review based on 115 cases. *Eur. J. Pediatr.* **138**, 105–9. [p. 132]
1564. Schaefer, H. E. and Fischer, R. (1968). Eine spezifische Farbung eosinophiler Granulozyten mit Biebricher Scharlach. *Klin. Wochenschr.* **46**, 396–7. [p. 38]
1565. Schaefer, H. E., Hellriegel, K. P., Hennekeuser, H. H., Hubner, G., Zach, J., Fischer, R., and Gross, R. (1973). Eosinophilenleukamie, eine unreifzellige Myelose mit chloroacetatesterase-positiver Eosinophilie. *Blut* **26**, 7–19. [p. 155]
1566. Schaefer, H. E., Hubner, G., and Fischer, R. (1973). Spezifische Mikrogranula in Eosinophilen. *Acta Haematol. (Basel)* **50**, 92–104. [p. 44]
1567. Schatz, M., Wasserman, S., and Patterson, R. (1981). Eosinophils and immunologic lung disease. *Med. Clin. North Am.* **65**, 1055–71. [p. 194, 324]
1568. Schatz, M., Wasserman, S., and Patterson, R. (1982). The eosinophil and the lung. *Arch. Intern. Med.* **142**, 1515–19. [p. 197]
1569. Schiffmann, E. and Gallin, J. I. (1979). Biochemistry of phagocyte chemotaxis. *Curr. Top. Cell. Regul.* **15**, 203–61. [p. 323]
1570. Schmelas, A., Drobnitsch, I., and Schneider, I. (1986). Hypereosinophilic dermatitis with response to ketotifen and sulfone. *Dermatol. Monatsschr.*, **172**, 397–402. [p. 298]
1571. Schmitz, N., Godde Salz, E., Gassmann, W., and Löffler, H. (1984). Acute myelomonocytic leukemia with involvement of eosinophils and inversion of chromosome 16. *Blut* **48**, 263–7. [p. 270]

1572. Schmitz, N., Maubach, P. A., Godde Salz, E., Gassmann, W., and Loffler, H. (1985). Acute eosinophilic leukemia: characterization by cytochemistry, chromosomal analysis, and in vitro colony formation. *Klin. Wochenschr.* **63**, 133–7. [p. 158]

1573. Schneider, H. A., Yonker, R. A., Katz, P., Longley, S., and Panush, R. S. (1985). Rheumatoid vasculitis: experience with 13 patients and review of the literature. *Semin. Arthritis Rheum.* **14**, 280–6. [p. 177]

1574. Schooley, R. T., Flaum, M. A., Gralnick, H. R., and Fauci, A. S. (1981). A clinicopathologic correlation of the idiopathic hypereosinophilic syndrome. II. Clinical manifestations. *Blood* **58**, 1021–6. [p. 290]

1575. Schooley, R. T., Parrillo, J. E., Wolff, S. M., and Fauci, A. S. (1980). Management of the idiopathic hypereosinophilic syndrome. In *The eosinophil in health and disease* (eds. A. A. Mahmoud, K. F. Austen, and A. S. Simon), pp 323–39. Grune and Stratton, New York. [p. 290]

1576. Schrader, J. W. (1983). Bone marrow differentiation in vitro. *CRC Crit. Rev. Immunol.* **4**, 197–277. [p. 325]

1577. Schuler, G., Stingl, G., Aberer, W., Stingl Gazze, L. A., Honigsmann, H., and Wolff, K. (1983). Histiocytosis X cells in eosinophilic granuloma express Ia and T6 antigens. *J. Invest. Dermatol.* **80**, 405–9. [p. 164]

1578. Schwartz, L. B. (1984). Hypereosinophilic syndrome: a review. *Va. Med.* III, 350–5. [p. 325]

1579. Schwartz, N. D., So, Y. T., Hollander, H., Allen, S., and Fye, K. H. (1986). Eosinophilic vasculitis leading to amaurosis fugax in a patient with acquired immunodeficiency syndrome. *Arch. Intern. Med.* **146**, 2059–60. [p. 135]

1580. Schwarz, E. (1914). Die Lehre von der allgemeinen und ortlichen 'Eosinophilie'. *Ergeb. Allge. Pathol. Pathol. Anat.* **17**, 137–789. [p. 8, 323]

1581. Scott, D. G., Bacon, P. A., Elliott, P. J., Tribe, C. R., and Wallington, T. B. (1982). Systemic vasculitis in a district general hospital 1972–1980: clinical and laboratory features, classification and prognosis of 80 cases. *Q. J. Med.* **51**, 292–311. [p. 231]

1582. Scott, D. W. (1987). Sterile eosinophilic pustulosis in dog and man: comparative aspects. *J. Am. Acad. Dermatol.* **16**, 1022–6. [p. 304]

1583. Scott, M. E. and Bruce, J. H. (1975). Löffler's endocardites. *Br. Heart J.* **37**, 534–8. [p. 239]

1584. Scott, R. E. and Horn, R. G. (1970). Fine structural features of eosinophil granulocyte development in human bone marrow: evidence for granule secretion. *J. Ultrastruct. Res.* **23**, 16–28. [p. 12, 13]

1585. Scudamore, H. H., Phillips, S. F., Swedlund, H. A., and Gleich, G. J. (1982). Food allergy manifested by eosinophilia, elevated immunoglobulin E level, and protein-losing enteropathy: the syndrome of allergic gastroenteropathy. *J. Allergy Clin. Immunol.* **70**, 129–38. [p. 184]

1586. Segal, A. W., Garcia, R., Goldstone, H., Cross, A. R., and Jones, O. T. (1981). Cytochrome b-245 of neutrophils is also present in human monocytes, macrophages and eosinophils. *Biochem. J.* **196**, 363–7. [p. 69]

1587. Seitz, H. M., Cottrell, B. J., and Sturrock, R. F. (1987). A histological study of skin reactions of baboons to Schistosoma mansoni schistosomula. *Trans. R. Soc. Trop. Med. Hyg.* **81**, 385–90. [p. 147]

1588. Sekiguchi, M., Yu, Z. X., Take, M., Hiroe, M., Hirosawa, K., Shirai, T.,

Ishide, T., and Takahashi, T. (1984). Ultrastructural features of the endomyocardium in patients with eosinophilic heart disease: an endomyocardial biopsy study. *Jpn. Circ. J.* **48**, 1375–82. [p. 242]

1589. Selsted, M. E., Harwig, S. S., Ganz, T., Schilling, J. W., and Lehrer, R. I. (1985). Primary structures of three human neutrophil defensins. *J. Clin. Invest.* **76**, 1436–9. [p. 119]

1590. Serhan, C. N., Hirsh, U., Palmblad, J., and Samuelsson, B. (1987). Formation of lipoxin A by granulocytes from eosinophilic donors. *FEBS Lett.* **217**, 242–6. [p. 70]

1591. Serke, S., Brenner, M., Zimmermann, R., and Lobeck, H. (1986). Malignant fibrous histiocytoma associated with peripheral blood eosinophilia. *In vitro* studies demonstrating tumor-derived eosinophilopoietic activity. *Oncology* **43**, 230–3. [p. 22, 23]

1592. Serratrice, G., Pellissier, J. F., Cros, D., Gastaut, J. L., and Brindisi, G. (1980). Relapsing eosinophilic perimyositis. *J. Rheumatol.* **7**, 199–205. [p. 179]

1593. Sewell, W. A. and Vadas, M. A. (1983). Evidence for the control of eosinophilia by the major histocompatibility complex in mice. *Immunogenetics* **17**, 167–77. [p. 26]

1594. Shafer, W. M., Martin, L. E., and Spitznagel, J. K. (1984). Cationic antimicrobial proteins isolated from human neutrophil granulocytes in the presence of diisopropyl fluorophosphate. *Infect. Immun.* **45**, 29–35. [p. 119]

1595. Shakir, A. A., Youngberg, G., and Alvarez, S. (1986). Strongyloides infestation as a cause of acute appendicitis. *J. Tenn. Med. Assoc.* **79**, 543–4. [p. 146]

1596. Shalev, O., Rubinger, D., Barlatzky, Y., Kopolovic, J., and Drukker, A. (1982). Eosinophilia associated with acute allograft kidney rejection. *Nephron* **31**, 182–3. [p. 225]

1597. Shaper, A. G. (1972). Cardiovascular disease in the tropics. II. Endomyocardial fibrosis. *Br. Med. J.* **3**, 743–6. [p. 250, 255]

1598. Shaper, A. G., Hutt, M. S., and Coles, R. M. (1968). Necropsy studies of endomyocardial fibrosis and rheumatic heart disease in Uganda 1950–1965. *Br. Heart. J.* **30**, 391–401. [p. 252]

1599. Shaper, A. G., Kaplin, M. H., Mody, N. J., and McIntyre, P. A. (1968). Malarial antibodies and autoantibodies to heart and other tissues in the immigrant and indigenous peoples of Uganda. *Lancet* **i**, 1342–4. [p. 255]

1600. Shapiro, L. G. (1919). Eosinophilic (polymorphonuclear) leukemia: report of a case with autopsy (abstracted). *Proc. New York Path. Soc.* **19**, 73–83. [p. 279]

1601. Sharma, O. P. (1973). Drug-induced pulmonary disease. *Ann. Intern. Med.* **78**, 616–19. [p. 309]

1602. Sharma, S. C. (1983). The hypereosinophilic syndrome. *Indian Pediatr.* **20**, 137–9. [p. 269, 270]

1603. Shaw, R. J., Cromwell, O., and Kay, A. B. (1984). Preferential generation of leukotriene C4 by human eosinophils. *Clin. Exp. Immunol.* **56**, 716–22. [p. 198]

1604. Shaw, R. J., Walsh, G. M., Cromwell, O., Moqbel, R., Spry, C. J., and Kay, A. B. (1985). Activated human eosinophils generate SRS-A leukotrienes following IgG-dependent stimulation. *Nature* **316**, 150–2. [p. 34, 71]

1605. Sheffer, A. L., Rocklin, R. E., and Goetzl, E. J. (1975). Immunologic components of hypersensitivity reactions to cromolyn sodium. *N. Engl. J. Med.* **293**, 1220–4. [p. 313]

1606. Sheikhzadeh, A. H., Tarbiat, S., Nazarian, I., Aryanpur, I., and Senning, A. (1979). Constrictive endocarditis: report of a case with successful surgery. *Br. Heart J.* **42**, 224–8. [p. 255]

1607. Sheperd, A. J., Walsh, C. H., Archer, R. K., and Wetherley Mein, G. (1971). Eosinophilia, splenomegaly and cardiac disease. *Br. J. Haematol.* **20**, 233–9. [p. 263]

1608. Shepherd, N. A., Blackshaw, A. J., Hall, P. A., Bostad, L., Coates, P. J., Lowe, D. G., Levison, D. A., Morson, B. C., and Stansfeld, A. G. (1987). Malignant lymphoma with eosinophilia of the gastrointestinal tract. *Histopathology* **11**, 115–30. [p. 163]

1609. Sher, R. and Glover, A. (1976). Isolation of human eosinophils and their lymphocyte-like rosetting properties. *Immunology* **31**, 337–41. [p. 76]

1610. Sher, R. and Wadee, A. A. (1981). Eosinophil degranulation: monitoring by interference contrast microscopy. *Inflammation* **5**, 37–53. [p. 92]

1611. Sheth, K. J., Casper, J. T., and Good, T. A. (1977). Interstitial nephritis due to phenytoin hypersensitivity. *J. Pediatr.* **91**, 438–41. [p. 309, 313]

1612. Shield, J. M., Scrimgeour, E. M., and Vaterlaws, A. L. (1980). Intestinal helminths in an adult hospital population in the Eastern Highlands of Papua New Guinea: relationship with anaemia, eosinophilia and asthma. *Papua New Guinea Med. J.* **23**, 157–64. [p. 202]

1613. Shields, C. L., Shields, J. A., and Rozanski, T. I. (1986). Conjunctival involvement in Churg-Strauss syndrome. *Am. J. Ophthalmol.* **102**, 601–5. [p. 218]

1614. Shields, J. A., Lerner, H. A., and Felberg, N. T. (1977). Aqueous cytology and enzymes in nematode endophthalmitis. *Am. J. Ophthalmol.* **84**, 319–22. [p. 140]

1615. Shimer, G. R. and Helwig, E. B. (1984). Inflammatory fibroid polyps of the intestine. *Am. J. Clin. Pathol.* **81**, 708–14. [p. 186]

1616. Shindoh, Y., Shimura, S., Tomioka, M., Aikawa, T., Sasaki, H., and Takishima, T., (1986). Cellular analysis in bronchoalveolar lavage fluids in infiltrative and fibrotic stages of idiopathic pulmonary fibrosis. *Tohoku, J. Exp. Med.* **149**, 47–60. [p. 209]

1617. Shoenfeld, Y., Tal, A., Berliner, S., and Pinkhas, J. (1986). Leukocytosis in non hematological malignancies – a possible tumor-associated marker. *J. Cancer Res. Clin. Oncol.* **111**, 54–8. [p. 170]

1618. Shub, M. D., Ulshen, M. H., Hargrove, C. B., Siegal, G. P., Groben, P. A., and Askin, F. B. (1985). Esophagitis: a frequent consequence of gastroesophageal reflux in infancy. *J. Pediatr.* **107**, 881–4. [p. 184]

1619. Shulman, L. E. (1975). Diffuse fasciitis with eosinophilia: a new syndrome? *Trans. Assoc. Am. Physicians* **88**, 70–86. [p. 181]

1620. Shult, P. A., Graziano, F. M., and Busse, W. W. (1986). Enhanced eosinophil luminol-dependent chemiluminescence in allergic rhinitis. *J. Allergy Clin. Immunol.* **77**, 702–8. [p. 68]

1621. Shult, P. A., Graziano, F. M., Wallow, I. H., and Busse, W. W. (1985). Comparison of superoxide generation and luminol-dependent chemiluminescence with eosinophils and neutrophils from normal individuals. *J. Lab. Clin. Med.* **106**, 638–45. [p. 68]

1622. Sibbett, S. S., Klebanoff, S. J., and Hurst, J. K. (1985). Resonance Raman characterization of the heme prosthetic group in eosinophil peroxidase. *FEBS Lett.* **189**, 271–5. [p. 58]

1623. Sidh, S. M., Smith, S. P., Silber, S. B., and Young, J. D. Jr. (1980). Eosinophilic cystitis: advanced disease requiring surgical intervention. *Urology* **15**, 23–6. [p. 223]

1624. Siebenschein, R. and Siebenmann, R. E. (1977). (Paraneoplastic eosinophilic leukemoid with eosinophilic parietal thromboendocarditis in malignant melanoma). *Schweiz Med. Wochenschr.* **107**, 1257–65. [p. 169, 173]

1625. Siegal, G. P., Dehner, L. P., and Rosai, J. (1985). Histiocytosis X (Langerhans' cell granulomatosis) of the thymus. A clinicopathologic study of four childhood cases. *Am. J. Surg. Pathol.* **9**, 117–24. [p. 164]

1626. Sigal, C. E., Valone, F. H., Holtzman, M. J. and Goetzl, E. J. (1987). Preferential human eosinophil chemotactic activity of the platelet-activating factor (PAF) 1–0-hexadecyl–2–acetyl-sn-glyceryl–3–phosphocoline (AGEPC). *J. Clin. Immunol.* **7**, 179–84. [p. 97, 101]

1627. Silberstein, D. S. and David, J. R. (1987). The regulation of human eosinophil function by cytokines. *Immunol. Today* **8**, 380–5. [p. 71, 105, 107, 109, 326]

1628. Silberstein, D. S., Dessein, A. J., Elsas, P. P., Fontaine, B., and David, J. R. (1987). Characterization of a factor from the U937 cell line that enhances the toxicity of human eosinophils to Schistosoma mansoni larvae. *J. Immunol.* **138**, 3042–50. [p. 107]

1629. Silberstein, D. S., Owen, W. F., Gasson, J. C., DiPersio, J. F., Golde, D. W., Bina, J. C., Soberman, R., Austen, K. F., and David, J. R. (1986). Enhancement of human eosinophil cytotoxicity and leukotriene synthesis by biosynthetic (recombinant) granulocyte-macrophage colony-stimulating factor. *J. Immunol.* **137**, 3290–4. [p. 108]

1630. Silberstein, D. S., Owen, W. F., Gasson, J. C., Golde, D. W., and David, J. R. Regulation of human eosinophil cytotoxicity by granulocyte-macrophage colony-stimulating factor (GM-CSF) and tumor necrosis factor (TNF) (abstract). Presented to the 6th International Congress of Immunology, Toronto, Canada, 1986. [p. 108]

1631. Silverman, R. A. and Rabinowitz, A. D. (1985). Eosinophils in the cellular infiltrate of granuloma annulare. *J. Cutan. Pathol.* **12**, 13–17. [p. 305]

1632. Sim, B. K., Kwa, B. H., and Mak, J. W. (1982). Immune responses in human Brugia malayi infections: serum dependent cell-mediated destruction of infective larvae in vitro. *Trans. R. Soc. Trop. Med. Hyg.* **76**, 362–70. [p. 116]

1633. Sim, B. K., Kwa, B. H., and Mak, J. W. (1987). Human in vitro immune reactions to animal filariids. *Trop. Med. Parasitol.* **38**, 11–14. [p. 141]

1634. Simon, J. W., Riddell, N. J., Wong, W. T., Au, A. C., Ko, R. C., and Templer, M. J. (1986). Further observations on the first documented outbreak of trichinosis in Hong Kong. *Trans. R. Soc. Trop. Med. Hyg.* **80**, 394–7. [p. 145]

1635. Simpson, D. G. and Walker, J. H. (1960). Hypersensitivity to para-aminosalicylic acid. *Am. J. Med.* **29**, 297–306. [p. 309]

1636. Singer, J. Z. and Wallace, S. L. (1986). The allopurinol hypersensitivity syndrome: unnecessary morbidity and mortality. *Arthritis Rheum.* **29**, 82–7. [p. 310]

1637. Singh, R. K., Chandra, R., Narang, R. K., Singh, S. K., Katiyar, S. K., Singh, R. P., Pandey, H. N., and Joshi, L. D. (1987). Circadian variations of the absolute eosinophil count and serum histaminase activity in tropical pulmonary eosinophilia. *Trop. Geogr. Med.* **39**, 49–52. [p. 141]
1638. Sivalingam, S., Corkill, G., Ellis, W. G., and Claiche, J. R. (1977). Focal eosinophilic granuloma of the temporal lobe: case report. *J. Neurosurg.* **47**, 941–5. [p. 217]
1639. Sklavounou, A. and Laskaris, G. (1984). Eosinophil ulcer of the oral mucosa. *Oral Surg. Oral Med. Oral Pathol.* **58**, 431–6. [p. 192]
1640. Skubitz, K. M., Weisdorf, D. J., and August, J. T. (1987). Identification and purification of the human myeloid differentiation antigen recognized by monoclonal antibody AHN-7. *J. Leukocyte Biol.* **41**, 104–10. [p. 87]
1641. Sladek, G. D., Vasey, F. B., Sieger, B., Behnke, D. A., Germain, B. F., and Espinoza, L. R. (1983). Relapsing eosinophilic myositis. *J. Rheumatol.* **10**, 467–70. [p. 180]
1642. Slater, E. E. (1978). Cardiac tamponade and peripheral eosinophilia in a patient receiving cromolyn sodium. *Chest* **73**, 878–9. [p. 309]
1643. Slater, J. M. and Swarm, O. J. (1980). Eosinophilic granuloma of bone. *Med. Pediatr. Oncol.* **8**, 151–64. [p. 323]
1644. Slavin, R. G. (1985). Allergic bronchopulmonary aspergillosis. *Clin. Rev. Allergy* **3**, 167–82. [p. 132]
1645. Slifman, N. R., Loegering, D. A., McKean, D. J., and Gleich, G. J. (1986). Ribonuclease activity associated with human eosinophil-derived neurotoxin and eosinophil cationic protein. *J. Immunol.* **137**, 2913–17. [p. 55]
1646. Slungaard, A., Ascensao, J., Zanjani, E., and Jacob, H. S. (1983). Pulmonary carcinoma with eosinophilia: demonstration of a tumor-derived eosinophilopoietic factor. *N. Engl. J. Med.* **309**, 778–81. [p. 22, 23]
1647. Slungaard, A., Vercellotti, G., Zanjani, E., Ascensao, J., and Jacob, H. S. (1982). Tumor-induced eosinophilia and endocardial fibrosis: evidence for ectopic eosinophilopoietin production and toxic O_2 metabolite-mediated endothelial damage. *Trans. Assoc. Am. Physicians* **95**, 8–11. [p. 247]
1648. Smith, D. H., Scott, D. L., and Zaphiropoulos, G. C. (1983). Eosinophilia in D-penicillamine therapy. *Ann. Rheum. Dis.* **42**, 408–10. [p. 307]
1649. Smith, D. M., Gerrard, J. M., and White, J. G. (1987). Comparison of arachidonic acid metabolism in nasal polyps and eosinophils. *Int. Arch. Allergy Appl. Immunol.* **82**, 83–8. [p. 69, 214]
1650. Smith, J. A. (1981). Molecular and cellular properties of eosinophils. (A review). *Ric. Clin. Lab.* **11**, 181–93. [p. 324]
1651. Smith, J. W. (1978). Hypoplastic right ventricle with eosinophilic endomyocarditis and patent foramen ovale. *West J. Med.* **129**, 64–7. [p. 236]
1652. Smith, L. H. Jr. and Boushey, H. (1969). Eosinophilia and eosinophilic carditis. *California Med.* **3**, 388–95. [p. 238, 272, 276]
1653. Smith, P. D., Keister, D. B., and Elson, C. O. (1983). Human host response to Giardia lamblia. II. Antibody-dependent killing in vitro. *Cell Immunol.* **82**, 308–15. [p. 117]
1654. Smith, P. M., Morgans, M. E., Clark, C. G., Lennard Jones, J. E.,

Gunnlaughsson, O., and Jonasson, T. A. (1975). Lipodystrophy, pancreatitis, and eosinophilia. *Gut* **16**, 230–4. [p. 191]

1655. Snider, G. L. (1985). Distinguishing among asthma, chronic bronchitis, and emphysema. *Chest* **87** (1 Suppl), 35S-39S. [p. 204]

1656. Snover, D. C., Sibley, R. K., Freese, D. K., Sharp, H. L., Bloomer, J. R., Najarian, J. S., and Ascher, N. L. (1984). Orthotopic liver transplantation: a pathological study of 63 serial liver biopsies from 17 patients with special reference to the diagnostic features and natural history of rejection. *Hepatology* **4**, 1212–22. [p. 190]

1657. Soeprono, F. F. and Schinella, R. A. (1986). Eosinophilic pustular folliculitis in patients with acquired immunodeficiency syndrome: report of three cases. *J. Am. Acad. Dermatol.* **14**, 1020–2. [p. 304]

1658. Soffer, T., Chan, W. C., Brynes, R. K., Vogler, W. R., and O'Neal, S. (1984). Myeloproliferative disorder with profound hypereosinophilia associated with chemotherapy for breast cancer. *Cancer* **54**, 2356–9. [p. 154]

1659. Sokol, R. J., Hudson, G., Brown, M. J., Wales, J., and James, N. T. (1988). Hypereosinophilic syndrome: case report and morphometric study. *Acta haematol. (Basel)* **79**, 107–11. [p. 40, 280]

1660. Sokol, R. J., James, N. T., Wales, J., and Hudson, G. (1987). Morphometry of eosinophils in human blood. *Acta Anat. (Basel)* **129**, 211–13. [p. 40]

1661. Solley, G. O., Maldonado, J. E., Gleich, G. J., Giuliani, E. R., Hoagland, H. C., Pierre, R. V., and Brown, A. L. Jr. (1976). Endomyocardiopathy with eosinophilia. *Mayo Clin. Proc.* **51**, 697–708. [p. 277, 281]

1662. Somers, K., Hut, M. S., Patel, A. K., and D'Arbela, P. G. (1971). Endomyocardial biopsy in diagnosis of cardiomyopathies. *Br. Heart J.* **33**, 822–32. [p. 252]

1663. Sonakul, D. (1978). Pathological findings in four cases of human angiostrongyliasis. *Southeast Asian J. Trop. Med. Public Health* **9**, 220–7. [p. 139]

1664. Songsiridej, V., Peters, M. S., Dor, P. J., Ackerman, S. J., Gleich, G. J., and Busse, W. W. (1985). Facial edema and eosinophilia: evidence for eosinophil degranulation. *Ann. Intern. Med.* **103**, 503–6. [p. 300]

1665. Sonkodi, S., Jarmay, K., Korom, I., Kemeny, E., Szabo, E., Abraham, G., Sonkodi, I., Ribari, O., and Mohacsi, G. (1987.) Membranous nephropathy accompanied by angiolymphoid hyperplasia of the skin. *Nephron* **47**, 32–5. [p. 168]

1666. Sorensen, H., Mygind, N., Tygstrup, I., and Winge Flensborg, E. (1977). Histology of nasal polyps of different etiology. *Rhinology* **15**, 121–8. [p. 214]

1667. Spada, C. S., Woodward, D. F., Hawley, S. B., and Nieves, A. L. (1986). Leukotrienes cause eosinophil emigration into conjunctival tissue. *Prostaglandins* **31**, 795–809. [p. 97]

1668. Sparrewohn, S. and Wulff, H. R. (1967). The nuclear segmentation of eosinophils under normal and pathological conditions. *Acta Haematol. (Basel)* **37**, 120–5. [p. 40]

1669. Speirs, R. S. (1958). Advances in the knowledge of the eosinophil in relation to antibody formation. *Ann. NY Acad. Sci.* **73**, 283–92. [p. 8]

1670. Spicer, B. A., Hatt, P. A., Laycock, S. M., and Smith, H. (1986). Effect of drugs on the increase in cell numbers in the peritoneal cavity of the actively sensitised mouse after intraperitoneal challenge with antigen. *Int. Arch. Allergy Appl. Immunol.* **81**, 81–4. [p. 95]

1671. Spicer, S. J. and Lillie, R. D. (1961). Histochemical idenficiation of basic proteins with Biebrich Scarlet at alkaline pH. *Stain Technol.* **36**. 365–70. [p. 38]

1672. Spiers, A. S., Bain, B. J., and Turner, J. E. (1977). The peripheral blood in chronic granulocytic leukaemia: study of 50 untreated Philadelphia-positive cases. *Scand. J. Haematol.* **18**, 25–38. [p. 159]

1673. Spinowitz, B. S., Golden, R. A. Rascoff, J. H., and Charytan, C. (1982). Eosinophilic peritonitis. *Clin. Exp. Dial. Apheresis* **6**, 187–91. [p. 220, 221]

1674. Spitzer, G. and Garson, O. M. (1973). Lymphoblastic leukemia with marked eosinophilia: a report of two cases. *Blood* **42**, 377–84. [p. 159]

1675. Spritz, R. A. (1985). The familial histiocytoses. *Pediatr. Pathol.* **3**, 43–57. [p. 166]

1676. Spry, C. J. (1971). Mechanism of eosinophilia. V. Kinetics of normal and accelerated eosinopoiesis. *Cell Tissue Kinet.* **4**, 351–64. [p. 14]

1677. Spry, C. J. (1971). Mechanism of eosinophilia. VI. Eosinophil mobilisation. *Cell Tissue Kinet.* **4**, 365–74. [p. 14]

1678. Spry, C. J. (1972). Mechanism of eosinophilia. VII. Eosinophilia in rats with lymphoma. *Br. J. Haematol.* **22**, 407–13. [p. 161]

1679. Spry, C. J. (1976). Eosinophilia in Addison's disease. *Yale J. Biol. Med.* **49**, 411–13. [p. 306]

1680. Spry, C. J. (1978). Eosinophils as effector cells in disease. *Schweiz Med. Wochenschr.* **108**, 1572–6. [p. 89, 323]

1681. Spry, C. J. (1980). Eosinophilia and allergic reactions to drugs. *Clin. Haematol.* **9**, 521–34. [p. 307, 323]

1682. Spry, C. J. (1981). Alterations in blood eosinophil morphology, binding capacity for complexed IgG and kinetics in patients with tropical (filarial) eosinophilia. *Parasite Immunol.* **3**. 1–11. [p. 142]

1683. Spry, C. J. (1982). The hypereosinophilic syndrome: clinical features, laboratory findings and treatment. *Allergy* **37**, 539–51. [p. 234, 324]

1684. Spry, C. J. (1983). Lung diseases associated with eosinophils. In *Current perspectives in allergy* (eds. E. J. Goetzl, and A. B. Kay), pp. 67–77. Churchill Livingstone, Edinburgh. [p. 194, 205]

1685. Spry, C. J. (1984). Eosinophilic gastroenteritis. In *Textbook of gastroenterology* (eds. I. A. Bouchier, R. N. Allan, H. J. Hodgson, and M. R. Keighley), pp. 596–8. Bailliere Tindall, London. [p. 184, 185]

1686. Spry, C. J. (1985). Visceral larva migrans and hypereosinophilia. *Clin. Notes On Line* **1**, 49. [p. 140]

1687. Spry, C. J. (1985). Synthesis and secretion of eosinophil granule substances. *Immunol. Today* **6**, 332–5. [p. 56, 325]

1688. Spry, C. J. (1986). Eosinophils in eosinophilic endomyocardial disease. *Postgrad Med. J.* **62**, 609–13. [p. 246]

1689. Spry, C. J. (1987). Eosinophilia and the heart. In *Immunological aspects of cardiovascular diseases. Clinical Immunology and Allergy*, 1 (ed. W. A. Littler), pp. 591–606. Bailliere Tindall, London. [p. 234]

1690. Spry, C. J. (1987) Neutrophils and myocardial injury. In *Immunology and Molecular Biology of Cardiovascular Diseases* (ed. C. J. Spry), pp. 129–42. MTP Press Ltd, Lancaster. [p. 229]

1691. Spry, C. J. (1987). Eosinophils amd endomyocardial fibrosis: a review of clinical and experimental studies 1980–86. In *Pathogenesis of myocarditis and cardiomyopathy: recent experimental and clinical studies: cardiomyopathy update.* 1. (eds. C. Kawai and W. A. Abelmann), pp. 293–310. University of Tokyo Press, Tokyo. [p. 234, 326]

1692. Spry, C. J., Davies, J., and Tai, P.-C. (1983). Eosinophils and endomyocardial fibrosis. *Contrib. Microbiol. Immunol.* **7**, 212–17. [p. 246]

1693. Spry, C. J., Davies, J., Tai, P.-C., and Fattah, D. (1983). The pathogenesis of eosinophilic endomyocardial disease. In *Immunobiology of the eosinophil* (eds. T. Yoshida and M. Torisu), pp. 229–44. Elsevier Biomedical, New York. [p. 233]

1694. Spry, C. J., Davies, J., Tai, P.-C., Olsen, E. G., Oakley, C. M., and Goodwin, J. F. (1983). Clinical feature of fifteen patients with the hypereosinophilic syndrome. *Q. J. Med.* **52**, 1–22. [p. 234, 242, 273, 288]

1695. Spry, C. J. and Kumaraswami, V. (1982). Tropical eosinophilia. *Semin. Hematol.* **19**, 107–15. [p. 141, 324]

1696. Spry, C. J. and Tai, P.-C. (1976). Studies on blood eosinophils. II. Patients with Löffler's cardiomyopathy. *Clin. Exp. Immunol.* **24**, 423–34. [p. 77, 78, 81, 104, 246]

1697. Spry, C. J., Tai, P.-C., and Barkans, J. (1985). Tissue localization of human eosinophil cationic proteins in allergic diseases. *Int. Arch. Allergy Appl. Immunol.* **77**, 252–4. [p. 50]

1698. Spry, C. J., Tai, P.-C., Davies, J., Olsen, E. G., and Goodwin, J. F. (1984). The role of eosinophils in myocarditis. In *Viral myocarditis* (ed. H. D. Bolte), pp. 83–6. Springer Verlag, Berlin. [p. 230]

1699. Spry, C. J., Tai, P.-C., and Ogilvie, B. M. (1980). Hypereosinophilia in rats with Trichinella spiralis infections. *Br. J. Exp. Pathol.* **61**, 1–7. [p. 267]

1700. Spry, C. J., Take, M., and Tai, P.-C. (1985). Eosinophilic disorders affecting the myocardium and endocardium: a review. *Heart Vessels Suppl.* **1**, 240–2. [p. 229]

1701. Spry, C. J., Weetman, A. P., Olsson, I., Tai, P.-C., and Olsen, E. G. (1985). The pathogenesis of eosinophilic endomyocardial disease in patients with carcinomas of the lung. *Heart Vessels* **1**, 162–9. [p. 246]

1702. Stanley, J. and Fallon Pellicci, V. (1978). Phenytoin hypersensitivity reaction. *Arch. Dermatol.* **114**, 1350–3. [p. 313]

1703. Stark, E. W., Garvin, D. F., Surana, R. B., Dale, N. L., Hummer, W., Clark, M., and Schumacher, H. R. (1985). Acute myelomonocytic leukemia (M-4 subtype) with abnormal marrow eosinophilia and a normal chromosome 16. *Am. J. Clin. Pathol.* **84**, 551–4. [p. 159]

1704. Stark, R. J. (1979). Eosinophilic polymyositis. *Arch. Neurol.* **36**, 721–2. [p. 179]

1705. Steffen, C. (1985). Eosinophilic pustular folliculitis (Ofuji's disease) with response to dapsone therapy. *Arch. Dermatol.* **121**, 921–3. [p. 304]

1706. Steigleder, G. K. and Inderwisch, R. (1975). Eosinophilic granulocytes in the skin lesions of psoriasis and neurodermatitis. *Arch. Dermatol. Res.* **254**, 253–6. [p. 304]

1707. Steinbach, K. H., Shick, P., Trepel, F., Raffler, H., Dohrmann, J., Heilgeist, G., Heltzel, W., Li, K., Past, W., van der Woerd de Lange, J. A., Theml, H., Fliedner, T. M., and Begemann, H. (1979). Estimation of kinetic parameters of neutrophilic, eosinophilic, and basophilic granulocytes in human blood. *Blut* **39**, 27–38. [p. 14, 28]

1708. Stephan, W. C., Parks, R. D., and Tempest, B. (1978). Acute hypersensitivity pneumonitis associated with carbamazepine therapy. *Chest* **74**, 463–4. [p. 309]

1709. Stern, J. B., Sobel, H. J., and Rotchford, J. P. (1984). Wells' syndrome: is there collagen damage in the flame figures? *J. Cutan. Pathol.* **11**, 501–5. [p. 168]

1710. Stevenson, H. C., Kimball, E., Schroff, R. W., Buescher, S., Clarke, G., Gregorio, T., Wilburn, S., and Foon, K. A. (1984). Two new monoclonal antibodies to human monocytes and granulocytes: isolation of membrane antigens and lack of effects of antibodies on leukocyte functions in vitro. *Hybridoma* **3**, 247–6. [p. 87]

1711. Stillman, R. G. (1912). A case of myeloid leukemia with predominance of eosinophile cells. *Med. Record* **81**, 594–5. [p. 263]

1712. Stockdill, G., Hartley, S. E., and Allan, N. C. (1980). Eosinophilic leukaemia in association with a double Philadelphia chromosome. *Postgrad. Med. J.* **56**, 268–70. [p. 157]

1713. Stoddart, R. W., Collins, R. D., and Jacobson, W. (1980). Lectin staining of carbohydrates of haemic cells; the cells of normal blood and bone marrow and of the myeloid leukaemias. *J. Pathol.* **131**, 321–32. [p. 72]

1714. Strath, M. and Sanderson, C. J. (1986). Detection of eosinophil differentiation factor and its relationship to eosinophilia in Mesocestoides corti-infected mice. *Exp. Hematol.* **14**, 16–20. [p. 284]

1715. Strath, M., Warren, D. J., and Sanderson, C. J. (1985). Detection of eosinophils using an eosinophil peroxidase assay: its use as an assay for eosinophil differentiation factors. *J. Immunol. Methods* **83**, 209–15. [p. 16]

1716. Strayer, D. R. and Bender, R. A. (1977). Eosinophilic meningitis complicating Hodgkin's disease: a report of a case and review of the literature. *Cancer* **40**, 406–9. [p. 216]

1717. Strydom, D. J., Fett, J. W., Lobb, R. R., Alderman, E. M., Bethune, J. L., Riordan, J. F., and Vallee, B. L. (1985). Amino acid sequence of human tumor derived angiogenin. *Biochemistry* **24**, 5486–94. [p. 51]

1718. Su, W. P. (1985). Angioimmunoblastic lymphadenopathy. *Dermatol. Clin.* **3**, 759–68. [p. 163]

1719. Sueblinvong, V. and Sanpradit, M. (1984). Endomyocardial fibrosis in Thai children. *J. Med. Assoc. Thai* **67**, 334–40. [p. 234]

1720. Sugane, K. and Matsuura, T. (1987). Eosinophilia in chimeric mice infected with Toxocara canis. *J. Helminthol.* **61**, 157–62.[p. 26]

1721. Sugane, K. and Oshima, T. (1980). Recovery of large numbers of eosinophils from mice infected with Toxocara canis. *Am. J. Trop. Med. Hyg.* **29**, 799–802. [p. 127]

1722. Sugane, K. and Oshima, T. (1985). Induction of a marked eosinophilia by cyclophosphamide in Toxocara canis infected SJL mice. *Parasite Immunol.* **7**, 255–63. [p. 24]

1723. Sugaya, H. and Yoshimura, K. (1988). T-cell-dependent eosinophilia in the cerebrospinal fluid of the mouse infected with Angiostrongylus cantonensis. Submitted. [p. 138]

1724. Sullivan, M. J., Wanger, G. P., Schonfeld, S. A., and Bashore, T. M. (1983). Cardiac rhabdomyosarcoma presenting as hypereosinophilic syndrome. *Am. J. Cardiol.* **51**, 909–10. [p. 170]

1725. Sullivan, T. J. (1979). The role of eosinophils in inflammatory reactions. *Prog. Hematol.* **11**, 65–82. [p. 323]
1726. Sun, X. H., Davis, W. B., Fukuda, Y., Ferrans, V. J. and Crystal, R. G. (1985). Experimental polymyxin B-induced interstitial lung disease characterized by an accumulation of cytotoxic eosinophils in the alveolar structures. *Am. Rev. Respir. Dis.* **131**, 103–8. [p. 209]
1727. Sutphin, M. and Middleton, A. W. Jr. (1984). Eosinophilic cystitis in children: a self-limited process. *J. Urol.* **132**, 117–19. [p. 224]
1728. Sutton, J. M. (1986). Urinary eosinophils. *Arch. Intern. Med.* **146**, 2243–4. [p. 224]
1729. Suvatte, V., Mahasandana, C., Tanphaichitr, V., and Tuchinda, S. (1979). Acquired platelet dysfunction with eosinophilia: study of platelet function in 62 cases. *Southeast Asian J. Trop. Med. Public Health* **10**, 358–67. [p. 262]
1730. Swirsky, D. M., Li, Y. S., Matthews, J. G., Flemans, R. J., Rees, J. K., and Hayhoe, F. G. (1984). 8;21 translocation in acute granulocytic leukaemia: cytological, cytochemical and clinical features. *Br. J. Haematol.* **56**, 199–213. [p. 159]
1731. Sylvester, R. A. and Pinals, R. S. (1970). Eosinophilia in rheumatoid arthritis. *Ann. Allergy* **28**, 565–8. [p. 177]
1732. Symmans, W. A., Beresford, C. H., Bruton, D., Despommier, D. D., Dickson, D., Linehan, B. J., Reeder, W. J., and Shepherd, C. S. (1986). Cyclic eosinophilic myositis and hyperimmunoglobulin-E. *Ann. Intern. Med.* **104**, 26–32. [p. 180]
1733. Tai, P.-C., Ackerman, S. J., Spry, C. J., Dunnette, S., Olsen, E. G., and Gleich, G. J. (1987). Deposits of eosinophil granule proteins in cardiac tissues of patients with eosinophilic endomyocardial disease. *Lancet* **1**, 643–7. [p. 248]
1734. Tai, P.-C., Bakes, D. M., Barkans, J. R., and Spry, C. J. (1985). Plasma membrane antigens on light density and activated human blood eosinophils. *Clin. Exp. Immunol.* **60**, 427–36. [p. 87, 281]
1735. Tai, P.-C., Capron, M., Bakes, D. M., Barkans, J., and Spry, C. J. (1986). Monoclonal antibodies to human eosinophil plasma membrane antigens enhance the secretion of eosinophil cationic protein. *Clin. Exp. Immunol.* **63**, 728–37. [p. 91]
1736. Tai, P.-C., Hayes, D. J., Clark, J. B., and Spry, C. J. (1982). Toxic effects of human eosinophil products on isolated rat heart cells in vitro. *Biochem. J.* **204**, 75–80. [p. 118, 248]
1737. Tai, P.-C., Holt, M. E., Denny, P., Gibbs, A. R., Williams, B. D., and Spry, C. J. (1984). Deposition of eosinophil cationic protein in granulomas in allergic granulomatosis and vasculitis: the Churg-Strauss syndrome. *Br. Med. J. (Clin Res)* **289**, 400–2. [p. 203]
1738. Tai, P.-C. and Spry, C. J. (1976). Studies on blood eosinophils. I. Patients with a transient eosinophilia. *Clin. Exp. Immunol.* **24**, 415–22. [p. 77, 81, 281]
1739. Tai, P.-C. and Spry, C. J. (1977). Purification of normal human eosinophils using the different binding capacities of blood leucocytes for complexed rabbit IgG. *Clin. Exp. Immunol.* **28**, 256–60. [p. 32]
1740. Tai, P.-C. and Spry, C. J. (1980). Enzymes altering the binding capacity of

human blood eosinophils for IgG antibody-coated erythrocytes (EA). *Clin. Exp. Immunol.* **40**, 206–19. [p. 78, 80, 81, 83, 87]

1741. Tai, P.-C. and Spry, C. J. (1981). The mechanisms which produce vacuolated and degranulated eosinophils. *Br. J. Haematol.* **49**, 219–26. [p. 66]

1742. Tai, P.-C., Spry, C. J., Peterson, C., Venge, P., and Olsson, I. (1984). Monoclonal antibodies distinguish between storage and secreted forms of eosinophil cationic protein. *Nature* **309**, 182–4. [p. 50, 56, 247, 283, 299]

1743. Take, M., Sekiguchi, M., Hiroe, M., Hirosawa, K., Mizoguchi, H., Kijima, M., Shirai, T., Ishide, T., and Okubo, S. (1985). Clinical spectrum and endomyocardial biopsy findings in eosinophilic heart disease. *Heart Vessels Suppl.* **1**, 243–9. [p. 234, 235]

1744. Takematsu, H., Nakamura, K., Igarashi, M., and Tagami, H. (1985). Eosinophilic pustular folliculitis: report of two cases with a review of the Japanese literature. *Arch. Dermatol.* **121**, 917–20. [p. 304]

1745. Takematsu, H., Terui, T., Torinuki, W., and Tagami, H. (1986). Incontinentia pigmenti: eosinophil chemotactic activity of the crusted scales in the vesiculobullous stage. *Br. J. Dermatol.* **115**, 61–6. [p. 304]

1746. Takenaka, T. and Nakamine, H. Regulation of eosinophilia and IgE production by suppressor T cells (abstract). Presented to the 6th International Congress of Immunology, Toronto, Canada, 1986. [p. 24]

1747. Takenaka, T., Okuda, M., Kawabori, S., and Kubo, K. (1977). Extracellular release of peroxidase from eosinophils by interaction with immune complexes. *Clin. Exp. Immunol.* **28**, 56–60. [p. 81]

1748. Takubo, T., Kikuchi, T., Harunari, H., Takeuchi, A., and Inai, S. (1987). A case of lowered eosinophilic leucocyte peroxidase activity found unexpectedly using an automated haematology analyser (the Technicon H6000 system). *Clin. Lab. Haematol.* **9**, 289–96. [p. 31]

1749. Tallgren, L. G., Wegelius, R., Andersson, L. C., and Jansson, E. (1974). Eosinophilic leukaemia: recovery of mycoplasma orale from the bone marrow. *Acta Med. Scand.* **195**, 87–92. [p. 153]

1750. Tallman, M. S., McGuffin, R. W., Higano, C. S., Starkebaum, G., Collins, S. J., Johnston, H., Singer, J. W., Perry, D. J., and Kunath, A. (1987). Bone marrow transplantation in a patient with myelodysplasia associated with diffuse eosinophilic fasciitis. *Am. J. Hematol.* **24**, 93–9. [p. 182]

1751. Tamura, N., Agrawal, D. K., Suliaman, F. A., and Townley, R. G. (1987). Effects of platelet activating factor on the chemotaxis of normodense eosinophils from normal subjects. *Biochem. Biophys. Res. Commun.* **142**, 638–44. [p. 101]

1752. Taniguchi, N., Mita, H., Saito, H., Yui, Y., Kajita, T., and Shida, T. (1985). Increased generation of leukotriene C4 from eosinophils in asthmatic patients. *Allergy* **40**, 571–3. [p. 198]

1753. Tanino, M., Kitamura, K., Ohta, G., Yamamoto, Y., and Sugioka, G. (1983). Hypereosinophilic syndrome with extensive myocardial involvement and mitral valve thrombus instead of mural thrombi. *Acta Pathol. Jpn.* **33**, 1233–42. [p. 242]

1754. Tanno, Y., Bienenstock, J., Richardson, M., Lee, T. D., Befus, A. D., and Denburg, J. A. (1987). Reciprocal regulation of human basophil and eosinophil differentiation by separate T-cell-derived factors. *Exp. Hematol.* **15**, 24–33. [p. 23]

1755. Tanno, Y., Stadler, B., and Denburg, J. A. (1987). Human interleukin-3-like activity, basophil and eosinophil growth promoting activities and colony stimulating factor derived from several cell lines. *Int. Arch. Allergy Appl. Immunol.* **83**, 1–5. [p. 23]

1756. Tantravahi, R., Schwenn, M., Henkle, C., Nell, M., Leavitt, P. R., Griffin, J. D., and Weinstein, H. J. (1984). A pericentric inversion of chromosome 16 is associated with dysplastic marrow eosinophils in acute myelomonocytic leukemia. *Blood* **63**, 800–2. [p. 158]

1757. Tauber, A. I., Goetzl, E. J., and Babior, B. M. (1979). Unique characteristics of superoxide production by human eosinophils in eosinophilic states. *Inflammation* **3**, 261–72. [p. 69]

1758. Tauro, G. P. (1966). Hodgkin's disease associated with raised eosinophil counts. *Med. J. Aust.* **2**, 604–6. [p. 162]

1759. Tavassoli, M. (1981). Eosinophil, eosinophilia, and eosinophilic disorders. *CRC Crit. Rev. Clin. Lab. Sci.* **16**, 35–83. [p. 324]

1760. Taylor, K. J. and Luksza, A. R. (1987). Peripheral blood eosinophil counts and bronchial responsiveness. *Thorax* **42**, 452–6. [p. 197]

1761. Tchernitchin, A. N. (1973). Fine structure of rat uterine eosinophils and the possible role of eosinophils in the mechanism of estrogen action. *J. Steroid. Biochem.* **4**, 277–82. [p. 9, 44]

1762. Tchernitchin, A. N., Barrera, J., Arroyo, P., Mena, M. A., Vilches, K., and Grunert, G. (1985). Degranulatory action of estradiol on blood eosinophil leukocytes in vivo and in vitro. *Agents Actions* **17**, 60–6. [p. 82]

1763. Tchernitchin, A. N., Mena, M. A., Rodriguez, A., and Maturana, M. (1985). Radioautographic localization of estrogen receptors in the rat uterus: a tool for the study of classical and nontraditional mechanisms of hormone action. In *Localization of putative steroid receptors*. (eds. L. P. Pertschuk and S. H. Lee), pp. 5–37. CRC Press, Florida. [p. 82]

1764. Tebbi, C. K., Mahmoud, A. A., Polmar, S., and Gross, S. (1980). The role of eosinophils in granulopoiesis. I. Eosinophilia in neutropenic patients. *J. Pediatr.* **96**, 575–81. [p. 14]

1765. Telerman, A., Amson, R. B., Delforge, A., Collard, E., and Stryckmans, P. A. (1982). A case of chronic aneosinocytosis. *Am. J. Hematol.* **12**, 187–97. [p. 316]

1766. Temmink, J. H. and Bayne, C. J. (1987). Ultrastructural characterization of leucocytes in the pronephros of carp (Cyprinus carpio, L.). *Dev. Comp. Immunol.* **11**. 125–37. [p. 125]

1767. Teo, C. G. and Ting, W. C. (1984). Thrombocytopathic purpura associated with eosinophilia. *Trans. R. Soc. Trop. Med. Hyg.* **78**, 335–8. [p. 262]

1768. Testa, J. R., Hogge, D. E., Misawa, S., and Zandparsa, N. (1984). Chromosome 16 rearrangements in acute myelomonocytic leukemia with abnormal eosinophils (letter). *N. Engl. J. Med.* **310**, 468–9. [p. 156]

1769. Thomas, J. R. (1963). Eosinophilic leukemia presenting with erythrocytosis. *Blood* **22**, 639–45. [p. 152]

1770. Thomas, K. A. (1987). Fibroblast growth factors. *Faseb. J.* **1**, 434–40. [p. 62]

1771. Thomas, R. J., Bascom, R., Yang, W. N., Fisher, J. F., Baser, M. E., Greenhut, J., and Baker, J. H. (1986). Peripheral eosinophilia and respiratory symptoms in rubber injection press operators: a case-control study. *Am. J. Ind. Med.* **9**, 551–9. [p. 204]

1772. Thompson, A. B., Barron, M. M., and Lapp, N. L. (1985). The hypereosinophilic syndrome presenting with eosinophilic mastitis. *Arch. Intern. Med.* **145**, 564–5. [p. 277]

1773. Thomsen, S. and Plum, P. (1939). Eosinophilic leukemia. *Acta. Med. Scand.* **101**, 116–37. [p. 153]

1774. Thomson, A. W., Mathie, I. H., and Sewell, H. F. (1987). Cyclophosphamide-induced eosinophilia in the rat: concomitant changes in T-cell subsets, B cells and large granular lymphocytes within lymphoid tissues. *Immunology* **60**, 383–8. [p. 24]

1775. Thorne, K. J. and Franks, D. (1984). Surface proteins of the human eosinophil. I. Isolation of eosinophil IgG binding proteins. *Clin. Exp. Immunol.* **56**, 464–72. [p. 77]

1776. Thorne, K. J., Free, J., Franks, D., and Oliver, R. C. (1982). The mechanism of Fc-mediated interaction of eosinophils with immobilized immune complexes. II. Identification of two membrane proteins, modified by the interaction. *J. Cell. Sci.* **56**, 357–69. [p. 78]

1777. Thorne, K. J., Glauert, A. M., Svvennsen, R. J., and Franks, D. (1979). Phagocytosis and killing of Trypanosoma dionisii by human neutrophils, eosinophils and monocytes. *Parasitology* **79**, 367–79. [p. 116]

1778. Thorne, K. J., Richardson, B. A., and Butterworth, A. E. Eosinophil activating factor (EAF) from human blood monocytes (abstract). Presented to the 6th International Congress of Immunology, Toronto, Canada, 1986. [p. 110]

1779. Thorne, K. J., Richardson, B. A., Taverne, J., Williamson, D. J., Vadas, M. A., and Butterworth, A. E. (1986). A comparison of eosinophil-activating factor (EAF) with other monokines and lymphokines. *Eur. J. Immunol.* **16**, 1143–9. [p. 106, 107, 108, 109, 120, 121]

1780. Thorne, K. J., Richardson, B. A., Veith, M. C., Tai, P.-C., Spry, C. J., and Butterworth, A. E. (1985). Partial purification and biological properties of an eosinophil-activating factor. *Eur. J. Immunol.* **15**, 1083–91. [p. 108]

1781. Thornfeldt, C. R. and Menkes, A. W. (1987). Bullous pemphigoid controlled by tetracycline. *J. Am. Acad. Dermatol.* **16**, 305–10. [p. 303]

1782. Tiedemann, K. and van Ooyen, B. (1978). Prenatal hematopoiesis and blood characteristics of the cat. *Anat. Embryol. (Berl.)* **153**, 243–67. [p. 11]

1783. Tiltman, A. J. (1978). Eosinophilic infiltrates in carcinoma of the urinary bladder unassociated with schistosomiasis. *J. Pathol.* **126**, 79–83. [p. 175]

1784. Ting, S., Zweiman, B., Lavker, R. M., and Dunsky, E. H. (1981). In vivo release of eosinophil chemoattractant activity in human allergic skin reactions. *J. Immunol.* **127**, 557–60. [p. 98]

1785. Tobin, M. C., Karns, B. K., Anselmino, L. M., and Thomas, L. L. (1986). Potentiation of human basophil histamine release by protamine: a new role for a polycation recognition site. *Mol. Immunol.* **23**, 245–53. [p. 48]

1786. Tomonaga, M., Gasson, J. C., Quan, S. G., and Golde, D. W. (1986). Establishment of eosinophilic sublines from human promyelocytic leukemia (HL-60) cells: demonstration of multipotentiality and single-lineage commitment of HL-60 stem cells. *Blood* **67**, 1433–41. [p. 27]

1787. Tomonaga, M., Golde, D. W., and Gasson, J. C. (1986). Biosynthetic (recombinant) human granulocyte-macrophage colony-stimulating factor: effect on normal bone marrow and leukemia cell lines. *Blood* **67**, 31–6. [p. 20, 21]

1788. Tono-oka, T., Sato, Y., Matsumoto, T., Ueno, N., Ohkawa, M., Shikano, T., and Takeda, T. (1984). Hypereosinophilic syndrome in acute lymphoblastic leukemia with a chromosome translocation (t(5q;14q)). *Med. Pediatr. Oncol.* **12**, 33–7. [p. 156]

1789. Torisu, M., Yoshida, T., Ward, P. A., and Cohen, S. (1973). Lymphocyte-derived eosinophil chemotactic factor. II. Studies on the mechanism of activation of the precursor substance by immune complexes. *J. Immunol* **111**, 1450–8. [p. 100]

1790. Toth, J., Dworak, O., and Sugar, J. (1977). Eosinophil predominance in Hodgkin's disease. *Z. Krebsforsch* **89**, 107–11. [p. 162]

1791. Toth, S. R., Nash, A. S., McEwan, A. M., and Jarrett, O. (1985). Chronic eosinophilic leukaemia in blast crisis in a cat negative for feline leukaemia virus. *Vet. Rec.* **117**, 471–2. [p. 157]

1792. Touze, J. E., Metras, D., Chauvet, J., Kacou, M., Adoh, A., and Bertrand, E. (1984). Right ventricular dysfunction after endocardiectomy for right ventricular endomyocardial fibrosis. *Thorac. Cardiovasc. Surg.* **32**, 304–6. [p. 254]

1793. Tracey, R. and Smith, H. (1978). An inherited anomaly of human eosinophils and basophils. *Blood Cells* **4**, 291–300. [p. 11, 261]

1794. Treusch, P. J., Swetnam, R. E., and Woelke, B. J. (1981). Eosinophilic joint effusion and intestinal nematodiasis (letter). *Ann. Emerg. Med.* **10**, 614–15. [p. 177]

1795. Trounce, J. Q. and Tanner, M. S. (1985). Eosinophilic gastroenteritis. *Arch. Dis. Child.* **60**, 1186–8. [p. 186]

1786. Troxell, M. L., Mills, G. M., and Allen, R. C. (1984). The hypereosinophilic syndrome in acute lymphocytic leukemia. *Cancer* **54**, 1058–61. [p. 160]

1797. Tsutsumi, Y., Ohshita, T., and Yokoyama, T. (1984). A case of gastric carcinoma with massive eosinophilia. *Acta Pathol. Jpn.* **34**, 117–22. [p. 171]

1798. Tummala, V., Barwick, K. W., Sontag, S. J., Vlahcevic, R. Z., and McCallum, R. W. (1987). The significance of intraepithelial eosinophils in the histologic diagnosis of gastroesophageal reflux. *Am. J. Clin. Pathol.* **87**, 43–8. [p. 184]

1799. Turk, J., Henderson, W. R., Klebanoff, S. J., and Hubbard, W. C. (1983). Iodination of arachidonic acid mediated by eosinophil peroxidase, myeloperoxidase and lactoperoxidase: identification and comparison of products. *Biochim. Biophys. Acta* **751**, 189–200. [p. 60]

1800. Turk, J., Maas, R. L., Brash, A. R., Roberts, L. J., and Oates, J. A. (1982). Arachidonic acid 15-lipoxygenase products from human eosinophils. *J. Biol. Chem.* **257**, 7068–76. [p. 69]

1801. Turk, J., Rand, T. H., Maas, R. L., Lawson, J. A., Brash, A. R., Roberts, L. J., Colley, D. G., and Oates, J. A. (1983). Identification of lipoxygenase products from arachidonic acid metabolism in stimulated murine eosinophils. *Biochim. Biophys. Acta* **750**, 78–90. [p. 69]

1802. Turner, J. C., Jackson, H. Jr, and Parker, F. Jr. (1938). The etiologic relation of the eosinophil to the Gordon phenomenon in Hodgkin's disease. *Am. J. Med. Sci.* **195**, 27–32. [p. 53]

1803. Turner, K. J. (1978). The conflicting role of parasitic infections in modulating the prevalence of asthma. *Papua New Guinea Med. J.* **21**, 86–104. [p. 201]

1804. Turner-Warwick, M. (1978). *Immunology of the lung: Current Topics in Immunology Series.* 10. Edward Arnold, London. [p. 205]

1805. Turner-Warwick, M., Assem, E. S., Lockwood, M. (1976). Cryoptogenic pulmonary eosinophilia. *Clin. Allergy* **6**, 135–46. [p. 206]

1806. Turner-Warwick, M. and Haslam, P. L. (1987). The value of serial bronchoalveolar lavages in assessing the clinical progress of patients with cryptogenic fibrosing alveolitis. *Am. Rev. Respir. Dis.* **135**, 26–34. [p. 209]

1807. Tydd, T. F. and Dyer, N. H. (1976). Sulphasalazine lung. *Med. J. Aust.* **1**, 570–3. [p. 309]

1808. Tzvetanova, E. M. and Tzekov, C. T. (1986). Eosinophilia in the cerebrospinal fluid of children with shunts implanted for the treatment of internal hydrocephalus. *Acta Cytol. (Baltimore)* **30**, 277–80. [p. 217]

1809. Udell, I. J., Gleich, G. J., Allansmith, M. R., Ackerman, S. J., and Abelson, M. B. (1981). Eosinophil granule major basic protein and Charcot–Leyden crystal protein in human tears. *Am. J. Ophthalmol.* **92**, 824–8. [p. 218]

1810. Undritz, E., Lang, E. M., and Van Oye, E. (1956). La reaction peroxydasique des eosinophiles comme moyen de taxonomie (classification) des mammiferes. *Le Sang* **27**, 513–5. [p. 123, 125, 259]

1811. Urabe, A., Tsuneyoshi, M., and Enjoji, M. (1987). Epithelioid hemangioma versus Kimura's disease: a comparative clinicopathologic study. *Am. J. Surg. Pathol.* **11**, 758–66. [p. 167]

1812. Urbano Marquez, A., Estruch, R., Grau, J. M., Granena, A., Martin Ortega, E., Palou, J., and Rozman, C. (1986). Inflammatory myopathy associated with chronic graft-versus-host disease. *Neurology* **36**, 1091–3. [p. 314]

1813. Urhoghide, G. E. and Falase, A. O. (1987). Degranulated eosinophils, eosinophil granule basic proteins and humoral factors in Nigerians with endomyocardial fibrosis. *Afr. J. Med. Med. Sci.*, **16**, 133–9. [p. 256]

1814. Uyama, T., Moriwaki, S., Aga, Y., and Yamamoto, A. (1981). Eosinophilic ureteritis? Regional ureteritis with marked infiltration of eosinophils. *Urology* **18**, 615–17. [p. 223]

1815. Vaage, J., Pepin, K. G., and Au, T. L. (1986). Immunospecific eosinophil infiltration of a mouse mammary carcinoma. *Cancer Res.* **46**, 5344–8. [p. 170]

1816. Vadas, M. A. (1981). Cyclophosphamide pretreatment induces eosinophilia to nonparasite antigens. *J. Immunol.* **127**, 2083–6. [p. 24]

1817. Vadas, M. A. (1982). Genetic control of eosinophilia in mice: gene(s) expressed in bone marrow-derived cells control high responsiveness. *J. Immunol.* **128**, 691–5. [p. 24]

1818. Vadas, M. A. (1984). Newer aspects of regulation of human granulocyte function. *Aust. NZ J. Med.* **14**, 71–4. [p. 20]

1819. Vadas, M. A., Butterworth, A. E., Sherry, B., Dessein, A., Hogan, M., Bout, D., and David, J. R. (1980). Interactions between human eosinophils and schistosomula of Schistosoma mansoni. I. Stable and irreversible antibody-dependent adherence. *J. Immunol.* **124**, 1441–8. [p. 112]

1820. Vadas, M. A. and Clark Lewis, I. (1985). Regulation of human granulocyte function by products derived from murine tumors. *Exp. Hematol.* **13**, 151–6. [p. 16]

1821. Vadas, M. A., David, J. R. Butterworth, A., Pisani, N. T., and Siongok, T. A. (1979). A new method for the purification of human eosinophils and neutrophils, and a comparison of the ability of these cells to damage schistosomula of Schistosoma mansoni. *J. Immunol.* **122**, 1228–36. [p. 33]

1822. Vadas, M. A., David, J. R., Butterworth, A. E., Houba, V., Sturrock, R. F., David, L., Herson, R., Siongok, T. A., and Kimani, R. (1980). Functional studies on purified eosinophils and neutrophils from patients with Schistosoma mansoni infections. *Clin. Exp. Immunol.* **39**, 683–94. [p. 105]

1823. Vadas, M. A., Lopez, A. F., Begley, C. G., Williamson, D. J., Warren, D. J., and Sanderson, C. J. Activation of human eosinophils by an eosinophil specific colony-stimulating factor (abstract). Presented to the 6th International Congress of Immunology, Toronto, Canada, 1986. [p. 19, 35, 82, 87, 109]

1824. Vadas, M. A., Varigos, G., Nicola, N., Pincus, S., Dessein, A., Metcalf, D., and Battye, F. L. (1983). Eosinophil activation by colony-stimulating factor in man: metabolic effects and analysis by flow cytometry. *Blood* **61**, 1232–41. [p. 20]

1825. Valcke, Y., Pauwels, R., and Van der Straeten, M. (1987). Bronchoalveolar lavage in acute hypersensitivity pneumonitis caused by sulfasalazine. *Chest* **92**, 572–3. [p. 309]

1826. Valenzuela, R., McMahon, J. T., Glassy, F. J., Golish, J. A., and Caggiano, V. (1987). An unusual ultrastructural neutrophil abnormality of unknown function. *Cleve. Clin. J. Med.* **54**, 49–54. [p. 244]

1827. Valiathan, M. S., Sankarkumar, R., Balakrishnan, K. G., and Mohansingh, M. P. (1983). Surgical palliation for endomyocardial fibrosis: early results. *Thorax* **38**, 421–7. [p. 254]

1828. Vallejo, J. L., Alvarez, E. F., Acedo, J. M., and Salem, F. M. (1982). Endomyocardial fibrosis with aortic, mitral, and tricuspid valve involvement. *Arch. Intern. Med.* **142**, 1925–7. [p. 234]

1829. Valnes, K. and Brandtzaeg, P. (1981). Selective inhibition of nonspecific eosinophil staining or identification of eosinophilic granulocytes by paired counterstaining in immunofluorescence studies. *J. Histochem. Cytochem* **29**, 595–600. [p. 37]

1830. Valone, F. H. (1980). Modulation of human neutrophil and eosinophil polymorphonuclear leukocyte chemotaxis: an analytical review. *Clin. Immunol. Immunopathol.* **15**, 52–65. [p. 324]

1831. Van Crombrugge, P., Pauwels, R., and Van der Straeten, M. (1983). Thyroid carcinoma and eosinophilia. *Ann. Clin. Res.* **15**, 128–30. [p. 172]

1832. van den Bergh, V., Tricot, G., Fonteyn, G., Dom, R., and Bulcke, J. (1987). Diffuse fasciitis after bone marrow transplantation. *Am. J. Med.* **83**, 139–43. [p. 182]

1833. Van den Bosch, J. M., Wagenaar, S. S., and Westermann, C. J. (1986). Asthma, eosinophilic pleuropneumonia, and pericarditis without vasculitis. *Thorax* **41**, 571–2. [p. 202]

1834. van den Hoogenband, H. M. (1982). Skin lesions as the first manifestation of the hypereosinophilic syndrome. *Clin. Exp. Dermatol.* **7**, 267–71. [p. 299]

1835. van den Hoogenband, H. M., van den Berg, W. H., and van Diggelen, M.

W. (1985). PUVA therapy in the treatment of skin lesions of the hypereosinophilic syndrome (letter). *Arch. Dermatol.* **121**, 450. [p. 299]

1836. van der Gaag, I. and van der Linde Sipman, J. S. (1987). Eosinophilic granulomatous colitis with ulceration in a dog. *J. Comp. Pathol.* **97**, 179–85. [p. 190]

1837. van Overveld, F. J., Bruijnzeel, P. L., Kreukniet, J., Raaijmakers, J. A., and Terpstra, G. K. (1987). The isolation of inflammatory cells from normal human lung tissue. *Int. J. Tissue React.* **9**, 61–7. [p. 32]

1838. van Rensburg, L. C., Keet, A. D., and Adams, G. (1986). Eosinophilic granuloma of the stomach. *J. Surg. Oncol.* **31**, 143–7. [p. 184, 185]

1839. Van Slyck, E. J. and Adamson, T. C. (1979). Acute hypereosinophilic syndrome: successful treatment with vincristine, cytarabine, and prednisone. *JAMA* **242**, 175–6. [p. 291]

1840. Varigos, G. A., Morstyn, G., and Vadas, M. A. (1982). Bullous pemphigoid blister fluid stimulates eosinophil colony formation and activates eosinophils. *Clin. Exp. Immunol.* **50**, 555–62. [p. 22, 37, 303]

1841. Varma, S., Sakhuja, V., Deodhar, S. D., and Jain, S. (1983). Hypereosinophilic syndrome. *J. Assoc. Physicians India* **31**. 789–90. [p. 270]

1842. Varon, D., Wetzler, M., and Berrebi, A., (1986). Hypereosinophilic syndrome associated with polycythemia vera. *Arch. Intern. Med.* **146**, 1440–1. [p. 285]

1843. Vaughan Hudson, B., Linch, D. C., Macintyre, E. A., Bennett, M. H., MacLennan, K. A., Vaughan Hudson, G., and Jelliffe, A. M. (1987). Selective peripheral blood eosinophilia associated with survival advantage in Hodgkin's disease (BNLI Report No 31). British National Lymphoma Investigation. *J. Clin. Pathol.* **40**, 247–50. [p. 162]

1844. Veevaete, F., van der Straeten, M., de Vos, M., and Roels, H. (1978). Allergic granulomatous angiitis. *Scand. J. Respir. Dis.* **59**, 287–96. [p. 210]

1845. Veith, M. C. and Butterworth, A. E. (1983). Enhancement of human eosinophil-mediated killing of Schistosoma mansoni larvae by mononuclear cell products in vitro. *J. Exp. Med.* **157**, 1828–43. [p. 107]

1846. Vejjajiva, A. (1978). Parasitic diseases of the nervous system in Thailand. *Clin. Exp. Neurol.* **15**, 92–7. [p. 138, 139, 146]

1847. Venge, P., Carlson, M., and Peterson, C. Secretion of eosinophil granule proteins (abstract). Presented to the 6th International Congress of Immunology, Toronto, Canada, 1986. [p. 95]

1848. Venge, P., Dahl, R., Fredens, K., Hallgren, R., and Peterson, C. (1983). Eosinophil cationic proteins (ECP and EPX) in health and disease. In *Immunobiology of the eosinophil* (eds. T. Yoshida and M. Torisu), pp. 163–79. Elsevier Biomedical, New York. [p. 54, 55]

1849. Venge, P., Dahl, R., and Hallgren, R. (1979). Enhancement of factor XII dependent reactions by eosinophil cationic protein. *Thromb. Res.* **14**, 641–9. [p. 53, 247]

1850. Venge, P., Dahl, R., Hallgren, R., and Olsson, I. (1980). Cationic proteins of human eosinophils and their role in the inflammatory reaction. In *The Eosinophil in health and disease* (eds. A. A. Mahmoud, K. F. Austen, and A. S. Simon), pp. 131–42. Grune and Stratton, New York. [p. 53, 63, 121]

1851. Venge, P., Roxin, L. E., and Olsson, I. (1977). Radioimmunoassay of human eosinophil cationic protein. *Br. J. Haematol.* **37**, 331–5. [p. 50, 51]

1852. Venge, P., Stromberg, A., Braconier, J. H., Roxin, L. E., and Olsson, I.

(1978). Neutrophil and eosinophil granulocytes in bacterial infection: sequential studies of cellular and serum levels of granule proteins. *Br. J. Haematol.* **38**, 475–83. [p. 131]

1853. Venge, P., Zetterstrom, O., Dahl, R., Roxin, L. E., and Olsson, I. (1977). Low levels of eosinophil cationic proteins in patients with asthma. *Lancet* **ii**, 373–5. [p. 55, 198]

1854. Veress, J. F., Koss, L. G., and Schreiber, K. (1979). Eosinophilic pleural effusions. *Acta Cytol. (Baltimore)* **23**, 40–4. [p. 212]

1855. Verhagen, J., Bruynzeel, P. L., Koedam, J. A., Wassink, G. A., de Boer, M., Terpstra, G. K., Kreukniet, J., Veldink, G. A., and Vliegenthart, J. F. (1984). Specific leukotriene formation by purified eosinophils and neutrophils. *FEBS Lett.* **168**, 23–8. [p. 70]

1856. Verma, S. and Kieff, E. (1975). Cephalexin-related nephropathy. *JAMA* **234**, 618–19. [p. 309]

1857. Vetto, J. T., Papa, M. Z., Lotze, M. T., Chang, A. E., and Rosenberg, S. A. (1987). Reduction of toxicity of interleukin-2 and lymphokine-activated killer cells in humans by the administration of corticosteroids. *J. Clin. Oncol.* **5**, 496–503. [p. 20]

1858. Vieira, V. G. and Prolla, J. C. (1979). Clinical evaluation of eosinophils in the sputum. *J. Clin. Pathol.* **32**, 1054–7. [p. 199]

1859. Vignon-Pennamen, M. D. and Wallach, D. (1986). Infantile acropustulosis: a clinicopathologic study of six cases. *Arch Dermatol.* **122**, 1155–60. [p. 304]

1860. Vijayaraghavan, G., Davies, J., Sadanandan, S., Spry, C. J., Gibson, D. G., and Goodwin, J. F. (1983). Echocardiographic features of tropical endomyocardial disease in South India. *Br. Heart J.* **50**, 450–9. [p. 251]

1861. Vijayaraghavan, G. and Sadanandan, S. (1984). Immunological phenomena in tropical endomyocardial fibrosis. *Indian Heart J.* **36**, 87–9. [p. 250]

1862. Vilanova, J. R., Burgos-Bretones, J., Simon, R., and Rivera-Pomar, J. M. (1980). Leukaemoid reaction and eosinophilia in 'inflammatory fibrous histiocytoma'. *Virchows Arch. (Pathol. Anat.)* **388**, 237–43. [p. 187]

1863. Villalta, F. and Kierszenbaum, F. (1984). Role of inflammatory cells in Chagas' disease. I. Uptake and mechanism of destruction of intracellular (amastigote) forms of Trypanosoma cruzi by human eosinophils. *J. Immunol.* **132**, 2053–8. [p. 116]

1864. Villalta, F., Pankratz, H. S., and Kierszenbaum, F. (1987). Extracellular killing of Trypanosoma cruzi amastigotes by human eosinophils. *J. Protozool.* **34**, 285–90. [p. 47, 116]

1865. Vincent, M. E., Gerzof, S. G., and Robbins, A. H. (1977). Benign transient eosinophilia following intravenous urography. *JAMA* **237**, 2629. [p. 310]

1866. Viola, M. V., Chung, E., and Mukhopadhyay, M. G. (1972). Eosinophilia and metastatic carcinoma. *Med. Annal Dist. Columbia* **41**, 1–3. [p. 22]

1867. Virmani, R., Chun, P. K., Dunn, B. E., Hartmen, D., and McAllister, H. A. (1984). Eosinophilic constrictive pericarditis. *Am. Heart. J.* **107**, 803–7. [p. 228]

1868. Volpi, A., Rovelli, G. E., and Maggioni, A. P. (1985). Benign course of endomyocardial fibrosis as a late complication of hypereosinophilic syndrome. *G. Ital. Cardiol.* **15**, 238–40. [p. 256]

1869. Wald, J. A., Friedman, B. F., and Farr, R. S. (1986). An improved protocol for the use of troleandomycin (TAO) in the treatment of steroid-requiring asthma. *J. Allergy Clin. Immunol.* **78**, 36–43. [p. 291]

1870. Waldmann, T. A., Strober, W., Blaese, R. M., and Strauss, A. J. (1967). Thymoma, hypogammaglobulinemia, and absence of eosinophils (abstract). *J. Clin. Invest.* **46**, 1127–8. [p. 315]

1871. Walle, A. J. and Parwaresch, M. R. (1979). Estimation of effective eosinopoiesis and bone marrow eosinophil reserve capacity in normal man. *Cell Tissue Kinet.* **12**, 249–55. [p. 14]

1872. Walls, R. S. and Beeson, P. B. (1972). Mechanism of eosinophilia. VIII. Importance of local cellular reactions in stimulating eosinophil production. *Clin. Exp. Immunol.* **12**, 111–19. [p. 313]

1873. Walsh, G. M. and Kay, A. B. (1986). Binding of immunoglobulin classes and subclasses to human neutrophils and eosinophils. *Clin. Exp. Immunol.* **63**, 466–72. [p. 77, 80]

1874. Wantzin, G. L., Philip, P., and Killmann, S. A. (1979). Cytoplasmic labelling of eosinophils with tritiated thymidine triphosphate. *Biomedicine* **31**, 10–11. [p. 42]

1875. Ward, R. A., Feldhoff, P. W., and Klein, E. (1984). Role of dialyzer contaminants in the allergic epiphenomena of hemodialysis. *Artif. Organs* **8**, 338–49. [p. 222]

1876. Wardlaw, A. J. and Kay, A. B. PAF-acether is a potent chemotactic factor for human eosinophils (abstract). Presented to the 6th International Congress of Immunology, Toronto, Canada, 1986. [p. 101]

1877. Wardlaw, A. J., Moqbel, R., Cromwell, O., and Kay, A. B. (1986). Platelet-activating factor: a potent chemotactic and chemokinetic factor for human eosinophils. *J. Clin. Invest.* **78**, 1701–6. [p. 101]

1878. Warhol, M. J., Pinkus, G. S., and Said, J. W. (1987). Ultrastructural localization of Leu M1 in Reed-Sternberg cells and normal myeloid cells. *Hum. Pathol.* **18**, 824–9. [p. 45]

1879. Warren, D. J. and Sanderson, C. J. (1985). Production of a T-cell hybrid producing a lymphokine stimulating eosinophil differentiation. *Immunology* **54**, 615–23. [p. 19]

1880. Wasmoen, T. L., Benirschke, K., and Gleich, G. J. (1987). Demonstration of immunoreactive eosinophil granule major basic protein in the plasma and placentae of non-human primates. *Placenta* **8**, 283–92. [p. 227]

1881. Wasmoen, T. L., Coulam, C. B., Leiferman, K. M., and Gleich, G. J. (1987). Increases of plasma eosinophil major basic protein levels late in pregnancy predict onset of labor. *Proc. Natl. Acad. Sci. USA* **84**, 3029–32. [p. 227]

1882. Wasmoen, T. L., McKean, D. J., Coulam, C. B., Benirschke, K., and Gleich, G. J. Evidence for eosinophil granule major basic protein in human placenta (abstract). Presented to the 6th International Congress of Immunology, Toronto, Canada, 1986. [p. 227]

1883. Wasserman, S. I., Austen, K. F., and Soter, N. A. (1982). The functional and physicochemical characterization of three eosinophilotactic activities released into the circulation by cold challenge of patients with cold urticaria. *Clin. Exp. Immunol.* **47**, 570–8. [p. 102]

1884. Wasserman, S. I., Goetzl, E. J., and Austen, K. F. (1975). Inactivation of slow reacting substance of anaphylaxis by human eosinophil arylsulfatase. *J. Immunol.* **114**, 645–9. [p. 61]

1885. Wasserman, S. I., Goetzl, E. J., Ellman, L., and Austen, K. F. (1974).

Tumor-associated eosinophilotactic factor. *N. Engl. J. Med.* **290**, 420–4. [p. 101]

1886. Wasserman, S. I., Seibold, J. R., Medsger, T. A. Jr, and Rodnan, G. P. (1982). Serum eosinophilotactic activity in eosinophilic fasciitis. *Arthritis Rheum.* **25**, 1352–6. [p. 102]

1887. Wassom, D. L., and Gleich, G. J. (1979). Damage to Trichinella spiralis newborn larvae by eosinophil major basic protein. *Am. J. Trop. Med. Hyg.* **28**, 860–3. [p. 115]

1888. Wassom, D. L., Loegering, D. A., and Gleich, G. J. (1979). Measurement of guinea pig eosinophil major basic protein by radioimmunoassay. *Mol. Immunol.* **16**, 711–19. [p. 46]

1889. Wassom, D. L., Loegering, D. A., Solley, G. O., Moore, S. B., Schooley, R. T., Fauci, A. S., and Gleich, G. J. (1981). Elevated serum levels of the eosinophil granule major basic protein in patients with eosinophilia. *J. Clin. Invest.* **67**, 651–61. [p. 47]

1890. Waters, L. S., Taverne, J., Tai, P.-C., Spry, C. J., Targett, G. A., and Playfair, J. H. (1987). Killing of Plasmodium falciparum by eosinophil secretory products. *Infect. Immun.* **55**, 877–81. [p. 117, 148]

1891. Wathen, C. W. and Harrison, D. J. (1987). Circulating anti-neutrophil antibodies in systemic vasculitis (letter). *Lancet* **i**, 1037. [p. 231]

1892. Watters, L. C., Schwarz, M. I., Cherniack, R. M., Waldron, J. A., Dunn, T. L., Stanford, R. E., and King, T. E. (1987). Idiopathic pulmonary fibrosis: pretreatment bronchoalveolar lavage cellular constituents and their relationships with lung histopathology and clinical response to therapy. *Am. Rev. Respir. Dis.* **135**, 696–704. [p. 209]

1893. Webb-Peploe, M. M. (1983). Eosinophilic heart disease. In *Specific heart muscle disease* (eds. C. Symons, T. Evans, and A. G. Mitchell), pp. 24–32. Wright PSG, Bristol. [p. 234]

1894. Weeks, A. M. and Glomski, C. A. (1978). Cytology of the bone marrow in the Mongolian gerbil. *Lab. Anim.* **12**, 195–202. [p. 126]

1895. Weil, G. J. and Chused, T. M. (1981). Eosinophil autofluorescence and its use in isolation and analysis of human eosinophils using flow microfluorometry. *Blood* **57**, 1099–104. [p. 37]

1896. Weil, S. C. and Hrisinko, M. A. (1987). A hybrid eosinophilic-basophilic granulocyte in chronic granulocytic leukemia. *Am. J. Clin. Pathol.* **87**, 66–70. [p. 11]

1897. Weiler, J. M., Loegering, D. A., and Gleich, G. J. (1986). Inhibition of the alternative-amplification pathway of complement by eosinophilic major basic protein (MBP) (abstract). *Fed. Proc.* **45**, 735. [p. 48]

1898. Weinberg, A. G., Rosenfeld, C. R., Manroe, B. L., and Browne, R. (1985). Neonatal blood cell count in health and disease. II. Values for lymphocytes, monocytes, and eosinophils. *J. Pediatr.* **106**, 462–6. [p. 294]

1899. Weinfeld, A., Westin, J., and Swolin, B. (1977). Phi-negative eosinophilic leukaemia with trisomy 8: case report and review of cytogenetic studies. *Scand. J. Haematol.* **18**, 413–20. [p. 25, 156]

1900. Weingarten, J. S., O'Sheal, S. F., and Margolis, W. S. (1985). Eosinophilic meningitis and the hypereosinophilic syndrome: case report and review of the literature. *Am. J. Med.* **78**, 674–6. [p. 217, 270, 275]

1901. Weir, M. R., Hall Craggs, M., Shen, S. Y., Posner, J. N., Alongi, S. V.,

Dagher, F. J., and Sadler, J. H. (1986). The prognostic value of the eosinophil in acute renal allograft rejection. *Transplantation* **41**, 709–12. [p. 225]

1902. Weiss, S. J., Test, S. T., Eckmann, C. M., Roos, D., and Regiani, S. (1986). Brominating oxidants generated by human eosinophils. *Science* **234**, 200–3. [p. 59, 120]

1903. Weiss-Carmine, S. (1957). Die Endocarditis parietalis fibroplastica mit Bluteosinophilie (Löffler) und ihre stellung im Rahman der Parietalendokardfibrosen. *Schweiz Med. Wchnschr.* **87**, 890–8. [p. 234]

1904. Welch, N. T., Hall, P. A., and Sprague, D. B. (1987). Angiolymphoid hyperplasia with eosinophilia. *J. R. Soc. Med.* **80**, 384–5. [p. 167]

1905. Weller, P. F. (1984). Eosinophilia. *J. Allergy Clin. Immunol.* **73**, 1–14. [p. 325]

1906. Weller, P. F., Ackerman, S. J., and Smith, J. A. (1988). Eosinophil granule cationic proteins: major basic protein is distinct from the smaller subunit of eosinophil peroxidase. *J. Leukocyte Biol.* **43**, 1–4. [p. 46, 58]

1907. Weller, P. F. and Austen, K. F. (1983). Human eosinophil arylsulfatase B. Structure and activity of the purified tetrameric lysosomal hydrolase. *J. Clin. Invest.* **71**, 114–23. [p. 61]

1908. Weller, P. F., Bach, D. S., and Austen, K. F. (1982). Human eosinophil lysophospholipase: the sole protein component of Charcot–Leyden crystals. *J. Immunol.* **128**, 1346–9. [p. 65]

1909. Weller, P. F., Bach, D. S., and Austen, K. F. (1984). Biochemical characterization of human eosinophil Charcot–Leyden crystal protein (lysophospholipase). *J. Biol. Chem.* **259**, 15 100–5. [p. 64, 66]

1910. Weller, P. F., Corey, E. J., Austen, K. F., and Lewis, R. A. (1986). Inhibition of homogeneous human eosinophil arylsulfatase B by sulfidopeptide leukotrienes. *J. Biol. Chem.* **261**, 1737–44. [p. 61]

1911. Weller, P. F. and Dvorak, A. M. (1985). Arachidonic acid incorporation by cytoplasmic lipid bodies of human eosinophils. *Blood* **65**, 1269–74. [p. 42]

1912. Weller, P. F. and Goetzl, E. J. (1979). The regulatory and effector roles of eosinophils. *Adv. Immunol.* **27**, 339–71. [p. 323]

1913. Weller, P. F. and Goetzl, E. J. (1980). The human eosinophil: roles in host defense and tissue injury. *Am. J. Pathol.* **100**, 793–820. [p. 324]

1914. Weller, P. F., Goetzl, E. J., and Austen, K. F. (1980). Identification of human eosinophil lysophospholipase as the constituent of Charcot–Leyden crystals. *Proc. Natl. Acad. Sci. USA* **77**, 7440–3. [p. 63, 65]

1915. Weller, P. F., Lee, C. W., Foster, D. W., Corey, E. J., Austen, K. F., and Lewis, R. A. (1983). Generation and metabolism of 5-lipoxygenase pathway leukotrienes by human eosinophils: predominant production of leukotriene C4. *Proc. Natl. Acad. Sci. USA* **80**, 7626–30. [p. 70, 282]

1916. Weller, P. F., Ottesen, E. A., and Goetzl, E. J. (1981). Sequential alterations in the human eosinophil content of arylsulfatase B during therapy of Bancroftian filariasis. *Clin. Immunol. Immunopathol.* **18**, 76–84. [p. 61]

1917. Weller, P. F., Wasserman, S. I., and Austen, K. F. (1980). Selected enzymes preferentially present in the eosinophil. In *The eosinophil in health and disease.* (eds. A. A. Mahmoud, K. F. Austen, and A. S. Simon), pp. 115–30. Grune and Stratton, New York. [p. 61, 62, 65, 66, 83]

1918. West, B. C., Gelb, N. A., and Rosenthal, A. S. (1975). Isolation and partial characterization of human eosinophil granules: comparisons to neutrophils. *Am. J. Pathol.* **81**, 575–86. [p. 40, 43]

1919. Wever, R., Hamers, M. N., de Graaf, C. J., Weening, R. S., and Roos, D. (1982). Characterization of the peroxidase in human eosinophils. *Adv. Exp. Med. Biol.* **141**, 501–9. [p. 59]

1920. Wever, R., Plat, H., and Hamers, M. N. (1981). Human eosinophil peroxidase: a novel isolation procedure, spectral properties and chlorinating activity. *FEBS Lett.* **123**, 327–31. [p. 58]

1921. Wharton-Jones, T. (1846). The blood-corpuscle considered in its different phases of development in the animal series. Memoir I Vertebrata. *Philos. Trans. R. Soc. Lond.* **136**, 63–87. [p. 4]

1922. Whitcher, B. L. and Webb, D. J. (1986). Treatment of recurrent eosinophilic granuloma of the mandible following radiation therapy. *J. Oral Maxillofac. Surg.* **44**, 565–70. [p. 165]

1923. Whitcomb, C. C., Sternheim, W. L., Borowitz, M. J., Davila, E., and Byrne, G. E. Jr. (1985). T-cell lymphoma mimicking granulocytic sarcoma. *Am. J. Clin. Pathol.* **84**, 760–3. [p. 12]

1924. Whitcomb, M. E., Schwarz, M. I., and Tormey, D. C. (1972). Methotrexate pneumonitis: case report and review of the literature. *Thorax* **27**, 636–9. [p. 309]

1925. White, C. J., Maxwell, C. J., and Gallin, J. I. (1986). Changes in the structural and functional properties of human eosinophils during experimental hookworm infection. *J. Infect. Dis.* **154**, 778–83. [p. 34, 69, 1440]

1926. Whittaker, S. J., Russell-Jones, R., and Spry, C. J. (1988). Lymphomatoid papulosis and its relationship to 'idiopathic' hypereosinophilic syndrome. *J. Am. Acad. Dermatol.* **18**, 339–44. [p. 12, 163, 274, 304]

1927. Whittingham, S., Morstyn, G., Wilson, J. W., and Vadas, M. A. (1981). An autoantibody reactive with nuclei of polymorphonuclear neutrophils: a cell differentiation marker. *Blood* **58**, 768–71. [p. 41]

1928. Wichman, A., Buchthal, F., Pezeshkpour, G. H., and Fauci, A. S. (1985). Peripheral neuropathy in hypereosinophilic syndrome. *Neurology* **35**, 1140–5. [p. 276]

1929. Wickramasinghe, S. N. and Hughes, M. (1978). High resolution autoradiographic studies of RNA, protein and DNA synthesis during human eosinophil granulocytopoiesis: evidence for the presence of RNA on or within eosinophil granules. *Br. J. Haematol.* **38**, 179–83. [p. 42]

1930. Wickramasinghe, S. N. and Moffatt, B. (1972). DNA synthesis during human eosinopoiesis. *Acta Haematol. (Basel)* **48**, 158–163. [p. 72]

1931. Wiktor Jedrzejczak, W. and Ratajczak, M. (1985). Eosinophilic granulocyte deficiency in mice mutant in sl and w loci. *Experientia* **41**, 1596–8. [p. 25]

1932. Williams, D. M., Linder, J. E., Hill, M. W., and Gillett, R. (1978). Ultrastructural localization of alkaline phosphatase in rat eosinophil leucocytes. *J. Histochem. Cytochem.* **26**, 862–4. [p. 43]

1933. Williams, H. J., Ziter, F. A., and Banta, C. A. (1986). Childhood eosinophilic fasciitis – progression to linear scleroderma. *J. Rheumatol.* **13**, 961–2. [p. 181]

1934. Williams, J. F., Ghalib, H. W., Mackenzie, C. D., Elkhalifa, M. Y., Ayuya, J. M., and Kron, M. A. (1987). Cell adherence to microfilariae of Onchocercavolvulus: a comparative study. *Ciba Found. Symp.* **127**, 146–63. [p. 116]

1935. Willoughby, C. P., Piris, J., and Truelove, S. C. (1979). Tissue eosinophils in ulcerative colitis. *Scand. J. Gastroenterol.* **14**, 395–9. [p. 190]

1936. Wimmer, R. S., Raney, R. B. Jr, and Naiman, J. L. (1978). Hypereosinophilia with acute lymphocytic and acute myelocytic leukemia in childhood. *J. Pediatr.* **92**, 244–6. [p. 629, 295]

1937. Winchester, R. J., Litwin, S. D., Koffler, D., and Kunkel, H. G. (1971). Observations on the eosinophilia of certain patients with rheumatoid arthritis. *Arthritis Rheum.* **14**, 650–65. [p. 177]

1938. Winkel, P., Statland, B. E., Saunders, A. M., Osborn, H., and Kupperman, H. (1981). Within-day physiologic variation of leukocyte types in healthy subjects as assayed by two automated leukocyte differential analyzers. *Am. J. Clin. Pathol.* **75**, 693–700. [p. 31]

1939. Winkelmann, R. K., Camp, R., English, J. S., and Greaves, M. W. (1986). The perivascular cell populations in human skin after tropical application of leukotriene B4. *Acta Derm. Venereol. (Stockh.)* **66**, 340–3. [p. 101]

1940. Winkelmann, R. K. and Frigas, E. (1986). Eosinophilic panniculitis: a clinicopathologic study. *J. Cutan. Pathol.* **13**, 1–12. [p. 297, 304, 309]

1041. Winkler, C. F., Snider, H. L., and Yam, L. T. (1981). Unusual manifestations of hypereosinophilia. *South Med. J.* **74**, 1401–3. [p. 152]

1942. Winqvist, I., Olofsson, T., and Olsson, I. (1984). Mechanisms for eosinophil degranulation; release of the eosinophil cationic protein. *Immunology* **51**, 1–8. [p. 92, 93, 94, 95]

1943. Winqvist, I., Olofsson, T., and Olsson, I. (1985). Mechanisms for adherence of eosinophils to an antibody-coated surface. *Scand. J. Haematol.* **35**, 88–95. [p. 75]

1944. Winqvist, I., Oloffson, T., Olsson, I., Persson, A. M., and Hallberg, T. (1982). Altered density, metabolism and surface receptors of eosinophils in eosinophilia. *Immunology* **47**, 531–9. [p. 34, 282]

1945. Winqvist, I., Olofsson, T., and Persson, E. (1985). Effect of zinc and other cations on the release of the eosinophil cationic protein. *Scand. J. Clin. Lab. Invest.* **45**. 671–7. [p. 95]

1946. Winqvist, I., Olsson, I., Werner, S., and Stenstam, M. (1981). Variations of cationic proteins from eosinophil leukocytes in food intolerance and allergic rhinitis. *Allergy* **36**, 419–23. [p. 188]

1947. Woessner, S., Lafuente, R., Florensa, L., Sans Sabrafen, J., and Antich, J. (1985). Acute myelomonocytic leukaemia with abnormal eosinophils and inversion of chromosome 16. *Blut* **50**, 45–50. [p. 11, 158]

1948. Wolford, S. T., Shroer, R. A., Gallo, P. P., Gohs, F. X., Brodeck, M., Falk, H. B., and Ruhren, R. (1987). Age-related changes in serum chemistry and hematology values in normal Sprague-Dawley rats. *Fundam. Appl. Toxicol.* **8**, 80–8. [p. 127]

1949. Wolford, S. T., Schroer, R. A., Gohs, F. X., Gallo, P. P., Brodeck, M., Falk, H. B., and Ruhren, R. (1986). Reference range data base for serum chemistry and hematology values in laboratory animals. *J. Toxicol. Environ. Health* **18**, 161–88. [p. 123]

1950. Wood, A. E., Byle, D., O'Hara, M. D., and Cleland, J. (1982). Mitral annuloplasty in endomyocardial fibrosis: an alternative to valve replacement. *Ann. Thorac. Surg.* **34**, 466–51. [p. 243]

1951. Wood, C., Miller, A. C., Jacobs, A., Hart, R., and Nickoloff, B. J. (1986).

Eosinophilic infiltration with flame figures: a distinctive tissue reaction seen in Wells' syndrome and other diseases. *Am. J. Dermatopathol.* **8**, 186–93. [p. 168]

1952. Wood, M. L. and Slater, D. N. (1984). Cutaneous manifestations of the hypereosinophilic syndrome treated with sodium cromoglycate. *Clin. Exp. Dermatol.* **9**, 139–42. [p. 273]

1953. Woodward, D. F., Spada, C. S., Hawley, S. B., and Nieves, A. L. (1986). Conjunctival eosinophil infiltration evoked by histamine and immediate hypersensitivity. Modification by H1- and H2- receptor blockade. *Invest. Ophthalmol. Vis. Sci.* **27**, 1495–503. [p. 219]

1954. Wright, J. L., Pare, P. D., Hammond, M., and Donevan, R. E. (1983). Eosinophilic pneumonia and atypical mycobacterial infection. *Am. Rev. Respir. Dis.* **127**, 497–9. [p. 131]

1955. Wright, R. and Truelove, S. C. (1966). Circulating and tissue eosinophils in ulcerative colitis. *Am. J. Dig. Dis.* **11**, 831–46. [p. 190]

1956. Wulfhekel, U., Dullmann, J., Bartels, H., and Hausmann, K. (1975). (On the ultrastructure and cytochemistry of eosinophil-myelomonocytic leukemias). *Virchows. Arch. (Pathol. Anat.)* **365**, 289–308. [p. 155]

1957. Wykoff, R. F. (1986). Eosinophilia. *South Med. J.* **79**, 608–12. [p. 310]

1958. Wynn, S. R., Sachs, M. I., Keating, M. U., Ostrom, N. K., Kadota, R. P., O'Connell, E. J., and Smithson, W. A. (1987). Idiopathic hypereosinophilic syndrome in a 5½-month-old infant. *J. Pediatr.* **111**, 94–7. [p. 296]

1959. Wysenbeek, A. J., Lahav, M., Aelion, J. A., and Kaufmann, L. (1985). Eosinophilic pleural effusion: a review of 36 cases. *Respiration* **48**, 73–6. [p. 212]

1960. Xipell, J. M., Beamish, M. R., and Clark, D. (1987). Case report 432: granulocytic sarcoma (GS), with hypereosinophilic syndrome (HES). *Skeletal Radiol.* **16**, 425–7. [p. 152]

1961. Yakulis, R. and Bedetti, C. D. (1983). Löffler's endocarditis: occurrence with malignant lymphoma with a high content of epithelioid histiocytes ('Lennert's lymphoma'). *Arch. Pathol. Lab. Med.* **107**, 531–4. [p. 247]

1962. Yam, L. T., Li, C. Y., Necheles, T. F., and Katayama, I. (1972). Pseudoeosinophilia, eosinophilic endocarditis and eosinophilic leukemia. *Am. J. Med.* **53**, 193–202. [p. 153, 233]

1963. Yamada, E. and Yamauchi, R. (1966). Some observations on the cytochemistry and morphogenesis of the granulocytes in the rat bone marrow as revealed by electron microscopy. *Acta Haematol. Jap.* **29**, 530–41. [p. 59]

1964. Yamaguchi, N., Takeuchi, T., Kobayashi, S., Tanabe, M., Miura, S., Asami, K., and Tateno, S. (1984). Health status of Indochinese refugees in Japan: statistical analyses on anemia, eosinophilia and serum alkaline phosphatase. *Southeast Asian J. Trop. Med. Public Health* **15**, 209–16. [p. 136]

1965. Yamashima, T., Kubota, T., and Yamamoto, S. (1985). Eosinophil degranulation in the capsule of chronic subdural hematomas. *J. Neurosurg.* **62**, 257–60. [p. 217]

1966. Yang, L. C., Lee, M. S., Tsai, C. L., Chang, C. C., Lin, Y. N., and Hsu, C. T. (1984). Uterine cervical cancer associated with eosinophilic infiltration. *Asia Oceania J. Obstet. Gynaecol.* **10**, 105–9. [p. 175]

1967. Yang, T. J. and Kennedy, J. R. (1976). Spontaneous eosinophil-erythrocyte rosette formation. *Lab. Invest.* **35**, 302–5. [p. 125]

1968. Yasuoka, S., Nakayama, T., Kawano, T., Ogushi, F., Doi, H., Hayashi, H., and Tsubura, E. (1985). Comparison of cell profiles of bronchial and bronchoalveolar lavage fluids between normal subjects and patients with idiopathic pulmonary fibrosis. *Tohoku J. Exp. Med.* **146**, 33–45. [p. 209]

1969. Yazdanbakhsh, M., Eckmann, C. M., De Boer, M., and Roos, D. (1987). Purification of eosinophils from normal human blood, preparation of eosinoplasts and characterization of their functional response to various stimuli. *Immunology* **60**, 123–9. [p. 34, 68, 92]

1970. Yazdanbakhsh, M., Eckmann, C. M., Koenderman, L., Verhoeven, A. J., and Roos, D. (1987). Eosinophils do respond to fMLP. *Blood* **70**, 379–83. [p. 34]

1971. Yazdanbakhsh, M., Eckmann, C. M., and Roos, D. (1985). Characterization of the interaction of human eosinophils and neutrophils with opsonized particles. *J. Immunol.* **135**, 1378–84. [p. 77, 81]

1972. Yazdanbakhsh, M., Eckmann, C. M., and Roos, D. Mechanism of action of monocyte supernatant on human eosinophil and neutrophil functions (abstract). Presented to the 6th International Congress of Immunology, Toronto, Canada, 1986. [p. 82, 95, 108]

1973. Yazdanbakhsh, M., Tai, P.-C., Spry, C. J., Gleich, G. J., and Roos, D. (1987). Synergism between eosinophil cationic protein and oxygen metabolites in killing of schistosomula of Schistosoma mansoni. *J. Immunol.* **138**, 3443–7. [p. 115]

1974. Yii, C. Y. (1976). Clinical observations on eosinophilic meningitis and meningoencephalitis caused by Angiostrongylus cantonensis on Taiwan. *Am. J. Trop. Med. Hyg.* **25**, 233–49. [p. 139]

1975. Yokota, S., Deimann, W., Hashimoto, T., and Fahimi, H. D. (1983). Immunocytochemical localization of two peroxisomal enzymes of lipid beta-oxidation in specific granules of rat eosinophils. *Histochemistry* **78**, 425–33. [p. 43]

1976. Yokota, S., Deimann, W., Hashimoto, T., and Fahimi, H. D. (1984). Specific granules of rat eosinophils contain peroxisomal acyl-CoA oxidase: possible involvement in production of H_2O_2. *Histochem. J.* **16**, 573–7. [p. 43]

1977. Yokota, S., Tsuji, H., and Kato, K. (1984). Localization of lysosomal and peroxisomal enzymes in the specific granules of rat intestinal eosinophil leukocytes revealed by immunoelectron microscopic techniques. *J. Histochem. Cytochem.* **32**, 267–74. [p. 43]

1978. Yonker, R. A., and Katz, P. (1984). Necrotizing granulomatous vasculitis with eosinophilic infiltrates limited to the prostate: case report and review of the literature. *Am. J. Med.* **77**, 362–4. [p. 224]

1979. Yonker, R. A. and Panush, R. S. (1985). Idiopathic eosinophilic myositis with preexisting fibromyalgia. *J. Rheumatol.* **12**, 165–7. [p. 179]

1980. Yoo, T. J., Orman, S. V., Patil, S. R., Dorminey, C., Needleman, S., Rajtora, D., Graves, N., Ackerman, L., and Taylor, W. W. (1984). Evolution to eosinophilic leukemia with a t(5:11) translocation in a patient with idiopathic hypereosinophilic syndrome. *Cancer Genet. Cytogenet.* **11**, 389–4. [p. 25, 156]

1981. Yoon, I. L. (1959). The eosinophil and gastrointestinal carcinoma. *Am. J. Surg.* **97**, 195–200. [p. 171]

1982. Yoshida, T. and Torisu, M., Eds. (1983). *Immunobiology of the eosinophil.* Elsevier Biomedical, New York. [p. 322]

1983. Yoshimura, K., Uchida, K., Sato, K., and Oya, H. (1984). Ultrastructural evidence for eosinophil-mediated destruction of Angiostrongylus cantonensis transferred into the pulmonary artery of non-permissive hosts. *Parasite Immunol.* **6**, 105–18. [p. 113]

1984. Young, D. K., Burton, M. F., and Herman, J. H. (1986). Multiple cholesterol emboli syndrome simulating systemic necrotizing vasculitis. *J. Rheumatol.* **13**, 423–6. [p. 230]

1985. Young, J. D., Peterson, C. G., Venge, P., and Cohn, Z. A. (1985). How human eosinophil cationic protein damages target membranes. In *Inflammation: basic mechanisms, tissue injurying principles and clinical models* (eds. P. Venge, and A. Lindblom pp. 351–8). Almqvist & Wibsell International, Stockholm, Sweden. [p. 119]

1986. Young, J. D., Peterson, C. G., Venge, P., and Cohn, Z. A. (1986). Mechanism of membrane damage mediated by human eosinophil cationic protein. *Nature* **321**, 613–16. [p. 119, 248]

1987. Young, M., Nuss, R., and Benrubi, G. (1985). Stromal and peripheral eosinophilia in cervical carcinom. *Eur. J. Gynaecol. Oncol.* **6**, 94–7. [p. 174]

1988. Yousem, S. A., Lifson, J. D., and Colby, T. V. (1985). Chemotherapy-induced eosinophilic pneumonia: relation to bleomycin. *Chest* **88**, 103–6. [p. 309]

1989. Yuen, E., Brown, R. D., Kronenberg, H., and Rickard, K. A. (1986). Human bone marrow progenitor cells stimulated by cord blood. *Exp. Hematol.* **14**, 771–5. [p. 294]

1990. Zabucchi, G., Menegazzi, R., Soranzo, M. R., and Patriarca, P. (1986). Uptake of human eosinophil peroxidase by human neutrophils. *Am. J. Pathol.* **124**, 510–18. [p. 60]

1991. Zabucchi, G., Skerlavaj, B., Menegazzi, R., Talarico Bidoli, L., and Patriarca, P. (1985). A simple method to obtain pure granule-rich eosinophil fragments (cytosomes) from normal human blood. *J. Immunol. Methods* **85**, 393–400. [p. 40]

1992. Zain, R., Abdul Hamid, J., and Awang, M. N. (1986). Traumatic granuloma/eosinophilic ulcer. *Ann. Acad. Med. Singapore* **15**, 451–3. [p. 192]

1993. Zeiger, R. S. and Colten, H. R. (1977). Histaminase release from human eosinophils. *J. Immunol.* **118**, 540–3. [p. 82]

1994. Zeiger, R. S., Twarog, F. J., and Colten, H. R. (1976). Histaminase release from human granulocytes. *J. Exp. Med.* **144**, 1049–61. [p. 62]

1995. Zeiger, R. S., Yurdin, D. L., and Colten, H. R., (1976). Histamine metabolism. II. Cellular and subcellular localization of the catabolic enzymes, histaminase and histamine methyl transferase, in human leukocytes. *J. Allergy Clin. Immunol.* **58**, 172–9. [p. 62]

1996. Zheutlin, L. M., Ackerman, S. J., Gleich, G. J., and Thomas, L. L. (1984). Stimulation of basophil and rat mast cell histamine release by eosinophil granule-derived cationic proteins. *J. Immunol.* **133**, 2180–5. [p. 52, 56]

1997. Zheutlin, L. M., Ackerman, S. J., Gleich, G. J., and Thomas, L. L. (1985). Donor sensitivity to basophil activation by eosinophil granule major basic protein. *Int. Arch. Allergy Appl. Immunol.* **77**, 216–17. [p. 48]

1998. Ziltener, H. J., Chavaillaz, P. A., and Jorg, A. (1983). Leukotriene formation by eosinophil leukocytes: analysis with ion-pair high pressure liquid chromatography and effect of the respiratory burst. *Hoppe Seylers Z. Physiol. Chem.* **364**, 1029–37. [p. 70]

1999. Zimmerman, H. J. (1972). Drug induced hepatic injury. In *International encyclopaedia of pharmacology and therapeutics.* 1, *Section 75: Hypersensitivity to drugs.* (eds. M. Samter and C. W. Parker), pp. 299–365. Oxford University Press, Oxford. [p. 310, 311]

2000. Zinkham, W. H. (1978). Visceral larva migrans. A review and reassessment indicating two forms of clinical expressions: visceral and ocular. *Am. J. Dis. Child.* **132**, 627–33. [p. 140]

2001. Zinkl, J. G. (1981). The leukocytes. *Vet. Clin. North Am. (Small Anim. Pract.)* **11**, 237–63. [p. 125]

2002. Zittoun, J., Farcet, J. P., Marquet, J., Sultan, C., and Zittoun, R. (1984). Cobalamin (vitamin B12) and B12 binding proteins in hypereosinophilic syndromes and secondary eosinophilia. *Blood* **63**, 779–83. [p. 62, 284]

2003. Zola, H., McNamara, P., Thomas, M., Smart, I. J., and Bradley, J. (1981). The preparation and properties of monoclonal antibodies against human granulocyte membrane antigens. *Br. J. Haematol.* **48**, 481–90. [p. 87]

2004. Zolov, D. M. and Levine, B. B. (1969). Correlation of blood eosinophilia with antibody classes: studies with the penicillin hypersensitivity system. *Int. Arch. Allergy Appl. Immunol.* **35**, 179–93. [p. 312]

2005. Zsebo, K. M., Cohen, A. M., Murdock, D. C., Boone, T. C., Inoue, H., Chazin, V. R., Hines, D., and Souza, L. M. (1986). Recombinant human granulocyte colony stimulating factor: molecular and biological characterization. *Immunobiology* **172**, 175–84. [p. 21]

2006. Zucker-Franklin, D. (1978). Eosinophil function related to cutaneous disorders. *J. Invest. Dermatol.* **71**, 100–5. [p. 297, 323]

2007. Zucker-Franklin, D. (1980). Eosinophil structure and maturation. In *The eosinophil in health and disease* (eds. A. A. Mahmoud, K. F. Austen, and A. S. Simon) pp. 43–59. Grune and Stratton, New York. [p. 13, 15, 44, 65, 125]

2008. Zucker-Franklin, D. (1981). Eosinophils. In *Atlas of blood cells: functions and pathology* (eds. D. Zucker-Franklin, M. F. Greaves, C. E. Grossi, and A. M. Marmont). pp. 255–84. [p. 324]

2009. Zucker-Franklin, D., Davidson, M., and Thomas, L. (1966). The interaction of mycoplasmas with mammalian cells. I. HeLa cells, neutrophils and eosinophils. *J. Exp. Med.* **124**, 521–31. [p. 89, 111]

2010. Zulian M., Bellome, J., and Deboom, G. W. (1987). Multiple linear ulcers on the dorsum of the tongue in a patient with Waldenström's macroglobulinemia. *J. Am. Dent. Assoc.* **114**, 79–80. [p. 192]

2011. (1977). What eosinophils do (editorial). *Lancet* **ii**, 388–9. [p. 315]

2012. (1977). Histiocytosis X (eosinophilic granuloma) (editorial). *Lancet* **ii**, 440–1. [p. 164]

2013. (1980). Case records of the Massachusetts General Hospital. Weekly clinicopathological exercises. Case 18–1980. *N. Engl. J. Med.* **302**, 456–60. [p. 165]

2014. (1980). Case records of the Massachusetts General Hospital. Weekly clinicopathological exercise. Case 18–1980. *N. Engl. J. Med.* **302**, 1077–83. [p. 237]

2015. (1981). Löffler's eosinophilic endocarditis (editorial). *Lancet* **ii**, 1028–9. [p. 246]

2016. (1983). Eosinophilia, heart failure, and adenopathy in a black man (clinical conference). *Am. J. Med.* **74**, 887–97. [p. 270]

2017. (1986). Case records of the Massachusetts General Hospital. Weekly clinicopathological exercises. Case 8–1986. A 39-year-old woman with bilateral pulmonary infiltrates. *N. Engl. J. Med.* **314**, 564–74. [p. 210]

2018. (1986). Case records of the Massachusetts General Hospital. Weekly clinicopathological exercises. Case 30–1986. A 74-year-old man with azotemia, eosinophilia, and peripheral cyanosis and mottling. *N. Engl. J. Med.* **315**, 308–15. [p. 224]

2019. (1987). Case records of the Massachusetts General Hospital. Weekly clinicopathological exercises. Case 47–1987: A 79-year-old cuban native with asthma, weight loss, vomiting, eosinophilia, and past meningitis. *N. Engl. J. Med.* **317**, 1332–42. [p. 145]

Index

A23187, *see* calcium ionophore A23187
abdominal eosinophilic pseudotumours 187
absence of eosinophils 315–6
  with thymoma 24, 316
acid phosphatase 43, 44, 57, 60–1, 126, 282
  masked, and unmasked 44, 60–1
Ackerman, Stephen and eosinophil research 54, 320
acquired immunodeficiency syndrome (AIDS) and eosinophils 135
  interleukin 2 treated eosinopoietic factors in serum 23–4
acquired platelet dysfunction with eosinophilia 262
acropustulosis and eosinophils 302
actinomycetales infections and eosinophils 131
actions of
  Charcot–Leyden crystal, and crystal protein 65
  eosinophil cationic protein 51
  eosinophil major basis protein 47
  eosinophil peroxidase 59
  eosinophil-derived neurotoxin/eosinophil protein-X 55
activation of eosinophils 103–11, *Fig. 5.1*
  activated eosinophils
    in asthma 199
    Churg-Strauss syndrome 203, *Plate 12*
    idiopathic hypereosinophilic syndrome 283
    in eosinophil endomyocardial fibrosis 248
    metabolism of 67
    oestrogen binding to 67
  eosinophil activating factors 105–11, *Fig. 6.2*
    actions on eosinophils 110–11
    endogenous factors, 106–10
      colony stimulating factors 108–9
      from endothelial cells 109
      platelet activating factor 109
      substance P 109
      T-lymphocyte-derived factors 107–8
      β-interferon 109
      interleukin 1, 3, and 5 19, 109–10
      mast-cell-, and basophil-derived factors 108
      mononuclear-cell-derived factors 107–8
    exogenous factors 110
      parasite-derived factors 110
    induction of leukotriene secretion 71
  assays for 103, *Plates 3, 4, 6, 7, 12*
  history 104
  in vivo studies 104–5
acute eosinophilic leukaemia, *see* eosinophilic leukaemia
acute nonlymphocytic leukaemia, *see* myeloblastic leukaemia
Adams' stain for eosinophils 38
Addison's disease and eosinophils 306
adenosine diphosphate (ADP) release from platelets
  in acquired platelet dysfunction with eosinophilia 262
adenosine triphosphate (ATP) synthesis in heart cells damaged by eosinophil secretion products 248
adenylate cyclase and eosinophil leukotriene synthesis 71
adult respiratory distress syndrome (ARDS) and eosinophil cationic protein 211
adults
  normal blood eosinophil counts 31
  with eosinophilic leukaemia 154–5
Africa, cardiac surgery for tropical endomyocardial fibrosis 254
agar colony cultures
  assays for eosinopoietic factors 15–6
  colonies of eosinophils and basophils 12
  in chronic eosinophilic leukaemia 156–7
  drugs inhibiting 16
  history 8
  normal findings 15
  stains for eosinophil colonies 15
  types of colony formed 15
age at presentation of idiopathic hypereosinophilic syndrome 268
AIDS, *see* acquired immunodeficiency syndrome
alcohol intolerance in idiopathic hypereosinophilic syndrome 270–1

alkaline phosphatase
absence in human eosinophil granules 43
presence in American alligator eosinophils 127
ALL, *see* lymphocytic leukaemia
allergic bronchopulmonary aspergillosis 133
allergic gastroenteritis and eosinophils 188–9
allergic granulomatosis and angiitis, *see* Churg–Strauss syndrome
allergic proctitis and eosinophils 189
allergic rhinitis and eosinophils 68
allergy to
cow's milk and eosinophils 188–9
soy protein and eosinophils 188–9
alligator, eosinophils in 127
3-amino-1,2,4-triazole inhibition of eosinophil peroxidase 59
ammonium chloride lysis of red cells 32
amoebiasis and eosinophils 148
entamoeba 148
naegleria 148
amphibia, eosinophils in 124
Amplictacum robertsi complexes degranulating rat eosinophils 80
anaphylatoxins C3a, and C5a binding, and receptors on eosinophils 82
ancylostomiasis and eosinophils 143–4
Ancylostoma braziliense, and *A. ceylanicum* infections 144
angioedema, *see* episodic angioedema
angiogenin relationship with eosinophil ribonucleases 51
angiography, fluorescent retinal 275
angioimmunoblastic lymphadenopathy and eosinophils 163
angiolymphoid hyperplasia with eosinophilia 167–9
angiostrongyliasis and eosinophils 138–9
Angiostrongylus cantonensis 113, 138
A. costaricensis 138
aniline blue for staining eosinophils 38
animal models of
conjunctival diseases with eosinophilia 219
endomyocardial fibrosis 257
idiopathic hypereosinophilic syndrome 267–8
animals
eosinophil major basis protein in 46
eosinophil peroxidase in 58
eosinophils in 123–7
with solid neoplasms and eosinophilia 175
ankylosing spondylitis and eosinophils 179
anthrax bacilli degranulation of frog eosinophils 90
anthropoidea, eosinophil in 126
anti-platelet drugs in the treatment of idiopathic hypereosinophilic syndrome 288
antibodies, monoclonal, *see* monoclonal antibodies
antibodies, polyclonal to
antigens in plasma membrane of eosinophils 84–5
guinea pig eosinophils 84
human eosinophils 85
mouse eosinophils 84
anticoagulants in
idiopathic hypereosinophilic syndrome 291–2
eosinophilic endomyocardial fibrosis 242
antigen presentation by eosinophils 88
antigens in plasma membrane of eosinophils 84–5, *Fig. 4.2*
antineoplastic drugs
drug hypersensitivity, reactions to 310
treatment of idiopathic hypereosinophilic syndrome 291
antinuclear antibodies to fixed eosinophils 40
disease occurrence 41
antiplatelet drug treatment of
eosinophilic endomyocardial fibrosis 242
idiopathic hypereosinophilic syndrome 291–2
appendicitis in strongyloidiasis 146
arachidonic acid metabolism by eosinophils 69–72
and glucose metabolism 67
and lipid bodies 42
Archer, G.T. and eosinophil research 6, 57, 60, 64, 80
Archer, R.K. and eosinophil research 6
arterial diseases, *see* vascular diseases
arteritis and eosinophils 230–1
polyarteritis nodosa 231
spontaneous dissection of the coronary artery 231
temporal arteritis 231
Wegener's granulomatosis 231
arthritic diseases, *see* musculo-skeletal diseases
artiodactyla, eosinophil in 125
arylsulphatase B in eosinophils 61
localization in
blood eosinophils 44
marrow eosinophils 57
small granules 43
secretion from 82, 92
ascariasis and eosinophils 139–40
toxocariasis 139
visceral larva migrans 139

ascites, *see* eosinophilic ascites
aspergillosis and eosinophils 132–3, 214
aspirin
  asthma and eosinophils 202
  drug hypersensitivity reactions to 310, 311
  treatment of
    eosinophilic endomyocardial fibrosis 242
    idiopathic hypereosinophilic syndrome 292
assays for
  Charcot–Leyden crystal protein 65
  eosinophil activation 103
  eosinophil cationic protein 50
  eosinophil major basic protein 46
  eosinophil peroxidase 58
  eosinophil-derived neurotoxin/eosinophil protein-X 54
  eosinopoietic factors 14–17
    agar colony cultures 15–16
    in vivo techniques 17
    liquid culture of bone marrow 16–17
  phospholipases in rodent tissues 29
asthma and eosinophils 195–202, *Fig. 15.1*
  activated eosinophils in lavage fluid 199
  aspirin-induced 202
  blood eosinophils 80, 197–8
  bronchial challenge 200
  bronchoalveolar lavage eosinophils 199–200
  Charcot-Leyden crystal protein in sputum 199
  eosinophil cationic protein levels in serum 198
  eosinophil-derived neurotoxin/eosinophil protein–X in serum 198
  eosinophil major basic protein in lung tissues 197
  eosinophil major basis protein in sputum 199
  histopathology 197
  history 5
  importance of leukotriene secretion 71
  intrinsic asthma 202
  sputum eosinophils 198–9
  tissue injury in 117–18
  with parasitic diseases 201–2
atherosclerosis and eosinophils 230
atopic dermatitis and eosinophils 298
atopic eczema 117
Austen, K. Frank and eosinophil research 6, 320
autofluorescence of eosinophils 37
autoimmune diseases and eosinophils 306

B_{12} in eosinophils, *see* vitamin B_{12}
babies, *see* infants
baboons 126, 147
bacterial endocarditis in eosinophilic endomyocardial fibrosis 277
bacterial infections and eosinophils 131–2
  actinomycetales infections 131
  chlamydial infections 132
  enterobacteriaceae infections 131
  staphylococcal infections 132
  streptococcal infections 132
BAL, *see* bronchoalveolar lavage
Balint's syndrome 274
Bancroftian filariasis 142
  blood eosinophils in 142
    arylsulphatase content after treatment 61
  serum levels of eosinophil granule proteins 142
basic orcein staining of eosinophils 38
basic proteins in cytotoxicity by eosinophils, and neutrophils 119
basophil granules
  in eosinophils in chronic myelocytic leukaemia 11
basophils 86
  Charcot–Leyden crystal protein content 45
  common origins with eosinophils 11–12
  eosinophil activating factors from 108
  eosinophil cationic protein actions on 52
  eosinophil major basic protein actions on 48
  eosinophil major basic protein content 45
  eosinophil peroxidase content 45
  eosinophil-derived neurotoxin/eosinophil protein-X actions on 56
Bass, David and eosinophil research 60, 321, 322
Basten, Anthony and T-lymphocytes in eosinopoiesis 7, 313
Baylisascaris procyonis cause of visceral larva migrans 139
B-cell growth factor II, *see* interleukin 5
Beeson, Paul and eosinophil research, forward 7, 137, 313, 321, 322
ϱ-benzoquinone inhibition of nonspecific eosinophil fluorescent staining 37
betamethasone inhibition of eosinophil secretion 95
Biebrich scarlet for staining eosinophils 38
biliary tract diseases, *see* liver and biliary tract diseases
biochemistry of eosinophils *see* constituents, metabolism, etc.
biopsy, cardiac in
  eosinophilic endomyocardial fibrosis 241–2

biopsy, cardiac in (*cont.*)
  pathogenesis of
    eosinophilic endomyocardial fibrosis 247
    tropical endomyocardial fibrosis 252–3
biosynthesis of
  Charcot–Leyden crystal protein 63
  eosinophil cationic protein 48
  eosinophil peroxidase 57
  ^{14}C-leucine pulse chase 48, 57
birds, eosinophils in 124
bladder neoplasms and eosinophils 175
blood diseases and eosinophils 259–62
  acquired platelet dysfunction with eosinophilia 262
  cyclical haematopoiesis 261
  Fanconi's anaemia 261
  inherited diseases 259–61
  see also idiopathic hypereosinophilic syndrome
blood eosinophil counts
  automated methods 30
  in cord blood 294
  differential counts 5
  diurnal variations 31
  and eosinophil numbers in tissues 5
  and exercise 31
  highest recorded 3
  history 5
  hypotonic solutions in 5
  manual methods 30
  in normal
    adults 31
    animals 123
    children 31
    ethnic groups 31
    infants 294
    neonates 294
    premature infants 294
  and pathogenesis of tropical endomyocardial fibrosis 256
  reduced in infections 28
blood eosinophilia non-allergic rhinitis syndrome (BENAR) 214
blood eosinophils
  constituents 40–66
  content of eosinophil major basic protein 45
  counts in normal people 29
  culture 35
  density 32
  electronmiscroscopy, transmission 38–40
  fractionation 40
  kinetics 27–8
    measured with ^{111}In-labelled blood eosinophils 284
  morphology 38–40
  separation 32–5
  stains 36
blood eosinophils in idiopathic hypereosinophilic syndrome 278–84, *Plates 5, 10*
  activation 283, *Plates 4, 5*
  chemotaxis 282–3
  cytotoxicity 283
  density 279
  granule constituents 281–2
  kinetics 284
  metabolism 282
  morphology 279–81, *Plates 1, 5*
  motility 282–3
  plasma membrane components 281
  secretion 283
blood transfusion, *see* exchange blood transfusion
blood vessel diseases, *see* vascular diseases
bone diseases and eosinophils 176
bone lesions in acute eosinophilic leukaemia 152
bone marrow
  eosinophil differentiation in 12
  eosinophil kinetics in man 14
  eosinophil kinetics in rats 14
bone marrow eosinophils 10–13
  density 16
  history 4, 5
  in idiopathic hypereosinophilic syndrome 284–6
    culture 285–6
    cytogenetic studies 286
    fibrosis in 285
    transplantation in idiopathic hypereosinophilic syndrome 293
  morphology 12–13
  receptors for immunoglobulin G 77
  stains 36–8
  see also eosinopoiesis
bone neoplasms and eosinophils 170
books on eosinophils 322
brain, *see* central nervous system
breast
  disease in idiopathic hypereosinophilic syndrome 277
  neoplasms and eosinophils 170
Breinlia booliati and tropical (filarial) eosinophilia 141
bronchial challenge in asthma 200–1
bronchial diseases and eosinophils 195–204
  acute, and chronic bronchitis 204
  asthma 195–202
  Churg–Strauss syndrome 202–3
  respiratory hypersensitivity 204
bronchitis and eosinophils 204

bronchoalveolar lavage fluid eosinophils 194–5
in asthma
eosinophil major basic protein levels in 199–200
in eosinophilic pneumonia 207–8
light density eosinophils 34
immunoglobulin E binding 80
in tropical (filarial) eosinophilia 141
Brugia pahangi and tropical (filarial) eosinophilia 141
buffalos, eosinophils in 125
bullous skin diseases and eosinophils 302–3
bullous pemphigoid 303
fluid
GM-CSF-like activity in 22
induction of eosinophil autofluorescence 37
dermatitis herpetiformis 303
linear IgA disease 303
Butterworth, Anthony and eosinophil research, 8, 107, 319

Clq, C3a, C3b, C3d, C5a *see* complement
caecal neoplasms *see* large intestinal neoplasms
calcium
content of stimulated eosinophils 95
requirement for secretion by eosinophils 94
hypercalcaemia in eosinophilic leukaemia 152
calcium ionophore A23187 effects on eosinophils
acid phosphatase staining 61
leukotriene synthesis 68, 70, 282
platelet activating factor synthesis 72
plasma membrane freeze-fracture appearances 75
prostaglandin, and thromboxane synthesis 71
protein phosphorylation 110
secretion 93, 94, 283
cancers, *see* neoplasms
Candida albicans endocytosis by eosinophils 89
Capillaria infections and eosinophils 144
Capron, Monique and eosinophil research 79, 318
carbohydrates in plasma membrane of eosinophils 83–4
carbohydrates in eosinophils 72
carbol chromotrope staining of eosinophils 37
carcinomas, *see* neoplasms
Cardbox-Plus reference database 321
cardiac allograft rejection and eosinophils 229
cardiac biopsy *see* biopsy, cardiac
cardiac catheterization *see* catheterization, cardiac
cardiac neoplasms and eosinophils 170
cardiac rupture after myocardial infarction, eosinophils in 229
cardiac surgery for
eosinophihlic endomyocardial fibrosis 243–5, *Plate 9*
in Europe 244
in USA 244
tropical endomyocardial fibrosis 253–5
in Africa 254
in Europe 254
in India 254–5
in South America 255
cardiac tissue susceptability to injury, in eosinophilic endomyocardial fibrosis 245, 249
cardiomyopathy, dilated and eosinophils, serum levels of eosinophil cationic protein 230
cardiovascular diseases and eosinophils 228–31
heart diseases 229–30
in idiopathic hypereosinophilic syndrome 271
pericardial diseases 228–9
vascular diseases 230
vasculitis 230–1
see also endomyocardial fibrosis, and heart disease
carnivora, eosinophils in 125
carp, eosinophils in 124
catalase
detection in eosinophils 62
detoxification of reactive oxygen products 119
differences from eosinophil peroxidase 58,
catheterization, cardiac of
eosinophilic endomyocardial fibrosis 240–1
tropical endomyocardial fibrosis 252
angiocardiography 252, 257
cationic protein *see* eosinophil cationic protein
cation resin exchange chromatography 51
cats
eosinophils in 125
eosinophils leukaemia in 157
eosinophilic enterocolitis in 190
idiopathic hypereosinophilic syndrome in 268
peroxidase staining in 123, 259

cattle
eosinophils in 125
eosinophilic myositis in 180
CD, *see* cluster of differentiation
cell fractionation, *see* fractionation
cell lines
A549 (human type 11 pneumocytes) 117
cat alveolar cell line AK-D 118
cytotoxicity by eosinophils 118
eosinophil 26–7
from eosinophilic leukaemia 27
EoL 25, 26–7
from HL-60 cell lines 26–7
eosinopoietic factors from 22–3
ESH 98, 107,
U 937 107
human lung fibroblasts HFL-1 118
cell mediated drug hypersensitivity reactions with eosinophilia 313
cell membrane, *see* plasma membrane
cell surface change on eosinophils 74
central nervous system diseases and eosinophils 216–17
cerebrospinal fluid eosinophils 216–17
eosinophil cationic protein actions on 52
eosinophil-derived neurotoxin/eosinophil protein-X action 55
in idiopathic hypereosinophilic syndrome 274–5
meningitis 217
neoplasms and eosinophils 172–3
subdural haematomas 217
cerebrospinal fluid (CSF) eosinophils 216–17
cervical neoplasms and eosinophils 174–5
cestode infections and eosinophils 137–8
cysticercosis 138
and eosinophilic meningitis 216
echinococcosis 137
and eosinophilic meningitis 216
taeniasis 138
CFUc, *see* progenitor cells
Chagas' heart disease 251
Charcot–Leyden crystal protein 63–6
actions on
lysophospholipids 66
parasites 66
assays 65
in basophils 45
biosynthesis 63
in eosinophils 63
content 65, 66
localization in eosinophils 65
lysophospholipase activity 65–6
plasma and serum levels 65
in Bancroftian filariasis 142
purification 63
secretion from dividing eosinophils 13
sputum levels of
in asthma 199
structure 63–4
Charcot–Leyden crystals 64–5
in separated eosinophils 32
Chediak–Higashi syndrome and eosinophils 260–1
chemokinesis of
eosinophils 96
light density eosinophils 101
chemoluminescence
by eosinophils 67, 68–9
by light density eosinophils 37–8, 68
chemotactic factors for eosinophils 99–102
complement components 101
histamine 99–100
history 7
leukotrienes 101
leukotriene B4 97
from lymphocytes 100
from macrophages 101–2
from mast cells 99–100; *see also* eosinophil chemotactic factor(s) of anaphylaxis (ECF-A)
from neoplasms 101
Kimura's disease 168
from parasites 100
platelet activating factor 97, 100–1
in serum 102
asthma 102
cold urticaria 102
eosinophilic fasciitis 102
in skin diseases 102
incontinentia pigmenti 304
chemotactic factors receptors in plasma membrane of eosinophils 83
chemotaxis of eosinophils 98–102
Boyden chamber technique 98
critical remarks 96
history 96
in idiopathic hypereosinophilic syndrome 282–3
light density eosinophils 101, 283
chest diseases, *see* respiratory tract diseases
chickens, eosinophils in 124
children
eosinophilic endomyocardial fibrosis in 236
eosinophilic leukaemia in 152
idiopathic hypereosinophilic syndrome in 268–70
normal blood eosinophil counts 31
chlamydial infections and eosinophils 132
chloradenosine inhibition of eosinophil secretion 95
Chlorazol black E stain for eosinophils 38

chlorpromazine inhibition of eosinophil secretion 95
cholesterol emboli syndrome and eosinophils 230
chondroitin 4-, and 6-sulphate in eosinophils 73
chromosome 5
and eosinopoiesis 25
in eosinophilic leukaemias 25
localization of genes for interleukins, and colony stimulating factors 25
chromosome 7
and eosinopoiesis 25
in eosinophilic leukaemias 25
chromosome 8
and eosinopoiesis 25
in eosinophilic leukaemias 25
chromosome 8:21 translocation in myeloblastic leukaemia (M4Eo) 159
chromosome 12
and eosinopoiesis 25, 266
in eosinophilic leukaemias 25
chromosome 16
abnormalities in myeloblastic leukaemia (M4Eo) 158
and eosinopoiesis 26
in eosinophilic leukaemias 26
chromotrope 2R for staining eosinophils 37
chronic eosinophilic leukaemia *see* eosinophilic leukaemia
chronic eosinophilic pneumonia 64, 80 206–9
blood eosinophil counts 207
bronchoalveolar lavage 207–8
clinical features 206–7
drug therapy 208–9
electronmicroscopy, transmission 208
eosinophil major basic protein 208
and eosinophil endomyocardial fibrosis 237
histopathology 208
pulmonary function tests 207
radiological investigation of the chest 207
chronic ganulomatous disease (CGD), eosinophils in 261
with defective parasite killing 119
chronic inflammatory bowel diseases, *see* individual diseases
chronic lymphocytic choriomeningitis with eosinophils 216
chronic myelocytic leukaemia 159
eosinophils used to make antisera 85
eosinopoietic factors in serum 23
with basophilia, and eosinophils in tissues 12
cells containing basophilic and eosinophilic granules 11
Churg–Strauss syndrome and eosinophils 80, 202–3, 237
cardiac complications in 203, *Plate 12*
clinical features 202–3
treatment 203
CLC, *see* Charcot–Leyden crystal
cluster of differentiation 9 (CD9) 86
CML, *see* chronic myelocytic leukaemia
coagulation
eosinophil cationic protein actions on 53
eosinophil major basic protein actions on 48
coagulation factor XII 53
studies in eosinophilic endomyocardial fibrosis 247–8
idiopathic hypereosinophilic syndrome 286–7
cobalt in eosinophils 63
coccidioidomycosis and eosinophils 133
coeliac disease and eosinophils 188
cocaine and eosinophils 204
collagenases in eosinophils 61
digestion of collagen types 1, and 3 61
Colley, Daniel and eosinophil research 100, 104, 114, 320
colonic diseases and eosinophils 189–90
eosinophilic gastroenteritis 185
neoplasms 171–2
ulcerative colitis 189–90
colony stimulating factors (CSFs), 17–18, 20–4
as eosinophil activating factors 108–9
colony stimulating factor α (CSF-α); *see* granulocyte-macrophage colony stimulating factor
colony stimulating factor β (CSF–β) 108–9; *see also* granulocyte colony stimulating factor effects on tissue cultures of mature eosinophils 35–6
in idopathic hypereosinophilic syndrome 286
multi-colony stimulating factor (M-CSF), 22; *see also* interleukin 3
complement
activation products and eosinophil secretion 92
coated particles 93
chemotactic factors 101
eosinophil cationic protein actions on 53
eosinophil major basic protein actions on 48
complement receptors (CR) in plasma membrane of eosinophils 75, 81–3, *Plate 1*
recycling of 76

complexes, *see* immune complexes
components in eosinophils, *see* constituents
concanavalin A (con A),
 binding sites on eosinophil plasma membrane 83–4
 stimulation of eosinophil secretion 93
Congo red staining of eosinophils 38
conjunctival diseases and eosinophils 218–19
conjunctival epithelium 97
constituents in eosinophils 40–66
 acid phosphatases 60
 arylsulphatase B 61
 arylsulphatases 61
 catalase 62
 Charcot–Leyden crystal protein 63
 collagenases 61
 cytoplasm 41
 cytoplasmic granules 42
 elastase 61
 eosinophil cationic protein 48
 eosinophil eosinophil-derived neurotoxin/eosinophil 53
 eosinophil major basic protein 45
 eosinophil peroxidase 57
 fibroblast growth factors 62
 glycosaminoglycans 63
 Golgi apparatus 42, *Fig. 3.2*
 in idiopathic hypereosinophilic syndrome 281–2
 lysosomal enzymes 60
 metals 63
 mitochondria 42
 nicotinamide–adenine dinucleotide phosphate (NADPH) oxidase 67
 nonspecific esterase 62
 nucleus 40
 phosphatases 60
 phospholipases B, and D 62
 proteases 61
 respiratory chain 69
 vitamin B_{12} binding proteins 62
constrictive pericarditis and eosinophils 228
content in eosinophils of
 Charcot–Leyden crystal protein 65
 eosinophil cationic protein 50
 eosinophil major basic protein 46, 47
 eosinophil peroxidase 59
 eosinophil-derived neurotoxin/eosinophil protein-X 55
continuous ambulatory peritoneal dialysis (CAPD) and eosinophils 222
copper in eosinophils 63
cord blood, normal blood eosinophil counts 294
corneal diseases and eosinophils 219
coronary heart disease and eosinophils 229
 spontaneous dissection of 231
Corynaebacterium pseudotuberculosis and eosinophils 131
coughing attacks in idiopathic hypereosinophilic syndrome 272
counting eosinophils, *see* methods, blood eosinophil counts
coxackie B meningitis with eosinophils in cerebrospinal fluid 135, 216
CR, *see* complement receptor
cricetidae, eosinophils in 126
Crohn's disease and eosinophils 117, 189
cromoglycate, sodium, *see* sodium cromoglycate
cryptococcosis and eosinophils 134
cryptogenic pulmonary fibrosis and eosinophils 209
crystalloid granules
 absence of crystalloids in some animals 124
 in eosinophil cytoplasm 43
 inclusion abnormality in eosinophils 261
 relationship to small granules 44
CSF, *see* colony stimulating factor, or cerebrospinal fluid
culture, *see* tissue culture
Curvularia lunata and eosinophils 133, 214
cyanide inhibition of eosinophil peroxidase 59
cyclical haematopoiesis and eosinophils 261
cyclo-oxygenase pathway inhibitors 202
cyclophosphamide effects on eosinopoiesis 24
cynomologus monkeys, eosinophil major basic protein in pregnancy 227
cysticercosis
 and eosinophils 138
 and eosinophilic meningitis 216
cystitis, *see* eosinophilic cystitis, and interstitial cystitis
cytarabine treatment of idiopathic hypereosinophilic syndrome 291
cytocentrifuge preparations and eosinophil morphology 37
cytochalasin-B inhibition of eosinophil secretion 62
cytochrome b-245 in eosinophil plasma membrane 69
cytogenetic studies
 and eosinopoiesis 25–6
 in acute eosinophilic leukaemia 155–6
 in chronic eosinophilic leukaemia 157
 in idiopathic hypereosinophilic syndrome 286
 in myeloblastic leukaemia (M4Eo) 158–9
cytokines, *see* interleukins

cytoplasmic constituents in eosinophils 41–66
  lipid bodies 41–2
  ribonucleic acid 42
cytoplasmic granules in eosinophils 42–5, *Figs 3.2, 3.3, 3.4*
  comparison with basophil, neutrophil, and mast cell granules 44–5
  crystalloid granules 43
  microgranules 44
  small granules 43–4
  organization of 41
  solubilization 94
cytoplasmic projections from eosinophils 74
cytoplasmic vacuoles in eosinophils 94
  in filariasis 142
  in histoplasmosis 133
  in idiopathic hypereosinophilic syndrome 279–80, *Plates 4, 5*
cytoplasts from eosinophils 68
cytotoxicity by eosinophils 111–21, *Fig. 6.3*
  in chronic granulomatous disease 119
  effector mechanism 118–20
  in eosinophilic endomyocardial fibrosis 246, 248
  factors increasing 120–1
  history 6, 8
  in idiopathic hypereosinophilic syndrome 283
  mammalian cells 117
  parasites 112–17
    filaria 116
    giardia 116
    leishmania 116
    malaria parasites 116–17
    Schistosoma mansoni 113–15
      eggs 114
      schistosomula 80, 113–15
    trichinella 115–16
    trypanosomes 116

dapsone and eosinophil secretion 95
database of references vii, 321
David, John and eosinophil research 105, 107, 320
deer, eosinophils in 125
defensins in neutrophils 119
Demodex brevis, and *D. folliculorum* and eosinophils 149
density gradient separation of eosinophils 33–5
  light density eosinophils in 34–5
  metrizamide method 33, *Fig. 3.1*
  Percoll methods 33–4
density of
  eosinophil granules 43
  blood eosinophils
    normal 32
    in idiopathic hypereosinophilic syndrome 279
^{3}H 2-deoxyglucose transport into eosinophils 67
deoxyribonuclease (DNAase) in eosinophil separation 33
deoxyribonucleic acid viruses and eosinophils 135
dermatan sulphate in eosinophils 73
dermatitis and eosinophils 297–9
  atopic dermatitis 298–9
  urticaria 299
dermatitis herpetiformis and eosinophils 303
dermatological diseases, *see* skin diseases
DeSimone, C. and eosinophil research 318
development of eosinophils, *see* differentiation of eosinophils
dexamethasone inhibition of eosinophil secretion 95
dextran in eosinophil separation 32
diabetes mellitus, eosinophils in the pancreas 306
dialysis, *see* renal dialysis
diamine oxidase, *see* histaminases
diarrhoea in idiopathic hypereosinophilic syndrome 273
diethylcarbamazine (DEC) treatment, and eosinophils in
  loiasis 257
  onchocerciasis 116, 143
  tropical (filarial) eosinophilia 141
  Mazzotti reaction 142
differential binding to surfaces
  for separation of eosinophils 32
differentiation of eosinophils 12–13
  electronmicroscopy of 12–13
digestive system diseases and eosinophils 183–91
  abdominal pseudotumours 187
  inflammatory fibroid polyps 186–7
  colonic diseases 189–90
  Crohn's disease 117, 189
  enteritis, and enterocolitis 188–9
  eosinophilic gastroenteritis 184–6
  idiopathic hypereosinophilic syndrome 272–3
  liver, and biliary tract diseases 190–1
  neoplasms and eosinophils 171–2
  oesophageal diseases 183–4
  pancreatic diseases 191
  peptic ulcers 184
  rectal diseases 190
  stomach diseases 184

ϱ-dimethylaminobenzaldehyde-nitrite staining of eosinophils 38
Diphyllobothrium and eosinophils 137
Dipylidium and eosinophils 137
dipyridamole treatment of idiopathic hypereosinophilic syndrome 242, 292
dirofilariasis and eosinophils 142
disease associations in
  eosinophilic endomyocardial fibrosis 246–7
    negative associations 248
    tropical endomyocardial fibrosis 255–7
    idiopathic hypereosinophilic syndrome 266
disodium cromoglycate inhibition of eosinophil
  complement receptors 82
  secretion 95
diurnal variations in blood eosinophil counts 31
DNA, *see* deoxyribonucleic acid
dogs
  blood eosinophils 125
  chronic myeloid leukaemia with eosinophilia 157
  eosinophilic enterocolitis 190
  epsonophilic myositis 180
  idiopathic hypereosinophilic syndrome 268
  solid tumours 175
Down's syndrome, eosinophil nuclear segmentation 295
drug effects on
  eosinophil secretion 95
  eosinopoiesis 24
drug hypersensitivity reactions and eosinophils 88, 306–14, *Fig. 29.1*
  clinical features 307–10
  drugs involved 310
    allopurinol 308, 309, 310, 311, 313
    ϱ-aminosalicyclic acid 309
    amoxicillin 310
    amphotericin B 309
    ampicillin 309, 310
    anti-inflammatory drugs 310
    antibiotics 308, 310
    anticoagulants 310
    antifungal agents 308
    antineoplastic drugs 310
    antituberculous drugs 313
    aspirin 310, 311
    aurothiomalate 307, 312
    azathioprine 309
    barbiturate 308
    bleomycin 309
    capreomycin sulphate 309
    carbamazepine 309, 310, 313
    cephalosporin 309, 310
    cephalothin 312
    chlorophenindione 310
    chlorpropamide 309, 310
    cimetidine 309
    sodium cromoglycate (cromolyn sodium), 309, 313
    dacarbazine 310
    fungicides 310
    gentamycin 217
    hydantoin groups of compounds 308
    hypoglycaemic agents 310
    isoniazid 309
    mephenesin 309
    methicillin 309
    methotrexate 309
    naproxen 309
    neoarsphenamine 237
    nitrofurantoin 309, 312, 313
    non-steroidal anti-inflammatory drugs 309
    paraaminosalicylic acid 309
    penicillins 308, 309, 310, 311, 312
    phenindione 310
    phenothiazines 310
    phenylbutazone 309
    phenytoin 308, 309, 310, 313
    potassium iodide 310
    radiographic contrast media 310
    rifampicin 269, 309
    streptomycin 237
    sulphasalazine 309
    sulphisalazole 292
    sulphonamides 309, 311
    tartrazine 311
    tolbutamide 310, 309
  pathogenesis of, 311–14
  roles of eosinophils in 314
  susceptibility to 310–11
  with heart involvement 309
  with kidney involvement 309
  with liver involvement 310
  with lung involvement 309
  with skin involvement 308–9
drug therapy of
  acute eosinophilic leukaemia 156
  eosinophilic pneumonia 208
  eosinophilic endomyocardial fibrosis 242–3
    anticoagulants 242
    antiplatelet drugs 242
    steroids 242–3
ducks, eosinophils in 124
duodenal ulcer, *see* peptic ulcer
Durack, David and eosinophil research 54

EAF, *see* eosinophil activating factor
ear, nose, and throat diseases and eosinophils 213–15
  neoplasms and eosinophils 173
Ebstein's anomaly compared with tropical endomyocardial fibrosis 250–1
ECEA (eosinophil cytotoxicity enhancing activity) 107, 120
ECEF (eosinophil cytotoxicity enhancing factor) 71
ECF-A *see* eosinophil chemotactic factor of anaphylaxis
echinococcosis and eosinophils 137, 191
echocardiograms
  in eosinophilic endomyocardial fibrosis 239–40
  in tropical endomyocardial fibrosis 251
ECP, *see* eosinophil cationic protein
ectoparasitic infestations and eosinophils 149
EDF (eosinophil differentiation factor), *see* interleukin 5
EDN/EPX, *see* eosinophil-derived neurotoxin/eosinophil protein-X
E-EMF, *see* endomyocardial fibrosis, eosinophilic
effector functions of
  eosinophils, *Fig. 6.1*
    history 6
    cytotoxic mechanisms 118–20
    basic proteins 119
    eosinophil peroxidase 120
  neutrophils, cytotoxic mechanisms 119
Ehrlich, Paul and the discovery of eosinophils 4
elasmobranchs, eosinophils in 124
elastase, absence in eosinophil 61
electrocardiogram (ECG) in,
  eosinophilic endomyocardial fibrosis 238–9
  tropical endomyocardial fibrosis 251
electronmicroscopy (EM)
  scanning (SEM), of plasma membrane of eosinophils 74
  stereo high voltage of blood eosinophils 41
  transmission of blood eosinophils
    normal 38–40
    in idiopathic hypereosinophilic syndrome 280–1
    chronic eosinophilic pneumonia 208
    eosinophil differentiation 12–13
    eosinophilic endomyocardial fibrosis 241–2, 247
    schistosomes killing by eosinophils 115
    tropical endomyocardial fibrosis 252–3
elutriation centrifugation separation of eosinophils 35, 172
emboli, *see* thromboemboli
EMF, *see* endomyocardial fibrosis
emphysema and eosinophils 211
endocardial fibrosis, *see* endomyocardial fibrosis
endocarditis, bacterial in eosinophilic endomyocardial fibrosis 243
endocrine diseases and eosinophils 306
  neoplasms 172
endocytosis 6, 89–90
  microendocytosis by rat eosinophils 90
  phagocytosis by
    human blood eosinophils of
      leishmania 117
      Trypanosoma cruzi 116
    tissue eosinophils of *Escherichia coli* 89, 105
endomyocardial fibrosis 232–58
  animal models of 257–8
  comparisons of tropical, and eosinophilic endomyocardial fibrosis 257–49
  cytotoxicity of eosinophil secretion products 118
  eosinophilic endomyocardial fibrosis 253–49
  history 232–5
  national incidences 234
  tropical endomyocardial fibrosis 249–57
endoplasmic reticulum
  association with nonspecific esterase 62
  and eosinophil peroxidase
    biosynthesis 57
    secretion 93
  seen as 'small granules' 44
endothelial cells, *see* vascular endothelial cells
endotoxin stimulation of eosinophil secretion 88
ENT diseases, *see* ear nose and throat diseases
entamoeba and eosinophils 148
enteritis, and enterocolitis and eosinophils 188–9
  coeliac disease 188
  milk, and soy allergy 188–9
enterobacteriaceae infections and eosinophils 131
Enterobius vermicularis, enterobiasis and eosinophils 146
eosin (tetrabromo-fluorescein, eosin-Y) 30, 36
  absorption spectrum 36
  for staining eosinophils 36
  history 4

eosin (*cont.*)
lack of staining of hyenas' eosinophils 123
structure 5
use with haematoxylin 5
eosinophil activating factor (EAF) 107
cytotoxicity enhancing activity 120
effect on leukotriene C4 secretion 71
eosinophil activation, *see* activation of eosinophils
eosinophil basic proteins in the heart in pathogenesis of eosinophilic endomyocardial fibrosis 248
eosinophil cationic protein (ECP) 48–53
actions on 51–3
basophils 52
central nervous system 52
coagulation 53
complement 53
lymphocytes 52–3
mast cells 52
parasites 51–2, 115, 116
respiratory system 52
suppressor lymphocytes 52
assays 50
biosynthesis 48
in blood eosinophils
content 50
localization 50–1, *Fig. 3.4*
normal levels 48
in idiopathic hypereosinophilic syndrome 281–2
in bronchoalveolar lavage fluid in
adult respiratory distress syndrome 211
bronchial challenge in asthma 201
in cerebrospinal fluid in meningitis 217
in heart tissues in
Churg–Strauss syndrome 203
eosinophilic endomyocardial fibrosis 248
history 7, 48
purification 48–9
relationship to
angiogenin 51
eosinophil-derived neurotoxin/eosinophil protein-X 56
pancreatic ribonuclease 51
ribonuclese activity 51
secreted form 49–50
secretion from eosinophils 91, 94
in serum in
asthma 198
dilated cardiomyopathy 230
haemodialysis 222
idiopathic hypereosinophilic syndrome 284
myocardial infarction 229
normal levels 51
patients without eosinophils 316
pneumonia 131
renal failure 220
rheumatoid arthritis 177
tropical endomyocardial fibrosis 256
in skin in urticaria 299
structure 49
in synovial fluid 177, 178
in tears 218
in urine 50, 223
zinc associated 49
eosinophil cell lines, *see* cell lines, eosinophil
eosinophil chemotactic factor(s) of anaphylaxis (ECF-A) 99
stimulation of eosinophil
immunoglobulin receptor expressions 78
complement receptor expression 82
cytotoxicity 120
history 7, 99
receptor for 83
see also chemotactic factors
eosinophil counts, *see* methods, blood eosinophil counts
eosinophil cytotoxicity enhancing activity (ECEA) 107, 120
eosinophil cytotoxicity enhancing factor (ECEF) 71
eosinophil-derived neurotoxin/eosinophil protein-X (EDN/EPX) 53–6, 91, 94, 116
actions on 55–6
basophils 56
central nervous system 55
lymphocytes 56
mast cells 56
parasites 55
assays for 54–5
content in blood eosinophils 55
history 53
in heart tissues in eosinophilic endomyocardial fibrosis 248
in nasal polyp eosinophils
localization 55
in plasma and serum
normal levels 55
in asthma 198
purification 54
relationship to eosinophil cationic protein 56
ribonuclease activity 55
structure 54
eosinophil differentiation factor (EDF) *see* interleukin 5

eosinophil growth factors, *see* eosinopoietic factors
eosinophil growth stimulating factor (eosinophil-GSF) 16
eosinophil major basic protein (MBP) 45–8
absence, in serum of patients with no eosinophils 316
actions on 47–8
basophils 48
coagulation, and complement systems 48
intestinal cells 48
mast cells 48
parasites 47
Schistosoma mansoni schistosomula 115
Trichinella spiralis newborn larvae 116
respiratory tissues 47–8
skin 47
skin cells in vitro 48
vascular endothelial cells 48
in animals 46
assays for 46–7
content in
blood eosinophils in
normal people 45, 46
idiopathic hypereosinophilic syndrome 4 , 281–2
bronchoalveolar lavage fluid in asthma 199–200
pleural fluid 47
serum and plasma in 47
treated Bancroftian filariasis 142
asthma with bronchial challenge 200–1
idiopathic hypereosinophilic syndrome 284
pregnancy 227
sputum in asthma 47, 199
basophils 45
tear fluid 218
in eosinophilic endomyocardial fibrosis 248
in guinea pigs 46
history 7, 46
localization in eosinophils 46, *Fig. 3.4*
purification 46
in rats 46
in respiratory tissues in
asthma 197
chronic eosinophilic pneumonia 208
secretion from 93, 94
bone marrow cells 13
blood eosinophils induced by immunoglobulin E complexes 81
mechanism 93
in skin
atopic dermatitis 298
episodic angioedema with eosinophils 300, 301
flame figures 168
onchocerciasis 143
urticaria 299
structure of 46
eosinophil peroxidase 57–60
actions 59–60
with chloride, bromide, and iodide ions 59
in cytotoxicity by eosinophils 120
on leukotrienes 60
on macrophages 60
on mast cells 60
on neutrophils 60
on parasites 59–60
peroxidation 59–60
on tumour cells 60
assays for 58–9
biosynthesis of 57
blood eosinophils 57
content 59
localization 43, 59, *Fig. 3.4*
in bone marrow eosinophils 57
comparisons with myeloperoxidase 57
deficiency of
in man 57, 259–60
in animals 123
and eosin staining of blood eosinophils 36
history 259–60
haemoprotein properties 58
histochemistry 59
history 57
immunocytochemistry 59
inhibition by 3-amino-1, 2, 4-triazole 59
in animals 58
guinea pigs 58
horses 58
rats 58
in basophils 45
in bullous pemphigoid 303
in Hodgkin's disease 59
purification 58
secretion from eosinophils
immunoglobulin E-induced 81, 91
in bone marrow 57
in idiopathic hypereosinophilic syndrome 283
pathways used 93
structure 58
eosinophil stimulation promoter (ESP) 18
cytotoxicity enhancing activity 120
eosinophilic ascites 186

eosinophilic cystitis 117, 223–4
eosinophilic endomyocardial fibrosis (E-EMF) 232, 235–249, *Plate 7, Fig. 22.1*
  bacterial endocarditis complicating 243, 277
  clinical features 237–8
  comparisons with tropical endomyocardial fibrosis 257–8, *Fig. 22.3*
  disease associations 235–7
    eosinophilic leukaemia 236
    eosinophilic pneumonia 237
    idiopathic hypereosinophilic syndrome 236
    hypersensitivity diseases 237
    neoplasms 237
    parasitic diseases 236
    vasculitic diseases 237
  history 232–5
  investigations in 238–42
    cardiac catheterization 240
    coagulation studies 247–8
    echocardiogram 239–40
    electrocardiogram 238–9
    histopathology 232, 241–2, *Fig. 22.2*
    radiological investigations 238
  pathogenesis of 233, 245–9
    experimental studies 248
  treatment of 242–5
    cardiac surgery 243–5, *Plate 9*
    drug therapy 242–3
eosinophilic fasciitis 181
eosinophilic gastroenteritis 67, 82, 184–6, *Fig. 13.1*
  colonic disease 185
  eosinophilic ascites 186
  histopathology of 185
  history 184
  investigations of 185
  oesophageal disease 185
eosinophilic granuloma and eosinophils 164–5
  Charcot–Leyden crystals in 64
  in lungs 210–11
eosinophilic granuloma of soft tissue 167–9
eosinophilic leukaemia 150–7, 246
  acute eosinophilic leukaemia 152–6
    in adults 154–5
    bone lesions 152
    in children 152
    drug therapy 156
    in infants 152–3, 295
    investigations 155–6
      cytogenetics 155–6
      histochemistry 155
      serum vitamin B_{12} 155
    in animals 157
    eosinophil cell lines from 27
    eosinophilic endomyocardial fibrosis in 236
  chronic eosinophilic leukaemia 156–7
    investigations of 156–7
      agar colony cultures 156–7
      cytogenetic studies 157
  history 4
eosinophilic meningitis 139
eosinophilic meningoencephalitis 139
eosinophilic panniculitis 297
eosinophilic pneumonia, *see* chronic eosinophilic pneumonia
eosinophilic pustular folliculitis 132, 304
eosinophilic spongiosis 302
eosinophilopoietin (EPP) and eosinophil production 16, 17, 18
eosinopenia induced by steroids, and infections 28, 290
eosinopoiesis 10–28
  and cytogenetic studies 25–6
  and marrow reticulum cells 10, 12
  blood eosinophil kinetics 27
  cell lines 26–7
  chromosome abnormalities and genetic factors affecting 25–6
  cyclophosphamide effects on 24
  defects in S1/S1, and Wv/Wv mice 25
  drugs affecting 24
  factors affecting 17–24
  genetic studies in mice 26
  granule protein secretion during 13
  kinetics 14
  lineages 11–12
  lithium effects on 24
  morphology 12
  ontogeny 10–11
  in rats 14, *Plate 2*
  serum inhibitors of 316
  steroid effects on 24, 28, 290
  suppression of granulocytopoiesis 24
  suppressor cells affecting 24–5
  T-lymphocyte dependency 7
  tissue eosinophil kinetics 28
eosinopoietic factors 17–24
  assays for 14–17
    agar colony cultures 15–16
    in vivo assays 17
    liquid cultures of bone marrow 16–17
  colony stimulating factors 20–4
  eosinophilopoietin (EPP) 16, 17, 18
  eosinophil growth stimulating factor (eosinophil-GSF) 16
  following interleukin 2 (IL-2) treatment 23–4
  from cell lines 22–3

from human immunodeficiency virus infected lymphocytes 22
from inflamed tissues 22
from neoplastic cells 22
from T-lymphocytes 18–20
in neoplasms 23
in serum 23–4
idiopathic hypereosinophilic syndrome 284
chronic myelocytic leukaemia 23
AIDS patients treated with interleukin 2 23
EPA (eosinophil promoting activity) 23
episodic angioedema
in loiasis 142
with eosinophilia 299, *Plate 14*
eosinophil cationic protein in 300, 301
EPO, *see* eosinophil peroxidase
EPP, *see* eosinophilopoietin
erythema annulare and eosinophils 305
erythema multiforme and eosinophils 309
erythema nodosum and eosinophils 304
erythema toxicum neonatorum and eosinophils 302
Escherichia coli
cytotoxicity by eosinophil peroxidase-halide system 120
endocytosis by eosinophil from
blood 89
tissues 105
ESP, *see* eosinophil stimulation promoter
esterases, nonspecific in eosinophils 62
ethnic groups, normal blood eosinophil counts in 31
ethylene diamine tetraacetic acid (EDTA)
as an anticoagulant 32
enhancement of eosinophil staining 36
Europe, cardiac surgery for
eosinophilic endomyocardial fibrosis 244
tropical endomyocardial fibrosis 254
Eustoma rotundum, and inflammatory fibroid polyps 187
exchange blood transfusions and eosinophils 295
exercise increasing blood eosinophil counts 31
exocytosis, *see* secretion
eye diseases and eosinophils 218–19
conjunctival diseases 218–19
corneal diseases 219
in idiopathic hypereosinophilic syndrome 275, *Plate 11*
orbital diseases 219
retinal diseases 219

factor VIII in idopathic hypereosinophilic syndrome 287
familial eosinophilia 295
familial reticuloendotheliosis and eosinophils 166
Fanconi's anaemia and eosinophils 261
fasciitis syndromes and eosinophils 180–2
eosinophilic fasciitis 181–2
Spanish toxic oil syndrome 182
Fasciola hepatica and eosinophils 147
fascioliasis 147
and eosinophilic endomyocardial fibrosis 236
fatty acids, *see* unsaturated fatty acids
Fauci, Anthony and eosinophil research 320
Fc receptors, and FcR *see* receptors for immunoglobulin
female genital tract diseases, pregnancy, and eosinophils 226–7
neoplasms 174–5
pregnancy 227
uterus, and uterine diseases 226
feminization in tropical endomyocardial fibrosis 253
fever in idiopathic hypereosinophilic syndrome 270
fibrinogen levels in serum, in idiopathic hypereosinophilic syndrome 248, 287
fibroblast growth factors in eosinophils 62–3
filariasis and eosinophils 140–3
Bancroftian filariasis 142
blood eosinophils
cytotoxicity 116
secretion 81
dirofilariasis 142
loiasis 142–3
onchocerciasis 143
tropical endomyocardial fibrosis 250, 256–7
tropical (filarial) eosinophilia 141–2
fingernails, in episodic angioedema, *Plate 16*
fishes, eosinophils in 124–5
fixatives for eosinophils 36
flame figures, eosinophil major basic protein localization in 168
fluorescein derivatives
fluorescein-isothiocyanate (FITC) 36
nonspecific staining of eosinophils 36–7
tetrabromo-fluorescein, *see* eosin
tetrabromo-tetrachloro-fluorescein (phloxin) 30, 36
formyl-methionyl-leucine-phenylalanine (fMLP) effects on eosinophils
calcium content 95
chemotactic activity 283

formyl-methionyl-leucine-phenylalanine (fMLP) effects on eosinophils (*cont.*)
complement receptor expression 82
cytotoxicity enhancing activity 120
respiratory burst 68
secretion 71
separation of eosinophils 33
fractionation of blood eosinophils 40
subcellular fractionation 50
freeze-fracture studies of
schistosomes killing by eosinophils 115
blood eosinophils
plasma membranes 74–5
in idiopathic hypereosinophilic syndrome 281
frogs, eosinophil secretion 90
functions of eosinophils 4, 6, 8, *Fig. 6.1*
fungal infections and eosinophils 132–3
lung infections 132–3
see also mycoses
Fura2 assay for eosinophil calcium 95

G-CSF, *see* granulocyte colony stimulating factor
galactose in eosinophils 72
gall bladder diseases, *see* liver and biliary tract diseases
gangliosidase deficiencies 259
gastric neoplasms and eosinophils 171
gastric ulcers, *see* peptic ulcers
gastroenteritis, eosinophilic, *see* eosinophilic gastroenteritis
gastrointestinal diseases, *see* digestive system diseases
gelatinase in neutrophils 45
genetic diseases, *see* inherited diseases
genetic factors affecting
eosinopoiesis 25–6
tropical endomyocardial fibrosis 255
geographical distribution of tropical endomyocardial fibrosis 255
gerbil, eosinophils in 126
GFA (granulocyte functional antigens) 81, 86, 87, 88
Giardia lamblia 117, 148
giardiasis and eosinophils 148
cytotoxicity by eosinophils 117
Gleich, Gerald and eosinophil research 7, 55, 84, 320
glioblastoma and eosinophilia 172–3
glucocorticoid receptors on eosinophils 83
glucose,
and lipoxygenase metabolism in eosinophils 67
metabolism by eosinophils 66–7
hexose monophosphate shunt 67
hexose transport 67
labelled glucose 67
labelled
metabolism by eosinophils 67
β-glucuronidase
in eosinophil granules 43
secretion from eosinophils 82, 92
glutathione peroxidase detoxification of oxygen radicals 119
glyceride (IpOCOC9) induction of eosinophil secretion 91
β-glycerophosphate in eosinophil granules 43
glycocalyx of eosinophils 83
glycosaminoglycans in eosinophils 61, 63
GM-CSF, *see* granulocyte macrophage colony stimulating factor
Gnathostoma spinigerum and eosinophils 146
gnathostomiasis and eosinophils 146
Goetzl, Edward and eosinophil research 320
Golgi apparatus in eosinophils 42
peroxidase biosynthesis 57
granule protein secretion 94
Gordon phenomenon 53; *see also* eosinophil cationic protein, and eosinophil-derived neurotoxin/eosinophil protein-X
gorilla, eosinophil major basic protein in pregnancy 227
graft-versus-host (GvH) disease, and eosinophils 314
granules, *see* cytoplasmic granules
granulocyte colony stimulating factor (G-CSF) 109
identity with colony stimulating factor β (CSF-β) 20
granulocyte functional antigens (GFA) 81, 86, 87, 88
granulocyte-macrophage colony stimulating factor,
(GM-CSF, colony stimulating factor α) 15, 20, 21–2, *Fig. 2.1*
blood eosinophils
activation 108
cytotoxicity enhancing activity 108, 120
maintenance *in vitro* 35
gene localization 25
HL-60 cell differentiation to eosinophils 21
identity with CSF-α 21
induction of eosinophilia in man 21
recombinant 20
secretion by
vascular endothelial cells 109
structure 20

granulocytopoiesis suppression by eosinophils 24–5
Griffonia simplicifolia binding to eosinophil granules 38
GSF (eosinophil growth stimulating factor), *see* eosinopoiesis
guaiacol assay for eosinophil peroxidase 59
guinea pigs
  blood eosinophils 126–7
    complement receptors 81
    eosinophil major basic protein 46
    eosinophil peroxidase 58
  immunoglobulin G1, 97
  pancreatic eosinophils in diabetes 306
  peritoneal eosinophils
    polyclonal antibodies to 84
    purification 126
    secretion 90
  uterine eosinophils
    oestrogen effects on 83
gynaecological diseases, *see* female genital tract diseases

haematological diseases, *see* blood diseases, and idiopathic hypereosinophilic syndrome
haemodialysis and eosinophils 222–3
  serum levels of eosinophil cationic protein 222
hamsters, eosinophils in 126, 157
Hand–Schüller–Christian disease and eosinophils 166
Hansel's stain for eosinophils in urine 37
hayfever conjunctivitis and eosinophils 218
heart diseases and eosinonophils 229–30
  allograft rejection 229
  myocyte injury by eosinophils 118
  coronary heart disease 229
  drug hypersensitivity reactions 309
  endomyocardial fibrosis 232–58
helminthiasis and eosinophils 136–48
  cestode infections 137–8
  nematode infections 138–46
  trematode infections 146–8
heparin
  anticoagulant *in vitro* 32
    inhibition by eosinophil cationic protein 53
    inhibition by eosinophil major basic protein 223
  treatment of eosinophilic endomyocardial fibrosis 242
  inhibition of cytotoxicity by
    eosinophil major basic protein 47, 116
    eosinophil cationic protein 121
heparin-Sepharose isolation of
  eosinophil cationic protein 49
  eosinophil-derived neurotoxin/ eosinophil protein-X 54
hepatic diseases, see liver and biliary tract diseases
hereditary eosinophilia 295
HES, *see* idiopathic hypereosinophilic syndrome
hexose monophosphate shunt metabolism by eosinophils 67
hexose transport by eosinophils 67
  ^{3}H-2-deoxyglucose transport 67
HILDA (human interleukin DA) and eosinophil activation 107
Hirashima, M. and eosinophil research 319
Hirsch, James and eosinophil research 6
histaminases in eosinophils 61–2
histamine 48, 52, 82, 282
  chemotactic factor for eosinophils 99–100
  cytotoxicity enhancing activity 120
histiocytosis-X and eosinophils 164–6
  Charcot–Leyden crystals in 64
  eosinophilic granuloma 164–5
  familial reticuloendotheliosis 166
  Hand–Schüller–Christian disease 166
  Letterer–Siwe disease 166
histochemistry of
  acute eosinophilic leukaemia 155
  eosinophil peroxidase 59
histones in eosinophil extracts 40
histopathology of
  angiolymphoid hyperplasia with eosinophilia 167–8
  asthma 197
  eosinophilic endomyocardial fibrosis 232, 241–2
    electronmiscroscopy 241–2
  tropical endomyocardial fibrosis 252–3
    electronmicroscopy 252–3
histoplasmosis and eosinophils 133
history of eosinophils and eosinophils in disease 4–9
  eosinophils
    activation 104
    agar colony cultures 8, 15
    Charcot–Leyden crystals 64
    chemotactic factors 7, 96, 99
    eosinophil cationic protein 7, 48
    eosinophil-derived neurotoxin/ eosinophil protein-X 53
    eosinophil major basic protein 7, 46
    eosinophil peroxidase 57
    eosinopoietic factors 18
    Gordon phenomenon 53
    light density eosinophils 35

history of eosinophils and eosinophils in disease (*cont.*)
eosinophil protein-X (*cont.*)
plasma membrane receptors for
complement 81
immunoglobulin G 77
secretion 90
unsaturated fatty acid metabolism 69–70
eosinophils in disease
asthma and eosinophils 5, 195
deficiency of eosinophils 259–60
endomyocardial fibrosis 232–5
eosinophilic endomyocardial fibrosis 245
tropical endomyocardial fibrosis 255–7
eosinophilic gastroenteritis 184
idiopathic hypereosinophilic syndrome 7, 263–6, 289
neoplasms and eosinophils 5, 169
eosinophilic leukaemia 150–1
lymphocytic leukaemia and eosinophils 159
myeloblastic leukaemia (M4Eo) and eosinophils 158
solid tissue neoplasms 169
parasitic diseases and eosinophils 5
pleural effusions containing eosinophils 212
HL-60 cell lines and eosinophils 26–7
HLA antigens on eosinophil plasma membranes 84
Hodgkin's disease and eosinophils 53, 162–3
eosinophil peroxidase in 59
in cerebrospinal fluid 216
small granules in tissue eosinophils 44
hookworm infections and eosinophils 69, 143–4, 210
ancylostomiasis 143–4
larva migrans 144
necatoriasis 144
horseradish peroxidase relationship to eosinophil peroxidase 58
horses 126
blood eosinophils 90
electronmicroscopy of secretion 94
granule enzymes 6
eosinophil peroxidase 6, 58
eosinophilic leukaemia 157
human immunodeficiency virus (HIV)
eosinopoietic factors from infected lymphocytes 22
infection, and eosinophilia 135
human interleukin DA (HILDA) and eosinophil activation 107
hydatid disease, and eosinophils 137
hydrocortisone inhibition of eosinophil secretion 95
hydrogen peroxide formation by eosinophils 59, 67, 69, 120
hydroxyethyl starch and leukapheresis 32
hydroxyurea treatment of the idiopathic hypereosinophilic syndrome 288, 291
hyenas, eosinophils in 123
hypochlorite ions
produced by eosinophil peroxidase 59
inhibited by eosinophil major basic protein 51
Hymenolepsis, and eosinophils 137
Hypaque in eosinophil separation 32
hypereosinophilic syndrome, *see* idiopathic hypereosinophilic syndrome
hypergammaglobulinaemia E and infection syndrome and eosinophils 316–17
hypersensitivity diseases
and eosinophilic endomyocardial fibrosis 237
and the pathogenesis of tropical endomyocardial fibrosis 256
hypertension in idiopathic hypereosinophilic syndrome 276–7
hypodense eosinophils, *see* light density eosinophils
hypogammaglobulinaemia and absence of eosinophils 315, 316
hypogranular blood eosinophils in
the pathogenesis of E-EMF 245, 246
histoplasmosis 135
drug hypersensitivity reactions 314
the idiopathic hypereosinophilic syndrome 279–80, *Plate 5*
tropical (filariae) eosinophilia 280

ibuprofen and eosinophilic meningitis 217
idiopathic hypereosinophilic syndrome 64, 69, 80, 263–93, *Plate 10*
age at presentation 268
in children, case reports 268–70
with eosinophilic endomyocardial fibrosis 236
in infants 295
animal models of 267–8
clinical features of 263–77, *Fig. 24.1*
alcohol intolerance 270–1
breast disease 277
cardiovascular complications 271, *Plate 7*
central nervous system disease 274–5
coughing attacks in 272
diarrhoea 273

digestive system complications 272–3
eye disease 275, *Plate 11*
fever 270
hypertension 276–7
joint disease 276
liver involvement 273
musculoskeletal complications 276
nervous system involvement 274–6
nonspecific symptoms 270–1
oro–genital ulcers 272
papules and macules 273
peripheral nerve disease 275–6
presentation 270
pulmonary infiltrates 272
renal complications 276–7
respiratory tract complications 272
skin complications 273–4
thromboembolic complications 271–2
urticaria 273
vascular complications 271–2
weight loss 270
course of the disease 288–93
diseases processes underlying 266
history of 7, 263–6
investigations in 278–87
blood eosinophils 278–84, *Plates 4, 5*
bone marrow features 284–6
coagulation studies 286–7
immunological investigations 286
serum and plasma constituents 284
patients affected 268–70
races affected 270
sex incidence 268
treatment of 288–93
anticoagulant drugs 291–2
antineoplastic drugs 291
antiplatelet drugs 292
bone marrow transplantation 293
history of 289
leukapheresis 292
plasma exchange 292
radiotherapy 289
splenectomy 289
steroids 289–91
troleandomycin 291
variants of 266–7
IL-1, -2, -3, -5, *see* interleukins
immune complexes and eosinophils 71, 91, 93
immunocytochemistry of eosinophil peroxidase 59
immunofluorescent non-specific staining of eosinophils 37
immunoglobulin A and interleukin 5 20
immunoglobulin E
complexes and eosinophil endocytosis 79
drug hypersensitivity reactions with eosinophilia 312
in idiopathic hypereosinophilic syndrome 286
immunoglobulin G
complexes and eosinophil
drug hypersensitivity reactions 312
endocytosis 79
secretion 94
stimulation 78
in idiopathic hypereosinophilic syndrome 286
subclasses binding to eosinophils 77, 79
immunoglobulin M
hyperglobulinaemia and eosinophilia 302
serum levels in idiopathic hypereosinophilic syndrome 286
immunoglobulin receptors in plasma membrane of eosinophils 75–81
immunoglobulin E (Fc ε R), 79–81
high affinity (Fc ε R1) 77
low affinity (Fc ε R11) 77, 79
immunoglobulin G (Fc γ R) 76–9, 105, 110
high affinity (Fc γ R1) 77
low affinity (Fc γ R11) 77
in eosinophilic endomyocardial fibrosis 245–6
immunoglobulin M (Fc μ receptors) 76
immunological diseases 306–17
absence of eosinophils 315–16
autoimmune diseases and eosinophils 306
drug hypersensitivity reactions and eosinophils 306–14
graft-versus-host disease and eosinophils 314
hyperimmunoglobulinaemia E and infection syndrome, and eosinophils 316–17
immunological deficiency syndromes and eosinophils 314–15
hypogammaglobulinaemia 315
severe combined immune deficiency syndrome 314–15
immunological investigations in idiopathic hypereosinophilic syndrome 286
incontinentia pigmenti and eosinophils 303–4
India, cardiac surgery for tropical endomyocardial fibrosis 254–5
infants
diseases and eosinophils 294–6
with eosinophilic leukaemia 152–3
normal blood eosinophil counts 294
skin diseases and eosinophils 302
infections
effects on blood eosinophil kinetics 28
in the aetiology of tropical endomyocardial fibrosis 255–7

inflamed tissues, eosinopoietic factors from 22
inflammatory fibroid polyps and eosinophils 186–7
information sources for the book, vii, 321
ingestion, *see* endocytosis
inherited diseases and eosinophils 259–61, 295
  Chediak–Higashi syndrome 260–1
  chronic granulomatous disease 261
  crystalloid inclusion abnormality 261
  Down's syndrome 295–60
  eosinophil peroxidase deficiency 259
  Pelger–Hüet abnormality 261
insect bites and eosinophils 149
interactions of eosinophil secretion products with
  mast cells 8
  normal cells and tissues 121–2, *Fig. 6.4*
α-interferon, stimulation of
  eosinophil secretion 109
  inhibition of eosinopoiesis 109
β-interferon stimulation of eosinophil
  activation 109
  cytotoxicity 121
  plasma membrane immunoglobulin receptor expression 78
interleukins 18–22
  interleukin-1 (IL-1) 109
    eosinophil activation by 109
    interleukin-2 (IL-2) 20, *Fig. 2.1*
    and GM-CSF production 20
    treatment with,
      and eosinophilia 20, 301
      and eosinopoietic factors in serum 23–4
  interleukin-3 (IL-3, multi-colony stimulating factor) 20, 22, *Fig. 2.1*
    gene location 25
    eosinophil activation 109–10
interleukin-5 (IL-5, eosinophil differentiation factor EDF) 18, 19–20, *Fig. 2.1*
  effects on
    blood eosinophils
      cytotoxicity 109
      complement receptor expression 82
      cytotoxicity 120
      GFA-1, and -2 antigen expression 88
      survival in culture 35
    bone marrow eosinophil growth 19–20
    pre-B-lymphocytes and platelets 19–20, 87
  gene location 25
  recombinant IL–5 19
  see also eosinopoiesis
interstitial cystitis and eosinophil cationic protein in urine 50
intestinal cells, eosinophil major basic protein actions on 48
intestinal peroxidase relationship to eosinophil peroxidase 58
intramembranous particles in eosinophils 75
intrinsic asthma and eosinophils 202
iodoacetate and eosinophil cytotoxicity 114
iron in eosinophils 63
Ison, Peter, vii
isoprenaline inhibition of eosinophil secretion 95

joint diseases and eosinophils 176–9
  ankylosing spondylitis 179
  rheumatoid arthritis 176–7
  synovial fluid 177–8
  synovitis 177–8
joint fluid, *see* synovial fluid
journals with papers on eosinophils and eosinophilic disorders 321

Kaposi's sarcoma with eosinophilia 169
Katayama syndrome and eosinophils 147
Kay, A. Barry and eosinophil research 7, 82, 319
ketotifen inhibition of eosinophil secretion 95
  treatment of dermatitis 298
kidney diseases
  allograft rejection and eosinophils 224–5
  in drug hypersensitivity reactions with eosinophilia 309
  and eosinophils 220
  in idiopathic hypereosinophilic syndrome 276–7
  in tropical endomyocardial fibrosis 253
killing, *see* cytotoxicity
Kimura's disease 167–9
kinetics of
  blood eosinophils 27–8
    assays wtih ^{3}H-thymidine 27–8
    effects of infections 28
    in idiopathic hypereosinophilic syndrome 284
  eosinopoiesis 14
  tissue eosinophils 28
Klebanoff, Seymour and eosinophil research 320

lactoferrin in neutrophils 45
lactoperoxidase relationship with eosinophil peroxidase 58

lagomorpha, eosinophil in 125
lamellipodia
  induced by eosinophil activating factors 110
  in fish eosinophils 124
Langerhans' cell
  eosinophils adjacent to, in atopic dermatitis 298–9
  origin of reticuloendotheliosis 164, 165
large intestinal neoplasms and eosinophils 171–2
larva migrans and eosinophils 144
laryngeal diseases and eosinophils 214–15
latex–IgG endocytosis by eosinophils 89–90
lectins binding to eosinophil granules 38
leishmaniasis and eosinophils 148
Leishmania mexicana amazonensis cytotoxicity by eosinophils 117
lemurs, eosinophils in 126
leprosy bacilli cytotoxicity by eosinophil peroxidase-halide system 120
Letterer-Siwe disease and eosinophils 166
leucine, ^{14}C-, and ^{3}H- uptake by eosinophils 48, 57, 72
leucocyte functional antigens (LFA) 81
leukaemias and eosinophils 150–62
  biclonal
    eosinophils and basophils 11
    eosinophils and lymphocytes 12
  cytogenetics 25–6
  eosinophilic leukaemia
    in man 150–7
    in animals 157
  lymphocytic leukaemia 159–61
  monocytic leukaemia 162
  myelocytic leukaemia 157–9
  plasma cell neoplasms 162
leukapheresis
  eosinophil separation from blood 32
  in the idiopathic hypereosinophilic syndrome 292
leukotrienes
  as chemotactic factors for eosinophils 101
  eosinophil peroxidase breakdown of 60
  from eosinophils 69–70
    factors decreasing 71
    factors increasing 71
    history 70
    stimuli inducing 70
  leukotriene B4 (LTB4) 69–70
  chemotactic properties
    for blood eosinophils 97, 101
    for idiopathic hypereosinophilic syndrome blood eosinophils 283
  eosinophil cytotoxicity enhancing activity 120
  inactivation by eosinophil peroxidase 60
  in incontinentia pigmenti 303–4
  induction of eosinophil chemoluminescence 68
  induction of eosinophil complement receptors 82
  secretion by neutrophils 69
  leukotriene C4 (LTC4) 69–70
    chemotactic properties for idiopathic hypereosinophilic syndrome blood eosinophils 283
    from blood eosinophils in idiopathic hypereosinophilic syndrome 282
    in asthma 195
    inactivation by eosinophil peroxidase 60
    inactivation of arylsulphatase 61
    production
      by idiopathic hypereosinophilic syndrome blood eosinophils 282
      increased by eosinophil activating factors 108, 109
    synthesis by bronchoalveolar lavage eosinophils 199
  leukotriene D4 (LTD4) 69
    chemotactic properties 97
    inactivation by eosinophil peroxidase 60
  leukotriene E4 (LTE4)
    chemotactic properties 97
LFA (leucocyte functional antigens) 81; *see also* granulocyte functional antigens
light density eosinophils 34–5
  chemoluminescense of 37–8, 68
  chemotaxis of 283
    and chemokinesis of 101
  content of eosinophil major basic protein 47
  cytotoxic capacity 80
  induced by endothelial cell culture 100
  plasma membrane antigens on 86
  platelet activating factor production of 72
  secretion by 81
  unsaturated fatty acid metabolism by 70
lineage pathways common to
  eosinophils, and basophils 11–12
  eosinophils, and lymphocytes 12
  eosinophils, basophils, and lymphocytes 11–12
linear IgA disease and eosinophils 303
lipid bodies in
  avian eosinophils 124
  human blood eosinophils in, 41–2, *Fig. 3.2*
    Spanish toxic oil syndrome 41
    idiopathic hypereosinophilic syndrome 281

lipodystrophy, pancreatitis, and eosinophilia 191
lipoxin A synthesis by eosinophils 70
lipoxygenase pathway products from eosinophils
  5-lipoxygenase pathway products, *see* leukotrienes
  11-HETE and hexose transport by eosinophils 67
  15-lipoxygenase pathway products 69–70
    15-HETE synthesis by bronchoalveolar lavage eosinophils 199
    5-HETE
      chemotactic properties for eosinophils 101
      induction of eosinophil complement expression 82
      stimulation of hexose transport by eosinophils 67
    5-HPETE
      chemotactic properties for eosinophils 101
      induction of eosinophil complement receptor expression 82
  see also unsaturated fatty acids
liquid cultures of bone marrow to assay eosinopoietic factors 16
literature on eosinophils and eosinophilic disorders 321–6
lithium effects on eosinopoiesis 24
liver
  disease in
    allograft rejection 190
    drug hypersensitivity reactions 310
    idiopathic hypereosinophilic syndrome 273
  and biliary
    neoplasms and eosinophils 172
    diseases and eosinophils 190–1
lizards, eosinophils in 127
Loa loa infections (loaiasis) and eosinophils 142–3
loach, eosinophils in 124
  in tropical endomyocardial fibrosis 236, 256
localization
  in eosinophils of *Fig. 3.4*
    Charcot–Leyden crystal protein 65
    eosinophil cationic protein 50
    eosinophil major basic protein 46
    eosinophil peroxidase 59
    eosinoiphil-derived neurotoxin/eosinophil protein-X 55
  of eosinophils *in vivo* 97–8
Löffler's syndrome and eosinophils 205–6
Löffler, W. and eosinophil research 232
LPS, *see* lipopolysaccharide
LTB4, C4, D4, and E4, *see* leukotriene B4, C4, D4, and E4
luminol-dependent chemoluminescence of eosinophils 68
lung diseases and eosinophils 205–12
  drug hypersensitivity reactions 309
  emphysema 211
  eosinophilic granuloma of the lung 210–11
  lymphomatoid granulomatosis 210
  obstructive lung diseases 211
  pulmonary eosinophilia 205–9
  pulmonary fibrosis 209
  respiratory distress syndrome in adults 211
  sarcoidosis 211
  Wegener's granulomatosis 209–10
Luxol fast blue staining of eosinophils 38
lymphangiomas with eosinophilia 169
lymphatic vessel neoplasms with eosinophilia 169
lymphocytes
  chemotactic factors from 100
  common origin with eosinophils 12
  eosinophil cationic protein actions on 52–3
  eosinophil-derived neurotoxin/eosinophil protein-X actions on 56
  products affecting tissue cultures of mature eosinophils 35
lymphocytic leukaemia and eosinophils 159–61
  case reports in
    children, and adults 161
    infants 295
  in cerebrospinal fluid 216
  eosinophilic endomyocardial fibrosis in 237
lymphomas and eosinophils 162–4, *Plate 6*
  angioimmunoblastic lymphadenopathy 163
  Hodgkin's disease 162–3
  lymphomatoid granulomatosis 164
  mycosis fungoides 164
  non-Hodgkin's lymphomas 163
  Sezary's syndrome 164
lymphomatoid granulomatosis and eosinophils 164, 210
lymphomatoid papulosis and eosinophils 274, 304–5, *Plate 13*
  similarities with non-Hodgkin's lymphoma 163
lymphosarcomas with eosinophilia 169
lysophospholipase
  activity of Charcot–Leyden crystal protein 65–6
  in stimulated mouse eosinophils 110

toxicity for *Trichinella spiralis* newborn larvae 116
lysophospholipids, Charcot–Leyden crystal protein actions on 66
lysosomal enzymes in eosinophils 60–2
lysozyme, absence in eosinophils 43

M-CSF (multi-colony stimulating factor, interleukin-3), *see* interleukins
M-mode echocardiogram, *see* echocardiogram, M-mode
M4Eo, *see* myeloblastic leukaemia (M4Eo)
macaque monkeys, eosinophils in 126
α 2-macroglobulin binding to eosinophil cationic protein 51, 121
macrophages
  chemotactic factors from 101–2
  eosinophil activating factors from 107–8
  eosinophil peroxidase actions on 60
magnesium
  in eosinophils 63
  requirement for eosinophil secretion 94
Maguire, Kathy vii
Mahmoud, Adel and eosinophil research 17
major basic protein, *see* eosinophil major basic protein
Makino, Sohei and eosinophil research 319
malaria parasite cytotoxicity by eosinophils 116–17, 148
male genital tract neoplasms and eosinophils 175
malignant diseases, *see* neoplasms
mammalian cells cytotoxicity by eosinophils 117–18
  cell lines 118
  vascular endothelial cells 118
  heart cells 118
  respiratory tissues 117–18
    tracheal cells 117
  tumour cells 118
mammals other than man, eosinophils in 125–7
  artiodactyla 125
  carnivora 125
  lagomorpha 125
  marsupials 125–6
  muridae 127
  perissodactyla 126
  primates 126
  rodentia 126–7
manganese, in eosinophils 63
mannose in eosinophils 72
marrow, *see* bone marrow
marsupials, eosinophil in 125–6
mast cells
  production of
    eosinophil activating factors 108
    eosinophil chemotactic factors 99–100
  stimulation by
    eosinophil cationic protein 52
    eosinophil-derived neurotoxin/eosinophil protein-X 56
    eosinophil major basic protein 48
    eosinophil peroxidase 60
Maxwell, M.H., and eosinophil research 319
Mazzotti reaction and eosinophils 142, 143
MBP (major basic protein), *see* eosinophil major basic protein
mebendazole treatment of
  helminthic infections 136
  Necator americanus infections 144
Medline reference sources for the book, vii 321
meetings' reports on eosinophils 322
melanomas and eosinophilia 173
mellitin damage to plasma membranes 119
membrane, *see* plasma membrane
meningitis, eosinophil cationic protein levels in cerebrospinal fluid 217
mercurochrome staining of eosinophils 38
Mesocestoides corti infections in mice 19, 127, 284
metabolism of blood eosinophils 66–73
  activated blood eosinophils 67
  comparison with neutrophils 67
  ^{14}C-fumarate metabolism 67
  glucose metabolism 66–7
    ^{14}C-glucose metabolism 67
    6-^{14}C-glucose 67
  in idiopathic hypereosinophilic syndrome 282
  ^{35}S-methionine incorporation 72
  ^{125}iodide incorporation 67
  oxidative metabolism 68–9
  protein phosphorylation 110
  protein synthesis 72
  proteoglycan synthesis 72
  unsaturated fatty acid metabolism 69–70
metals in eosinophils 63
Metcalf, Donald, and eosinophil research 20, 318
methods 14–17, 29–38
  blood eosinophil counts 29–31
    automated methods 30–1
    comparisons of absolute counts, and 'per cent eosinophils' 29, 30
    manual methods 30
  chemotaxis of eosinophils 98
  leukapheresis 32
  preparation of eosinophil cytoplasts 68
  schistosomes killing by eosinophils 114
  separation of eosinophils 32–5, *Fig. 3.1*

methods (*cont.*)
  stains for eosinophils 36–8
  tissue culture of mature eosinophils 35–6
  see also assays
methylcellulose for eosinophil separation 32
methylene blue staining of cell nuclei 30
metrizamide for density gradient separation of eosinophils 33, *Fig. 3.1*
MEZZ database of references 321
mice
  eosinophils in 127
    activated in trichinosis 104
  fungal antigens, and eosinophilia 132
  genetic studies on eosinopoiesis 26
  heart damage produced by eosinophil cationic protein 118
  infected with *Mesocestoides corti* 19, 127
  with defective eosinopoiesis, S1/S1, and Wv/Wv, 25
microendocytosis by rat eosinophils 90
microfilaments, requirements in eosinophil cytotoxicity 114
microgranules in eosinophil cytoplasm 44
microvilli on rat peritoneal eosinophils 74
milk, and soy allergy, and eosinophils 188–9
  allergic gastroenteritis 188–9
  allergic proctitis 189
mites and eosinophils 149
mitochondria
  in eosinophils 42
    non-specific esterase in membrane of 62
monensin inhibition of
  eosinophil cationic protein synthesis 48
  eosinophil peroxidase synthesis 57
Moniliformis dubius infections in rats 111
mono-sup, *see* monocyte-derived activating factors
monoclonal antibodies to
  eosinophil membrane antigens 85–88, *Fig. 4.2*
    immunoglobulin receptors
      antibody 3G8 77
      antibody BB10 79
      antibody CLB-FcR-1 77
      antibody IV3 77
    which do not bind to neutrophils
      antibodies to CD1-CD9 88
      antibody Eo-1 85
      antibody TP82 86
    which also bind to neutrophils
      antibody AHN-7 87
      antibody EoN1-7 87
      antibody FMC10 87
      antibodies to GFA–1, GFA-2 87
      antibody MEL-14 98
      antibody Mo95 87
      antibody PM-81 87
      antibody TG1 87
    which also bind to T-lymphocytes
      antibodies to CD1-CD9 88
      antibody MLR4 88
  eosinophil cationic protein, and eosinophil-derived neurotoxin/ eosinophil protein-X
    antibody EG1 50, *Plate 4 (b)*
    antibody EG2 50, 94, 103, 248, 298, *Plates 3, 4, 6, 12*
  eosinophil-derived neurotoxin/eosinophil protein-X 54, 55
  eosinophil and neutrophil granules
    antibody LEU M1 45
  eosinophil peroxidase 59
monocyte-derived activating factors 107–8
  cytotoxicity enhancing activity 120
  cytotoxicity-enhancing factor (M-ECEF) 107
  supernatant (mono-sup) 82
monocytic leukaemia and eosinophils 162
mononuclear cell injury by eosinophil major basic protein 48
morphology of normal blood eosinophils 38–40, *Plate 1*
morphology of blood eosinophils in
  idiopathic hypereosinophilic syndrome 279–81 *Plates 4, 5*
    light microscopy 279–80
    transmission electronmicroscopy 280–1 *Fig. 3.2*
  the pathogenesis of E-EMF 245
    hypogranular eosinophils 245
morphometric studies on
  human blood eosinophils
    normal 39, 40
    in idiopathic hypereosinophilic syndrome 280–1
  rat eosinophil granules 13
motility of eosinophils 95–102
  localization *in vivo* 97–8, *Fig. 5.3*
  in idiopathic hypereosinophilic syndrome 282–3
  in vitro 98–102
mouse eosinophils, polyclonal antibodies to 84
mouth
  diseases and eosinophils 192
    chronic (traumatic) inflammatory ulcer 192
  neoplasms and eosinophils 172
movement, directional of eosinophils 95–102

mucus
impaction in asthma, caused by eosinophil major basic protein 48
secretion, induced by leukotriene C4 70
multi-CSF (multi-colony stimulating factor, interleukin-3), *see* interleukins
muridae, eosinophil in 127
muscle diseases and eosinophils
myositis, and polymyositis 179–80
in tropical endomyocardial fibrosis 253
musculo-skeletal diseases and eosinophils 176–82
bone diseases 176–9
complicating idiopathic hypereosinophilic syndrome 276
fasciitis syndromes 180–2
joint diseases 176–9
muscle diseases 179–80
Sjögren's syndrome 182
mycobacterial infections and eosinophils 131
mycoses and eosinophils 132–3
aspergillosis 132–3
coccidioidomycosis 133
fungal lung diseases 132
histoplasmosis 133
paranasal sinus infections 214
mycosis fungoides and eosinophils 164
myelocytic leukaemia and eosinophils 157–9
myeloblastic leukaemia and eosinophils 158–9
myeloblastic leukaemia (M4Eo) 158
chromosome 16 abnormalities in 158
chromosome 8:21 translocation in 159
chronic myelocytic leukaemia 159
myelofibrosis in idiopathic hypereosinophilic syndrome 285
myelography, and eosinophils in cerebrospinal fluid 216
myeloperoxidase 57
comparisons with eosinophil peroxidase 57
myocardial diseases 229–30
Churg–Strauss syndrome 203, *Plate 15*
myocardial infarction and eosinophils
cardiac rupture 229
serum levels of eosinophil cationic protein 229
myocarditis, necrotizing eosinophilic 229
myositis, and polymyositis and eosinophils 179–80
myristic acid and Charcot–Leyden crystal protein biosynthesis 63

N-nitrosomorpholine induction of endomyocardial fibrosis in rats 257
nicotinamide-adenine dinucleotide phosphate (NADPH) oxidase in eosinophils 67
Naegleria infections with eosinophils in the heart 148
nasal polyps
colony stimulating factor production in epithelial cells 22
eosinophil major basic protein in eosinophil granules 46
eosinophils in 214
National Library of Medicine USA, Medline database 321
Necator americanus and eosinoiphils 144
nedocromil inhibition of eosinophil secretion 95
nematode infections and eosinophils 138–46
angiostrongyliasis 138–9
ascariasis 139–40
capillaria infections 144
enterobiasis 146–53
filariasis 140
gnathostomiasis 146
hookworm infections 143–4
strongyloidiasis 145–6
toxocariasis 139–40
trichinosis 144–5
trichostrongyloidiasis 146
trichuris infections 145
neonates
diseases and eosinophils 294–6
normal blood eosinophil counts 294
neoplasms
eosinophil chemotactic factors from 101
eosinopoietic factors detected in 22, 23
associated with eosinophilic endomyocardial fibrosis 237
and eosinophils 150–175, *Fig. 11.1*
history 5, 150
leukaemias 150–62
lymphomas 162–4
neoplasms of solid tissues 169–75
reticuloendotheliosis 164–6
vascular tissue neoplasms 166–9
of solid tissues and eosinophils 169–75
animals with solid neoplasms 175
bone neoplasms 170
breast neoplasms 170
cardiac neoplasms 170
digestive system neoplasms 171–2
ear, nose, and throat neoplasms 173
endocrine neoplasms 172
history 169
incidence 170
nervous system neoplasms 172–3
respiratory tract neoplasms 173–4

neoplasms (*cont.*)
skin neoplasms 173
squamous cell carcinomas of the skin 173
urogenital neoplasms 174–5
nervous system
and eosinophils 216–17
peripheral nervous system diseases 217
schizophrenia 217
disease in idiopathic hypereosinophilic syndrome 274–6
eye disease 275
peripheral nervous system 275–6
neoplasms and eosinophils 172–3
neuraminidase action on eosinophil plasma membrane glycocalyx 78, 83
neurotoxins from eosinophils, *see* eosinophil-derived neurotoxin, and eosinophil cationic protein
neutrophils
compared with eosinophils v, 3, 4
eosinophil peroxidase ingestion by 60
granule proteins compared with eosinophil granule proteins 43, 44–5
metabolism compared with eosinophil metabolism 67
unsaturated fatty acid metabolism 70
monoclonal antibodies to, which also bind to eosinophils 87–8
suppression of production by eosinophils 14
ninhydrin for staining eosinophils 38
Nippostrongylus brasiliensis infections in rats 80
nitroblue tetrazolium salts, reduction by eosinophils 67
non-Hodgkin's lymphomas and eosinophils 163
non-allergic rhinitis and eosinophilia syndrome (NARES) 213
nose diseases and eosinophils 213–14
nasal polyps 214
paranasal sinus fungal infections 214
rhinitis 213–14
5′-nucleotidase
in eosinophil plasma membrane 75
in Omenn's syndrome 166
nucleus of eosinophils 40–1
nuclear membrane 72
segmentation (nuclear index) of blood eosinophils
compared to tissue eosinophils 40
in idiopathic hypereosinophilic syndrome 279–80
in Down's syndrome 295

obstructive lung diseases and eosinophils 211
oesophageal diseases and eosinophils 183–4
eosinophilic gastroenteritis 185
neoplasms and eosinophils 171
reflux oesophagitis 183–4
oestrogen binding by
eosinophils in man and animals 83
activated human peritoneal eosinophils 67
Ofuji's disease (eosinophilic pustular folliculitis) 132, 304
okapi, eosinophils in 123
Olsson, Inge and eosinophil research 7, 319
Omenn's syndrome (familial reticuloendotheliosis) 166
Onchocerca volvulus
cytotoxicity by eosinophils 116
eosinophill peroxidase interaction with 113
onchocerciasis and eosinophils 143
ontogeny of eosinophils 10–11
ophthalmological diseases, *see* eye diseases
opossums, eosinophils in 125
opsonized zymosan, *see* zymosan-C3b
oral diseases, *see* mouth diseases
orangutan, and eosinophilic enterocolitis 190
orbital diseases and eosinophils 219
oro-genital ulcers in idiopathic hypereosinophilic syndrome 272
otorhinolaryngological diseases, *see* ear nose and throat diseases
Ottesen, Eric and eosinoiphil research 320
Ottolenghi, A, and eosinophil research 29
oxidative metabolism
of eosinophils 68–9
chemoluminescence 68–9
inhibition of 2-oxoglutarate dehydrogenase 118, 248
reactive oxygen species 69
respiratory burst 68
oxygen radicals (reactive oxygen species) in
eosinophil cytotoxicity 69, 118–19
Trichinella spiralis newborn larvae killing 115
Schistosoma mansoni schistosomula killing 115
neutrophil cytotoxicity 119

P150,95 glycoprotein in neutrophil plasma membrane 81
PAF-acether, *see* platelet activating factor
paediatric diseases, *see* neonatal diseases and infant diseases
Palade, G. E. and eosinophil research 38

palladium chloride and electronmicroscopy of eosinophil granules 38
pancreatic diseases and eosinophils 191
  neoplasms and eosinophils 172
pancreatic ribonuclease 51
papers on eosinophils and eosinophilic disorders
  journals, involved 321
  numbers published per year 321
papules and macules in idiopathic hypereosinophilic syndrome 273
paranasal sinus fungal infections and eosinophils 214
parasites
  chemotactic factors from 100
  cytotoxicity by
    Charcot–Leyden crystal protein 66
    eosinophils 112–17
    eosinophil cationic protein 51–2
    eosinophil major basic protein 47
    eosinophil peroxidase 59
    eosinophil-derived neurotoxin/ eosinophil protein-X 55
  eosinophil activating factor from 110
  see also individual parasites
parasitic diseases and eosinophils 136–49, *Fig. 10.1*
  in South East Asian refugees, and visitors to the tropics 136
  induction of eosinophilia 137
  with asthma and eosinophils 201–2
  in eosinophilic endomyocardial fibrosis 236
  see also individual parasitic diseases
passive cutaneous anaphylaxis and eosinophils 84, 97
pathogenesis of
  eosinophilic endomyocardial fibrosis 233
  drug hypersensitivity reactions with eosinophilia 311–14
  eosinophilic endomyocardial fibrosis 245–9
  tropical endomyocardial fibrosis 255
Pelger–Hüet abnormality in eosinophils 261
pemphigoid, *see* bullous skin diseases
pemphigus vegetans and Charcot–Leyden crystals 64
peptic ulcers and eosinophils 184
percentage eosinophils *vs* absolute eosinophil counts 29, 30
Percoll density gradient separation of blood eosinophils from
  dogs 125
  man 33–4
perennial allergic conjunctivitis and eosinophils 218
pericardial diseases and eosinophils 228–9
  constrictive pericarditis 228
  effusions 228–9
perinuclear cisternae, nonspecific esterase in 62
peripheral nerve diseases and eosinophils 217
  idiopathic hypereosinophilic syndrome 275–6
Perissodactyla (horses), eosinophil in 126
peritoneal dialysis and eosinophils 221–2
peritoneal neoplasms and eosinophils 172
peroxidase, *see* eosinophil peroxidase
peroxidation, by eosinophil peroxidase 59
peroxisomal enzymes in rat eosinophils 43
pertussoid eosinophilic pneumonia 295
PGE, *see* prostaglandins
PHA (phytohaemagglutin) stimulation of lymphocytes, inhibition by eosinophil cationic protein, and eosinophil-derived neurotoxin/ eosinophil protein-X 52, 56
phagocytosis, *see* endocytosis
Pharmacia, and eosinophil cationic protein assay kit 50
pharyngeal diseases and eosinophils 214–15
ϱ-phenylenediamine assay for eosinophil peroxidase 59
Philadelphia (Phi) chromosome in chronic eosinophilic leukaemia 157
phloxin (tetrabromo-tetrachloro-fluorescein) staining of eosinophils 30, 36
phorbol myristate acetate (PMA), stimulation of blood eosinophil
  chemoluminescence 68
  protein phosphorylation 110
  respiratory burst 68–9
  secretion 92
phosphatases in eosinophils 60–1
phosphodiesterase inhibitors, and leukotriene synthesis by eosinophils 71
phospholipases A2, and C, and eosinophil secretion 94, 95
phospholipases B, and D in eosinophils 62
  assays in rodent tissues 29
phospholipid–exchange protein in plasma membrane of eosinophils 83
phylogeny of eosinophils 123–4
PIE (pulmonary infiltrates with eosinophilis) syndrome 206
pigs, eosinophilic leukaemia in 157
pigeons, eosinophils in 124
Pincus, Stephanie and eosinophil research 320
placenta, presence of eosinophil major basic protein in man and primates 227
plasma cell neoplasms and eosinophils 162

plasma exchange in idiopathic hypereosinophilic syndrome 292
plasma membrane of eosinophils 72, 74–88, *Fig. 3.2*
  alterations in 88
  antigens in
    blood eosinophils 84–8
      in idiopathic hypereosinophilic syndrome 281
    bone marrow eosinophil progenitor cells 16
  carbohydrates in 83–4
  electronmicroscopy, scanning of 74
  freeze-fracture studies 74–75
  pits induced by calcium ionophore A23187 75
  proteins in 75–83
plasminogen activation inhibited by eosinophil cationic protein 53
Plasmodium berghei infections in mice 257
platelet activating factor (PAF-acether)
  synthesis by blood eosinophils 71–2, 282
  stimulation of blood eosinophil
    cytotoxicity 109
    chemoluminescence 68–9
    chemotaxis 97, 100–1
    leukotriene secretion 71
platelet dysfunction with eosinophilia 262
platelet factor 4 serum levels in idiopathic hypereosinophilic syndrome 248, 287
platelets, monoclonal antibodies to 86
pleural diseases and eosinophils 212
  pleural effusions 212
    Charcot–Leyden crystals in 64
    content of eosinophil major basic protein 47
PMA, *see* phorbol myristate acetate
pneumococcal meningitis and eosinophils 216
Pneumocystis carinii infections and eosinophilia in infants and children with immunodeficiency diseases 148, 315
pneumocyte cytotoxicity by
  eosinophil major basic protein 47
  eosinophil peroxidase, hydrogen peroxide, halide system 47
pneumonia, eosinophil cationic protein levels in serum 131
polyarteritis nodosa and eosinophilia, 80, 206, 231
polymyositis and eosinophilia 179–80
polyps and eosinophils
  inflammatory fibroid 186–7
  nasal 214
pre-B lymphocytes, plasma antigens shared with eosinophils 85–7
pregnancy
  eosinophil major basic protein levels in plasma and serum 227
  skin diseases and eosinophils 302
  see also placenta
premature infants, blood eosinophil counts in 294
presentation of antigens by eosinophils 88
primates, eosinophil in 126
progenitor cells, (colony forming cells in culture, CFUc) eosinophil 15–16
  with two cell lineages 11
  numbers in blood 16
propranolol, inhibition of eosinophil secretion 95
propylene glycol, use in blood eosinophil counting 30
Prosimii, eosinophil in 126
prostaglandins (PG), synthesis by eosinophils of prostaglandins E1 (PGE1), and E2 (PGE2), and 6-keto-prostaglandin F1 (6-keto-PGF1) 71
prostatic diseases and eosinophils 224
proteases in eosinophils 61
protein kinase C, and eosinophil activation 95
protein synthesis
  of eosinophil plasma membrane proteins 78
  by blood eosinophils 72
    assayed with ^{35}S-methionine 72
  by bone marrow eosinophils, assayed with
    ^{14}C-leucine 48, 57
    ^{3}H-leucine 72
    ^{3}H-lysine 42
  see also metabolism of eosinophils
proteins in plasma membrane of eosinophilia 75–83
  phospholipid-exchange protein 83
  receptors for chemotactic factors 83
  receptors for immunoglobulins, and complement components 75–83
  receptors for steroids 83
proteoglycan synthesis by eosinophils 72–3
protozoan infections and eosinophils 148–9
  amoebiasis 148
  giardiasis 148
  leishmaniasis 148
  malaria 148
  Pneumocystis carinii 148, 315
  toxoplasmosis 148–9
  and eosinophilic meningitis 216
  trypanosomiasis 149
pseudopodia on eosinophils 38

psoriasis and eosinophils 304
pulmonary eosinophilia 205–9
  chronic eosinophilic pneumonia 206
  classification 205
  Löffler's syndrome 205–6
  pulmonary infiltrates with eosinophilia (PIE) sydrome 206
pulmonary fibrosis and eosinophils 34–5, 209
pulmonary infiltrates in idiopathic hypereosinophilic syndrome 272
purification of
  Charcot–Leyden crystal protein 63
  eosinophil cationic protein 48
  eosinophil major basic protein 46
  eosinophil peroxidase 58
  eosinophil-derived neurotoxin/eosinophil protein-X 54
  eosinophils 32–5
Purkinje cells loss in animals injected with eosinophil neurotoxins 55
PUVA therapy of urticaria in idiopathic hypereosinophilic syndrome 299
pyruvate dehydrogenase inhibition by eosinophil secretion products 118, 248
rabbits
  eosinophils in 125
  Gordon phenomenon induced by eosinophil cationic protein 52
racial occurrence of idiopathic hypereosinophilic syndrome 270
radiological investigation of the chest in
  chronic eosinophilic pneumonia 207
  eosinophilic endomyocardial fibrosis 238
  tropical endomyocardial fibrosis 251
radiotherapy in idiopathic hypereosinophilic syndrome 289
ragweed antigen-immunoglobulin IgE complexes, endocytosis by eosinophils 79
rats
  eosinophils 127
    eosinophil major basic protein in 46
    eosinophil peroxidase in 58
    eosinopoiesis in 14, *Plate 2*
    in intestine during space flight 183
    microendocytosis by 90
    morphometric studies on granules 13
    parasite killing by 111, 117
    peroxisomal granules in 43
    secretion 90
    steroid receptors on 83
  eosinopoenia induced by steroids, and infections 28, 290
  eosinopoiesis and T-lymphocytes 313
  hypereosinophilia during *Trichinella spiralis* infection 267
  pancreatic eosinophils in diabetic BB rats 306
  spontaneously high peritoneal eosinophil counts in 127
receptors in eosinophil plasma membrane for *Fig. 4.1*
  chemotactic factors 83
  complement components (CR) 75, 81–3, *Plate 1*
  immunoglobulins (Fc receptors) 75–81
    immunoglobulin E (Fc ε R) 79–81
    immunoglobulin G (Fc γ R) 76–9, 105, 110
    immunoglobulin M (Fc μ receptors) 76
  sheep red cells (E) 76
  steroids 83
    glococorticoids 83
    oestrogens 83
rectal diseases and eosinophils 190
  neoplasms 171–2
reference sources for the book, vii, 321
reflux oesophagitis and eosinophils 183–4
rejection, *see* kidney allograft rejection; cardiac allograft rejection; liver allograft rejection
renal dialysis and eosinophils 220–3
  haemodialysis 222–3
  peritoneal dialysis 221–3
renal diseases, *see* kidney diseases
reports of meetings on eosinophils 322
reptiles, eosinophils in 127
research groups, addresses of 318–20
respiratory burst by eosinophils 68
respiratory chain constituents in blood eosinophils 69
respiratory distress syndrome in adults, and eosinophils 211
respiratory tissue injury induced by
  eosinophils 117–18
  eosinophil cationic protein 52
  eosinophil major basic protein 47–8
respiratory tract diseases and eosinophils 193–212
  bronchial diseases 195–204
  bronchoalveolar lavage 194–5
  carcinomas and eosinophils 173–4
  hypersensitivity and eosinophils 204
    extrinsic allergic alveolitis 204
    hayfever 204
  in idiopathic hypereosinophilic syndrome 272
  lung diseases 205–12
  pleural diseases 212
  sputum 194
reticuloendotheliosis and eosinophils 164–6

reticulum cells in bone marrow and eosinopoiesis 10
retinal diseases and eosinophils 219, 275, *Plate 11*
reviews on eosinophils 322–6
rhabdomyosarcoma, and eosinophils 170
rhesus monkeys, eosinophil major basic protein in pregnancy 227
rheumatoid arthritis and eosinophils 176–7
  eosinophil cationic protein levels in serum 177
  rheumatoid vasculitis 177
  with lung involvement 177
  with vasculitis 177
  see also musculo-skeletal diseases
rhinitis and eosinophils 213–14
rhinocerous, eosinophils in 123
ribonuclease activity
  of eosinophil cationic protein 51
  of eosinophil-derived neurotoxin/ eosinophil protein-X 55
ribonucleic acid in eosinophils 42
ribonucleic acid viruses and eosinophils 135
  human immunodeficiency virus-1 (HIV-1) 135
rickettsial infections and eosinophils 133–4
Rocky Mountain spotted fever and eosinophilic meningitis 216
rodentia, eosinophil in 126–7
roles of eosinophils *see* functions of eosinophils
Romanowsky stains
  for eosinophils 36, 37
  enhanced by ethylenediaminetetraacetic acid (EDTA) 36
Royal Society of Medicine, London 321

Saito, H. and eosinophil research 318
SANBIO bv., supply of monoclonal antibodies EG1, and EG2 50
Sanderson, Colin and eosinophil research 19, 111, 284, 319
saponin in eosinophil fractionation 40
Sarcocystis in animals with eosinophilic myositis 180
sarcoidosis and eosinophils 211
scabies and
  eosinophils 149
  absence of eosinophils 315
scanning electronmicroscopy (SEM), of eosinophil plasma membrane 74
schistosome-released products (SRP) and eosinophil cytotoxicity 110
Schistosoma haematobium and eosinophils 148
Schistosoma japonicum schistosomula eosinophil cytotoxicity using IgE antibody 80
Schistosoma mansoni
  schistosomula cytotoxicity by eosinophils *in vitro* 111, 112–15
    activated blood eosinophils 105–7, 108, 109, 110
    eosinophil major basic protein 47
    eosinophil cationic protein 51–2
    eosinophil-derived neurotoxin/ eosinophil protein-X 55
    eosinophil peroxidase-halide system 60, 120
    light density eosinophils and IgE 81
    oxygen metabolites from 115, 119
  eggs 104–5
schistosomiasis and eosinophils 147–8, 266
schizophrenia and eosinophils 217
scleroderma syndromes and eosinophils 302; *see also* fasciitis syndromes and eosinophils
sclerosing cholangitis and eosinophils 191
seasonal allergic conjunctivitis and eosinophils 218
secreted form of eosinophil cationic protein 49, *Plates 3, 4, 6, 12*
secretion by eosinophils 90–5, *Figs 5.1, 5.2*
  drugs affecting 95
  during eosinopoiesis 13
  in idiopathic hypereosinophilic syndrome 283
  induced by immunoglobulin E-immune complexes 80
separation of eosinophils 32–5
  autofluorescence in a cell sorter 37
  density gradient separation 33
  differential binding to surfaces 32
  elutriation centrifigation 35
  methylcellulose and Hypaque 32
Sephadex-C3b, and -IgG, and sepharose-C3b induction of eosinophil
  phagocytosis 89
  secretion of
    granule proteins 82, 92, 94, 95
    leukotriene C4 71
serine esterases in eosinophil cytotoxicity 114
severe combined immune deficiency syndrome and eosinophils 314–15
sex incidence of idiopathic hypereosinophilic syndrome 268
Sezary's syndrome and eosinophils 164
sharks, eosinophils in 124
sheep
  eosinophils 180
  erythrocytes (E) 76
sialic acid in eosinophils 72

Sjögren's syndrome and eosinophils 182
skeletal muscle, *see* muscle
skin
  chemotactic factors extracted from 102
  eosinophil major basic protein actions on 47
skin cells, eosinophil major basic protein actions on 48
skin diseases and eosinophils 297–305, *Fig. 28.1*
  bullous diseases 302–3
  dermatitis 297–9
  drug hypersensitivity reactions 308–9
  episodic angioedema with eosinophilia 299–302
  erythema annulare 305
  erythema nodosum 304
  history 5
  idiopathic hypereosinophilic syndrome 273–4
  infants 302
  pregnancy 302
  incontinentia pigmenti 303–4
  lymphomatoid papulosis 304–5
  psoriasis 304
  pustular folliculitis 304
  scleroderma syndromes 302
  neoplasms and eosinophils 173
small granules
  in eosinophil cytoplasm 43–4
  in Hodgkin's disease tissue eosinophils 44
  relationship to crystalloid granules 44
small intestinal neoplasms and eosinophils 171
Smith, Harry and eosinophil research 95, 319
sodium cromoglycate
  and eosinophils 82, 95
  drug hypersensitivity reactions to 309, 313
solid tissue neoplasms, *see* neoplasms of solid tissues
South America, cardiac surgery for tropical endomyocardial fibrosis 255
soy protein allergy and eosinophils 188–9
soybean lectin binding to eosinophil
  granules 38
  plasma membrane 84
space travel and eosinophilia 183
Spanish toxic oil syndrome and eosinophils 182
Spirometra infections and eosinophilia 137
spinal cord, *see* central nervous system
spleen cells, cytotoxicity by eosinophil major basic protein 48
splenectomy in idiopathic hypereosinophilic syndrome 289
Spry, Christopher and eosinophil research 319
sputum
  content of eosinophil major basic protein in asthma 47, 199
  eosinophils 194
    in asthma 198–9
squamous cell carcinomas of the skin and eosinophils 173
SRP (schistosome released products) and eosinophil cytoxicity 110
SRS-A (slow reacting substance of anaphylaxis), *see* leukotrienes
stains for eosinophils in
  blood, and tissue preparations 36–8
  agar colonies 15
staphyloccocal infections and eosinophils 132
staphylococci and eosinophils
  phagocytosis, studied by interference contrast microscopy 91
  killing 89
steroids and eosinophils
  receptors for 83
  inhibition of eosinopoiesis 24, 290
    secretion 95
  treatment of idiopathic hypereosinophilic syndrome 288–91
    eosinophilic endomyocardial fibrosis 242–3
stomach diseases and eosinophils 184
  neoplasms 171
streptococcal infections and eosinophils 132
striped bass, eosinophils in 124
strongyloidiasis and eosinophils 145–6
structure of blood eosinophils in
  animals 123
  man 38–40
  see also morphology
structure of eosinophil constituents
  Charcot–Leyden crystal protein 63
  eosinophil cationic protein 49
  eosinophil major basic protein 46
  eosinophil peroxidase 58
  eosinophil peroxidase light chain 58
  eosinophil-derived neurotoxin/eosinophil protein-X 54
subcellular fractionation of eosinophils 50
subdural haematomas and eosinophils 217
substance P and eosinophil activation 109
superoxide production by eosinophils 69
  compared to neotrophils 67, 69
  stimulated with
    eosinophil activating factor 108
    interleukin 1 109
  cytotoxic properties 119

superoxide production by eosinophils (*cont.*)
  in idiopathic hypereosinophilic syndrome 282
  destruction by superoxide dismutase 119
suppressor lymphocytes and
  eosinophil-derived neurotoxin/eosinophil protein-X 56
  eosinopoiesis 24
suramin inhibition of eosinophil secretion 95
synovial fluid and eosinophils 177–8
  eosinophil cationic protein levels 178
synovitis and eosinophils 177–8

T-EMF, *see* tropical endomyocardial fibrosis
T-lymphocytes
  eosinophil activating factors from 106–8
  eosinophil cytotoxicity enhancing factors from 120
  eosinopoietic factors from 18–20
  membrane antigens shared with eosinophils 88
Tai, Po–Chun vii, 87
taeniasis and eosinophils 138
  in eosinophilic endomyocardial fibrosis 236
tamarins, eosinophils in 126
Tchernitchin, Andrei, and eosinophil research 83, 226, 318
teleosts, eosinophils in 124
temporal arteritis and eosinophils 231
tench, eosinophils in 124
tetracycline treatment of bullous pemphigoid 303
thiabendazole treatment of toxocariasis 140
6-thioguanine treatment of idiopathic hypereosinophilic syndrome 291
thromboembolic complications of idiopathic hypereosinophilic syndrome 271–2
β–thromboglobulin in serum in
  eosinophilic endomyocardial fibrosis 248
  idiopathic hypereosinophilic syndrome 287
thromboxane B2 (TXB2) secretion from eosinophils 71
^{3}H-thymidine
  assays of blood eosinophil kinetics 27
  assays of human bone marrow eosinophil kinetics 14
  assays of rat bone marrow eosinophil kinetics 14, *Plate 2*
thymidine-5-triphosphate and cytoplasmic granules 42
thymoma, absence of eosinophils in patients with 24, 316
tick immunity in guinea pigs 84
tissue culture of
  blood eosinophils, prolonged by
    colony stimulating factors 35–6
    endothelial cell products 35
    lymphocyte products 35
  bone marrow, in idiopathic hypereosinophilic syndrome 285
tissue eosinophils
  electronmicroscopy, transmission 38
  kinetics 28
  morphology 38–40
  small granules in 43–4
  stains 36–8
TNF, *see* tumour necrosis factor
toxic oil syndrome and eosinophils 182
Toxocara canis, resistance to eosinophil cytotoxicity 113
toxocariasis and eosinophils 127, 139–40
  retinal lesions 219
Toxoplasma gondii, cytotoxicity by eosinophil peroxidase-halide system 60, 120
toxoplasmosis and eósinophils 148–9
TPE (tropical (filarial) eosinophilia) 141–2
tracheal cells damaged by eosinophil major basic protein 47, 117
transplant rejection, *see* renal, and cardiac allograft rejection
trematode infections and eosinophils 146–8
  fascioliasis 147
  schistosomiasis 147–8
triacyglycerides, induction of eosinophil secretion 95
Trichinella spiralis
  infections in
    man 144–5
    mice
      lysophospholipase levels in 66
      cytotoxic capacity of peritoneal eosinophils 104
    rats
      intravascular injection and eosinophilia 137
      hypereosinophilia in 267
      requirement for T-lymphocytes in eosinopoiesis 313
  newborn larvae
    cytotoxicity by
      eosinophils 115–16
      eosinophil cationic protein 52, 55, 116
      eosinophil-derived neurotoxin/eosinophil protein-X 55, 116
      eosinophil major basic protein 47, 55, 116

eosinophil peroxidase-halide system 60
lysophospholipase 66
oxygen metabolites 115
destruction in the heart 113, 230
trichostrongyloidiasis, *see* trichuris
Trichostrongylus colubriformis infections in guinea pigs, effects of antieosinophil serum 84
trichuris infections and eosinophils 145
tRNA, degraded by eosinophil-derived neurotoxin/eosinophil protein-X 55
tropical (filarial) eosinophilia 141–2
Charcot–Leyden crystals in 64
hypogranular blood eosinophils in 280
tropical endomyocardial fibrosis and eosinophils 249–57, *Plate 8*
clinical features 250–251
feminization 253
kidney disease 253
muscle disease 253
compared to eosinophilic endomyocardial fibrosis 257–8, *Fig. 22.3*
histopathology 252
history 232, 249
investigations 251–3
cardiac catheterization 252
echocardiograms 251
electrocardiograms 251
radiological investigations 251
pathogenesis 255–7
treatment 253–5
cardiac surgery 253–5
tropical pulmonary eosinophilia (TPE), *see* tropical (filarial) eosinophilia
Trypanosoma cruzi phagocytosis and killing by
eosinophils 89
eosinophil major basic protein 116
eosinophil peroxidase
hydrogen peroxide system 60, 120
with macrophages 113
secretion of eosinophil cationic protein 94
Trypanosoma dionisii and eosinophils 116
trypanosomiasis and eosinophils 149
tryptase of mast cell type, absence in eosinophils 45
tuatara, eosinophils in 127
tuberculosis, avian, and eosinophilia 131
tuberculous meningitis and eosinophils in cerebrospinal fluid 216
tubulo-vesicular structures in eosinophils 78
tumour cells
cytotoxicity by eosinophils 118
eosinophil peroxidase actions on 60
tumour necrosis factor (TNF)
cytotoxicity enhancing activity 121
eosinophil activation by 108, 109
component in M-ECEF 107
tumours, *see* neoplasms
turtles, eosinophils in 127
TX, *see* thromboxane

ulcer, chronic (traumatic) inflammatory, of the mouth, and eosinophils 192
ulcerative colitis and eosinophils 64, 189–90
unsaturated fatty acid metabolism by eosinophils 69–70
compared with neutrophils 69
history of 69
leukotrienes 69–70
light density eosinophils 70
15-lipoxygenase pathway products 69
platelet activating factor 71–2
prostaglandins, and thromboxane 71
^{3}H-uridine, bone marrow uptake of 72
urine
eosinophils in 224
content of eosinophil cationic protein 50, 223
urogenital neoplasms and eosinophils 174–5
bladder neoplasms 175
female genital tract neoplasms 174–5
male genital tract neoplasms 175
urological diseases and eosinophils 220–4, *Fig. 19.1*
eosinophilic cystitis 223–4
eosinophils in urine 224
kidney diseases 220
prostatic diseases 224
renal allograft rejection 224–5
renal dialysis 220–3
urticaria and eosinophils 299
in idiopathic hypereosinophilic syndrome 273
USA, cardiac surgery for eosinophilic endomyocardial fibrosis 244
uterine diseases and eosinophils 226
neoplasms and eosinophils 174
uterus, eosinophils in
man 226
rodents 83, 226

vacuolated blood eosinophils *see* cytoplasmic vacuoles
Vadas, Matthew and eosinophil research 20, 26, 33, 318

vascular diseases and eosinophils 230
complicating the idiopathic hypereosinophilic syndrome 271–2
cardiac ventricular thrombi 271
large vessel occlusions 271–2
small vessel occlusions 271–2
multiple cholesterol emboli syndrome 230
vascular endothelial cells
cytotoxicity by
eosinophils 118
eosinophil major basic protein 48
increased permeability and eosinophils 121
products inducing
increased survival of blood eosinophils in tissue culture 35
increased eosinophil leukotriene C4 secretion 109
eosinophil activation 109
vascular tissue neoplasms and eosinophils 166–9
angiolymphoid hyperplasia with eosinophilia 167–9
case reports 166–7
lymphatic vessel neoplasms 169
vasculitis and eosinophils 230–1
arteritis 230–1
associated with eosinophilic endomyocardial fibrosis 237
Venge, Per and eosinophil research 319
vernal conjunctivitis and eosinophils 218
vesical diseases, *see* bladder diseases
vincristine treatment of idiopathic hypereosinophilic syndrome 288, 291
viral diseases and eosinophils 135
viruses, cytotoxicity by eosinophil peroxidase–halide system 120
visceral larva migrans and eosinophils 139
visitors to tropical countries, tropical endomyocardial fibrosis in 257
vitamin B_{12}
binding proteins in eosinophils 62
raised serum levels in
acute eosinophilic leukaemia 155
idiopathic hypereosinophilic syndrome 284
warfarin treatment in eosinophilic endomyocardial fibrosis 242
Wegener's granulomatosis and eosinophils 209–10
antineutrophil antibodies in 231
Weller, Peter and eosinophil research 65, 320
Wells' syndrome 167–9
Wharton Jones, T., and discovery of eosinophils 4
wheal-and-flare reaction induced by
leukotriene C4 70
eosinophil major basic protein 122
wheat germ agglutinin effects on guinea pig eosinophils 84
Wolff, Sheldon, and eosinophil research 7, 265

X-ray investigation, *see* radiological investigation

yak, nematode infections and eosinophilia in 125
yeast (cryptococcal) infections and eosinophils in cerebrospinal fluid 134

zinc
in eosinophils 63
content of purified eosinophil cationic protein 49
zinc-chelate Sepharose for purifying eosinophil cationic protein 49
zymosan-C3b induction of eosinophil
phagocytosis 89
freeze-fracture appearances 75
IL-3 stimulation of 110
respiratory burst 68
secretion 92
of granule enzymes 109
of histaminase 62
in idiopathic hypereosinophilic syndrome 283
of leukotriene C4, 69, 70, 71